A Companion to Specialist Surgical Practice
Third Edition

Series Editors
O. James Garden
Simon Paterson-Brown

Vascular and Endovascular Surgery

Third Edition

Edited by
Jonathan D. Beard
Consultant Vascular Surgeon
Sheffield Vascular Institute
Sheffield Teaching Hospitals NHS Trust
and
Peter A. Gaines
Consultant Vascular Radiologist
Sheffield Vascular Institute
Sheffield Teaching Hospitals NHS Trust

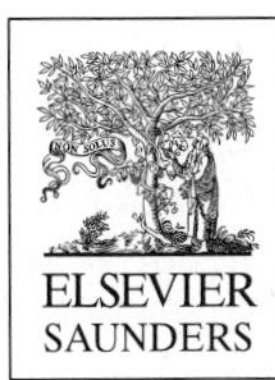

ELSEVIER
SAUNDERS

An imprint of Elsevier Limited

First edition 1997
Second edition 2001
Third edition 2006
Reprinted 2006, 2007

EAN 9780702027345

ISBN 0 7020 2734 0

British Library Cataloguing in Publication Data
A catalogue record for this book is available from the British Library

Library of Congress Cataloging in Publication Data
A catalog record for this book is available from the Library of Congress

Printed in The Netherlands
Last digit is the print number: 9 8 7 6 5 4 3

Commissioning Editor: Laurence Hunter
Project Development Manager: Sheila Black
Editorial Assistants: Kathryn Mason, Liz Brown
Project Manager: Cheryl Brant
Design Manager: Jayne Jones
Illustration Manager: Mick Ruddy
Illustrator: Martin Woodward
Marketing Managers: Gaynor Jones (UK), Ethel Cathers (USA)

Contents

Contributors

Raymond J. Ashleigh BSc MB BS FRCS(Ed) FRCR
Consultant Vascular Radiologist
Wythenshawe Hospital
Manchester, UK

Gillian Atkinson MCSP
Senior Physiotherapist
Mobility and Specialised Rehabilitation Centre
Northern General Hospital
Sheffield, UK

Jill J.F. Belch MB ChB MD FRCP(Glasg) FRCP(Ed) FRCP
Professor of Vascular Medicine
The Institute of Cardiovascular Research
University of Dundee;
Honorary Consultant Physician
Ninewells Hospital and Medical School
Dundee, UK

Jonathan D. Beard BSc ChM FRCS
Consultant Vascular Surgeon
Sheffield Vascular Institute
Sheffield Teaching Hospitals NHS Trust
Sheffield, UK

Andrew J.M. Boulton MD FRCP
Professor of Medicine
University of Manchester;
Consultant Physician
Manchester Royal Infirmary
Manchester, UK

Andrew W. Bradbury BSc MB ChB MD MBA FRCS(Ed)
Professor of Vascular Surgery and Head of Surgery
University of Birmingham;
Consultant Vascular Surgeon and Director of Research and Development
Heart of England NHS Foundation Trust
Birmingham, UK

Trevor Cleveland BMedSci BM BS FRCS FRCR
Consultant Vascular Radiologist
Sheffield Vascular Institute
Sheffield Teaching Hospitals NHS Trust
Sheffield, UK

Deborah J. Collinson MB BS MRCS
Clinical Research Fellow
University of Nottingham
Nottingham, UK

Jean-Michel Cormier MD
Emeritus Professor of Surgery
University of Paris
Paris, France

Dipak Datta MB BS FRCS(Ed) FRCS(Glasg) FRCP
Consultant in Rehabilitation Medicine
Specialised Rehabilitation Services
Northern General Hospital;
Honorary Senior Clinical Lecturer
University of Sheffield
Sheffield, UK

Richard Donnelly MB ChB(Hons) MD PhD FRCP FRACP
Professor of Vascular Medicine
University of Nottingham;
Honorary Consultant Physician
Derby City General Hospital
Derby, UK

Jonothan J. Earnshaw MB BS DM FRCS
Consultant Surgeon
Gloucestershire Royal Hospital
Gloucester, UK

Duncan F. Ettles MD FRCP FRCR
Consultant Cardiovascular and Interventional Radiologist
Hull Royal Infirmary;
Honorary Senior Lecturer in Radiology
Hull York Medical School
Kingston-upon-Hull, UK

Peter A. Gaines FRCP FRCR
Consultant Vascular Radiologist
Sheffield Vascular Institute
Sheffield Teaching Hospitals NHS Trust
Sheffield, UK

Christopher P. Gibbons MA DPhil MCh FRCS
Consultant Vascular Surgeon
Morriston Hospital
Swansea, Wales

George Hamilton MB ChB MD FRCS
Professor of Vascular Surgery
Royal Free and University College School of Medicine;
Consultant Vascular Surgeon
Royal Free Hospital
London, UK

Peter L. Harris MB ChB MD FRCS EBSQ(Vasc)
Consultant Vascular Surgeon
Royal Liverpool University Hospital
Liverpool, UK

Michael J.H.M. Jacobs MD PhD
Chief and Professor of Surgery
University Hospital Maastricht
Maastricht, The Netherlands

Edward B. Jude MB BS MD MRCP
Consultant Physician
Tameside General Hospital
Ashton-under-Lyme, UK

Philip A. Kalra MA MB BChir FRCP MD
Consultant Nephrologist
Hope Hospital
Salford, UK

Timothy A. Lees MD FRCS
Consultant Vascular Surgeon
Northern Vascular Centre
The Freeman Hospital
Newcastle upon Tyne, UK

Charles N. McCollum MB ChB FRCS ND
Professor of Surgery
University of Manchester;
Honorary Consultant Surgeon
Manchester University Hospital
Manchester, UK

Richard McWilliams MB FRCS FRCR
Consultant Interventional Radiologist
Royal Liverpool University Hospital
Liverpool, UK

Jacobus van Marle MB ChB MMed(Surg) FCS(SA)
Consultant Vascular Surgeon
Vascular Society of Southern Africa
Centurion, South Africa

Jonathan G. Moss MB ChB FRCS(Ed) FRCR
Consultant Interventional Radiologist
Gartnavel General Hospital
Glasgow, UK

Michael Murphy MB FRCSI DMRD FRCR
Consultant Interventional Radiologist
Royal Liverpool University Hospital
Liverpool, UK

Ahmed Nassef MD FRCS(Ed) FRCS(GenSurg)
Consultant in Vascular Surgery
The Sheffield Vascular Unit
Sheffield Teaching Hospitals NHS Trust
Sheffield, UK

A. Ross Naylor MB ChB MD FRCS
Professor of Vascular Surgery
University of Leicester;
Consultant Vascular Surgeon
Leicester Royal Infirmary
Leicester, UK

Dean Patterson MB ChB MRCP
Clinical Lecturer
The Institute of Cardiovascular Research
Ninewells Hospital and Medical School
Dundee, UK

Andrew Platts MB BS FRCS FRCR
Consultant Radiologist
The Royal Free Hospital
London, UK

Eric Preston MD FRCP FRCPath
Emeritus Professor of Haematology
University of Sheffield
Sheffield, UK

Nicholas F.W. Redwood MB BS FRCS
Consultant Vascular and General Surgeon
The Queen Elizabeth Hospital
King's Lynn, UK

Dirk A. le Roux MB ChB FCS(SA) CVS(SA)
Consultant Vascular Surgeon
Johannesburg General Hospital;
Lecturer in Vascular Surgery
University of the Witwatersrand
Johannesburg, South Africa

Jean-Baptiste Ricco MD PhD
Professor of Vascular Surgery and Head of Vascular Surgery Service
University of Poitiers
Poitiers, France

Rachel C. Sam MB ChB MA MRCS
Specialist Registrar in Vascular Surgery
Heart of England NHS Foundation Trust;
Honorary Research Fellow
University of Birmingham
Birmingham, UK

Peter R. Taylor MA MChir FRCS
Consultant Vascular Surgeon
Guy's and St Thomas' NHS Foundation Trust
London, UK

Steven M. Thomas MB BS MSc MRCP FRCR
Consultant Vascular Radiologist
Sheffield Vascular Institute
Sheffield Teaching Hospitals NHS Trust;
Senior Lecturer
University of Sheffield
Sheffield, UK

Matthew Thompson MA MB BS MD FRCS
Professor of Vascular Surgery
University of London;
Consultant Vascular Surgeon
St George's Hospital
London, UK

Anthony Watkinson MB BS MSc FRCS FRCR
Professor of Interventional Radiology
Peninsula Medical School;
Consultant Radiologist
The Royal Devon and Exeter Hospital
Exeter, UK

Preface

The *Companion to Specialist Surgical Practice* series was designed to meet the needs of surgeons in higher training and practising consultants who wish up-to-date and evidence-based information on the subspecialist areas relevant to their surgical practice. In trying to meet this aim, we have recognised that the series will never be as all-encompassing as many of the larger reference surgical textbooks. However, by their very size, it is rare that the latter are completely up to date at the time of publication. The first edition of this series was published in 1997, with the second following in 2001. In this third edition, we have been able to bring up to date the relevant specialist information that we and the individual volume editors consider important for the practising subspecialist surgeon. Where possible, all contributors have attempted to identify evidence-based references to support key recommendations within each chapter. These should all be interpreted with the help of the guidance summary 'Evidence-based practice in surgery', which follows this preface.

We are extremely grateful to all volume editors and to their contributors to this third edition. It is thanks to their enthusiasm and hard work that the relatively short time frame between each of the editions has been maintained, thereby providing to the reader the most accurate and up-to-date information possible. We were all immensely saddened by the sudden and tragic death of Professor John Farndon, who edited the first and second editions of the volumes *Breast Surgery* and *Endocrine Surgery*. While recognising that he was a unique and talented individual, we are pleased to welcome the additional editorial skills of Mike Dixon and Tom Lennard for this third edition.

We are also grateful for the support and encouragement of Elsevier Ltd and hope that our aim – of providing up-to-date and affordable surgical texts – has been met and that all readers, whether in training or in consultant practice, will find this third edition a valuable resource.

A modern vascular service encompasses many disciplines and success depends upon a team approach. Whilst the vascular surgeon often remains in overall charge of the patient, management may involve diagnostic and interventional radiology, the vascular laboratory, and medical disciplines – including haematology, angiology, diabetology and neurology – plus rehabilitation services. Our choice of authors reflects this diversity. We have retained many of the chapters from the second edition, although all of them have been extensively revised and updated in line with the increasing need for evidence-based practice. There is an increasing emphasis on the endovascular management of many conditions such as chronic leg ischaemia, abdominal aortic aneurysms and carotid stenosis. Therefore, many chapters are co-authored by a vascular surgeon and a vascular radiologist. The chapters have been rearranged into a more logical order in light of the reviews of the second edition. We are grateful to all our authors for the hard work that they have put into their respective chapters.

O. James Garden BSc, MB, ChB, MD, FRCS(Glasg), FRCS(Ed), FRCP(Ed)
Regius Professor of Clinical Surgery, Clinical and Surgical Sciences (Surgery), University of Edinburgh, and Honorary Consultant Surgeon, Royal Infirmary of Edinburgh

Simon Paterson-Brown MB, BS, MPhil, MS, FRCS(Ed), FRCS
Honorary Senior Lecturer, Clinical and Surgical Sciences (Surgery), University of Edinburgh, and Consultant General and Upper Gastrointestinal Surgeon, Royal Infirmary of Edinburgh

Jonathan D. Beard BSc, ChM, FRCS
Consultant Vascular Surgeon, Sheffield Vascular Institute, Sheffield Teaching Hospitals NHS Trust

Peter A. Gaines FRCP, FRCR
Consultant Vascular Radiologist, Sheffield Vascular Institute, Sheffield Teaching Hospitals NHS Trust

EVIDENCE-BASED PRACTICE IN SURGERY

The third edition of the *Companion to Specialist Surgical Practice* series has attempted to incorporate, where appropriate, **evidence-based practice in surgery**, which has been highlighted in the text and relevant references. A detailed chapter on evidence-based practice in surgery, written by Kathryn Rigby and Jonathan Michaels, has been included in the volume *Core Topics in General and Emergency Surgery*, to which the reader is referred for further information on assessing levels of evidence. We are grateful to them for providing this summary for each volume.

Critical appraisal for developing evidence-based practice can be obtained from a number of sources, the most reliable being randomised controlled clinical trials, systematic literature reviews, meta-analyses and observational studies. For practical purposes three grades of evidence can be used, analogous to the levels of 'proof' required in a court of law:

1. **Beyond reasonable doubt** – such evidence is likely to have arisen from high-quality randomised controlled trials, systematic reviews, or high-quality synthesised evidence such as decision analysis, cost-effectiveness analysis or large observational data sets. The studies need to be directly applicable to the population of concern and have clear results. The grade is analogous to burden of proof within a crimimal court and may be thought of as corresponding to the usual standard of 'proof' within the medical literature (i.e. $P<0.05$).
2. **On the balance of probabilities** – in many cases a high-quality review of literature may fail to reach firm conclusions owing to conflicting or inconclusive results, trials of poor methodological quality or the lack of evidence in the population to which the guidelines apply. In such cases it may still be possible to make a statement as to the best treatment on the 'balance of probabilities'. This is analogous to the decision in a civil court where all the available evidence will be weighed up and the verdict will depend upon the balance of probabilities.
3. **Not proven** – insufficient evidence upon which to base a decision or contradictory evidence.

Depending on the information available three grades of recommendation can be used:

a. strong recommendation, which should be followed unless there are compelling reasons to act otherwise;
b. a recommendaton based on evidence of effectiveness but where there may be other factors to take into account in decision-making, for example the user of the guidelines may be expected to take into account patient preferences, local facilities, local audit results or available resources;
c. a recommendation made where there is no adequate evidence as to the most effective practice, although there may be reasons for making a recommendation in order to minimise cost or reduce the chance of error through a locally agreed protocol.

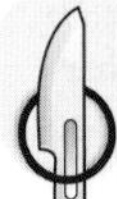

The text and references that are considered to be associated with reasonable evidence are highlighted in this volume with a 'scalpel code', leaving the reader to reach his or her own conclusion.

Further reading

This volume, by definition, cannot encompass the whole of vascular surgery. The books listed below will provide more detail when required:

Atlas of Vascular Surgery: Operative Procedures
Ouriel K, Rutherford RB (eds), WB Saunders, 1998
An ideal companion to Vascular and Endovascular Surgery. *Clear line diagrams of vascular surgical techniques and exposures.*

Vascular Surgery, 6th edn
Rutherford RB (ed.), WB Saunders, 2004
The 'bible' of vascular surgery. Encyclopaedic but expensive, with a strong US influence.

Comprehensive Vascular and Endovascular Surgery
Hallet JW, Mills JL, Earnshaw JJ, Reekers JA (eds), Mosby, 2004
A more affordable comprehensive textbook with a transatlantic flavour. Excellent colour illustrations and diagrams.

Pathways of Care in Vascular Surgery
Beard JD, Murray S (eds), tfm Publishing, 2002
An excellent book produced by the Joint Vascular Research Group. Evidence-based, multidisciplinary approach to the management of common vascular conditions.

ABC of Arterial and Venous Disease
Donnelly R, London NJM (eds), BMJ Books, 2000
An inexpensive, well-illustrated, soft-cover book suitable for junior doctors, students and nurses.

Endovascular Intervention: Current Controversies
Wyatt MG, Watkinson AF (eds), tfm Publishing, 2004
Up-to-date review of all aspects of arterial and venous imaging and intervention.

Epidemiology of Peripheral Vascular Disease
Fowkes FGR (ed.), Springer, 1991

An Introduction to Vascular Biology, 2nd edn
Hunt BJ, Poston L, Schachter M, Halliday AW (eds), Cambridge University Press, 2002

Connective Tissue Diseases
Belch JJF, Zurier RB (eds), Chapman & Hall, 1995

Disorders of Thrombosis
Hull R, Pimco GF (eds), WB Saunders, 1996

The Foot in Diabetes, 3rd edn
Boulton AJM, Connor H, Cavanagh PRC (eds), John Wiley, 2000

Atlas of Amputations and Limb Deficiencies: Surgical, Prosthetic, and Rehabilitation Principles, 3rd edn
Smith DG, Michael JN, Bowker JH (eds), American Academy of Orthopedic Surgeons, 2004

Introduction to Vascular Sonography, 4th edn
Zweibel W (ed.), WB Saunders, 2000

3D Contrast MR Angiography
Prince MR, Grist TM, Debatin JE (eds), Springer-Verlag, 1999

Spiral CT: Principles, Technique and Clinical Application
Fishman EK, Jeffrey RB (eds), Lippincott-Raven, 1998

Carotid Artery Surgery: A Problem-Based Approach
Naylor AR, Mackey WC (eds), WB Saunders, 2000

Varicose Veins, Venous Disorders and Lymphatic Problems in the Lower Limbs
Tubbs DJ, Sabiston DC, Davies MG, Mortimer PS, Scurr JH (eds), Oxford University Press, 1997

Handbook of Venous Disorders, Guidelines of the American Venous Forum, 2nd edn
Gloviczki P, Yao JST (eds), Arnold, 2001

Rare Vascular Disorders
Parvin SD, Earnshaw JJ (eds), tfm Publishing, 2005
A fascinating, well-illustrated collection of rare vascular conditions.

CHAPTER

One

Epidemiology and risk factor management of peripheral arterial disease

Deborah J. Collinson and
Richard Donnelly

INTRODUCTION

Peripheral arterial disease (PAD) involving one or more major vessels of the lower limb is a common manifestation of atherosclerosis, especially in Western societies where the interaction between environmental and genetic factors accentuates the development and progression of occlusive vascular disease. PAD may be asymptomatic in the early stages but is always associated with shortened survival due to the invariable association with atherosclerosis in other arterial territories, especially the coronary, carotid and cerebral circulation. This is highlighted by observational studies showing a clear relationship between ankle–brachial pressure index (ABPI, a marker of disease severity in PAD) and reduced survival (**Fig. 1.1**).[1] PAD is not a 'benign' form of atherosclerosis but indicates an increased risk of acute limb-threatening and/or life-threatening ischaemia. Thus patients with symptomatic PAD benefit from evidence-based, disease-modifying therapies (alone or in conjunction with surgical treatments) that retard the progression of atherosclerotic plaques and improve lower limb outcomes and patient survival.[2]

This chapter considers the epidemiology of PAD, the observational studies identifying reversible and irreversible risk factors for disease progression, and the evidence from randomised controlled trials, which underpins clinical use of disease-modifying therapies as part of multiple risk factor intervention.

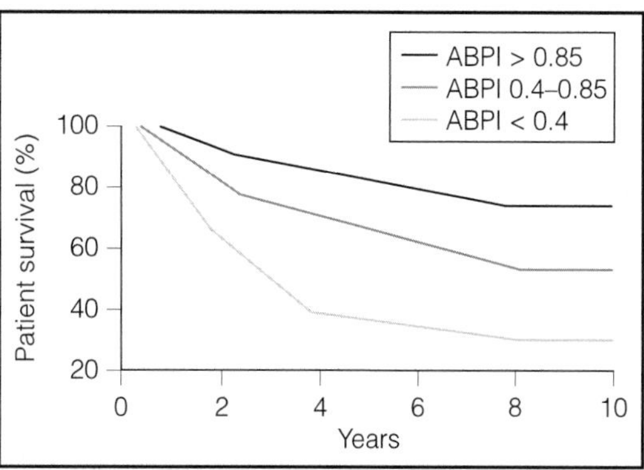

Figure 1.1 • Relationship between ankle–brachial pressure index (ABPI) and survival in patients with symptomatic peripheral arterial disease (PAD). The ABPI is simple to measure using a hand-held Doppler (in the normal setting, ankle and brachial systolic blood pressures are equal, i.e. ABPI = 1.0). This clearly illustrates how cardiovascular mortality increases in proportion to the severity of PAD. Adapted from McKenna M, Wolfson S, Kuller L. The ratio of ankle and arm arterial pressure as an independent predictor of mortality. Atherosclerosis 1991; 87:119–28, with permission.

EPIDEMIOLOGY OF PAD

The prevalence and incidence of PAD is difficult to define. Several epidemiological studies have focused on specific groups, e.g. in the workplace setting or referrals to hospital, which may not be truly representative of the wider population. Thus, workplace screening studies for PAD have excluded those who have retired and those who may be unfit for work. Similarly, epidemiological studies based on inpatient or outpatient referrals tend to underestimate the prevalence of PAD in the community. One of the largest and most reliable sources of information about the overall prevalence of symptomatic and asymptomatic PAD is the Edinburgh Artery Study, which screened large random samples of the general population using age/sex registers from general practices.[3]

Another challenge for epidemiological studies has been that many patients with PAD may be asymptomatic or have symptoms that go unrecognised. For example, intermittent claudication is sometimes dismissed as part of the slowing-down of normal ageing, or sometimes the impaired walking distance due to PAD is obscured by other exercise-induced symptoms, e.g. chronic lung disease or angina. Thus, only a minority of patients with atherosclerosis of the lower limb ever present with lower limb symptoms, and an even smaller proportion will show progression of occlusive vascular disease to the stage of critical limb ischaemia or amputation. Although PAD may cause few symptoms in the lower limb, the major impact of the disease (even when relatively silent in terms of the leg) is on cardiovascular complications such as acute limb-threatening or life-threatening ischaemia.[4]

Investigative techniques for epidemiological screening

Clearly, the technique used to establish the presence or absence of PAD will also affect the results of epidemiological surveys. Questionnaires have often been used to establish the nature and severity of symptomatic PAD, e.g. the WHO/Rose questionnaire designed in 1962.[5] The original questionnaire developed by Rose was shown to be highly sensitive but only moderately specific, and therefore in 1985 the tool was modified in a way that increased the specificity, albeit at the expense of a small decrease in sensitivity.[6] The Edinburgh Artery Questionnaire is designed to be self-administered and has a sensitivity of 91% and a specificity of 99% for symptoms of PAD.[7] In general, all questionnaires appear to underestimate the true prevalence of intermittent claudication, and the Transatlantic Inter-Society Consensus (TASC) group recommend great caution in interpreting epidemiological studies of symptomatic PAD based solely on questionnaires.

Physical examination to establish the presence or absence of peripheral pulses has also been used in epidemiological surveys to confirm a history of intermittent claudication. However, the absence of a peripheral pulse is not necessarily due to PAD, and at least one pulse may be undetectable in up to 10% of the adult population even though only 3% have symptomatic arterial disease.[8]

Establishing the prevalence of asymptomatic PAD in the general population is equally important. The most useful non-invasive test for this purpose is the ABPI, which is quick and painless and has excellent sensitivity and specificity. An ABPI less than 0.9 is 95% sensitive and 100% specific for detecting angiogram-positive disease.[9] At the more severe end of the spectrum, the prevalence of critical limb ischaemia has rarely been assessed from population-based studies or using ABPI criteria. Most of the data on critical limb ischaemia have been obtained from inpatient records.

Prevalence and incidence of PAD

Evidence from epidemiological studies using ABPI suggests that the prevalence of asymptomatic PAD in the middle-aged and elderly population is around 7–15%.[3,10] However, in the British Regional Heart Study, direct assessment of the femoral artery with ultrasound found that 64% of people aged 56–77 years had significant femoral atherosclerosis but only 10% of these were symptomatic.[11] Autopsy studies have found similar results, suggesting that the true incidence of asymptomatic PAD may be much higher than previously recognised.

Population studies have varied widely in reporting the incidence of intermittent claudication. Most of these are based on questionnaire surveys and therefore prone to some degree of over-reporting. Nevertheless, it is clear that the incidence of intermittent claudication increases steeply with age (**Fig. 1.2**).

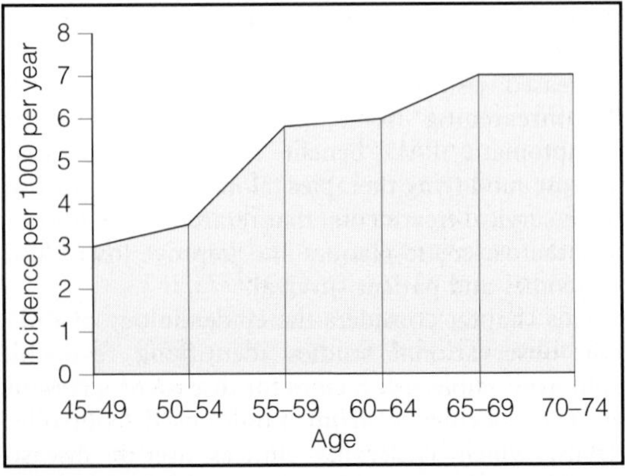

Figure 1.2 • Weighted mean incidence of intermittent claudication by age group from 45 to 74 years. Adapted from Transatlantic Inter-Society Consensus (TASC) Document. Management of peripheral arterial disease. J Vasc Surg 2000; 31:S5–S35, with permission.

Similarly, the prevalence of intermittent claudication has been reported differently according to the age group studied and the methods used. The Scottish Heart Study, for example, found a prevalence of 1.1% in subjects aged 40–59 years.[12] However, in the Limburg study the reported prevalence varied between 1.4 and 6.1% (depending on the criteria used) in individuals aged 40–79 years.[13] Figures from the Edinburgh Artery Study indicate a higher prevalence of 4.5%, but in a slightly older age group (55–74 years).[3]

The incidence of critical limb ischaemia has been estimated to be around 400 cases per million population per year, which equates to a prevalence of 1 in 2500 of the population annually.[14] For every 100 patients with intermittent claudication, approximately one new patient per year will develop critical ischaemia.[9]

NATURAL HISTORY OF PAD: CARDIOVASCULAR AND LOWER LIMB OUTCOMES

It is important in discussing the natural history of PAD to consider both the progression of the disease in the legs and the fate of the patient as a whole in terms of systemic cardiovascular complications.

Asymptomatic disease

The Edinburgh Artery Study is one of the few studies to have examined the pattern of progression among asymptomatic patients with abnormal ABPI and rate of development of symptoms. Of subjects with asymptomatic PAD, 7–15% developed intermittent claudication over a 5-year period, depending on the initial severity of the disease.[4] A more recent study from the Netherlands reported similar conversion rates, with 27 of 177 asymptomatic patients (15%) developing lower limb symptoms during a 7-year follow-up period.[15]

There is considerable evidence, however, that asymptomatic patients with PAD have a much higher risk of systemic cardiovascular complications. The risk of death or disability from cardiac or cerebral events may be higher than the risk of lower limb symptoms (claudication or acute limb ischaemia). The Edinburgh Artery Study showed that asymptomatic PAD patients have an increased risk of acute myocardial infarction (AMI) and stroke; in fact they have almost the same increased risk of cardiovascular events and death as that reported among patients with claudication.[3] The reverse also applies; for example in men with asymptomatic carotid stenosis, ABPI was the strongest predictor of stroke risk.[16]

Intermittent claudication

Large population follow-up studies suggest that up to 50% of patients with intermittent claudication will remain relatively stable (i.e. no deterioration in walking distance) or experience some spontaneous improvement in symptoms during a 5-year period; only 25% of claudicants will develop significant deterioration in walking distance.[17,18] The Basle study[18] is typical of several observational follow-up reports in showing that although two-thirds of patients surviving at 5 years reported no limiting intermittent claudication (i.e. their symptoms had resolved), 63% actually had angiographic progression of the disease. This suggests that although PAD is pathologically progressive, other factors contribute to symptomatology, e.g. collateral vessel formation or physiological and psychological adaptation. Although one-quarter of patients with intermittent claudication have symptoms that worsen over time, only 5% deteriorate sufficiently to merit revascularisation and only 1–2% will require major amputation (**Fig. 1.3**).[9]

Although lower limb outcomes are mostly very good for patients with uncomplicated intermittent claudication, the major concern for these patients relates to a heightened risk of cardiovascular complications due to silent or symptomatic atherosclerosis in other vascular territories. Patients with intermittent claudication have a 2–4% risk of undergoing a non-fatal cardiovascular event within the first year of diagnosis and a 1–3% yearly incidence thereafter.[9] For most patients, however, the absolute risk of coronary heart disease is greater than 30% over 10 years, and all-cause mortality rates are similar to those associated with many forms of cancer. During the CASS study, patients with PAD had a 25% greater likelihood of mortality than patients without PAD.[19]

Critical limb ischaemia

A national survey conducted in 1993 by the Vascular Surgical Society of Great Britain and Ireland found that around 70% of patients with critical ischaemia were offered some form of revascularisation procedure, with a 75% chance of limb salvage. However, the overall amputation rate was still 21.5% and the mortality rate was 13.5%.[14] Thus, the overall long-term prognosis for these patients is very poor. Mortality rates vary in different studies, but may be as high as 50% at 5 years. Randomised trials provide some information about outcomes if no revascularisation is attempted: possibly 40% will lose their leg within 6 months[20,21] and 80% will be dead within 10 years.[22]

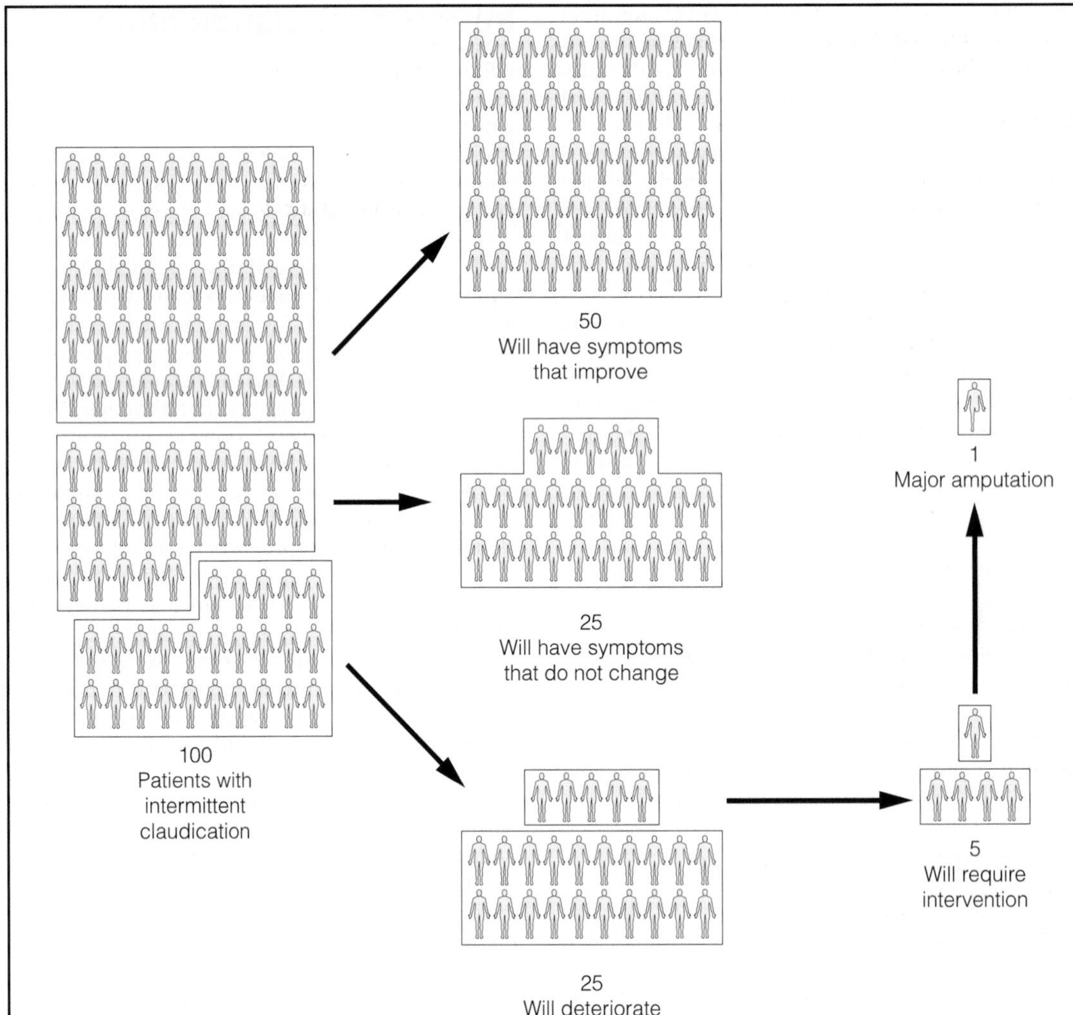

Figure 1.3 • Lower limb outcomes among 100 patients with intermittent claudication followed for 5 years.

EPIDEMIOLOGICAL RISK FACTORS FOR PAD AND RANDOMISED TRIALS OF DISEASE-MODIFYING THERAPY FOR SECONDARY PREVENTION

It is important to make a clear distinction between cardiovascular risk factors and their relationship with PAD, and the evidence that intervention to modify a risk factor improves clinical outcomes (i.e. symptoms or survival). Longitudinal follow-up studies have identified several cardiovascular risk factors (i.e. clinical or demographic characteristics) that are associated with a higher incidence of PAD in a population. Some risk factors (e.g. age and gender) cannot be modified, but others are amenable to therapeutic intervention. However, because a parameter is identified as a risk factor in observational follow-up studies in a population does not necessarily mean that intervention to lower that risk factor in an individual will result in a lower risk of a clinical endpoint. For example, there are many cardiovascular risk factors, and therefore selective intervention to lower one risk factor while others remain unchanged might have no significant effect on clinical outcome or disease progression. Thus, epidemiology (i.e. observational studies) can identify risk factors in a population, but randomised placebo-controlled trials are needed to establish whether therapeutic intervention to lower the risk factor translates into clinical benefit for individual patients. Factors such as high serum homocysteine[23] or fibrinogen levels may be weak risk factors for PAD, but for surgical practice this is largely meaningless without evidence from randomised prospective trials that homocysteine-lowering or fibrinogen-lowering therapy affects disease outcome.

The term 'secondary prevention' in cardiovascular management generally refers to those (evidence-based) treatments that, in patients with symptomatic cardiovascular disease, alter the atherosclerotic process (e.g. by causing plaque stabilisation and regression and/or by reducing the risk of plaque rupture with superimposed thrombus formation) and thereby improve survival.[2] This is best thought of as 'disease-modifying' therapy, rather than 'risk factor management', and the evidence in support of secondary prevention usually comes from long-term, randomised, placebo-controlled trials with hard clinical endpoints (e.g. death or major cardiovascular events).[2]

In patients with PAD, there is good evidence that long-term medical therapy appropriate to an individual patient can provide effective secondary prevention to modify atherosclerotic disease progression and reduce the risk of acute thrombotic complications such as acute limb ischaemia, AMI or sudden death. This evidence, however, is often derived from PAD subgroups in larger secondary prevention trials.[2]

Age and gender

There is clear evidence from several studies that increasing age is associated with an increased risk of PAD in both men and women (see **Fig. 1.2**).[3,24] The evidence for a gender difference is slightly less clear. Several studies, including the Framingham Heart Study, have suggested that men have nearly double the risk of developing intermittent claudication compared with women,[24] but the Edinburgh Artery Study failed to show any significant difference between the sexes,[3] and a follow-up to the Limburg study suggested that the incidence of both symptomatic and asymptomatic PAD was greater in women.[15] Family history is an independent risk factor for premature coronary heart disease,[25] but studies have failed to show the same (presumably genetic) association for PAD.

Cigarette smoking

Smoking is undoubtedly the most important modifiable risk factor for PAD. The relationship between smoking and lower limb arterial disease was first recognised as early as 1911, when Erb[26] reported a threefold increase in the incidence of claudication among smokers. Smoking affects not only the development of PAD[24,27] but also the clinical outcome in those patients who continue to smoke. Smokers with PAD are much more likely to progress to critical ischaemia, and more likely to require amputation or vascular intervention.[28,29] Furthermore, smoking increases the overall mortality rate among claudicants 1.5–3.0-fold.[7]

Smoking cessation reduces overall cardiovascular risk to the level of non-smokers within 2–4 years,[30] unlike the excess cancer risk associated with smoking, which often takes 10 years to subside after smoking cessation. Thus, smoking cessation for cardiovascular prevention is highly cost-effective: the benefits appear quickly.

In terms of helping motivated patients to quit smoking, nicotine replacement therapy (NRT) ameliorates the unpleasant symptoms of nicotine withdrawal following abrupt smoking cessation.

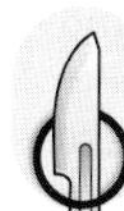

Several large randomised trials have shown that NRT in various forms achieves, on average, a twofold increase in quit rates at 1 year compared with placebo (**Fig. 1.4**).[31]

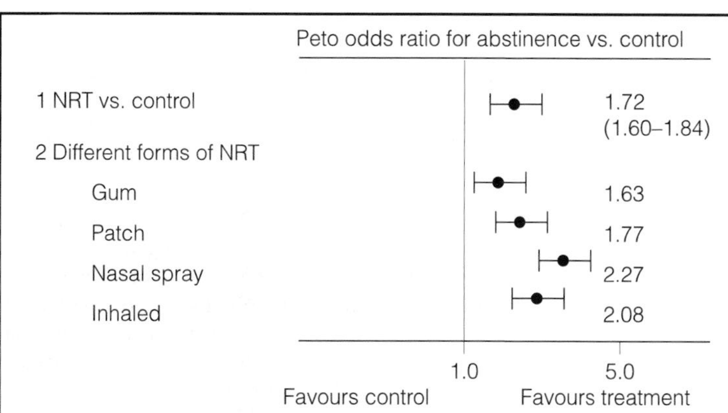

Figure 1.4 • Results of a Cochrane meta-analysis of over 50 randomised controlled trials of nicotine replacement therapy (NRT) showing that, in motivated patients, NRT roughly doubles quit rates at 1 year. From Silagy C. Meta-analysis on efficacy of nicotine replacement therapies in smoking cessation. Elsevier (The Lancet 1994; 343:139–42), with permission.

Physicians should recognise that nicotine is addictive and that spontaneous quit rates are very low even among genuinely motivated patients. NRT is an evidence-based intervention, suitable for motivated but nicotine-dependent patients, that assists with smoking cessation.[32]

Diabetes

Diabetes mellitus is well recognised as an important risk factor for cardiovascular disease and, apart from smoking, is probably the single most important risk factor in the development of PAD.[33] Lower limb arterial disease tends to be more diffuse and distal in diabetics, and ischaemic ulceration is common. Diabetes is a syndrome that includes many features in addition to hyperglycaemia, and in general patients with diabetes have a two- to four-fold increased risk of intermittent claudication and a 10–16-fold increased lifetime risk of lower limb amputation.[33–36] Diabetics with critical ischaemia fare less well than their non-diabetic counterparts, e.g. higher amputation rates and less success in revascularisation procedures.[37] The risks of lower limb ulceration are exacerbated by coexistent microvascular disease and peripheral neuropathy.

Several recent studies in both type 1 and type 2 diabetes have identified the glucose level as an independent risk factor for PAD.[38–40]

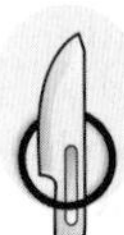

The UK Prospective Diabetes Study (UKPDS) identified a strong association between HbA_{1c} and risk of PAD: each 1% increase in HbA_{1c} was associated with a 28% increased risk of PAD.[39]

However, other important features of the 'metabolic syndrome' of type 2 diabetes include insulin resistance, hypertension, obesity and dyslipidaemia (typically low HDL-cholesterol and high triglycerides). Type 2 diabetes is thought to be preceded by a long period of insulin resistance during which compensatory increases in insulin secretion maintain glucose at near-normal levels.[41] There is already an increased risk of cardiovascular disease during this 'pre-diabetic' period, suggesting that insulin resistance per se may also promote atherosclerosis.[42] Indeed, epidemiological data have suggested that both insulin resistance and hyperinsulinaemia are independent risk factors for PAD in diabetic and non-diabetic individuals.[43,44]

Hypertension also plays a significant role in the development of PAD in diabetic subjects. In the UKPDS, for every 10 mmHg reduction in systolic blood pressure there was a 12% reduction in overall cardiovascular risk but, more specifically, a 16% reduction in risk of lower limb amputation or peripheral vascular disease-related mortality.[45] Hansson[46] showed that vigorous blood pressure control had a greater effect in reducing cardiovascular events in those patients with diabetes than in those without, and effective control of hypertension may limit vascular events even more effectively than tight glycaemic control.[47] The major benefits of glycaemic control appear to be in microvascular protection and prevention of neuropathy and secondary foot complications such as ulceration and infection.

Blood pressure

The Framingham study has provided good evidence that hypertension is a powerful predisposing risk factor in the development of intermittent claudication. A blood pressure above 160/95 mmHg increased the risk by 2.5-fold in men and fourfold in women during 26 years of follow-up.[24]

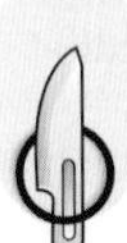

Large placebo-controlled intervention trials have shown that even modest reductions in blood pressure (e.g. 10/5 mmHg) reduce mortality from stroke (40%), coronary heart disease (16%) and all cardiovascular causes (30%).[48]

Aggressive target levels of blood pressure have been adopted in recent clinical guidelines, especially among patients with coexistent diabetes and/or proteinuria.

Most blood pressure-lowering trials have not included PAD as a primary endpoint, but it is clear that hypertension, and in particular isolated systolic hypertension (which is common in elderly patients), is an important risk factor for intermittent claudication. Thus, tight control of blood pressure in patients with PAD, mainly to reduce the risk of stroke and coronary heart disease, is an important aspect of secondary prevention. A target blood pressure below 140/85 mmHg should be the aim among treated hypertensives, and the choice of antihypertensive agent is less important than achieving the target blood pressure goal.[48] The British Hypertension Society recommends an 'ABCD' approach to treatment selection: first-line therapy with an angiotensin-converting enzyme (*A*CE) inhibitor (or angiotensin receptor antagonist) or *B*eta-blocker for those patients under 55 years of age (and non-black), and a *C*alcium channel blocker or *D*iuretic for older patients. Most patients will require combination therapy (e.g. A + B or C + D).[49]

ACE inhibitors for secondary prevention: beyond blood pressure reduction

The Heart Outcomes Prevention Evaluation (HOPE) study was a large international randomised controlled trial comparing long-term treatment with ramipril to placebo as add-on to other

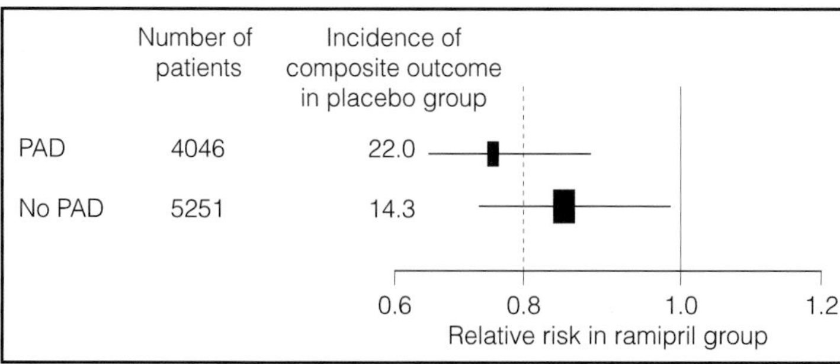

Figure 1.5 • In the HOPE study, analysis of subgroups according to baseline cardiovascular disease status shows that patients with peripheral arterial disease (PAD) gain at least as much benefit from the angiotensin-converting enzyme inhibitor ramipril as the study group overall. From Heart Outcomes Prevention and Evaluation Study Investigators. N Engl J Med 2000; 342:145–53.

cardiovascular therapies for secondary prevention in a diverse group of patients with established cardiovascular disease or diabetes. The actively treated group showed significant reductions in morbidity and mortality, and those patients with PAD at baseline achieved above-average benefit from ramipril (**Fig. 1.5**).[50]

Patients in the HOPE study were already treated with various blood pressure-lowering therapies and their blood pressure control at the start of the study was relatively good. Although adding ramipril produced a further small reduction in blood pressure (no more than 3/2 mmHg), it seems likely that the protective effects of the ACE inhibitor were not solely due to blood pressure reduction. The notion of non-blood pressure-dependent cardiovascular protection with ACE inhibitors is also supported by the PROGRESS study, which showed that patients (stroke survivors) with relatively normal blood pressure benefited from ACE inhibitor therapy in terms of reduced risk of stroke recurrence and other major cardiovascular events.[51]

These studies indicate (albeit indirectly, based largely on the PAD subgroup of HOPE) that patients with intermittent claudication should be treated with ACE inhibitor therapy, in addition to any other blood pressure-lowering medication, unless there is good medical reason not to do so, e.g. bilateral renal artery stenosis or unilateral renal artery stenosis with a single functioning kidney.

Cholesterol

The epidemiological evidence relating cholesterol levels to the incidence and progression of PAD is mixed. The Framingham study showed that a fasting cholesterol greater than 7 mmol/L doubled the risk of intermittent claudication,[52] but not all observational studies have reached the same conclusion. The ratio of low-density lipoprotein (LDL) cholesterol to high-density lipoprotein (HDL) cholesterol is at least as important as total cholesterol levels in determining risk of PAD. Nevertheless, the epidemiological relationship between total cholesterol levels and atherothrombotic disease in the coronary circulation is unequivocally strong, although the relationship between cholesterol and total stroke incidence is somewhat diluted since haemorrhagic stroke (accounting for 15–20% of strokes) is unrelated to serum lipid levels.

Circulating cholesterol (unlike triglyceride) is mainly derived from endogenous biosynthesis in the liver (<20% of cholesterol is derived from the diet). LDLs carry cholesterol from the liver to peripheral tissues, whereas HDLs are protective in transferring cholesterol back to the liver from the peripheral tissues, including the vessel walls (**Fig. 1.6**). Low HDL cholesterol, or an increased LDL to HDL ratio, appears to be an independent risk factor for PAD in epidemiological studies.[3] More recent studies also suggest that circulating levels of apolipoproteins A and B (proteins contained within LDL particles) are independent risk factors for PAD.[53,54]

Although these various lipid parameters have been implicated as risk factors in population studies, the only intervention trials have so far focused on total cholesterol lowering; there have been no trials that have examined, for example, increases in HDL or changes in apolipoproteins A and B (largely because specific pharmacological tools are unavailable). Thus, in clinical practice, the mainstay of intervention is total cholesterol lowering with statins, drugs that inhibit the rate-limiting enzyme in cholesterol biosynthesis in the liver, i.e. hydroxymethylglutaryl (HMG)-CoA reductase.

The original randomised controlled trials of statins in secondary prevention focused on patients post-AMI, and these studies (e.g. 4S[55] and CARE[56]) demonstrated the benefits of lipid-lowering therapy in reducing cardiovascular morbidity and mortality. The 4S study with simvastatin and the CARE study with pravastatin showed 30–40% reductions in fatal and non-fatal cardiac events and stroke.[55,56] There is little published about subgroups of patients in these studies, but only 4% of participants in the 4S study had intermittent claudication at baseline. However, the incidence of new-onset or worsening claudication during the 4S trial was significantly lower in the statin-treated group (**Fig. 1.7**).[57]

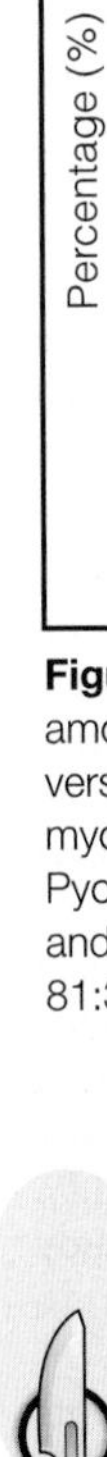

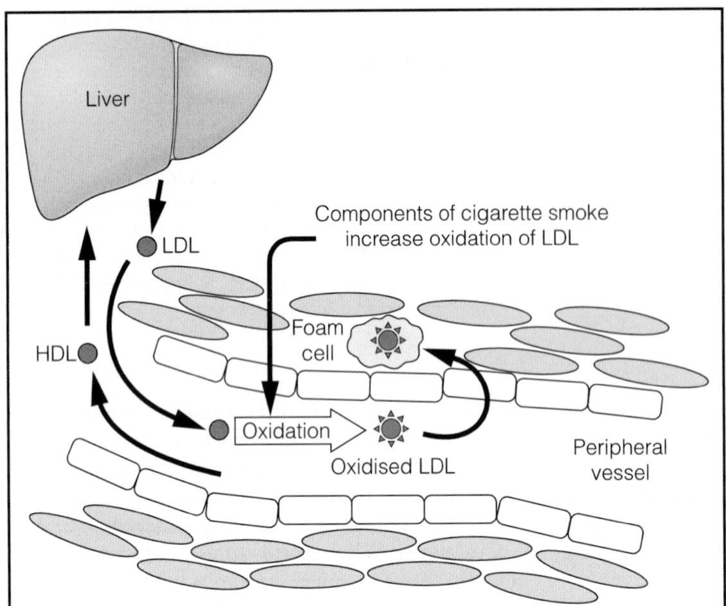

Figure 1.6 • Role of lipoproteins in atherosclerosis. High-density lipoproteins (HDL) transport cholesterol from peripheral tissues to the liver and low-density lipoproteins (LDL) transport from the liver to vascular tissues. Oxidised LDL is more readily taken up by macrophages in the vessel wall to form foam cells, a key step in plaque formation. The components of cigarette smoke increase the oxidation of LDL cholesterol.

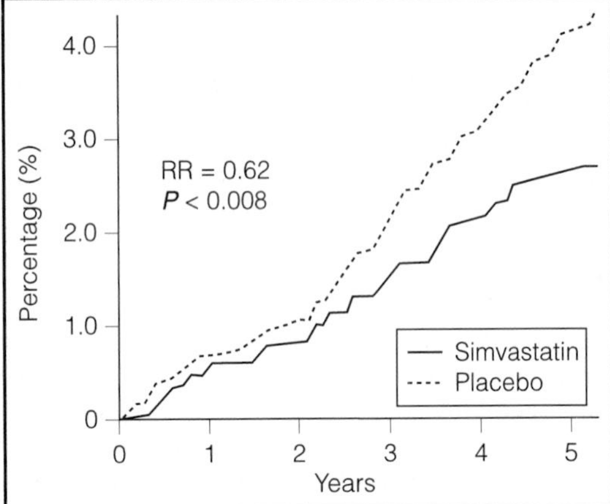

Figure 1.7 • Incidence of new or worsening claudication among 4000 participants in the 4S study of simvastatin versus placebo in patients recovering from acute myocardial infarction. From Pederson TR, Kjekshus J, Pyorala K et al. Effect of simvastatin on ischaemic signs and symptoms in the 4S study. Am J Cardiol 1998; 81:333–5, Excerpta Medica Inc., with permission.

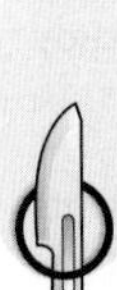

A Cochrane review of studies of lipid-lowering therapy in patients with PAD concluded that 'lipid-lowering therapy may be useful in preventing deterioration of underlying disease and alleviating symptoms' and found a marked, although non-significant, reduction in mortality.[58]

Patients with symptomatic PAD and hypercholesterolaemia should receive lipid-lowering therapy with a statin as the initial drug of choice.

In the light of the recent Heart Protection Study (HPS),[59] patients requiring secondary prevention are commenced on statins at even lower threshold levels of total cholesterol (e.g. >3.5 mmol/L) which, in practice, amounts to virtually everyone with PAD (**Fig. 1.8**). Thus statin use is based on levels of cardiovascular risk, not levels of cholesterol.

Antiplatelet therapy and warfarin

There is some evidence that PAD is associated with a hypercoagulable state. For example, it has been suggested that patients with intermittent claudication have a higher haematocrit and blood viscosity than the general population, but the Framingham study found no association between haematocrit and symptomatic PAD.[27] Several studies have confirmed that there is an association between high plasma fibrinogen levels and PAD, and that fibrinogen is a marker of thrombotic risk,[27] but of course there have been no intervention studies of fibrinogen lowering to establish whether selective modification of this risk factor improves clinical outcomes.

There have been numerous large randomised trials of antiplatelet therapy in patients with cardiovascular disease.

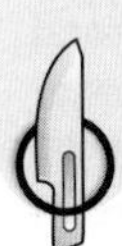

A meta-analysis by the Antiplatelet Trialists' Collaboration showed that antiplatelet therapy, mainly with low-dose aspirin, reduced the risk of non-fatal AMI, non-fatal stroke and vascular death in high-risk patients, including those with intermittent claudication.[60]

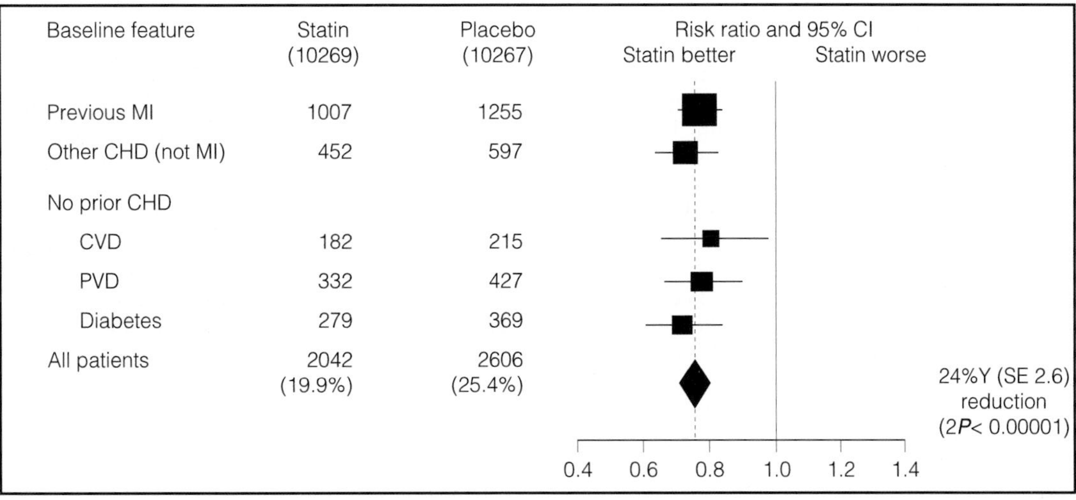

Figure 1.8 • Results of the Heart Protection Study showing that cholesterol reduction is of benefit to various subgroups, including those with peripheral arterial disease. CHD, coronary heart disease; CVD, cerebrovascular disease; PVD, peripheral vascular disease; MI, myocardial infarction. From Heart Protection Study Collaborative Group. MRC/BHF Heart Protection Study of cholesterol-lowering with simvastatin in 20,536 high-risk individuals. Elsevier (The Lancet 2002; 360:7–22), with permission.

Aspirin has no effect on symptoms of claudication, but some trials have shown that aspirin alone or in combination with dipyridamole delays the angiographic progression of PAD and reduces surgical intervention rates.[61,62] The standard dose of aspirin for secondary prevention, 75–100 mg daily, is effective in inhibiting platelet function but does not cause the excessive number of gastrointestinal adverse effects associated with higher doses.[63]

The CAPRIE study compared aspirin and clopidogrel and found a small net benefit with clopidogrel relative to aspirin (relative risk reduction of 9% for clopidogrel over aspirin). However, in the subgroup of patients with PAD enrolled in the CAPRIE study there was a more significant difference between the two groups.[2,64] Clopidogrel may therefore be preferred over aspirin as secondary prevention in patients with PAD, or reserved for use when aspirin cannot be tolerated. More recently, at least in acute coronary syndromes, the combination of clopidogrel and aspirin may be superior to either agent as monotherapy.[65]

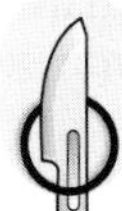

Guidelines for the use of antiplatelet therapy in PAD have recently been published.[66] These guidelines consider antiplatelet therapy in different common clinical scenarios and summarise the evidence to date.

Anticoagulation with warfarin is superior to aspirin in patients with PAD who are in atrial fibrillation, especially for reducing the risks of embolic stroke and acute limb ischaemia,[67] but there is no evidence to support the use of warfarin for secondary prevention in patients in sinus rhythm. Warfarin is maximally protective against acute embolic events in patients with atrial fibrillation when the international normalised ratio (INR) is optimised between 2 and 3; the risk of serious bleeding increases at INR levels greater than 4.

Physical exercise

A sedentary lifestyle may be an important risk factor for developing PAD.[68] The role of exercise in patients with chronic lower limb ischaemia is considered in detail in Chapter 3, but of course physical exercise has many beneficial health effects in secondary prevention. The importance of exercise and cardiac rehabilitation in post-AMI patients has been well established in randomised controlled trials, and regular exercise has favourable effects on body weight, insulin sensitivity and blood pressure in patients at high cardiovascular risk.

There is good evidence from randomised trials that exercise is of significant benefit to patients with established claudication. Indeed, a Cochrane review of 10 trials involving 250 patients found that supervised exercise programmes improved overall walking ability by approximately 150%, a significant improvement compared with both angioplasty and antiplatelet therapy[69] (see Chapter 3).

CONCLUSIONS

Occlusive arterial disease of the lower limbs is common and disabling; the prevalence increases steeply with age. Intermittent claudication affects 4–5% of the middle-aged population, but asymptomatic PAD is much more common and under-recognised. Although lower limb symptoms and outcomes are variable and generally benign, the associated excess risks of cardiovascular disease (i.e. AMI, stroke or sudden death) among patients with PAD are considerable and merit aggressive secondary prevention with atherosclerotic disease-modifying medical therapies.

Epidemiological studies have identified numerous risk factors that, in longitudinal follow-up studies in large populations, are associated with a higher incidence and more rapid progression of PAD. However, identifying a risk factor in a population does not necessarily imply that intervention in individuals to lower that risk factor will necessarily improve clinical outcomes. Such evidence only comes from randomised placebo-controlled trials.

The major modifiable risk factors are smoking, hyperlipidaemia, hypertension and diabetes. All patients with PAD merit secondary prevention with disease-modifying therapies to lower blood pressure and cholesterol levels, assist with smoking cessation and improve glycaemic control. The term 'conservative therapy', often favoured by surgeons, should be abandoned because it implies little or no intervention. Medical therapies are far from conservative, and will improve both patient and lower limb survival. Irrespective of whether the patient is offered revascularisation, everyone with PAD should receive 'best medical therapy' tailored to individual patients.

Cardiovascular risk factors have a greater-than-additive effect on overall risk. Most patients with PAD have more than one modifiable risk factor, and multiple risk factor intervention is likely to have a greater impact on risk reduction than targeted therapy for single risk factors.

Key points

- The prevalence of intermittent claudication in the middle-aged population is around 4–5%, but the prevalence of asymptomatic PAD may be nearer 50%.
- The incidence of PAD increases with increasing age and may be slightly more common in men.
- Among patients with intermittent claudication, around half will remain stable or improve and one-quarter will get worse over time. Only 5% will require surgical or radiological intervention and only 1–2% will end up having a major amputation.
- The risks of a fatal or non-fatal cardiovascular event are significantly increased in patients with intermittent claudication (similar risks are also present in asymptomatic PAD).
- Once patients have progressed to critical ischaemia, the overall mortality may be as high as 50% over 5 years.
- Risk factors for the development of PAD are similar to those for atherosclerotic disease elsewhere in the circulation, but smoking and diabetes may have a more significant impact in the legs.
- Smoking cessation reduces the excess cardiovascular risk within a relatively short period (2 years). Patients should be supported in smoking cessation via use of NRT to ameliorate nicotine withdrawal symptoms. NRT doubles quit rates at 1 year, relative to placebo, among motivated patients.
- Glycaemic control in diabetics is important in the prevention of microvascular complications, but other factors in the diabetes syndrome, such as hypertension and dyslipidaemia, may be more important in the development of PAD.
- Other important secondary prevention strategies to consider in any patient with PAD include statin therapy, blood pressure control, ACE inhibition, antiplatelet therapy and exercise.

REFERENCES

1. McKenna M, Wolfson S, Kuller L. The ratio of ankle and arm arterial pressure as an independent predictor of mortality. Atherosclerosis 1991; 87:119–28.
2. Donnelly R, Yeung JMC. Management of intermittent claudication: the importance of secondary prevention. Eur J Vasc Endovasc Surg 2002; 23:100–7.
3. Fowkes F. Edinburgh Artery Study: prevalence of asymptomatic and symptomatic peripheral arterial disease in the general population. Int J Epidemiol 1991; 20:384–92.
4. Leng GC. Incidence, natural history and cardiovascular events in symptomatic and asymptomatic peripheral arterial disease in the general population. Int J Epidemiol 1996; 25:1172–81.
5. Rose G. The diagnosis of ischaemic heart pain and intermittent claudication in field surveys. Bull WHO 1962; 27:645–58.
6. Criqui MH. The sensitivity, specificity, and predictive value of traditional clinical evaluation of peripheral arterial disease: results from noninvasive testing in a defined population. Circulation 1985; 71:516–22.
7. Leng GC, Fowkes FG. The Edinburgh Claudication Questionnaire: an improved version of the WHO/Rose Questionnaire for use in epidemiological surveys. J Clin Epidemiol 1992; 45:1101–9.
8. Schroll M, Munck O. Estimation of peripheral arteriosclerotic disease by ankle blood pressure measurements in a population study of 60-year-old men and women. J Chron Dis 1981; 34:261–9.
9. Transatlantic Inter-Society Consensus (TASC) Document. Management of peripheral arterial disease. J Vasc Surg 2000; 31:S5–S35.
10. Newman AB. Ankle–arm index as a marker of atherosclerosis in the Cardiovascular Health Study. Cardiovascular Heart Study (CHS) Collaborative Research Group. Circulation 1993; 88:837–45.
11. Leng GC. Femoral atherosclerosis in an older British population: prevalence and risk factors. Atherosclerosis 2000; 152:167–74.
12. Smith W, Woodward M, Tunstall-Pedoe H. Intermittent claudication in Scotland. In: Fowkes FGR (ed.) Epidemiology of peripheral vascular disease. London: Springer-Verlag, 1991; pp. 109–15.
13. Stoffers HE. The prevalence of asymptomatic and unrecognized peripheral arterial occlusive disease. Int J Epidemiol 1996; 25:282–90.
14. Critical limb ischaemia: management and outcome. Report of a national survey by the Vascular Surgical Society of Great Britain and Ireland. Eur J Vasc Endovasc Surg 1995; 10:108–13.
15. Hooi JD. Incidence of and risk factors for asymptomatic peripheral arterial occlusive disease: a longitudinal study. Am J Epidemiol 2001; 153:666–72.
16. Ogren M. Ten year cerebrovascular morbidity and mortality in 68 year old men with asymptomatic carotid stenosis. Br Med J 1995; 310:1294–8.
17. Bloor K. Natural history of arteriosclerosis of the lower extremities. Ann R Coll Surg Engl 1961; 28:36–51.
18. Da Silva A. The Basle longitudinal study: report on the relation of initial glucose level to baseline ECG abnormalities, peripheral artery disease, and subsequent mortality. J Chron Dis 1979; 32:797–803.
19. Eagle KA. Long-term survival in patients with coronary artery disease: importance of peripheral vascular disease. The Coronary Artery Surgery Study (CASS) Investigators. J Am Coll Cardiol 1994; 23:1091–5.
20. Lowe GD. Double-blind controlled clinical trial of ancrod for ischemic rest pain of the leg. Angiology 1982; 33:46–50.
21. Belch JJ. Epoprostenol (prostacyclin) and severe arterial disease. A double-blind trial. Lancet 1983; i:315–17.
22. De Weese J, Rob C. Autologous vein grafts ten years later. Surgery 1962; 6:775–84.
23. Boers G. Moderate hyperhomocysteinaemia and vascular disease: evidence, relevance and the effect of treatment. Eur J Pediatr 1998; 157(suppl. 2): S127–S130.
24. Murabito JM, D'Agostino RB, Silbershatz H et al. Intermittent claudication. A risk profile from the Framingham Heart Study. Circulation 1997; 96:44–9.
25. Phillips AN. Parental death from heart disease and the risk of heart attack. Eur Heart J 1988; 9:243–51.
26. Erb W. Klinische Beitrage zur Pathologie des intermittierenden hinkens. Munch Med Wochenschr 1911; 2:2487.
27. Kannel WB, McGee DL. Update on some epidemiologic features of intermittent claudication: the Framingham Study. J Am Geriatr Soc 1985; 33:13–18.
28. Jonason T, Ringqvist I. Factors of prognostic importance for subsequent rest pain in patients with intermittent claudication. Acta Med Scand 1985; 218:27–33.
29. Hirsch AT. The role of tobacco cessation, antiplatelet and lipid-lowering therapies in the treatment of peripheral arterial disease. Vasc Med 1997; 2:243–51.
30. Rosenberg L, Palmer JR, Shapiro S. Decline in the risk of myocardial infarction among women who stop smoking. N Engl J Med 1990; 322:213–17.
31. Silagy C. Meta-analysis on efficacy of nicotine replacement therapies in smoking cessation. Lancet 1994; 343:139–42.

This meta-analysis combines results of over 50 randomised trials of different forms of NRT and shows that active NRT (relative to placebo) doubles quit rates at 1 year among motivated patients.

32. Raw M, McNeill A, West R. Smoking cessation guidelines for health professionals. A guide to effective smoking cessation interventions for the health care system. Thorax 1998; 53(suppl. 5):S1–S19.

33. Cimminiello C. PAD: epidemiology and pathophysiology. Thromb Res 2002; 106:295–301.

34. Uusitupa M. 5-year incidence of atherosclerotic vascular disease in relation to gender, risk factors, insulin level and abnormalities in lipoprotein composition in non-insulin dependent diabetic and non-diabetic individuals. Circulation 1990; 82:27–36.

35. Kannel W, Wilson P, Zhang T. The epidemiology of impaired glucose tolerance and hypertension. Am Heart J 1991; 121:1268–73.

36. Fowkes FG. Epidemiological research on peripheral vascular disease. J Clin Epidemiol 2001; 54:863–8.

37. da Silva A. The management and outcome of critical limb ischaemia in diabetic patients: results of a national survey. Audit committee of the Vascular Surgical Society of Great Britain and Ireland. Diabetic Med 1996; 13:726–8.

38. Beks P. Peripheral arterial disease in relation to glycaemic level in an elderly caucasian population: the Hoorn study. Diabetologia 1995; 38:86–96.

39. Adler A. UKPDS 59: hyperglycaemia and other potentially modifiable risk factors for peripheral arterial disease in type 2 diabetes. Diabetes Care 2002; 25:894–9.

A large study conducted in the UK that showed a strong association between glycaemic control and PAD.

40. Forrest KY. Are predictors of coronary heart disease and lower-extremity arterial disease in type 1 diabetes the same? A prospective study. Atherosclerosis 2000; 148:159–69.

41. Haffner SM. Cardiovascular risk factors in confirmed prediabetic individuals. Does the clock for coronary heart disease start ticking before the onset of clinical diabetes? JAMA 1990; 263:2893–8.

42. Wheatcroft SB. Pathophysiological implications of insulin resistance on vascular endothelial function. Diabetic Med 2003; 20:255–68.

43. Price J, Lee A, Fowkes F. Hyperinsulinaemia: a risk factor for peripheral arterial disease in the non-diabetic population. J Cardiovasc Risk 1996; 3:501–5.

44. Orchard T. Insulin resistance-related factors, but not glycaemia, predict coronary artery disease in type 1 diabetes. Diabetes Care 2003; 26:1374–9.

45. Adler A. Association of systolic blood pressure with macrovascular and microvascular complications of type 2 diabetes (UKPDS 36): prospective observational study. Br Med J 2000; 321:412–19.

46. Hansson L. Effects of intensive blood-pressure lowering and low-dose aspirin in patients with hypertension: principal results of the Hypertension Optimal Treatment (HOT) randomised trial. HOT Study Group. Lancet 1998; 351:1755–62.

47. Beckman J, Creager M, Libby P. Diabetes and atherosclerosis: epidemiology, pathophysiology and management. JAMA 2002; 287:2570–81.

48. Neal B, MacMahon S, Chapman N. Effects of ACE inhibitors, calcium antagonists, and other blood-pressure-lowering drugs: results of prospectively designed overviews of randomised trials. Blood Pressure Lowering Treatment Trialists' Collaboration. Lancet 2000; 356:1955–64.

49. Brown MJ, Cruickshank JK, Dominiczak AF et al. Better blood pressure control: how to combine drugs. J Hum Hypertens 2003; 17:81–6.

50. Heart Outcomes Prevention Evaluation (HOPE) Study Investigators. Effects of ramipril on cardiovascular outcomes in people with diabetes mellitus: results of the HOPE Study and MICRO-HOPE Substudy. Lancet 2000; 355:253–9.

51. PROGRESS Collaborative Group. Randomised trial of perindopril-based blood pressure-lowering regimen among 6,105 individuals with previous stroke or transient ischaemic attack. Lancet 2001; 358:1033–41.

52. Kannel WB. Intermittent claudication. Incidence in the Framingham Study. Circulation 1970; 41:875–83.

53. Cheng SW, Ting AC, Wong J. Lipoprotein (a) and its relationship to risk factors and severity of atherosclerotic peripheral vascular disease. Eur J Vasc Endovasc Surg 1997; 14:17–23.

54. Pilger E. Risk factors for peripheral atherosclerosis. Retrospective evaluation by stepwise discriminant analysis. Arteriosclerosis 1983; 3:57–63.

55. Scandinavian Simvastatin Survival Study (4S). Randomised trial of cholesterol lowering in 4444 patients with coronary heart disease. Lancet 1994; 344:1383–9.

56. Sacks FM. The effect of pravastatin on coronary events after myocardial infarction in patients with average cholesterol levels. Cholesterol and Recurrent Events Trial Investigators. N Engl J Med 1996; 335:1001–9.

57. Pederson TR, Kjekshus J, Pyorala K et al. Effect of simvastatin on ischaemic signs and symptoms in the 4S study. Am J Cardiol 1998; 81:333–5.

58. Leng GC, Price JF, Jepson RG. Lipid-lowering for lower limb atherosclerosis. Cochrane Database Syst Rev 2000(2); CD000123.

Analysis of currently available data suggests that lipid-lowering therapy is of benefit for PAD patients in reducing morbidity and possibly mortality.

59. Heart Protection Study Collaborative Group. MRC/BHF Heart Protection Study of cholesterol-lowering with simvastatin in 20,536 high-risk individuals. Lancet 2002; 360:7–22.

60. Antiplatelet Trialists' Collaboration. Collaborative overview of randomised trials of antiplatelet therapy. I. Prevention of death, myocardial infarction, and stroke by prolonged antiplatelet therapy in various categories of patients. Br Med J 1994; 308:81–106.

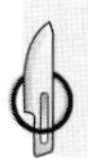

Evidence of the benefits of antiplatelet therapy in high-risk patients, including those with PAD.

61. Goldhaber SZ. Low-dose aspirin and subsequent peripheral arterial surgery in the Physicians' Health Study. Lancet 1992; 340:143–5.

62. Hirsh J. Aspirin and other platelet-active drugs. The relationship between dose, effectiveness, and side effects. Chest 1992; 102(4 suppl.):327S–336S.

63. Patrono C. Clinical pharmacology of platelet cyclooxygenase inhibition. Circulation 1985; 72:1177–84.

64. CAPRIE Steering Committee. A randomised, blinded trial of clopidogrel versus aspirin in patients at risk of ischaemic events (CAPRIE). Lancet 1996; 348:1329–39.

65. Yusuf S. Effects of clopidogrel in addition to aspirin in patients with acute coronary syndromes without ST-segment elevation. N Engl J Med 2001; 345:494–502.

66. Peripheral Arterial Disease Antiplatelet Consensus Group. Antiplatelet therapy in peripheral arterial disease: consensus statement. Eur J Vasc Endovasc Surg 2003; 26:1–16.

Recent evidence-based consensus guidelines for use of antiplatelet therapy in different clinical scenarios related to PAD.

67. Stroke Prevention in Atrial Fibrillation II Study. Warfarin versus aspirin for prevention of thromboembolism in atrial fibrillation. Lancet 1994; 343:687–91.

68. Housley E. Physical activity and risk of peripheral arterial disease in the general population: Edinburgh Artery Study. J Epidemiol Community Health 1993; 47:475–80.

69. Leng GC, Fowler B, Ernst E. Exercise for intermittent claudication. Cochrane Database Syst Rev 2000(2); CD000990.

CHAPTER

Two

Assessment of chronic lower limb ischaemia

Charles N. McCollum and
Raymond J. Ashleigh

INTRODUCTION

Atherosclerosis frequently results in stenosis or occlusion, which may involve either a single or multiple segments of the arteries supplying the leg. Stenosis, or even occlusion at the aortic bifurcation or in the superficial femoral artery at the adductor canal, is common and in isolation will usually cause the patient to suffer only intermittent claudication. More generalised disease involving proximal and distal arteries, or severe stenosis/occlusion in critical locations where the collaterals are poor, may result in critical ischaemia with rest pain, ulceration or gangrene involving the toes or forefoot.

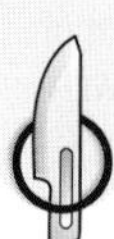

The prognosis for intermittent claudication is benign but critical ischaemia implies a threat of amputation unless an adequate blood supply can be restored to the involved tissues. Recognising the clinical features of critical ischaemia and understanding that all patients with lower limb arterial disease are also at risk of myocardial infarction, stroke or other cardiovascular events is the key to managing peripheral arterial disease (PAD).

Intermittent claudication

This symptom describes pain, analogous to angina, experienced by a patient when the arterial (or venous) supply to the leg muscles is insufficient to meet the metabolic needs on exercise. The blood supply required by resting muscles is relatively small and students are frequently surprised to hear that the total flow in the superficial femoral artery at rest is only 130–150 mL/min. This modest blood flow may easily be supplied through an arterial stenosis, or via collaterals in the event of occlusion. The blood supply to the foot may therefore appear normal at rest, although distal pulses are frequently absent. Occlusions are usually well tolerated when surrounded by muscle. Examples include the superficial femoral artery at the adductor canal, which is well collateralised by the profunda femoral artery through the thigh muscles, or occlusions of the iliac arteries where collaterals through the pelvis and buttock may perfuse the limb by reversing flow in the internal iliac or profunda femoral arteries (**Fig. 2.1**). In the latter example, collateral flow at rest may be sufficient to produce easily palpable pulses throughout the leg and feet, even in the presence of severe claudication. An exercise challenge will reveal a femoral bruit with the disappearance of the leg pulses.

The benign prognosis for claudication is based on the up to tenfold increase in blood flow required by exercising muscles. A flow of more than 1 L/min can no longer be delivered through a stenosis in the superficial femoral artery or via collaterals through the thigh (**Fig. 2.2**). As a result, the exercising calf muscle becomes profoundly ischaemic and this causes pain, which is rapidly relieved when the patient stops to rest. Although collaterals around distal aortic or common iliac occlusions may easily perfuse the lower limb at rest (**Fig. 2.1**), the ability to compensate for exercise is particularly poor as the flow demands of exercising calf, thigh and buttock muscles are much greater than can be supplied via collaterals. For this reason, conservative treatment with regular exercise may substantially improve

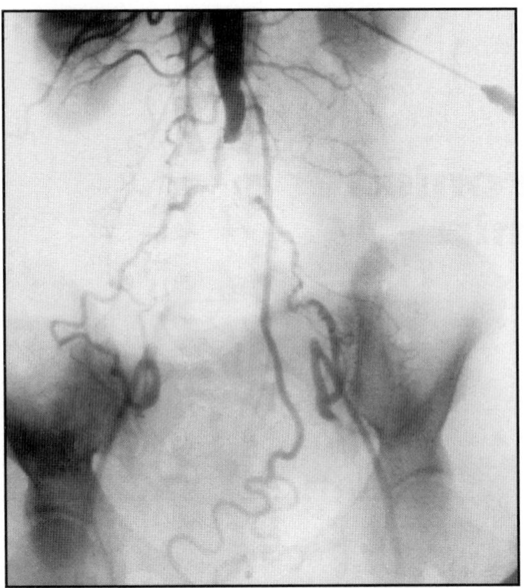

Figure 2.1 • Aortogram demonstrating complete occlusion of the distal aorta and common iliac arteries with collaterals from the lumbar and inferior mesenteric arteries retrogradely filling the internal iliac arteries to perfuse the legs. Despite a clear history of calf, thigh and buttock claudication with impotence (Leriche's syndrome), this 53-year-old man had palpable pulses at rest.

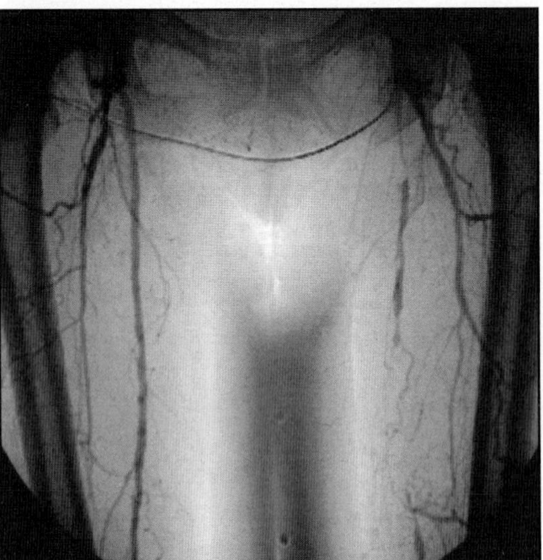

Figure 2.2 • Bilateral femoral angiogram demonstrating complete occlusion of the left superficial femoral artery at its origin and above the adductor canal, with well-developed thigh collaterals from the profunda femoral artery filling the proximal popliteal artery.

claudication distances in patients with calf claudication only but has little effect when claudication involves the entire leg.

Critical ischaemia

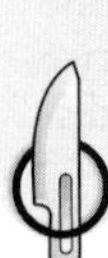

The diagnosis of ischaemic rest pain, and the appearance of either ischaemic ulceration or gangrene of the toes, imply the need for urgent revascularisation in order to avoid progressive tissue necrosis leading ultimately to amputation. The prognosis is entirely different to that for claudication and the recognition of rest ischaemia is a key skill for vascular surgeons.

In an attempt to standardise the diagnosis, there have been European consensus documents on critical leg ischaemia that include a requirement that the ankle arterial pressure be less than 50 mmHg.[1] However, this figure is arbitrary as at least one-third of patients presenting with a history of rest pain or even tissue necrosis may have an ankle systolic pressure greater than this.[2] Rest pain, or ischaemic gangrene of the toes, with higher than expected ankle arterial pressures implies either distal small-vessel disease in the foot or embolisation from proximal atherosclerosis.

The importance of critical ischaemia is that the blood supply to the involved tissue is insufficient to meet the metabolic demands of that tissue, even at rest: the ischaemic changes will progress unless an adequate blood supply can be restored. Frequently this is due to arterial occlusion at a site when there are no muscles to carry collaterals from above to below the occlusion, such as in the groin or popliteal fossa (**Fig. 2.3**) Transient improvement may occur with rest, by stimulating vasodilatation in the collaterals or by reducing blood viscosity. However, these patients frequently have multi-segment arterial occlusions or severe proximal disease that may be a source of embolisation into the feet. Unless this proximal disease is addressed, the majority of such patients will suffer progressive tissue necrosis leading to ischaemic gangrene and ultimately to amputation.

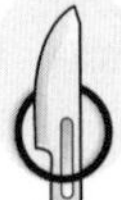

Although a conservative approach with management of risk factors may be ideal for claudication, patients with critical ischaemia require urgent investigation with a view to revascularisation.

CLINICAL ASSESSMENT

History

The diagnosis of both claudication and critical ischaemia can usually be made from the history supported by minimally invasive investigations. It is also important to take a full cardiovascular history and to document risk factors because the majority

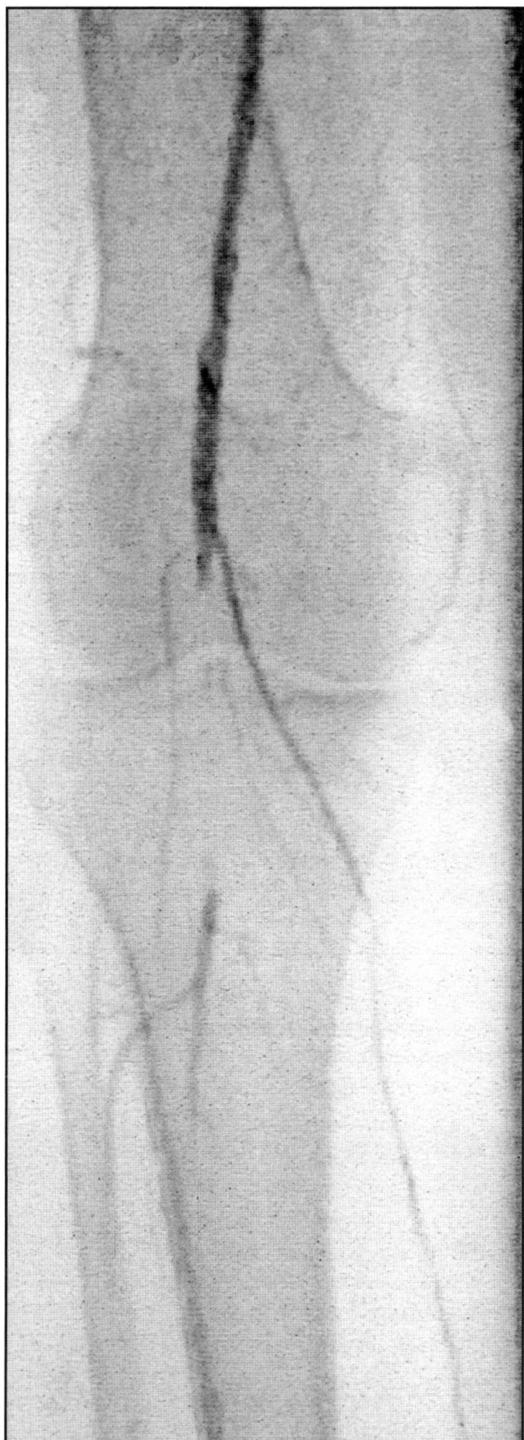

Figure 2.3 • Complete occlusion of the popliteal artery at the knee will usually cause severe ischaemia of the foot, as there are no muscles arising from above the knee and passing to below the knee in which collaterals may run.

of patients with PAD will ultimately die of myocardial infarction, stroke or other cardiovascular events.[3] The patient's lifestyle and quality of life are also important as arterial reconstruction for intermittent claudication is only appropriate when quality of life is significantly impaired.

INTERMITTENT CLAUDICATION

This is a frequent symptom in the elderly, occurring in 14% of men over the age of 65 years,[4] increasing to 21% in those over the age of 85 years. The differential diagnosis includes osteoarthritis of the hip or knee with referred pain down the leg and lumbar nerve route irritation causing sciatica. Occasionally, patients with symptoms very similar to claudication may have spinal stenosis, leading to neurological symptoms in the legs on walking.[5] Although the diagnosis can usually be established on history and examination alone, minimally invasive investigations to exclude arterial disease may be reassuring for the general practitioner (GP).

The classic features of intermittent claudication are that the pain develops within a muscle (usually the calf but often the thigh or buttock) on walking (**Box 2.1**). This pain is not felt at rest or when the first few steps are taken while setting out for a walk. The pain develops progressively on walking and is described as an ache, cramp or tightening in the muscle that usually forces the patient to stop. Occasionally, mild claudication may be felt only while walking uphill or quickly. In most cases, the patient stops to rest and experiences relief within minutes. The symptoms then return after walking a similar distance.

Patients with osteoarthritis of the hip with referred pain down the leg and a history similar to claudication are often referred by their GP. These patients usually experience some pain in the buttock or groin when turning in bed at night or when rising from an armchair. They can often continue walking with a limp despite the severity of their pain (which severe claudicants cannot). The pain is not relieved by standing still as the patient needs to take weight off the involved joint. This latter feature is also typical of osteoarthritis in the knee. Such patients

Box 2.1 • Key features of intermittent claudication

- No pain at rest or during the first few steps
- A relatively consistent walking distance
- Relief on standing for 1–3 minutes
- No need to sit or lie
- Recurrence on walking a similar distance
- Worse on walking quickly or uphill

complain of a severe pain in the leg while walking that can only be relieved when they sit or lie down.

Lumbar nerve route irritation may also cause aching in the calf or down the back of the leg from buttock to ankle. The sensation appears to be very similar to that of claudication, particularly when confined to the calf. Again, patients may experience symptoms in bed or particularly when descending stairs or stepping off curbs (jarring the back). Direct enquiry for these symptoms is helpful, but the key feature is again the need to sit or lie to obtain relief; spinal flexion may release the involved nerve routes (or reduce venous engorgement in spinal stenosis).[5] As both sciatica and claudication are common in the elderly, they may coexist in the same patient.

The history should include the duration of symptoms and the mode of onset. Most patients gradually become aware of pain on walking, which is typical in progressive arterial disease. The first, and apparently sudden, onset of symptoms while walking an unaccustomed distance (perhaps on holiday) is also consistent with PAD.

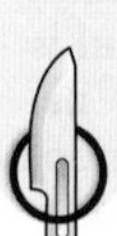

However, the sudden development of pain and numbness of the leg resolving over a period of hours but followed by severe claudication suggests femoral embolism or thrombosis. A history of sudden onset of this type, particularly if claudication is severe initially but improves over days or weeks, suggests the need to investigate for a proximal source of embolus.

CRITICAL ISCHAEMIA

'Cold feet' is a frequent and usually insignificant complaint in claudicants. Critical ischaemia in its mildest form starts with numbness in the toes at night sufficient to disturb the patient's sleep. This progresses to a burning pain, which occurs most nights when the feet are warm in bed. This warmth increases the metabolic rate of the involved tissues such that the blood supply is no longer able to meet the metabolic needs. In common with any chemical reaction, the metabolic rate approximately doubles when the temperature increases by 10°C. Patients with ischaemic rest pain obtain relief by hanging the involved leg out of bed or by getting up and walking around, thereby cooling the foot.

Students frequently describe 'rest pain' involving the ankle, calf or more proximal leg. Although this may be 'pain at rest', this clearly needs to be distinguished from ischaemic rest pain, which in PAD will almost always be experienced in the most distal part of the limb (toes or fingers). It is inconceivable that the arterial supply to the toes will be adequate while at the same time being inadequate to meet the metabolic needs of resting tissues proximally. The exceptions are acute compartment syndromes or where tissue necrosis is due to a combination of factors such as venous hypertension or compression. Thankfully, the diagnosis of ischaemic rest pain is usually made easy by a colour change, with pallor in the acute situation and cyanosis with chronic ischaemia.

Patients with rest ischaemia usually hang their feet out of bed or even sleep sitting in a chair. The limb swells with dependency oedema, which may be sufficiently severe to cause ankle ulceration of the mixed arterial–venous type (**Fig. 2.4**, see also Plate 1, facing p. 116). Oedema also increases the distance that oxygen and metabolites have to diffuse from the microcirculation to the relevant tissues, aggravating tissue damage.

Ulceration in critical ischaemia almost always involves a bony high point such as the head of the first or fifth metacarpal, a medial or lateral malleolus or the back of the heel where the foot rests while lying in bed (**Fig. 2.5**, see also Plate 2, facing

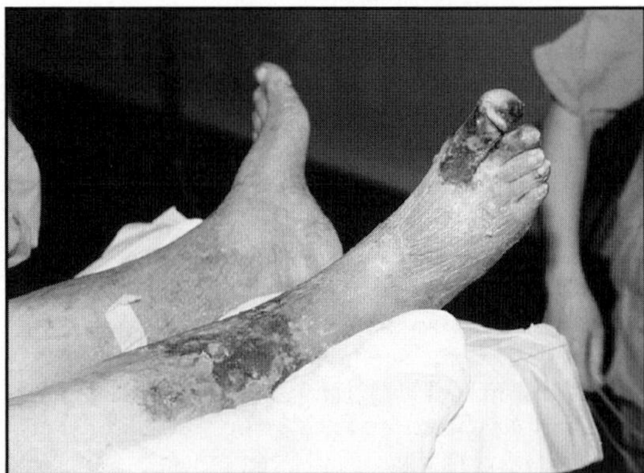

Figure 2.4 • Severe ischaemia over 3 months has resulted in gangrene of the great toe and ulceration of the venous type above the ankle as this man has been sleeping overnight in a chair.

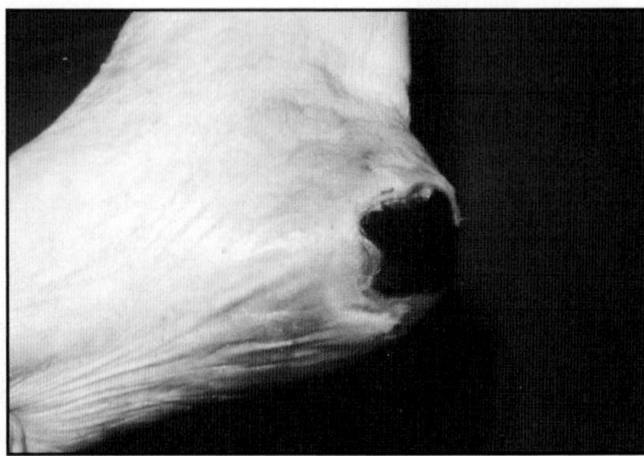

Figure 2.5 • Pressure necrosis of the type illustrated over this heel occurs easily in rest ischaemia of the foot, as tissue perfusion pressures are low and easily overwhelmed by compression within a shoe or against the mattress at night.

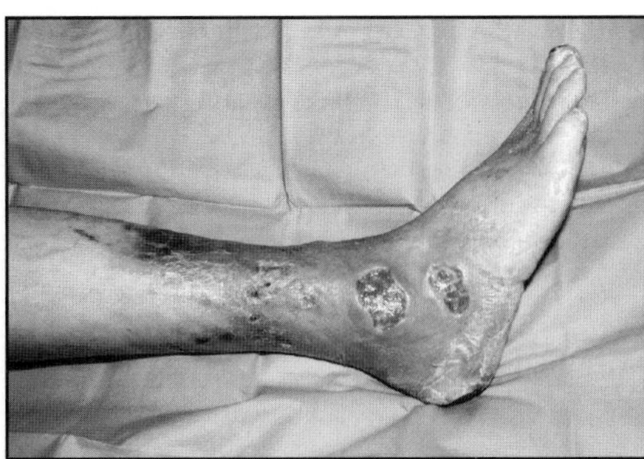

Figure 2.6 • Typical features of venous ulceration are apparent with pigmentation and lipodermatosclerosis. However, these atypical ulcers on the lateral aspect suggest mixed arterial and venous ulceration with an ankle pressure in this patient of only 65 mmHg (ABPI 0.4).

p. 116). Ulceration is due to pressure necrosis where the relatively mild pressures involved are sufficient to cause ischaemia when the arterial perfusion pressure is low. Ulceration may also occur in the lower leg just above the ankle, often atypical ulcers on the lateral aspect of the leg, with the position being a clue to the underlying diagnosis of mixed arterial–venous ulceration (**Fig. 2.6**, see also Plate 3, facing p. 116).

Digital gangrene may develop in a single toe initially, which perhaps emphasises the importance of embolisation. The great and little toes are most frequently involved (**Fig. 2.4**) but gangrene may develop in any of the toes in isolation or all the toes may become severely ischaemic, with necrosis from the tip progressing towards the base.

CARDIOVASCULAR HISTORY AND RISK FACTORS

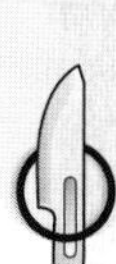

As all patients with PAD are at risk of myocardial infarction or stroke, a full history for other cardiovascular diseases and for risk factors is essential. In addition to previous myocardial infarction, stroke, coronary artery bypass grafting and arterial surgery, direct enquiry should cover symptoms suggestive of angina or transient cerebral ischaemia.

Although approximately 30% of patients with symptoms of limb ischaemia will also have a history of angina or myocardial infarction,[6] it is not uncommon for angina or transient ischaemic attack to be diagnosed for the first time. The investigation and treatment of these symptoms usually have a higher priority than PAD. The enquiry for cardiovascular risk factors is equally important and obviously covers smoking, diabetes, hypertension, cholesterol or other lipid abnormalities and a detailed drug history. This history alone, or supported by lipid analysis, allows the clinician to construct a relatively accurate risk score for subsequent cardiovascular events.[7,8]

Examination

Patients with PAD are usually elderly and often smoke. They are at risk of conditions such as cancer in addition to cardiovascular problems and deserve a full physical examination. This should focus on identifying risk factors, on the cardiovascular system generally and then specifically on clinical features to establish the severity and site of PAD.

CARDIOVASCULAR RISK FACTORS

The outpatient nursing staff should measure height and weight in order to calculate body mass index (BMI), test the urine for sugar and proteins and record blood pressure and pulse. The clinician examines the pulse for arrhythmias such as atrial fibrillation and looks for features of hypertension. The abdomen should be palpated for aortic aneurysm; where the aorta cannot be felt easily in patients aged over 65, an ultrasound examination should be requested. Although carotid bruits may originate from the common, internal or external carotid arteries, the detection of significant internal carotid stenosis is important and bruits should be investigated. Nicotine staining of the fingers and the typical smell of smoking is surprisingly frequent in patients who deny smoking. Clinicians should record the level of fitness in addition to the BMI.

THE LOWER LIMB

The general appearance is important; good hair growth on the foot or lower leg is unusual in patients with PAD. Tissue healing is impaired in critical ischaemia and small sores or non-healing wounds on the foot and lower leg are frequent. Clinicians should be aware of the microcirculation in the foot: a foot that appears redder than the other side, particularly associated with cyanosis, may demonstrate vasodilatation of the microcirculation due to tissue ischaemia (**Fig. 2.7**, see also Plate 4, facing p. 116).

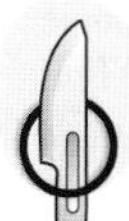

Buerger's test, with pallor on elevation and abnormal rubor on dependency, is perhaps the most important physical sign in PAD as it is the first reliable clinical warning of rest ischaemia.

Unfortunately, GPs are frequently reassured by the hyperaemic appearance of a pink or red vasodilated foot and may be unaware that the term 'sunset foot' covers both the appearance and the prognosis. Both feet should be examined with the legs elevated to at least 45° and then with the patient sitting on

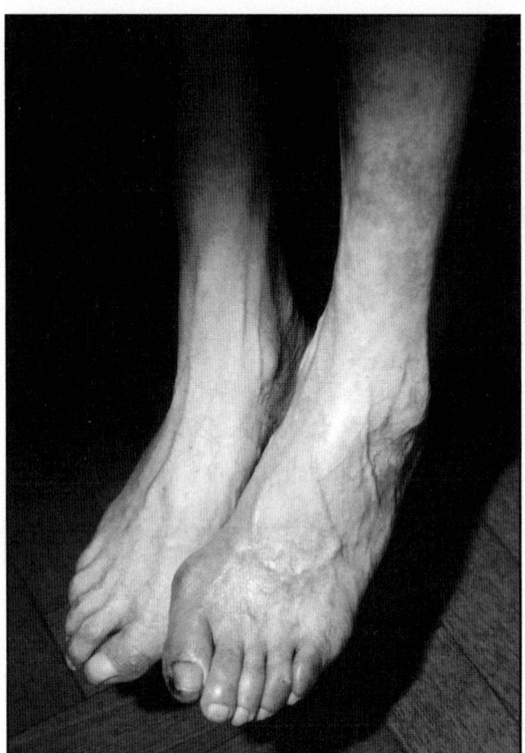

Figure 2.7 • There is profound vasodilatation of the toes and forefoot on the left typical of severe ischaemia. The appearances may be red or even cyanosed in dependency but on elevation this foot would become pale with venous guttering.

the edge of the couch with the feet in dependency (**Fig. 2.7**). Enthusiasts may record capillary and venous refilling times, but the severity and extent of vasodilatation involving the toes, forefoot or entire foot and ankle are more important

Every doctor knows it is essential to record the pulses, but palpation of pulses is subjective and influenced by both the sensitivity of the fingers and the experience of the examiner. If there is any doubt, arterial waveform and pressure can be established using hand-held Doppler, which should now be routine in clinical examination (**Fig. 2.8**). The femoral pulse should always be palpable and auscultation will reveal whether there is a bruit typical of iliac or common femoral stenosis. The popliteal pulse is more difficult, particularly in a well-muscled man. If a student feels a popliteal pulse easily, the possibility of popliteal aneurysm should be considered! Palpation of the foot pulses is only easy where the pulses are obvious. Describing a pulse as 'weak' is subjective and only appropriate when clearly different from the contralateral pulse. The absence of one foot pulse may have little clinical significance and, although it should be

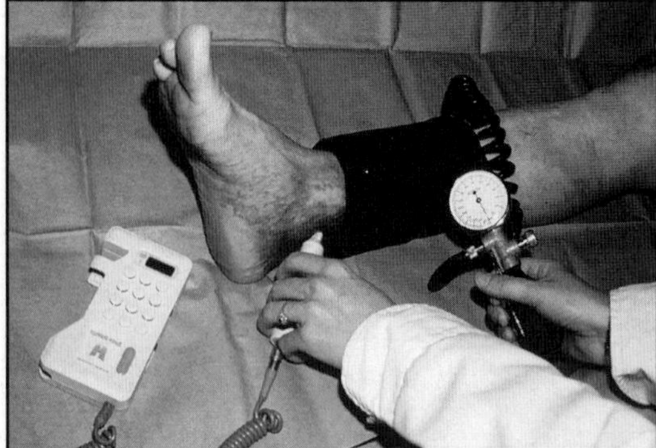

Figure 2.8 • Auscultation by hand-held Doppler establishes arterial flow waveforms at rest and allows measurement of the ankle arterial pressure.

recorded, is not an indication for more detailed investigation.

If foot pulses cannot be palpated, then insonation by hand-held Doppler will identify any abnormality. This is particularly useful in patients with reflex sympathetic dystrophy due to immobility of a limb following injury or paralysis. Those with long-standing paralysis, due to polio in childhood or previous stroke, may develop a swollen foot with cyanosis of the toes and absent pulses. On Doppler insonation there is a healthy biphasic or triphasic Doppler signal and normal arterial pressures. Although the foot may appear ischaemic, the cause is merely atrophy of the microcirculation due to reduced metabolic demands. Exercise if possible or massage tends to restore warmth and improve the colour.

EXERCISE CHALLENGE

Patients present occasionally with a history of intermittent claudication but with adequate pulses throughout the leg. These patients may have been investigated previously for joint disease or lumbar nerve route irritation or may even have been referred to pain clinics or psychiatrists. Typically, there is proximal aorto-iliac disease with collaterals through the pelvis sufficient to produce adequate or even normal pulses at rest. In patients who complain of symptoms only on exercise, it is surprising how rarely doctors examine the leg following an exercise challenge. This can be done quite simply in the consulting room. Even elderly patients find it easy to exercise the calf muscle by a repeated 'tip toe' while leaning on the couch (**Fig. 2.9**). The patient returns to the couch so that the pulses can be examined immediately after exercising for 1 minute. Absent or 'tapping' femoral pulses with overlying bruits confirm the diagnosis of aorto-iliac disease.

(a)

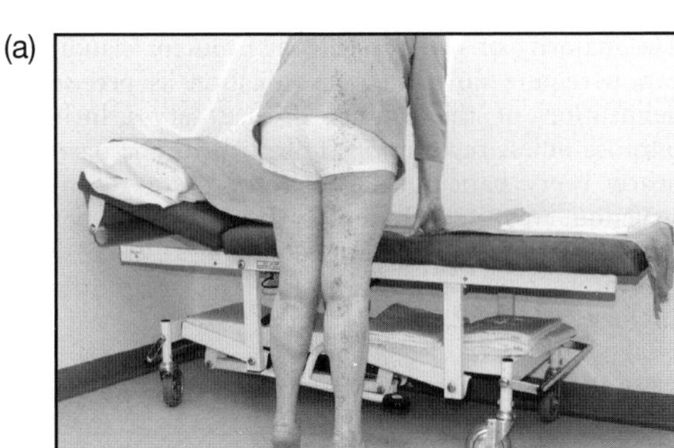

(b)

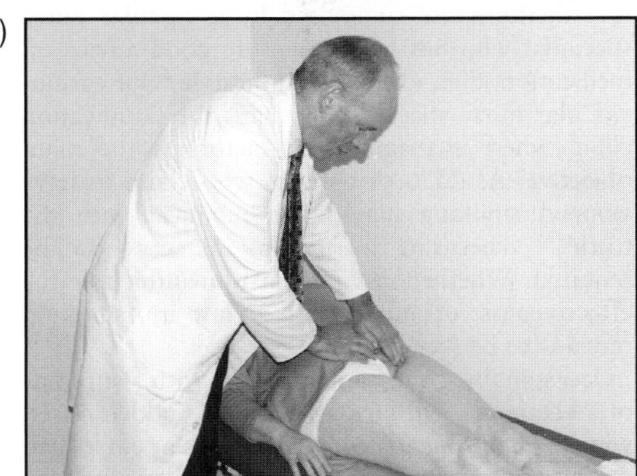

Figure 2.9 • Simple 'tip-toe' exercise of the calf muscle **(a)** causes vasodilatation with **(b)** disappearance of pulses and the emergence of bruits on examination immediately after the exercise.

EXAMINATION BY HAND-HELD DOPPLER

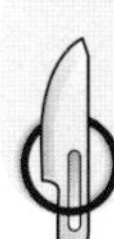

A hand-held Doppler with 4- and 8-MHz continuous-wave Doppler probes (**Fig. 2.8**) should be routine in vascular examination, but measuring ankle arterial pressures is not essential in every patient with intermittent claudication.

Most such patients have well-perfused feet and investigation of the arteries is entirely unnecessary as treatment will be conservative initially. Patients with aorto-iliac disease are the exception as little improvement in claudication distance can be expected with conservative therapy.

ANKLE–BRACHIAL PRESSURE INDEX

The perfusion pressure at the ankle can be measured using a tourniquet and insonation of the pedal arteries by continuous-wave Doppler (see **Fig. 2.8**). The patient should be lying supine and should rest for a few minutes prior to the application of a standard blood pressure tourniquet just above the ankle. This tourniquet should be 50% wider than the limb diameter. The tourniquet cuff is inflated above systolic pressure, when the pedal Doppler signal should disappear. On gradually lowering the cuff pressure, the Doppler signal reappears at the ankle systolic pressure. Ideally, two pedal pressures should be taken (dorsalis pedis and posterior tibial arteries) but more frequent cuff inflation will result in an exercise effect. The systolic blood pressure is taken from the brachial artery using the same 8-MHz Doppler probe and the ankle–brachial pressure index (ABPI) calculated as the ratio of the ankle to the brachial systolic pressures. As cardiac ejection generates pulses of kinetic energy in blood flowing down the aorta into the limb arteries, the systolic pressure at the ankle is normally higher than at the wrist, with an ABPI of 1.0–1.2. An ABPI of less than 0.9 suggests arterial disease, with 0.8 being the lower limit of normal. An ABPI of less than 0.3 is associated with critical ischaemia.

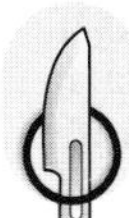

In practice, absolute pressures of more than 60 mmHg are rarely associated with foot ischaemia unless the distal foot arteries are diseased or have been embolised from a proximal source.

As falsely high ankle arterial pressures may be measured if the calf arteries are rigid due to calcification, the pedal signal is examined first for at least a biphasic waveform. Monophasic and damped waveforms clearly imply a resistance to flow proximal to the artery being examined. A clear cut-off on inflating a tourniquet with signal resumption on gradual deflation suggests that the pressure at which flow resumes is accurate. However, when the Doppler signal in the foot is monophasic, pressures above the brachial pressure suggest falsely high readings. Triphasic waveforms demonstrate considerable elasticity in the arterial system with no abnormal resistance to flow proximally. Even a biphasic waveform excludes significant resistance to flow proximally, although the elasticity in the arterial system may be impaired.

Hand-held Doppler is clearly indicated for patients with leg ulceration, foot ulcers or ischaemic lesions on the feet. The technique is particularly important in diabetic 'neuropathic' ulcers or infection involving the toes or feet where missed proximal arterial disease may lead to amputation due to rapidly progressing infection. Measuring the ABPI is also useful in elderly patients referred with foot symptoms that do not appear to be vascular. Their GPs can be reassured by an adequate ABPI and reasonable waveform (even if abnormal).

TOE PRESSURES

Toe pressure measurements may be useful when the calf arteries are incompressible or when severe distal arterial disease in the foot is suspected.[9] A

2–3 cm occlusion cuff is placed around the proximal phalanx of the great, second or third toe with a photoelectric cell on the toe distally. The toe pressure can be measured using photoplethysmography to detect the disappearance and reappearance of the pulse as the cuff is inflated and deflated. A warm room is essential to avoid vasospasm. Expressed as a ratio to brachial artery pressure, toe pressures are normally lower than ABPI at 0.8–0.9. Critical ischaemia is unusual with toe–brachial pressure ratios greater than 0.3 or absolute toe pressures greater than 30 mmHg.[10]

THE ISCHAEMIC ANGLE

As a refinement to Buerger's test, the level at which a pedal Doppler signal disappears on elevation of the foot may be taken as a crude measure of ankle arterial pressure when the calf arteries are incompressible.[10] This technique has been called the 'pole test' as the foot is raised alongside a calibrated pole marked in mmHg (0.73 mmHg = 1 cmH_2O). This technique is only useful in severe ischaemia as it is not possible to raise the foot high enough for normal pressures.

INVESTIGATION

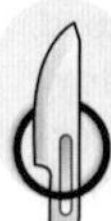

All patients should be investigated for risk factors as modification reduces both the risk of fatal cardiovascular events and the need for arterial reconstruction.[11,12]

The majority of patients with intermittent claudication require no further investigation as precise delineation of the arterial disease serves little purpose unless reperfusion is planned. In the past, nearly every patient being considered for reconstruction was investigated by angiography, but minimally invasive investigations in a vascular laboratory have progressively replaced diagnostic angiograms (**Fig. 2.10**).

Cardiovascular risk factors

The investigation of cardiovascular risk factors is summarised in **Box 2.2**. In our practice, these investigations are supervised by a vascular nurse specialist who has time to ensure good advice on medication, diet, exercise and lifestyle. Our cardiovascular nurse specialist also runs the claudication clinic where managing risk factors is the main objective. As 25% of patients who claim to have stopped smoking may be 'economical with the truth',[13] measuring a smoking marker may be required. Whether this information influences the effectiveness of advice on giving up smoking remains to be seen.

Occasionally, young adults attend with symptoms of PAD; some will give a history of sudden onset, which may be due to acute thrombosis or embolism. As thromboembolism is relatively frequent in patients under the age of 50, a thrombophilia screen is justified. Antiphospholipid antibodies are often found in sudden unexplained arterial thrombosis.

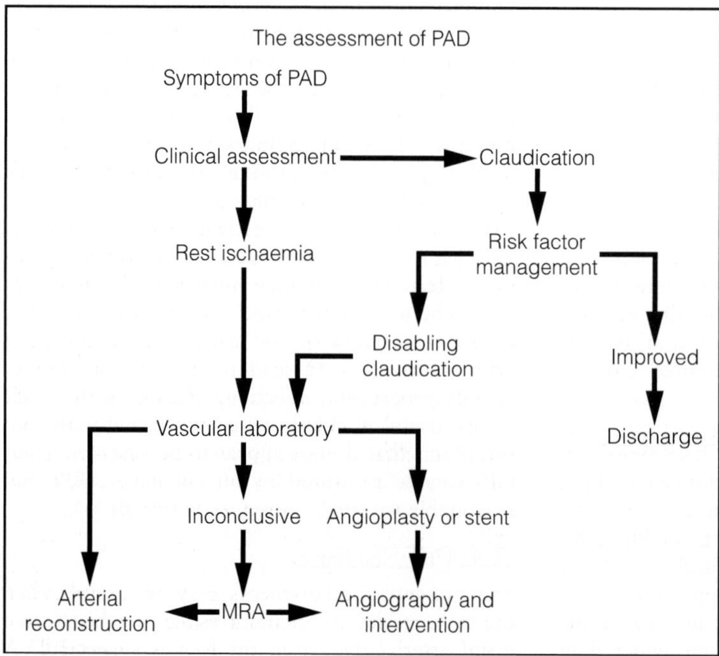

Figure 2.10 • Flow chart depicting our usual assessment of patients with peripheral arterial disease (PAD). Only claudicants with severe proximal disease or continued disabling claudication following months of conservative treatment undergo arterial investigations. MRA, magnetic resonance angiography.

Box 2.2 • Investigation of cardiovascular risk factors

ALL PATIENTS
Full blood count
Anaemia
Polycythaemia
Thrombocythaemia
Biochemical profile
Diabetes
Renal impairment
Paraproteinaemias
Fasting lipid profile
Total cholesterol
HDL cholesterol
LDL cholesterol
VLDL cholesterol
Triglycerides
SELECTED PATIENTS
Age <50 years or acute unusual thrombosis
Thrombophilia screen: antithrombin 3 deficiency, lupus anticoagulant, antiphospholipid antibodies
Ex-smokers
Thiocyanate or carboxyhaemoglobin

The failure to detect antiphospholipid antibodies or antithrombin III deficiency may lead to repeated rethrombosis following either angioplasty or reconstruction.

Vascular laboratory

A vascular laboratory staffed by specialist vascular technologists has become the ideal approach for the initial investigation of arterial disease. The number of minimally invasive vascular laboratory investigations at South Manchester University Hospital increased from 1500 in 1993 to 8000 in 2003. Our vascular laboratory has virtually replaced diagnostic angiography in PAD, allowing our vascular radiologists to concentrate on interventional procedures (**Fig. 2.10**).

WAVEFORM ASSESSMENT AND SEGMENTAL PRESSURES

Continuous-wave Doppler still has an important role in the investigation of PAD, although the clinician can perform this as part of the examination. A fall in pressure of 20% following an exercise challenge confirms significant arterial disease in patients with palpable pulses at rest.[14] It is valuable in confirming the presence or absence of PAD as a cause of leg symptoms. The elasticity in normal arteries gives a characteristic triphasic Doppler waveform. The blood pressure reduces distal to a stenosis and therefore the resistance from the capillary beds is reduced, changing the shape of this waveform. Distal to a 50% stenosis the waveform is biphasic, and with a greater than 70% stenosis the waveform becomes monophasic.[14] Waveform shape can be affected by distal disease, dilatation of arteries, multisegment disease, complete occlusion of an artery and also ambient temperature. Waveform shape can only give an indication of disease and should be used in conjunction with segmental pressures to determine which segments in the leg are diseased.

If the ABPI is reduced to less than 0.8, disease can be localised by placing the blood pressure cuff around the high calf, low thigh and final high thigh and repeating pressure measurements using the same pedal signal. The ratio can be calculated by dividing these pressures by the brachial pressure. A significant segment of disease is characterised by a fall in this ratio of 0.2 between two consecutive cuffs. These techniques can be used to guide further investigation and predict the outcome of intervention.

Segmental arterial pressures have value in both determining the level of disease and predicting whether proximal arterial reconstruction will be adequate to treat critical ischaemia in the foot. Clinicians frequently see patients with multisegment disease involving the iliac and superficial femoral arteries supplying the same leg (**Fig. 2.11**, see also Plate 5, facing p. 116). A proximal procedure (angioplasty or ilio-profunda bypass) is clearly essential but may fail to adequately reperfuse the foot when the superficial femoral artery is occluded. In this example, the brachial pressure is 160 mmHg, with a high thigh pressure of 80 mmHg, a low thigh pressure of 60 mmHg and an ankle pressure of 35 mmHg. Following proximal bypass to the profunda, we anticipate that the high thigh pressure would be corrected to 160 mmHg and the low thigh and ankle pressures to 120 and 70 mmHg respectively. This should be entirely sufficient to correct rest ischaemia and encourage healing of a foot wound in most patients. Had the high and low thigh pressures been considerably higher (perhaps 130 and 110 mmHg respectively) then the improvement in ankle pressure following a proximal reconstruction would almost certainly be inadequate. If the proximal procedure could be done by angioplasty, then it would be reasonable to

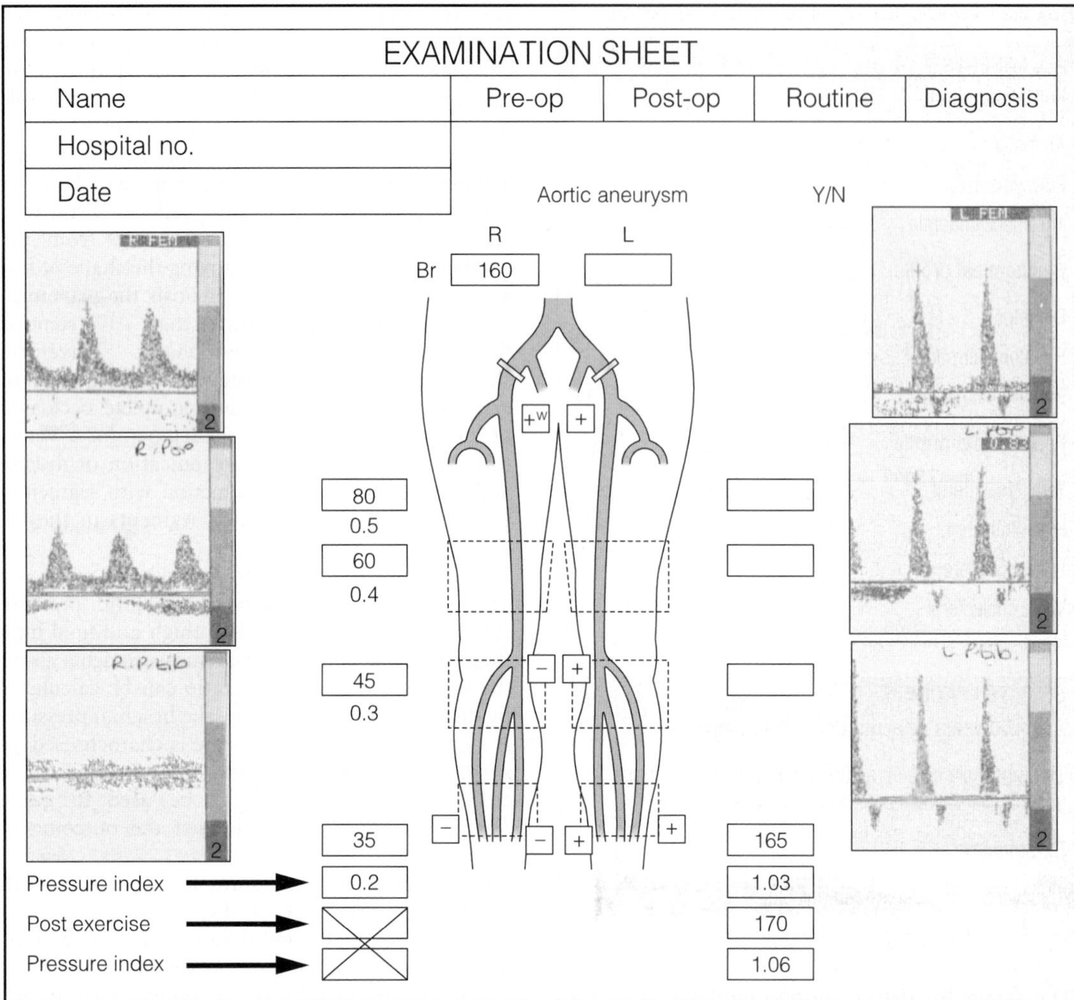

Figure 2.11 • Segmental arterial waveforms may help discriminate the functional significance of multisegment disease, such as the right iliac and superficial femoral occlusions in this patient. Theoretically, correcting the high thigh pressure to normal will approximately double the ankle arterial pressure to a level that should relieve ischaemic rest pain.

delay a decision on femoro-distal reconstruction until the result of this angioplasty could be assessed. Where surgical reconstruction is required, then it would be better to proceed immediately to simultaneous ilio-profunda and femoro-distal bypass.

DUPLEX IMAGING

Colour-flow duplex ultrasound allows the visualisation and haemodynamic assessment of arteries using grey-scale imaging, colour-flow Doppler mapping and pulse Doppler velocity profiles. In experienced hands, it can be used to accurately map the length of an artery and identify the severity of disease.

The value of duplex is that the diseased artery may be imaged clearly using grey-scale ultrasound, which visualises echogenic plaques and the anatomy of the artery/disease. Real-time colour-flow Doppler is used to identify blood flow through the ultrasound field. Colour filling will only occur where blood is moving and can therefore be used to enhance the grey-scale image by identifying 'soft' atheroma or thrombus as an area of absent colour filling. Colour flow also allows rapid identification of increased blood velocity by a change in colour within the lumen of the artery (**Fig. 2.12**, see also Plate 6, facing p. 116). Combining grey-scale and colour-flow mapping, a severe stenosis can be seen as grey echoes reducing the diameter of the colour filling and a 'mosaic' of colours indicating increased velocity and turbulence. Grey scale and colour flow do not provide a quantitative means of determining the severity of a stenosis.

(a)

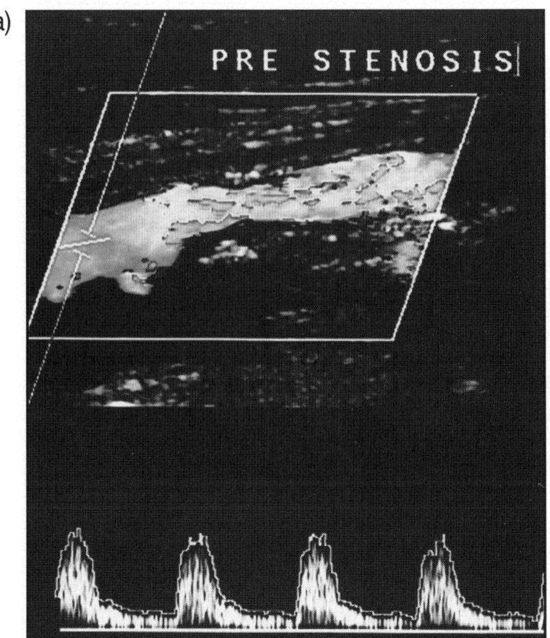

(b)

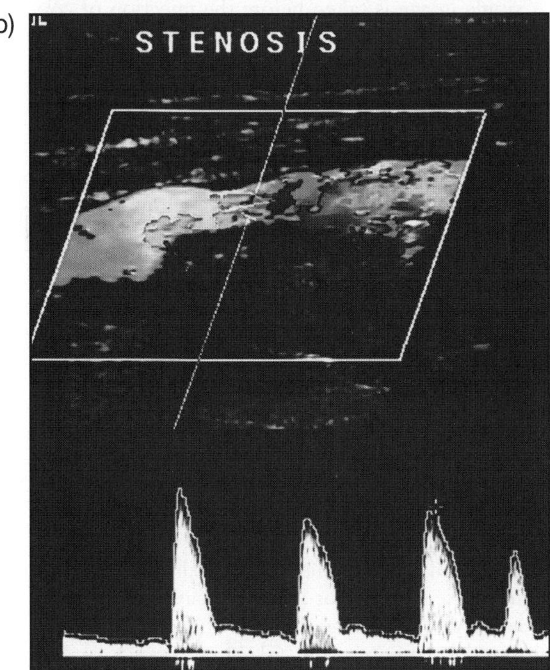

Figure 2.12 • Duplex imaging demonstrating the measurement of peak flow velocities **(a)** above and **(b)** within a stenosis allows the ratio of peak flow velocity to be calculated as an indication of the severity of stenosis.

In pulsed or gated Doppler, the ultrasound signal is pinpointed to a specific depth; the change of frequency in this reflected signal is determined by the transmitted frequency, angle of insonation and the velocity of blood. Modern colour-flow duplex instruments automatically calculate blood velocity but accuracy relies heavily on correct position and angling of the pulsed Doppler cursor. The peak systolic velocity is measured in the normal artery proximal to a stenosis and then in the stenosis identified by colour flow (**Fig. 2.12**). A twofold increase in the peak systolic velocity indicates a 50% narrowing of the artery while a 2.5-fold increase indicates a narrowing of greater than 50%.[15] Distal to a stenosis the Doppler waveform shape changes and the velocity is usually reduced.

Diagnosis of complete occlusion of an artery can be difficult and depends heavily on the experience of the sonographer. The shape of the Doppler signal proximally and distally, the absence of colour-flow and Doppler signals within the occlusion, and the presence of collaterals help the sonographer. Difficulties can arise with deep or tortuous arteries, where signal return is reduced and optimum angles of insonation are difficult to obtain.

Calcification or bowel gas may completely obscure imaging of the iliac or visceral arteries; varying the plane of insonation occasionally helps. Multiple stenoses along the length of an artery reduce the accuracy of flow velocity measurements in the distal stenoses. The sonographer must use judgement based on grey scale, colour flow and smaller increases in blood velocity to determine the severity of tandem stenosis.

AORTO-ILIAC ASSESSMENT

This can be difficult due to the depth of arteries, overlying bowel gas and calcification. Bowel preparation prior to assessment may reduce the effects of bowel gas but may not be well tolerated.[14] However, without any preparation aorto-iliac assessment matches angiography, with a sensitivity of 0.89 and specificity of 0.90.[16]

An experienced vascular technologist will report any limitations of an assessment. Changes in the Doppler waveform before and after an inadequately viewed segment give an indication of disease and the need for further investigation.

FEMORO-DISTAL ARTERIES

In experienced hands, duplex is accurate at identifying disease from the common femoral to the distal popliteal artery, with sensitivity of 84–87% and specificity 92–98% compared with angiography.[16–18]

The calf arteries can be more difficult, especially when there is severe proximal disease.[19,20] Calf blood flow can be improved by imaging with the legs dependent or by pulse generated run-off, which involves placing a cuff around the lower thigh or upper calf and inflating to 250 mmHg at a rate of 50/min.[21]

In large calves, the depth of insonation attenuates the signal return, making it difficult to visualise the proximal calf arteries.[20] Accuracy can be improved by using a 4.2-MHz curved-array abdominal probe, which allows deeper penetration. In most cases duplex detects the optimum calf artery for revascularisation.[22,23]

SURVEILLANCE FOLLOWING ANGIOPLASTY OR RECONSTRUCTION

Duplex imaging may also be used following arterial reconstruction to detect restenosis before thrombosis occurs. Restenosis is frequent following transluminal angioplasty of the superficial femoral or distal arteries and follow-up imaging at 1 month and then every 3 months throughout the first year is indicated. A doubling in flow velocity from that recorded shortly after the procedure may be taken as an indication for more frequent surveillance or intervention. Changes in the ABPI tend to occur later, occasionally after thrombosis. Detecting a severe stenosis at the distal anastomosis following aorto-bifemoral reconstruction suggests the need for early intervention to prevent that limb of the graft occluding.

Vein graft surveillance was widely recommended 10 years ago on the basis that 15% of grafts would develop a restenosis that predicts subsequent graft failure.[24] More recently, a randomised clinical trial questioned the overall benefit of surveillance. However, as clinical follow-up has little value, our policy is for surveillance in the vascular laboratory supervised by a nurse specialist.

LASER DOPPLER AND TRANSCUTANEOUS OXIMETRY

These are both techniques used to assess the viability of skin perfusion. Laser Doppler measures the Doppler shift in light emitted by a diode and measures overall skin perfusion to a depth of approximately 1.5 mm. It is most appropriately used as a trend instrument and has failed to gain any useful clinical applications in PAD. Transcutaneous oximetry can be used to measure the partial pressure of oxygen diffusing through the surface of the skin as an indirect measure for oxygen tension in the underlying tissue. It was hoped that $tcPo_2$ measurements of calf skin might be used to determine whether healing would occur following below-knee amputation.[25] Unfortunately, neither $tcPo_2$ nor ABPI is reliable for this as the changes in skin perfusion after the distal limb has been removed cannot be predicted. Where there is severe proximal disease, removing the distal limb is unlikely to have significant effect; however, with distal disease, removing this tissue reduces significantly the demands on the available blood supply. If there is a femoral pulse and the calf skin is viable, below-knee amputation using a long posterior flap and excision of the soleal muscle will usually heal.

Radiological investigations

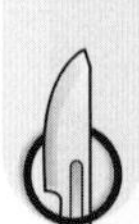

Our practice is to plan radiological investigation and treatment only following duplex imaging (see **Fig. 2.10**). The patient can then be appropriately counselled and consent obtained for a therapeutic procedure at the same time as angiography if technically possible. This requires close cooperation between surgeon, vascular laboratory and radiologist.

CATHETER ANGIOGRAPHY

This is still considered the ‘gold standard’ technique for the investigation of PAD. Over the last 15 years ‘conventional’ angiography has been almost completely superseded by digital subtraction angiography, where the output from the image intensifier is digitised and the images are stored on computer. A single image is taken before the injection of contrast (the mask image); following contrast injection, further images are taken that can be subtracted from the mask. This removes bony detail, leaving a clear image of the arterial tree (**Fig. 2.13**). With the introduction of small catheters (3 and 4 Fr) this has become an outpatient procedure in many departments. Non-ionic contrast agents should be used and there is growing evidence that the risk of nephrotoxicity can be further reduced by non-ionic dimers.[26]

Angiography is invasive and requires informed consent. A full explanation of the procedure, together with the potential risks and benefits, will reassure most patients, who then generally do not need sedation. However, in ischaemia, good-quality images of the calf arteries and plantar arch are important in planning distal bypass. These distal images are prone to movement artefact in the critical limb and adequate analgesia is therefore essential. Occasionally, opiate analgesia is still inadequate in which case epidural or general anaesthesia may be necessary. There is no need to shave the groin or starve the patient, as the risk of emergency surgery due to a complication of angiography is now remote.

Contrast media

Intravascular iodinated contrast medium is potentially nephrotoxic, although usually transient (reaching a maximum at approximately 48 hours) and of no clinical significance for patients with normal renal function.[27] If renal function is impaired, this short-term deterioration may be clinically important and irreversible. If serum creatinine is raised but is

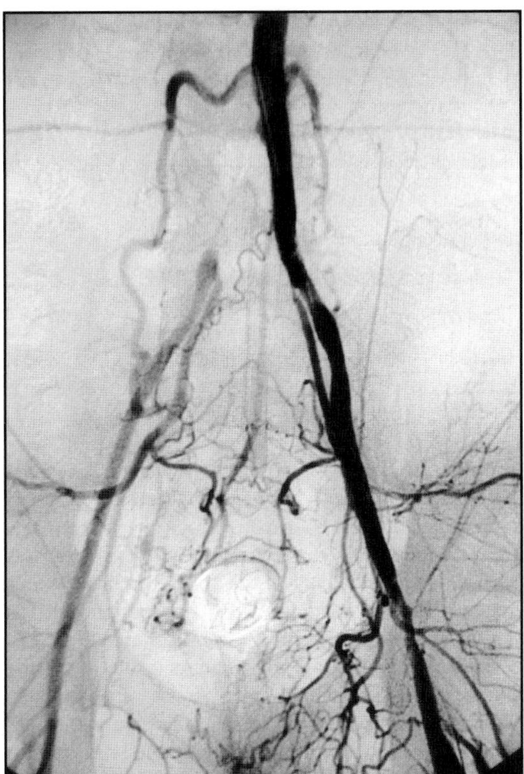

Figure 2.13 • The subtraction of bony detail in digital subtraction angiography leaves a clearer image of the arterial anatomy (compare with Fig. 2.1). Complete occlusion of the right common iliac artery with stenosis of the internal and external iliac and common femoral arteries on the left are clearly shown.

below 300 mmol/L, then intravenous fluids should be commenced at a rate of 100 mL/hour starting at least 6 hours before and continuing for 12 hours after the investigation to ensure an adequate diuresis. Fluid balance must be monitored and the serum creatinine checked until renal function returns to the pre-angiographic level.[28] Non-steroidal anti-inflammatory drugs (with the exception of aspirin) should be stopped as these may contribute to nephrotoxicity.

If the patient's creatinine exceeds 300 mmol/L, either alternative imaging techniques should be considered or non-toxic contrast media such as gadolinium[28] or carbon dioxide[29] should be used. The advice of a nephrologist should also be sought on how to safely manage the peri-angiographic period.

There is growing evidence that the risk of nephrotoxicity can be reduced by non-ionic dimers (e.g. iodixanol) compared with conventional non-ionic media.[26] Recently, attention has focused on an interaction between iodinated contrast media and metformin (Glucophage) because of a transient
impairment of renal function induced by this type 10
of contrast medium. If this causes a reduction in the renal excretion of metformin, then lactic acidosis may result. Guidelines issued by the Royal College of Radiologists[30] advise that metformin should be stopped in patients with high creatinine levels prior to contrast injection.

Technique

Basic angiographic access is by the modified Seldinger technique[31] using a hollow puncture needle, a floppy guidewire usually with a J-tip, and a catheter passed over the wire. Most angiograms for lower limb ischaemia require the injection of contrast by mechanical pumps using catheters with multiple side holes. This ensures that the contrast is distributed evenly within the circulating blood and that the catheter remains stable in position. Usually, diagnostic angiograms involve placing a pigtail catheter in the abdominal aorta with images from the renal arteries to the foot. More detailed images of the calf and foot arteries may be obtained by either withdrawing the catheter into the ipsilateral iliac or advancing the catheter across the aortic bifurcation for the contralateral limb. Such selective imaging allows more definition of the crural vessels, particularly below arterial occlusion proximally. Intra-arterial pressure gradients can also be measured across stenoses of uncertain significance.[32]

It has been traditional to use the femoral artery opposite to the symptomatic leg. The haematoma that may follow arterial puncture using large catheter systems may lead to infection following surgery performed soon after. This is less of an issue with the newer small catheters; the minimal benefit of a 'virgin' groin must be balanced against (i) better below-knee images and (ii) angioplasty of iliac disease when appropriate.

Anticoagulants

Anticoagulation should be reversed prior to angiography. With care, diagnostic angiography is safe with 3 or 4 Fr catheters in patients with international normalised ratios of prothrombin time up to 3.0, provided the blood pressure is well controlled.

Risks and limitations

The risks of conventional catheter angiography may be related to contrast or technique.

Contrast-related[33]

- Allergic: these are not dose related and probably result from mast cell degranulation. The incidence of severe anaphylactic reactions due to ionic contrast media is 0.01–0.02%, but the modern non-ionic low-osmolar compounds are five to ten times safer than their predecessors. Patients with asthma or hay fever are more likely to have an allergy and steroid prophylaxis should be used. Patients with known contrast allergy should be imaged using alternative techniques.

- Toxic: these are dose related and manifest themselves as a metallic taste in the mouth, feelings of warmth, nausea or vomiting, cardiac arrhythmias and pulmonary oedema. They are more likely to occur in patients with severe vascular disease.
- Renal (see above).

Technique-related

- Haematoma around the puncture site is inevitable. This can be reduced by smaller catheters and manual pressure for at least 5–10 minutes.
- Arterial spasm: relatively uncommon when access is from the femoral artery but may be a problem in smaller arteries, such as the brachial. It is avoided by careful technique and small catheters. Spasm may be treated by vasodilators such as papaverine or glyceryl trinitrate.
- Subintimal dissection: a dissection flap is usually caused by either undue force or hydrophilic guidewires. Although small flaps are rarely a problem, larger or antegrade flaps occlude the artery.
- Infection is rare with good aseptic technique.
- Arteriovenous fistula: as the femoral artery and vein are close neighbours they may both be punctured by the angiogram needle, although fistulas are infrequent.
- Embolisation: if atheromatous material lining the artery is inadvertently dislodged, it will embolise to lodge in an artery of smaller diameter.

These complications are uncommon and can usually be avoided. The Royal College of Radiologists has issued guidelines indicating the upper limit of acceptable complication rates (**Box 2.3**).[34] As catheter angiography is invasive, it should be limited to patients in whom a form of therapeutic intervention is planned.

Box 2.3 • Royal College of Radiologists recommendations for upper limit of complications arising from diagnostic angiography

Haematoma (requiring transfusion, surgery or delayed discharge)	3.0%
Occlusion of the artery	0.5%
Pseudoaneurysm	0.5%
Arteriovenous fistula	0.1%
Distal embolisation	0.5%
Occlusion of distal arteries	2.0%

COMPUTED TOMOGRAPHIC ANGIOGRAPHY

Originally, computed tomography (CT) involved a series of discrete sections through the body 4–10 mm apart. As each of these slices took time to image and process, the number of slices was limited by overheating of the X-ray tube. Thick sections (8–10 mm) had to be used for scanning over any distance and produced poor-quality reconstructions with low spatial resolution and movement artefacts. CT angiography was limited to small discrete areas such as the circle of Willis.

Over the last 10 years, helical (or spiral) CT has been developed where the tube continuously rotates and acquires information as the patient is fed through the machine. The volume scanned is then divided into many volume elements (voxels) and the computer reconstructs slices from this dataset. Because a *volume* of tissue has been scanned, these slices can be reconstructed in any plane (multiplanar reconstructions). Computer technology also allows more complex reconstructions, with the subtraction of bone or other detail that may obscure the arteries.

Maximum intensity projection (MIP) images are constructed by the computer selecting the highest density voxel along a given plane or planes (**Fig. 2.14**). This produces an angiographic-like image that can be displayed rotating in real time. A variety of three-dimensional reconstructions can also be displayed. The voxels nearest the observer appear whiter in surface-shaded three-dimensional reconstructions, as if the image was lit from behind the observer's head (**Fig. 2.15**). With the exception of complex vascular anatomy, such as arteriovenous malformations or intracranial aneurysms, little additional information is gained. In volume-rendered three-dimensional reconstructions the different elements of the vessel, such as calcification, thrombus and flowing blood in the lumen, are represented as different colours on the screen. This may be useful in the evaluation of abdominal aneurysms for endovascular repair. Finally, an intraluminal view of the vessel can be depicted (**Fig. 2.16**). The value of this technique in vascular disease is uncertain but in the gut is being used for 'virtual endoscopy'.

Recent tube technology allows up to 16 helices to be acquired simultaneously (multislice CT).[35] High heat capacity tubes can scan large volumes of tissue during a single acquisition. Following the intravenous

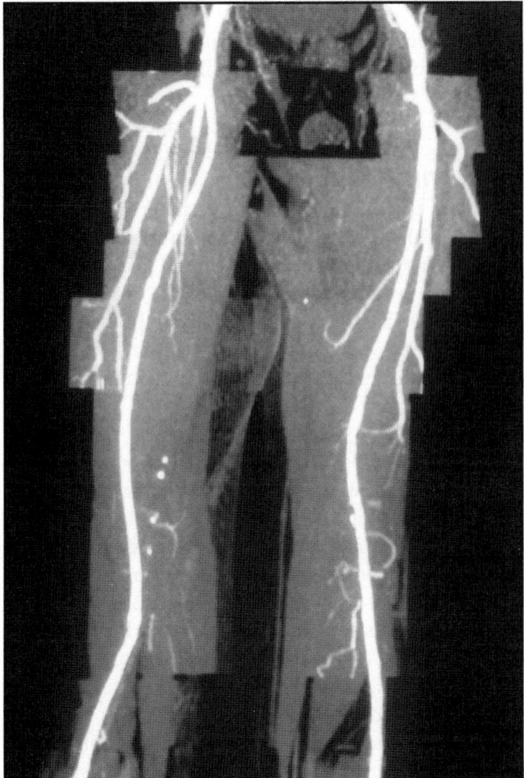

Figure 2.14 • CT angiography reconstructed to show the anatomy of the arteries in the thigh. These images can be rotated to demonstrate the origin of the profunda arteries and to exclude posterior plaques.

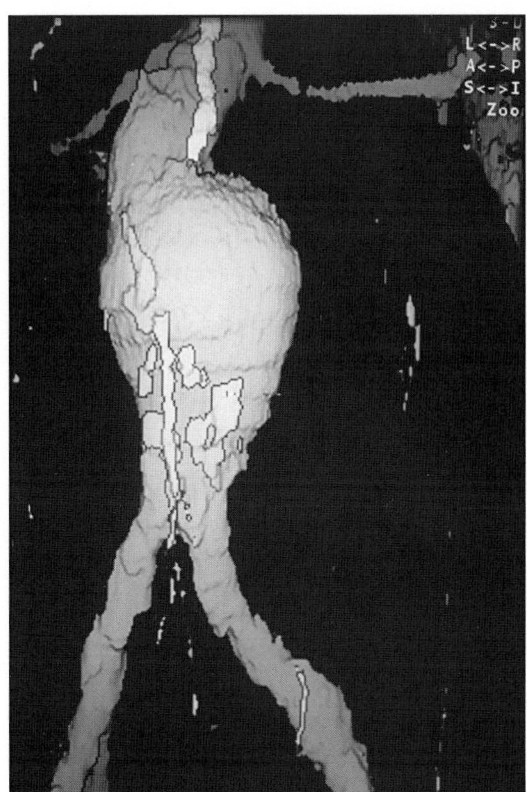

Figure 2.15 • This three-dimensional reconstruction of an aortic aneurysm from spiral CT gives a clear impression of tortuosity; multiplanar reconstructions are used to obtain measurements of aneurysm size and length.

injection of contrast, thin sections can be obtained rapidly from the abdomen to the ankles while the arterial concentration of contrast is at its peak.

Technique for PAD

The patient is scanned from the upper abdomen to the feet. A single transaxial section is taken towards the superior extent of the volume to be scanned (e.g. at the level of the renal arteries). With modern systems an area of interest can be placed over the aorta. Contrast injection is started (100–150 mL at 3 mL/s) and serial axial scans are taken at the level of the renal arteries. When the aortic attenuation rises to 120 Hounsfield units, the helical scan is automatically started.

Disadvantages

CT angiography (CTA) uses ionising radiation and requires iodinated contrast agents with their associated risks. Heavy calcification makes it difficult to identify whether an artery is stenosed or occluded (**Fig. 2.17**). The images are extensively processed by computer and when bones are

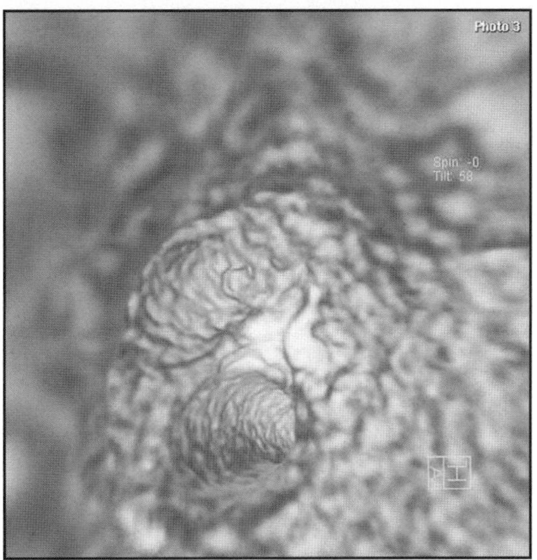

Figure 2.16 • This reconstruction of a spiral CT demonstrates the lumen of the aorta looking towards the bifurcation.

(a)

(b)

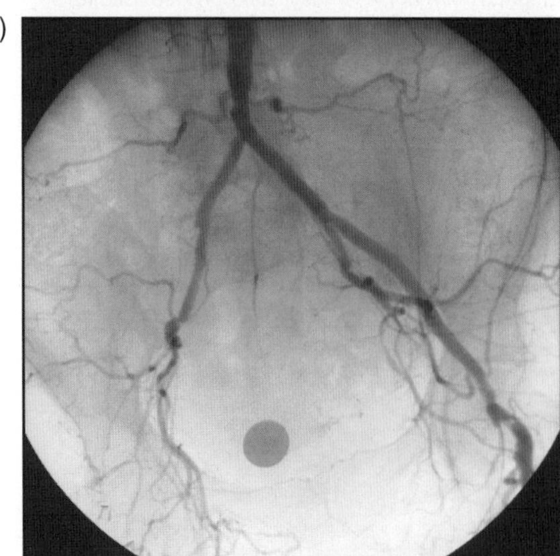

Figure 2.17 • **(a)** CT angiogram demonstrating heavy arterial calcification, which makes interpretation difficult. **(b)** The aorto-iliac segment is clearly displayed by conventional digital subtraction angiography.

subtracted adjacent arterial segments may be erased, mimicking an occlusion. The radiologist must therefore review the original transaxial slices as well as the reconstructions.

CTA is capable of obtaining images of a similar quality to those of conventional angiography but its role in PAD is uncertain as it has been inadequately validated in comparison with catheter angiography (**Table 2.1**). The radiation and contrast doses are also less appealing than those used with magnetic resonance angiography (MRA). It may be used when MRA is contraindicated by implanted metal or permanent pacemakers. CT remains the mainstay for the preoperative assessment of aortic aneurysm.[36]

MAGNETIC RESONANCE ANGIOGRAPHY

A detailed review of magnetic resonance physics is beyond the scope of this chapter, but the basic principles are important. Essentially, the distribution of hydrogen ions is imaged throughout the body. These ions are effectively protons and behave as minute magnets spinning on their axis. If the patient is placed in a strong homogeneous magnetic field, these small magnets align themselves with that field. In magnetic resonance imaging (MRI), a radiofrequency pulse of energy changes the spin of the magnets. When the radiofrequency pulse is turned off, the magnets flip back to their original alignment, emitting radio waves that can be detected as a signal by coils placed on the surface of the patient. The characteristics of the signal depend on the tissue being interrogated and the tissue water content.

The flow of blood can be utilised in MRI as activated protons within flowing blood are removed from the image. Arteries and veins appear black, known as signal voids. Repeatedly stimulating a block of tissue saturates the protons so that no signal is emitted. Arterial blood flowing into this tissue is then the only source of signals (time-of-flight angiography). Alternatively, differences in the phase of spin between the saturated and unsaturated protons can be detected (phase-contrast angiography). Both these methods produce 'white' blood vessels, suppress signal from stationary tissues and tend to overestimate the severity of stenosis due to turbulence. This turbulence results in dephasing of the protons and subsequent loss of signal from immediately distal to a stenosis; the resulting black area appears as an occlusion.[37]

These techniques have now been superseded by gadolinium-enhanced MRA.[38] Gadolinium is a paramagnetic element that shortens the T1 relaxation time of blood. Angiograms are obtained by

Table 2.1 • Sensitivity and specificity of CT angiography compared with catheter angiography

Reference	Segments	N	Sensitivity (%)	Specificity (%)
Martin et al.[38]	All stenoses	41	89	98
Martin et al.[39]	All occlusions	41	92	97
Ofer et al.[40]	All segments	18	91	92
Willman et al.[41]	Aorto-iliac	46	91	99

T1-weighted gradient echo sequences as gadolinium infused intravenously reaches the arteries. As gadolinium-enhanced MRA is less prone to artefacts due to turbulence, it is less inclined to overestimate stenoses. Acquisition times are much shorter, allowing greater patient throughput and reduced motion artefacts. Peripheral MRA may be completed within 20–30 minutes.

Technique

MRA is usually performed using a 'bolus chase' technique. The patient is placed on a movable table that allows the peripheral arteries, from aorta to feet, to be imaged during a single injection of contrast. This maximises the contrast between blood and stationary tissue. A time-of-flight acquisition is obtained in each table position to ensure the vessels are included in the image volume (**Fig. 2.18**). Images are then taken of the lower legs, thighs, abdomen and pelvis before and during contrast infusion. These sets of images can be subtracted from each other to increase the signal ratio between moving blood and stationary tissues.

The images produced can be viewed as either coronal images or MIP images. As in CTA, MIP images are highly processed and radiologists must review the source images for artefacts.

Sensitivities and specificities of over 90% have been reported in a number of small studies (**Table 2.2**).[41–44] Dedicated phased-array coils produce more accurate results than the general purpose body coils.[43] While acceptable results can be obtained down to the calf, there is often contrast within the veins that may obscure the arterial anatomy at this level. This can be overcome by reviewing the source images or by further image processing. For patients with critical limb ischaemia being assessed for distal bypass, the more proximal circulation can be assessed by duplex imaging allowing static MRA of the calf.

There are a number of pitfalls to MRA. The 'scout' images must be checked to ensure that the whole arterial tree is included. Stainless steel stents produce a signal void that mimics occlusion. Although nitinol stents are better, it is still difficult to assess intrastent stenoses. Duplex would be more appropriate in this situation. Similarly, clips used during previous bypass surgery may mimic stenoses (**Fig. 2.19**). Mistiming the contrast injection or incompletely filling the vessel with contrast may produce a black line in the centre of vessels that mimics dissection.

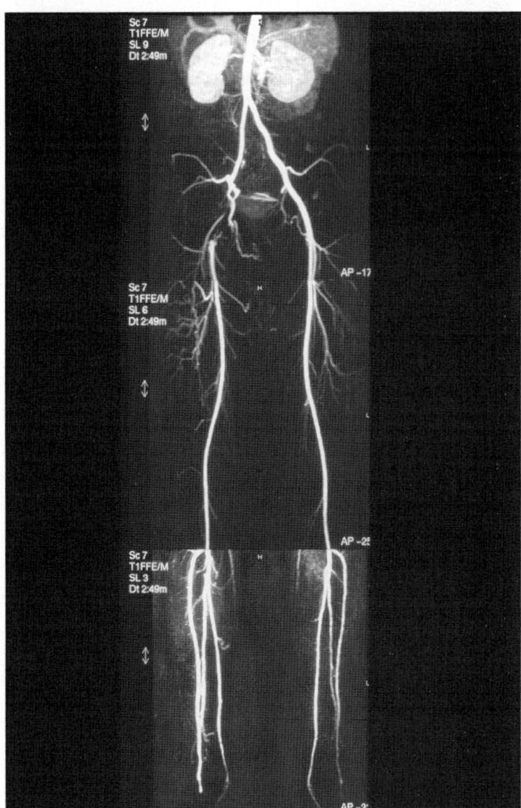

Figure 2.18 • This magnetic resonance angiogram is a composite of three table positions where the contrast between blood and stationary tissue has been maximised by the 'bolus chase' technique with gadolinium-enhanced MRA. This technique allows the arteries to be visualised from the abdominal aorta down to the ankles in a single acquisition.

Contraindications to MRA include the presence of a pacemaker or certain types of prosthetic cardiac

Table 2.2 • Sensitivity and specificity of magnetic resonance angiography compared with catheter angiography

Reference	Segments	*N*	Sensitivity (%)	Specificity (%)
Cronberg et al.[40]	Infrapopliteal	35	92	64
Willmann et al.[39]	Aorto-iliac	46	92	99
Huber et al.[41]*	Iliac	20	100	96
Huber et al.[41]*	Femoral	20	100	98
Huber et al.[41]*	Infrapopliteal	20	100	96
Loewe et al.[42]	Iliac	106	100	98–99
Loewe et al.[42]	Femoro-popliteal	106	88–99	92–98
Loewe et al.[42]	Infrapopliteal	106	94–98	87–98

*Dedicated phased-array coil.

(a)

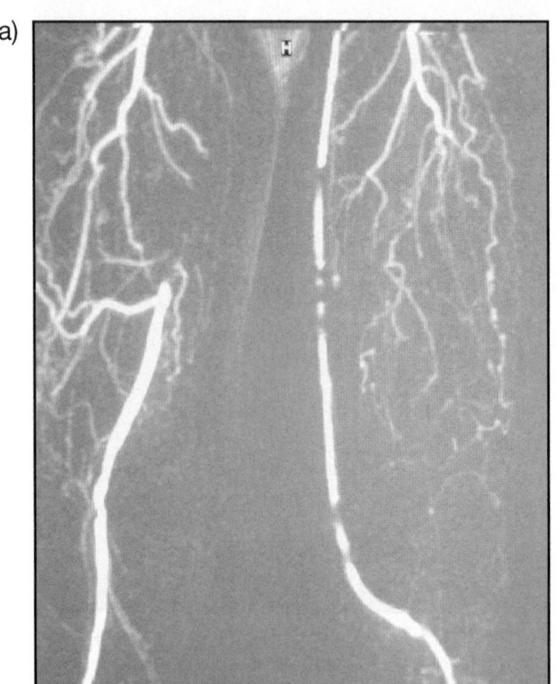

(b)

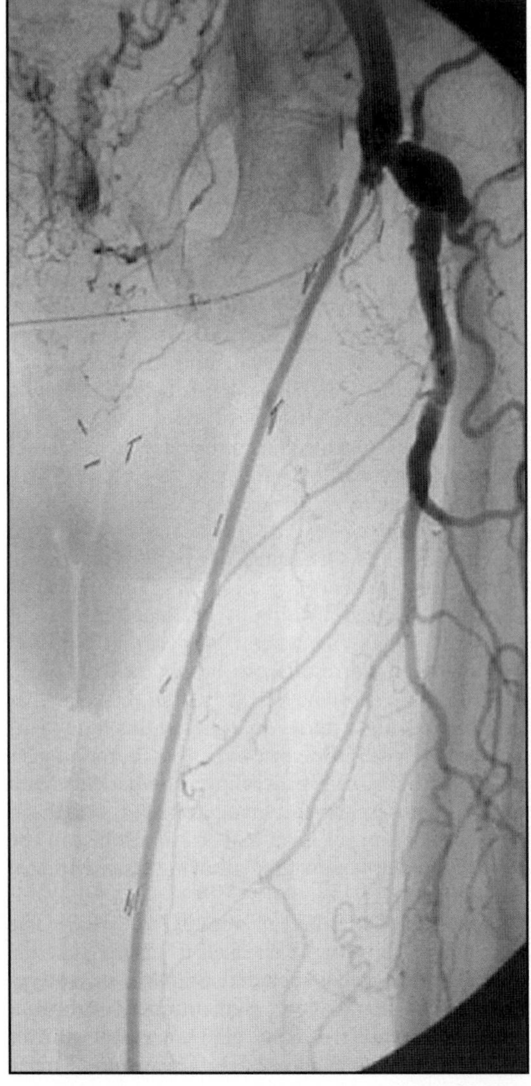

Figure 2.19 • **(a)** Magnetic resonance angiogram of both legs showing a saphenous vein bypass graft that appears to have multiple stenoses. **(b)** On catheter angiogram these stenoses are shown to be artefacts due to metallic clips used to occlude side branches from the vein.

valve implants that contain metal,[45] intracranial aneurysm clips, cochlear implants or metallic intraocular foreign bodies. MRA should be avoided within 8 weeks of inserting metal stents. Up to 10% of patients are too claustrophobic to tolerate the scanner.

SUMMARY

Chronic lower limb ischaemia is common, particularly in patients who smoke or who have cardiovascular risk factors. Most patients with claudication are managed by controlling risk factors and no investigation is needed. Arterial investigation should be limited to those patients requiring intervention. Initial assessment is clinical with resting and exercise Doppler studies; duplex imaging may be adequate to plan intervention. Catheter angiography is invasive but complications are rare. Intervention planned following duplex imaging can often be performed at the same time. MRA or CTA may be used for diagnosis to avoid the arterial puncture needed for conventional angiography.

Key points

- The prognosis for intermittent claudication is benign.
- Recognising critical ischaemia is a key clinical skill.
- Patients with symptoms on exercise should be examined after exercise.
- Minimally invasive investigation by ultrasound has largely replaced diagnostic angiography.
- The vascular radiologist has become an interventionist.
- Arterial puncture may be avoided by MRA or CTA.

REFERENCES

1. Second European Consensus Document on Chronic Critical Leg Ischaemia. Eur J Vasc Surg 1992; 6:1–4.
2. Thompson MM, Sayers RD, Varty K et al. Chronic critical leg ischaemia must be redefined. Eur J Vasc Surg 1993; 7:420–6.
3. Newman AB, Shemanski L, Manolio TA et al. Ankle–arm as a predictor of cardiovascular disease and mortality in the cardiovascular health study. Arterioscler Thromb Vasc Biol 1999; 19:538–45.
4. Hale WE, Marks RG, May FE et al. Epidemiology of intermittent claudication: evaluation of risk factors. Age Ageing 1988; 17:57–60.
5. Porter RW. Spinal stenosis and neurogenic claudication. Spine 1996; 21:2046–52.
6. Dumville JC, Lee AJ, Smith FB, Fowkes FGR. The health-related quality of life of people with peripheral arterial disease in the community: the Edinburgh Artery Study. Br J Gen Pract 2004; 54:826–31.
7. Dawber TR. The Framingham Heart Study: the epidemiology of atherosclerotic diseases. Cambridge, MA: Harvard University Press, 1980.
8. Haq IU, Jackson PR, Yeo WW, Ramsay LE. Sheffield risk and treatment table for cholesterol lowering for primary prevention of coronary heart disease. Lancet 1995; 346:1467–71.
9. Ubbink DT. Toe blood pressure measurements in patients suspected of leg ischaemia: a new laser Doppler device compared with photoplethysmography. Eur J Vasc Endovasc Surg 2004; 27:629–34.
10. Smith FCT, Shearman CP, Simms MH, Gwynn BR. Falsely elevated ankle pressures in severe leg ischaemia. The pole test: an alternative approach. Eur J Vasc Surg 1994; 8:408–12.
11. Hansson L, Zanchetti A, Carruthers SG et al. Effects of intensive blood-pressure lowering and low-dose aspirin in patients with hypertension: principal results of the Hypertension Optimal Treatment (HOT) randomised trial. HOT Study Group. Lancet 1998; 351:1755–62.
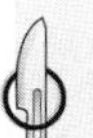
12. Heart Protection Study Collaborative Group. MRC/BHF Heart Protection Study of cholesterol lowering with simvastatin in 20,536 high risk individuals: a randomised placebo-controlled trial. Lancet 2002; 360:7–22.
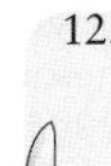
13. Silagy C, Mant D, Fowler G, Lodge M. Meta analysis on efficacy of nicotine replacement therapies in smoking cessation. Lancet 1994; 343:139–42.
14. Cole SEA, Walker RA, Norris R. Vascular Laboratory Practice IPEM Part III. York: Institute of Physics and Engineering in Medicine, 2001.
15. Legemate DA, Teeuwen C, Hoeneveld H, Ackerstaff RG, Eikelboom BC. Spectral analysis criteria in duplex scanning of aorto-iliac and femoropopliteal arterial disease. Ultrasound Med Biol 1991; 17:769–76.
16. Kohler TR, Nance DR, Cramer MM, Vandenburghe N, Strandness DE Jr. Duplex scanning for the diagnosis of aortoiliac and femoropopliteal disease: a prospective study. Circulation 1987; 76:1074–80.
17. Cossman DV, Ellison JE, Wagner WH et al. Comparison of contrast arteriography to arterial mapping with color-flow duplex imaging in the lower extremities. J Vasc Surg 1989; 10:522–9.

18. Moneta GL, Yeager RA, Antonovic R et al. Accuracy of lower extremity arterial duplex mapping. J Vasc Surg 1992; 15:275–84.
19. Larch E, Minar E, Ahmadi R et al. Value of color duplex sonography for evaluation of tibioperoneal arteries in patients with femoropopliteal obstruction: a prospective comparison with anterograde intra-arterial digital subtraction angiography. J Vasc Surg 1997; 25:629–36.
20. Grassbaugh JA, Nelson PR, Rzucidlo EM et al. Blinded comparison of preoperative duplex ultrasound scanning and contrast arteriography for planning revascularization at the level of the tibia. J Vasc Surg 2003; 37:1186–90.
21. Scott DJ, Horrocks EH, Kinsella D, Horrocks M. Preoperative assessment of the pedal arch using pulse generated runoff and subsequent femorodistal outcome. Eur J Vasc Surg 1994; 8:20–5.
22. Wain RA, Berdejo GL, Delvalle WN et al. Can duplex scan arterial mapping replace contrast arteriography as the test of choice before infra-inguinal revascularization? J Vasc Surg 1999; 29:100–9.
23. Ligush J Jr, Reavis SW, Preisser JS, Hansen KJ. Duplex ultrasound scanning defines operative strategies for patients with limb-threatening ischemia. J Vasc Surg 1998; 28:482–91.
24. Moody P, Gould PA, Harris PL. Vein graft surveillance improves patency in femoro-popliteal bypass. Eur J Vasc Surg 1990; 4:117–21.
25. de Graaff JC, Ubbink DT, Legemate DA, Tijssen JG, Jacobs MK. Evaluation of toe pressure and transcutaneous oxygen measurements in management of chronic critical leg ischaemia: a diagnostic randomised clinical trial. J Vasc Surg 2003; 38:528–34.
26. Aspelin P, Aubry P, Fransson S-G et al. Nephrotoxic effects in high-risk patients undergoing angiography. N Engl J Med 2003; 348:491–9.
27. Scherberich JE. Do contrast media affect renal function? In: Dawson P, Claub W (eds) Contrast media in practice. Berlin: Springer-Verlag, 1993; pp. 61–3.
28. Waybill MM, Waybill PN. Contrast media-induced nephrotoxicity: identification of patients at risk and algorithms for prevention. J Vasc Intervent Radiol 2001; 12:3–9.
29. Spinosa DJ, Matsumoto MH, Hagspiel KD, Angle JF, Hardwell GD. Gadolinium based contrast agents in angiography and interventional radiology. Am J Roentgenol 1999; 173:1403–9.
30. Royal College of Radiologists' guidelines with regard to metformin-induced lactic acidosis and X-ray contrast medium agents. London: Royal College of Radiologists (Board of the Faculty of Clinical Radiology), 1999; pp. 1–2.
31. Seldinger S. Catheter replacement of the needle in percutaneous angiography. Acta Radiol 1953; 39:368–76.
32. Vesely TM. General percutaneous transluminal angioplasty techniques: clinical aspects. In: LaBerge JM, Darcy MD (eds) Peripheral vascular interventions. London: Society of Cardiovascular and Interventional Radiologists, 1994; pp. 13–23.
33. Ansell G. Complications of intravascular iodinated contrast media. In: Ansell G (ed.) Complications in diagnostic imaging and interventional radiology, 3rd edn. Oxford: Blackwell, 1996; pp. 245–303.
34. Standards in vascular radiology. London: Royal College of Radiologists (Board of the Faculty of Clinical Radiology), 1999; pp. 1–3.
35. Rubin GD. MDCT imaging of the aorta and peripheral vessels. Eur J Radiol 2003; 45:S42–S49.
36. Errington ML, Ferguson JM, Gillespie IN et al. Complete pre-operative imaging assessment of abdominal aortic aneurysm with spiral CT angiography. Clin Radiol 1997; 52:369–77.
37. Snidow JJ, Aisen AM, Harris VJ et al. Iliac artery MR angiography: comparison of three-dimensional gadolinium-enhanced and two-dimensional time-of-flight techniques. Radiology 1995; 196:371–8.
38. Prince MR, Grist TM, Debatin JF. 3D contrast MR angiography, 3rd edn. Berlin: Springer-Verlag, 2003.
39. Martin ML, Tay KH, Flak B et al. Multidetector CT angiography of the aortoiliac system and lower extremities: A prospective comparison with digital subtraction angiography. Am J Roentgenol 2003; 180:1085–1091.
40. Ofer A, Nitecki SS, Linn S et al. Multidetector CT angiography of peripheral vascular disease: A prospective comparison with intraarterial digital subtraction angiography. Am J Roentgenol 2003; 180:719–724.
41. Willmann JK, Wildermuth S, Pfammatter T et al. Aortoiliac and renal arteries: prospective intra-individual comparison of contrast-enhanced three-dimensionl MR angiography and multi-detector row CT angiography. Radiology 2003; 226:798–811.
42. Cronberg CN, Sjoberg S, Albrechtsson U et al. Peripheral arterial disease. Contrast enhanced 3D MR angiography of the lower leg and foot compared with conventional angiography. Acta Radiol 2003; 44:59–66.
43. Huber A, Scheidler J, Wintersperger B et al. Moving-table MR angiography of the peripheral runoff vessels. Comparison of body coil and dedicated phase array coil systems. Am J Roentgenol 2003; 180:1365–73.
44. Loewe C, Schoder M, Rand T et al. Peripheral vascular occlusive disease: evaluation with contrast enhanced moving-bed MR angiography versus digital subtraction angiography in 106 patients. Am J Roentgenol 2003; 179:1013–21.
45. Edwards M-B. 25 years of heart valve replacements in the United Kingdom. A guide to types, models and MRI safety. United Kingdom Heart Valve Registry. London: Hammersmith Hospital, 2000.

CHAPTER

Three

Treatment of chronic lower limb ischaemia

Steven M. Thomas and
Ahmed Nassef

INTRODUCTION

Chronic lower limb ischaemia is common in the Western world, and with a growing elderly population the number of cases requiring treatment will continue to rise. The aim of treatment is to obtain the best outcome for the patient and to optimise the use of resources. This chapter examines the treatment strategies for patients with chronic ischaemia of the lower limb and includes an algorithm that summarises a care pathway (**Fig. 3.1**). We can divide such patients into those with intermittent claudication (IC) where the limb is not threatened and those with a significant risk of limb loss without intervention, i.e. critical limb ischaemia (CLI). The previous chapter on assessment of chronic lower limb ischaemia outlines the definitions, diagnosis and assessment of these patients.

AETIOLOGY

The vast majority of cases of chronic lower limb ischaemia are caused by atherosclerotic arterial disease, but some rarer conditions exist that tend to affect a younger age group. A good history of IC in a young patient should be taken seriously, as some of these conditions may progress rapidly to CLI. Resting Doppler ankle–brachial pressure index (ABPI) should be measured in all patients with leg pain on exercise, especially if foot pulses are absent. Those with a good history of IC and palpable foot pulses should undergo a treadmill test.

Persistent sciatic artery

In this congenital anomaly, the embryonic axial limb artery, the sciatic artery, does not obliterate and remains continuous with the popliteal artery, providing the major blood supply to the lower limb. The anomaly is bilateral in 22% of cases and is commonly associated with failure of the iliofemoral vessels to develop properly.[1] The presenting symptoms include pain and a pulsatile mass in the buttock due to aneurysmal degeneration of the artery as it emerges from the sciatic foramen. Thrombosis or distal embolism may lead to acute ischaemia.[2] Although pedal pulses may be present, the femoral pulse will be reduced or absent if the iliofemoral vessels are hypoplastic (Cowie's sign) and IC will result if neither system has developed properly (**Fig. 3.2**). Symptomatic patients should be treated by bypass grafting and aneurysm exclusion. Asymptomatic patients should be monitored for aneurysm development.

Cystic adventitial disease

Cystic adventitial disease, caused by a cystic abnormality of the adventitia of the popliteal artery, occasionally presents with IC. The contents resemble that of a ganglion and the cysts may be connected to the synovium of the knee joint. IC may be severe and of rapid onset. The condition should be particularly suspected in young patients without significant risk factors for peripheral arterial disease. Pedal pulses sometimes disappear on knee flexion. Arteriography may show an

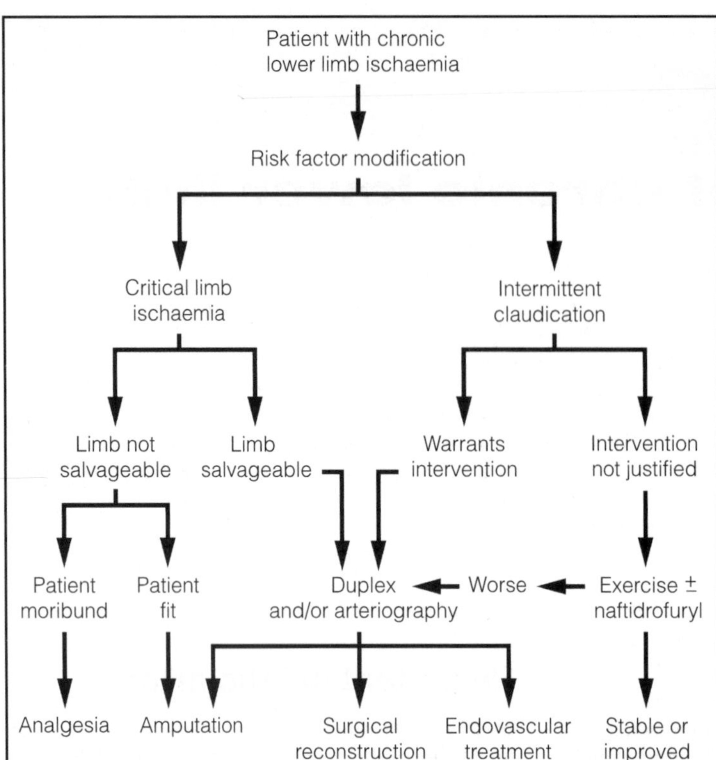

Figure 3.1 • Treatment pathway for patients with chronic lower limb ischaemia.

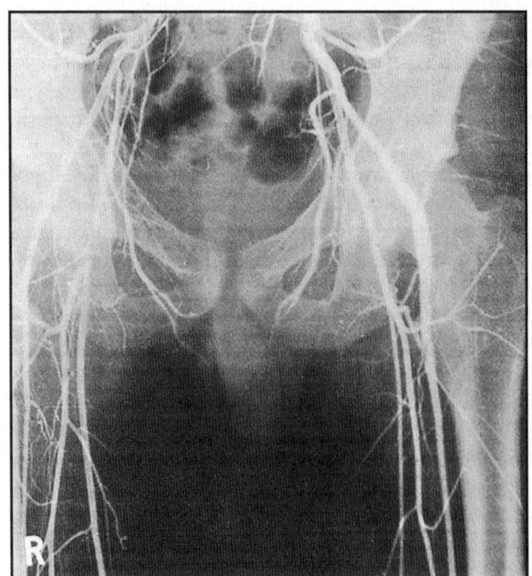

Figure 3.2 • Persistent bilateral sciatic arteries arising from the common iliac arteries with dilatation and intimal irregularity of the left sciatic artery at the level of the acetabulum.

unusually smooth 'hourglass' or eccentric stenosis (**Fig. 3.3**). Duplex will demonstrate the cystic abnormality as will computed tomography (CT) or magnetic resonance imaging (MRI). Angioplasty should not be attempted as the cyst contents may embolise distally. The affected segment of artery often requires resection and repair with an interposition vein graft via a posterior approach.[3]

Popliteal artery entrapment

Popliteal artery entrapment is more common than previously recognised. The condition can be anatomical or functional. In the anatomical variant, the artery courses around the medial head of gastrocnemius rather than between the two heads or, more rarely, passes deep to the popliteus muscle. Compression of the artery occurs during flexion resulting in IC, classically in athletes. Aneurysmal degeneration and/or thrombosis may develop. Two-thirds of cases are bilateral and the popliteal vein is involved in 10%.[4] Examination may reveal reduction or obliteration of pedal pulses during active plantar flexion. Duplex scanning or arteriography using this manoeuvre may also demonstrate kinking or

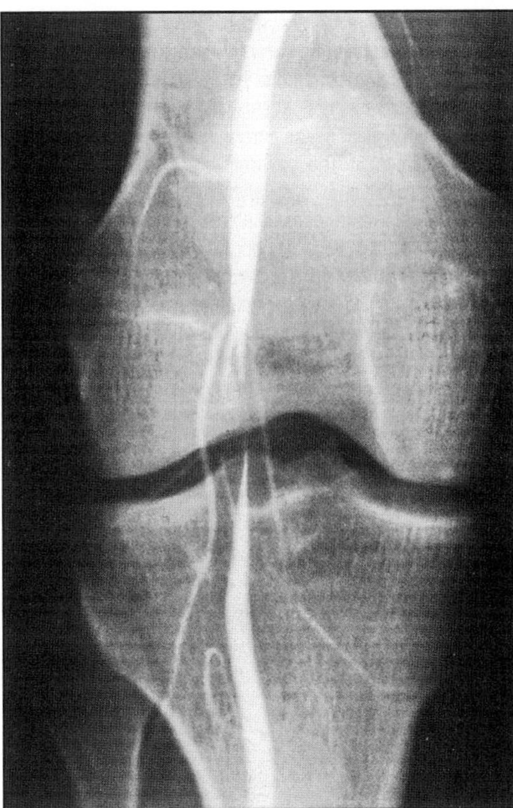

Figure 3.3 • Smooth 'hourglass' stenosis of popliteal artery due to cystic adventitial disease. A similar appearance may be seen in popliteal entrapment, especially during active plantar flexion.

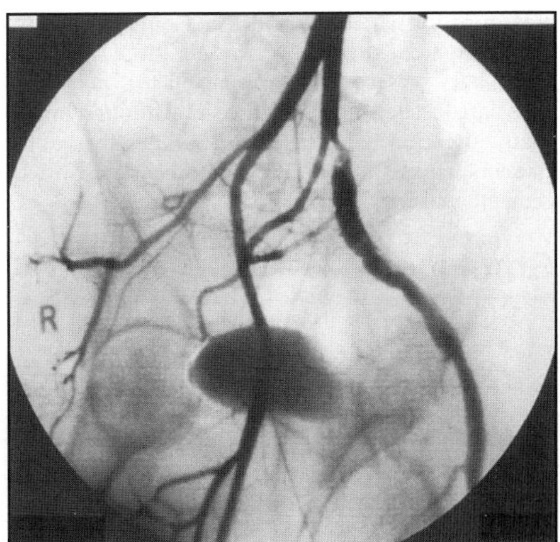

Figure 3.4 • Fibromuscular dysplasia affecting the left external iliac artery of a 12-year-old boy.

compression of the popliteal artery. CT or MRI can also demonstrate the anatomical abnormality. Symptomatic patients should be treated by division of the medial head of gastrocnemius and/or reconstruction of the popliteal artery. Surgery is also indicated for an asymptomatic contralateral limb whenever anatomical entrapment is detected.[5] In the functional variant of the condition, an anatomically normally positioned artery is compressed against a hypertrophied gastrocnemius or the soleal muscle ring. Unlike the anatomical variant, functional entrapment should only be treated when symptomatic.[6]

Fibromuscular dysplasia

Although fibromuscular dysplasia usually affects the renal and carotid arteries, it can affect the proximal upper and lower limb arteries in young people, causing IC. The external iliac artery appears the commonest site of involvement and arteriography may demonstrate a classic beaded appearance (**Fig. 3.4**). Patients with iliac fibromuscular dysplasia should be screened for renal involvement. Symptomatic stenoses usually respond well to angioplasty.

Buerger's disease

Buerger's disease should be considered in any young male claudicant who is a heavy smoker, especially if they are of Middle or Far Eastern origin.[7] Associated vasospastic symptoms commonly occur and patients may progress rapidly to, or present with, CLI. The pathophysiology and management of this condition are covered in Chapter 12.

RISK-FACTOR MODIFICATION

The risk factors associated with peripheral arterial occlusive disease (PAOD) are essentially the same as those for ischaemic heart disease, and include smoking, hyperlipidaemia, diabetes and hypertension (see Chapter 1). In addition to non-invasive Doppler assessment, all patients with PAOD require urinalysis, a full blood count and measurement of blood pressure, erythrocyte sedimentation rate (ESR) or viscosity, urea and electrolytes, random blood glucose, and lipids. Anaemia can present with symptoms of leg ischaemia, as can polycythaemia. An elevated ESR or viscosity may indicate a raised fibrinogen, which seems an important factor in the development of PAOD and vascular thrombosis. Renal impairment is often associated with PAOD and requires detection before contemplating arteriography (see Chapter 2). Identification and modification of risk factors should form the first line of treatment for patients with IC, not only to improve the outcome of treatment for their PAOD but also as primary or secondary prevention for their often associated ischaemic heart disease. Although immediate attention is focused on limb salvage for patients with CLI, risk-factor modification must be remembered for the future.

Smoking

Smoking remains the single most important risk factor for PAOD, and is associated with a threefold increased risk of the disease.[8] Cessation of smoking seems the most beneficial action the patient can take. This is likely to improve the claudication as well as reduce the general cardiovascular risk to the patient.

Stopping smoking will also improve the success of any subsequent intervention.[9] Patients often have great difficulty in giving up smoking. The official organisations that encourage smoking cessation are undoubtedly useful as they can give detailed advice and support; however, probably the most important aspect of this service is the provision of nicotine replacement therapy. This has been shown to be effective and will generally increase the odds of quitting by about 1.5–2-fold, regardless of setting.[10]

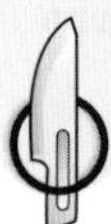

Hyperlipidaemia

Hyperlipidaemia is associated with between a one- and two-fold increase in the risk of PAOD.[11] Elevated levels of both cholesterol and triglycerides show a strong association with PAOD. However, the association with triglycerides seems largely due to the correlation between triglyceride and cholesterol levels.[12]

A systematic review of seven randomised trials of lipid-lowering therapy in PAOD found that the changes in ABPI and walking distance were inconsistent, although there was a general improvement in symptoms.[13] Two of the trials showed a significant reduction in peripheral arterial disease progression assessed by angiography. These trials used a combination of diet and drugs, such as fish oil, cholestyramine, fibrates and nicotinates. Attempting to reduce lipid levels by dietary means alone achieves reductions of only 5–10% and these older drugs cause considerable side effects, resulting in poor patient compliance. The newer statins (HMG-CoA reductase inhibitors) produce reductions in serum cholesterol of about 25–30% and appear well tolerated. It seems probable that these powerful agents will have more effect on PAOD. However, the main reason for using them is the 30% reduction in cardiovascular events as shown by several large prospective secondary intervention studies, including the Scandinavian Simvastatin Survival Study[14] and the Cholesterol and Recurrent Events Study.[15] Most of the patients in these studies had established ischaemic heart disease, but patients with symptomatic PAOD have a similar risk of cardiac events and obtain the same benefit. The joint British recommendations on the prevention of coronary heart disease state that patients with a total cholesterol in excess of 5 mmol/L and/or a low-density lipoprotein (LDL) cholesterol in excess of 3 mmol/L and symptomatic vascular disease should receive treatment with a statin. Current aims are reduction of total cholesterol to less than 5 mmol/L or by 20–25%, reduction of LDL cholesterol to less than 3 mmol/L or by 30%, and to achieve a triglyceride level of less than 1.7 mmol/L.[16] Evidence is lacking for beginning treatment over the age of 75 years, but once started treatment should continue beyond this age.

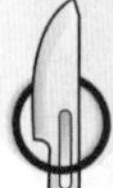

Atorvastatin 10 mg daily achieves cholesterol reductions greater than the milligram equivalents of other statins.[17] Furthermore, over 90% of patients do not require dose titration, which simplifies clinical management.[18] Atorvastatin interacts with clopidogrel, and as the price of simvastatin has fallen dramatically with the expiry of its patent, there is a case for returning to natural statins. Patients with very high cholesterol levels (>8 mmol/L) should be referred to a specialist lipid clinic as they may have familial hyperlipidaemia, which requires screening of other family members, and needs combination therapy. 5

Hypertension and diabetes

Hypertension is a strong predictor of stroke and ischaemic heart disease and the Framingham study found a strong association with the presence of PAOD, with the risk of claudication increased threefold in hypertensive patients.[19] PAOD may also cause hypertension due to reduced arterial compliance. Treating hypertension can reduce the stroke rate by 38%, cardiovascular deaths by 14% and peripheral vascular events by 26%.

Some have expressed concern that treatment, especially with beta-blockers, might adversely affect claudication due to reduced blood flow. A systematic review has failed to find any association between beta-blocker therapy and worsening claudication.[20]

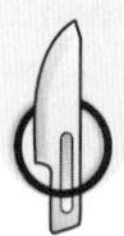

Beta-blockers are therefore safe in most patients with PAOD. However, if symptoms deteriorate after starting such therapy or if the patient complains of cold feet (a common occurrence) and as beta-blockers can cause vasospastic symptoms, it seems sensible to avoid them in patients with PAOD and use a calcium antagonist such as nifedipine instead.

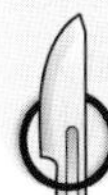

Patients with type 1 (insulin-dependent) and type 2 (non-insulin-dependent) diabetes have a threefold to fivefold increased risk of developing PAOD. Intensive blood-glucose control appears to reduce the risk of microvascular complications such as neuropathy, but has little impact on macrovascular disease including PAOD. However, control of the associated risk factors will reduce the risk of cardiovascular events.[21,22]

Homocysteine and antioxidants

In a case–control study of 100 patients with PAOD, patients with hyperhomocysteinaemia had a fourfold increase in the risk of disease compared with a normal level.[23] About one-third of patients with PAOD have mildly raised homocysteine levels. The mechanism of homocysteine-induced atheroma seems multifactorial but it probably impairs endothelial production of nitric oxide. Plasma levels can be lowered by dietary supplementation with folate and vitamin B_6.[24] There have been no randomised studies of this treatment in PAOD.[25] However, it seems sensible to measure plasma homocysteine and instigate treatment in young claudicants, especially if they have no other risk factors.

Oxidative damage plays a significant role in PAOD and patients have less antioxidant capacity. It seems possible that antioxidants such as vitamins C and E could reduce this damage. A systematic review concluded that, while inexpensive and probably safe, there was little evidence that vitamins were an effective treatment.[26] Chelation therapy entails repeated injections of ethylenediamine tetra-acetic acid (EDTA), often combined with the administration of vitamins, trace elements and iron supplements. Proponents of this popular therapy claim that EDTA reduces the calcium content of atherosclerotic plaques, reduces LDL oxidation, increases the effectiveness of hydroxyl radical scavengers, limits reperfusion injury and diminishes platelet adhesiveness. Only four randomised controlled trials have been undertaken and a systematic review concluded that the observed clinical effects are due to a powerful placebo response.[27]

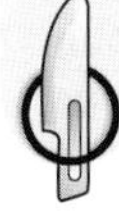

Antiplatelet therapy

There is now unequivocal evidence for the use of antiplatelet therapy as secondary prevention against cardiovascular events in patients with PAOD, and this is their major role.[28–30] The Antithrombotic Trialists' Collaboration analysed 287 randomised placebo-controlled studies and found that antiplatelet therapy in various forms reduced the odds of a 'serious vascular event' by 23% in patients with PAOD.[30] Aspirin, which irreversibly blocks cyclooxygenase-mediated production of thromboxane A_2, a powerful promoter of platelet aggregation, is cheap and should be the first-line agent. However, up to 20% of patients cannot take aspirin because of a history of allergy or gastrointestinal intolerance. Other antiplatelet agents should then be considered. Though there is probably a small additional benefit from the use of dipyridamole in combination with aspirin, there is little evidence to support its use alone. The CAPRIE study compared clopidogrel (a thienopyridine that blocks the ADP-dependent activation of platelets) with aspirin in patients suffering from stroke, myocardial infarction or IC.[31] Clopidogrel was found to be more effective than aspirin, with a relative risk reduction for vascular events of 8.7%, although the absolute risk reduction was only 0.51%. Therefore, to prevent one additional event 196 patients would need to be treated with clopidogrel, as opposed to aspirin, at an annual cost of £460 compared with £2 for aspirin. Such additional expense for this small benefit makes it hard to justify using clopidogrel as a first-line agent, but it is a very effective alternative in those who are aspirin intolerant. The recommendations contained in a consensus statement on the use of antiplatelet therapy in peripheral arterial disease, the latest paper by the Antithrombotic Trialists' Collaboration and the Trans-Atlantic Inter-Society Consensus (TASC) document reflect this and state that all patients with PAOD be considered for long-term antiplatelet therapy with aspirin 75–150 mg daily or clopidogrel 75 mg daily.[28–30]

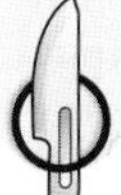

TREATMENT OF INTERMITTENT CLAUDICATION

The decision to intervene for IC depends upon how much the patient's symptoms impinge on the quality of life and day-to-day activity, rather than the actual walking distance. The effects of IC need to be determined on an individual basis. The patient's own assessment of walking distance is often unreliable and a treadmill test may not simulate their normal walking pace. IC may have considerably greater impact on the quality of life than either the doctor or the patient may perceive. Several studies have shown that IC has a major impact on sleep, emotional behaviour and social interaction as well as mobility.[32,33] Questionnaires and scoring systems may help to identify patients with IC, as well as monitoring the efficacy of therapy.[34,35] However, the interpretation of such questionnaires requires care, as other conditions may influence the results.

IC is a relatively benign condition as far as the leg is concerned, and the standard advice to patients remains 'stop smoking and keep walking'.[36] Approximately 50% of patients improve, 30% remain stable and 25% deteriorate, with less than 5% progressing to CLI (see Chapter 1).[37] However, many patients find their condition handicapping and get little comfort from the assurance that they are unlikely to lose their leg. The limitation of walking may have work and social implications for the patient, and cost implications for society if social services become necessary. Unfortunately, the evidence for the long-term efficacy of intervention is often lacking, particularly when the risks and costs are taken into account. Although the outlook for most patients with IC is good, some factors are associated with a worse prognosis. This may influence the selection of patients for treatment. Diabetics are more likely to deteriorate, as are those with ankle pressures less than 70 mmHg.[38] Patients who continue to smoke and those who have had previous vascular surgery also fare less well.[39] It seems best to treat IC of recent onset expectantly, as spontaneous improvement may pre-empt the need for intervention.

The risks from generalised vascular disease are more important than the actual complaint (see Chapter 1). Patients with IC have a risk of death 1.6–3.8 times that of age-matched control subjects.[40,41] This is largely due to ischaemic heart disease (50%), cerebrovascular disease (15%) and intra-abdominal vascular disease (10%).[42,43] Coronary angiography in patients undergoing peripheral vascular surgery reveals coronary artery disease in 90%, unsuspected from routine preoperative screening in many cases and significant in 36% of cases.[44] This has implications not only for the long-term survival of the patient but also for the risk of intervention in this group. Therefore, patients with IC require attention to their general cardiovascular condition as well as their presenting problem. There also seems little point in treating IC if shortness of breath or angina limits the patient's ability to walk.

Exercise

Telling patients to walk more has little effect,[45] but structured exercise training seems useful.

In 1995, a meta-analysis of 21 exercise training programmes showed that training for at least 6 months, by walking to near-maximum pain tolerance, produced a significant improvement in pain-free and maximum walking distance.[46] More recently, a systematic Cochrane review found ten good-quality randomised trials of exercise regimens in stable claudicants.[47] The trials were all small with a total of almost 250 patients. The conclusions of the review were that exercise therapy can achieve an overall improvement in walking ability of approximately 150%, with a thrice weekly programme of walking to near-maximal pain producing the best results. Exercise produced significant improvement in walking time compared with angioplasty at 6 months and compared with antiplatelet therapy alone. Surgery may be more effective, but must be weighed against the attendant increased morbidity and mortality. A trial from Oxford that compared exercise with transluminal angioplasty also found exercise to be better than angioplasty in prolonging the distance walked at 1 year.[48] However, only one-third of patients in the exercise group still undertook exercise after 70 months, and by this time there was no longer any difference between the two groups. Subgroup analysis suggested that patients with iliac lesions fared better with angioplasty, whereas those with superficial femoral disease did better with exercise. Another trial from Edinburgh showed that angioplasty was superior at 6 months but the advantage disappeared after 2 years.[49,50] The likely explanation for these differences is that both trials were too small, and a large, multicentre, randomised trial of exercise versus angioplasty versus surgery seems required, something that has now been addressed with the onset of the MIMIC trial in the UK.

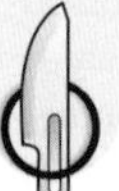

Exercise programmes appear relatively cheap compared with surgery or angioplasty and are certainly safer, although the optimum method of exercise has not been established. Encouraging regular exercise also has general health and cardiovascular benefits,[51] although compliance may be a problem in the long term. Obesity reduces the walking distance of patients with claudication, and so alternative forms of exercise plus dieting that helps weight reduction will improve the walking distance.

Drug treatment

The role of vasoactive drugs in claudication remains the subject of debate. No drug has been shown to be sufficiently effective in the treatment of PAOD to gain widespread acceptance. Five oral drug therapies have a licence for treatment of IC in the UK: naftidrofuryl, cilostazol, pentoxifylline, inositol nicotinate and cinnarizine. These drugs all have vasodilator and other haemorheological properties.

A retrospective single-patient data analysis of five randomised controlled trials looked at the effectiveness of naftidrofuryl, the most commonly used agent.[52] This confirmed a significant improvement in pain-free walking distance, although the clinical effect was not large. A trial of naftidrofuryl 200 mg t.d.s. for 3 months appears worthwhile in patients with moderate IC, when intervention is not possible and where exercise and risk-factor modification have had little benefit.[53,54]

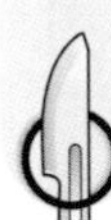

Cilostazol is a phosphodiesterase inhibitor with both antiplatelet and direct vasodilator effects. In four randomised placebo-controlled trials, cilostazol 50–100 mg twice daily has been shown to increase both pain-free walking distance and maximum walking distance. Cilostazol has also been shown to improve physical function and quality of life.[55–59]

The effect of these drugs on PAOD were reviewed in the TASC document on the management of peripheral arterial disease. The conclusions were that, currently, there are insufficient data to recommend the routine use of pharmacotherapy in IC and this is backed up by more recent reviews.[28,60]

Endovascular treatment

Successful endovascular treatment of claudication results in a significant improvement in the patient's quality of life and helps more than unsupervised exercise programmes.[45] It seems likely that supervised exercise programmes are helpful for claudicants (see above), but there is some evidence that angioplasty is cost-effective management for patients with IC.[61] That said, with regard to the relatively benign natural history of IC, endovascular techniques must be safe and focused on those likely to obtain long-term benefit.

The TASC recommendations classify lesions in the aorto-iliac and femoro-politeal segments into types A–D, depending on lesion morphology, with those classed type A (shorter focal disease) more amenable to endovascular treatment and those classed type D (longer more complex lesions) better treated by surgery.[28] However, in claudicants it is difficult to justify the potential complications of surgery, and hence endovascular techniques are often used even if the long-term results may be inferior to surgery. In general, claudicants have single-level disease restricted to the aorto-iliac or femoro-popliteal segments and this is the focus of this section. It is generally believed that treatment for crural disease should be restricted to cases with CLI (see later).

SUPRAINGUINAL INTERVENTION

Aorto-iliac intervention has the highest primary and long-term success, and when combined with relatively normal distal vessels results in a marked improvement in quality of life.[62,63] Femoro-popliteal intervention has a higher primary failure rate and a poorer long-term patency. Endovascular intervention should then be limited to those patients with focal disease and good run-off (see below).

Symptomatic infrarenal aortic stenoses usually occur in women, often in association with hyperlipidaemia. Simple lesions seem best treated by balloon dilatation, with primary success in greater than 90% of cases and long-term patencies of 70–90% at 4 years.[64,65] There are no randomised data to suggest that stent placement is superior and neither is there likely to be, since the prevalence of this disease pattern is small. If stents restrict distal embolisation, they may well have a role in bulky or eccentric stenoses (**Fig. 3.5**). The initial technical success with stent is in the region of 90–100%, with patencies at 4 years of around 90%.[66,67]

Simple iliac stenoses are relatively easy to treat by balloon dilatation. Reported primary success rates are 88–99%, with an average complication rate of 3.6% and reported long-term patencies of approximately 67–95% at 1 year, 60–80% at 3 years and 55–80% at 5 years.[28] Better results can be expected for short-segment disease, for those with good run-off and in claudicants.[28,68]

Despite the lack of good evidence for the use of stents in iliac stenoses, the custom has continued. In clinical practice it is generally accepted that stents in the aorto-iliac segment are indicated when there is failure of angioplasty as a result of residual stenosis, obstructing dissection or residual pressure drop across the lesion (though there is no consensus as to what constitutes haemodynamic significance when measuring iliac pressures).[69] Stents are also used in the treatment of lesions thought to be at high risk of primary failure (e.g. eccentric stenosis, chronic iliac occlusions) or when it is perceived there is an increased risk of distal embolisation. Large series of stents used mainly for iliac stenoses have shown a primary technical success of 95–100%, with an average complication rate of 6.3% and long-term patencies of 78–95% at 1 year, 53–95% at 3 years and 72% at 5 years.[28] These results appear to be slightly better than those of angioplasty alone, but the studies are non-randomised.

A meta-analysis of the results of angioplasty and stent placement for aorto-iliac occlusive disease, much of which is observational data, concluded that compared with angioplasty, stents have:

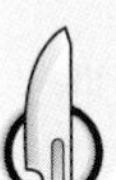

- an improved technical success rate;
- a similar complication rate;
- a 39% reduction in the risk of long-term failure.[70]

There is a paucity of randomised data. A widely known randomised trial by Richter has not been published in a peer-reviewed journal, although abstracts have been presented. Patients with iliac stenoses were randomised between angioplasty and stent placement. There was a significantly improved primary success rate in the stent group and a better 5-year angiographic patency (64.6% vs. 93.6%). Similarly, the 5-year clinical success rates rose from

(a)

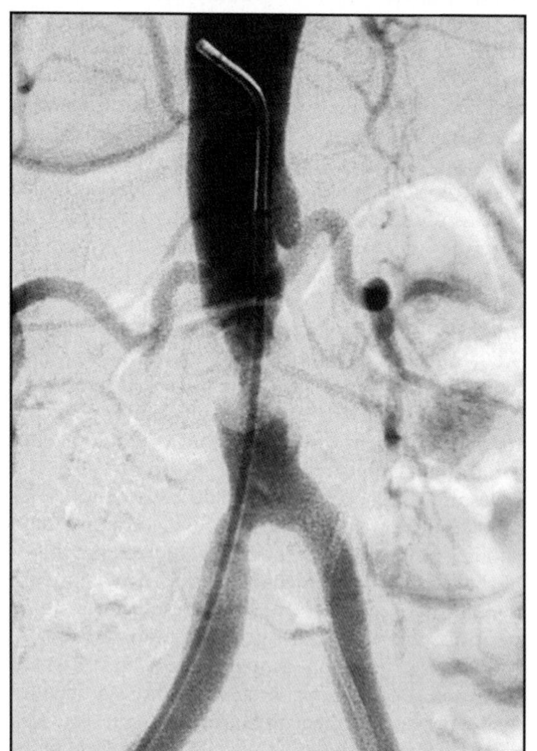

(b)

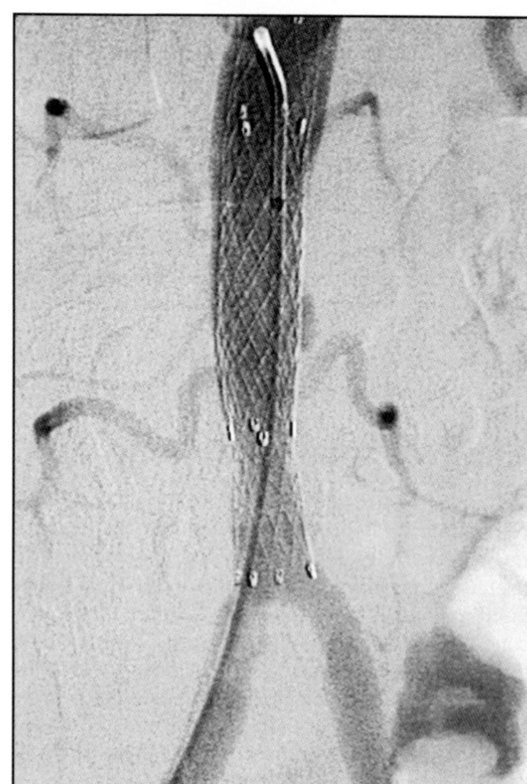

Figure 3.5 • Localised infrarenal aortic stenosis **(a)** successfully treated with self-expanding nitinol stents **(b)**.

69.7% to 92.7% in the stent group.[71,72] However, the non-publication of the data questions the validity of these results.

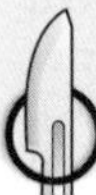

The Dutch Iliac Stent Trial Group has published a randomised trial of primary stent placement versus selective stent placement in patients with iliac artery occlusive disease.[73] In this study, 279 patients with IC and iliac artery disease (including only 12 iliac occlusions) were randomised to either primary stent placement or stent placement after angioplasty if there was a residual mean gradient of greater than 10 mmHg. The researchers found no difference in the two strategies at short- and long-term follow-up except that a policy of selective stent placement was cheaper than blanket stent placement. They concluded that for claudicants a policy of selective stent placement was superior to primary stenting for iliac lesions. However, the trial was based on the premise that a residual gradient following angioplasty predicts poor outcome, something for which there is no good scientific basis, and there are no published randomised data comparing angioplasty alone with stenting, selective or otherwise, to clearly show that stenting is superior.

In summary, angioplasty for iliac stenoses is effective and relatively safe. Stents should only be used for suboptimal angioplasty or a flow-limiting dissection, although more data are required.

Iliac occlusions can also be treated by balloon angioplasty. The review of the results of angioplasty for iliac occlusions in TASC reported technical success in an average of 83% of cases, an average complication rate of 6%, and 1-year and 3-year patency rates of 68 and 60% respectively, although if primary technical failures are excluded these rise to 85 and 77% respectively.[28] Another series by Leu et al., not included in the TASC review, reported a higher rate of distal embolisation of 24% of chronic iliac occlusions treated by angioplasty alone;[74] a perception that the use of stents to scaffold the high bulk of disease reduces this risk is one of the reasons these lesions are often primarily stented (**Fig. 3.6**). There are only limited data to support this or that stenting improves patency. TASC gives an average technical success rate of 82% for stents in iliac occlusions, an average complication rate of 5.6%, and average 1-year and 3-year patency rates of 75 and 64%, rising to 90 and 82% if primary technical failures are excluded.[28] These results are

(a)

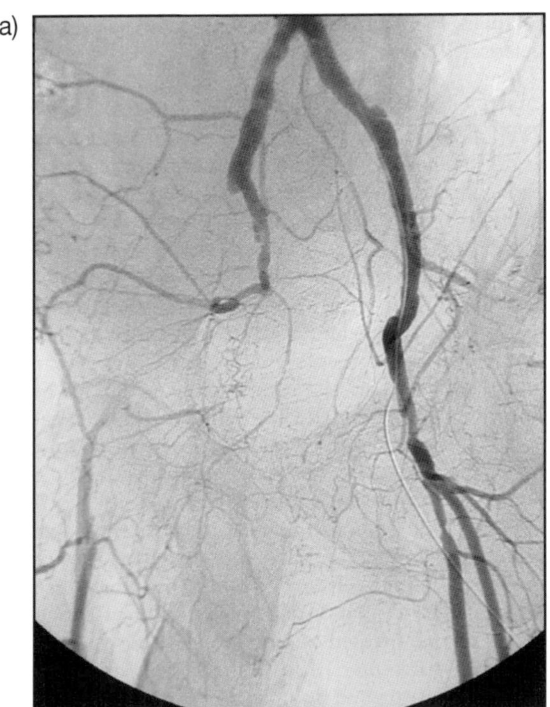

(b)

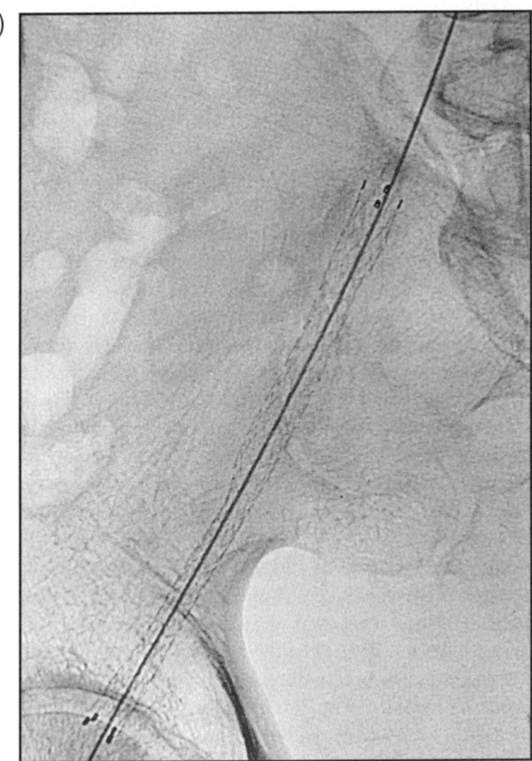

(c)

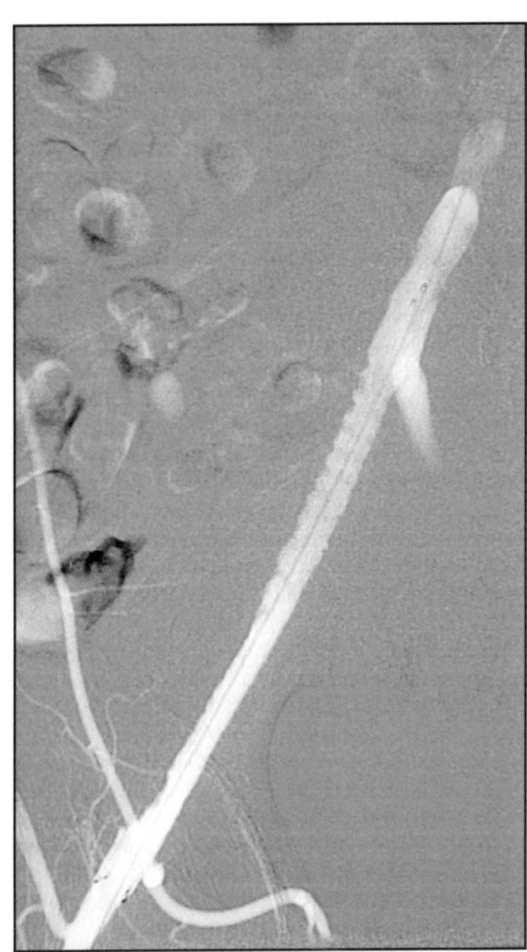

Figure 3.6 • Long right iliac occlusion **(a)** successfully treated with a self-expanding nitinol stent **(b)**, showing appearance after percutaneous transluminal angioplasty of the stent **(c)**.

little different from angioplasty alone and we await the result of a randomised trial from Sheffield.

INFRAINGUINAL INTERVENTION

Endovascular intervention for claudication due to femoro-popliteal disease appears more controversial because the early results from supervised exercise programmes are encouraging. In addition, the early and late results from angioplasty are less successful compared with the aorto-iliac system although, as in the aorto-iliac segment, the extent, bulk and type of disease affect the outcome and durability of the intervention. The reported overall primary success of angioplasty is 90%, with an average complication rate of 4.3% and patencies at 1, 3 and 5 years of 61, 51 and 48% respectively, rising to 71, 61 and 58% respectively if primary technical failures are excluded.[28] As in the aorto-iliac segment, stents have been assessed to try to improve these results. However, though technical success seems better at 98%, complications are higher at an average of 7.3%, and patency rates are no better, being on average 67% at 1 year and 58% at 3 years.[28] A more recent meta-analysis including observational data suggested that in patients with more severe disease and more complex lesions stenting may confer a benefit, though the authors conceded that this could be due to publication bias.[75] In general, even randomised trials[76,77] have failed to show any benefit for conventional stents and (unlike the coronary circulation) there is no convincing evidence for using drug-eluting stents.[76] Therefore stents do not usually have a role in treating femoro-popliteal disease, except as a bail-out following angioplasty complicated by flow-limiting dissection or thrombosis.

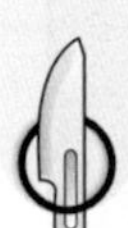

Taking these factors into consideration, along with the complications of intervention, TASC indicated that the choice of endovascular or surgical treatment for femoro-popliteal disease in IC should be based on the morphology of the disease, with less severe type A lesions best treated using angioplasty and more severe and complex type D lesions treated using surgical bypass. Stents had no place in the routine treatment of femoro-popliteal disease.[28]

There is no evidence to support the use of other endovascular techniques, such as lasers, atherectomy devices and stentgrafts, as there is no evidence that they confer any benefit over angioplasty/stenting for occlusive disease in either the aorto-iliac or femoro-popliteal segment. However, there is some limited evidence that brachytherapy may improve outcomes following angioplasty/stenting, but further research is required on its role in everyday clinical practice.[78,79]

Surgical treatment

The role of surgical bypass in claudication remains poorly defined, especially for infrainguinal disease. Initial enthusiasm has become tempered by the realisation that the morbidity and mortality associated with operating on a group of patients with a high prevalence of ischaemic heart disease, combined with the significant failure rate of bypass grafting, may be little better than the natural history of the condition. Every vascular surgeon knows of a patient who ended up with an amputation following occlusion or infection of a bypass graft performed for claudication.

SUPRAINGUINAL BYPASS

The initial results of inflow procedures such as aorto-bifemoral bypass are excellent, with reported 5-year patency rates of 85–90% and an associated mortality of 1–4%, with the best results in claudicants.[80,81] There is also the risk of graft infection and postoperative impotence. Cross-femoral and iliofemoral bypass provide technically satisfactory ways of dealing with unilateral iliac disease and in claudicants these should achieve 90% 1-year patency rates.[82,83] They also have the advantage of lower mortality rates and less risk of causing neurogenic impotence. Iliofemoral bypass may have a better patency compared with an extra-anatomical femoro-femoral crossover. However, iliofemoral bypass requires a patent non-calcified common iliac artery for inflow and a more extensive retroperitoneal incision. Inflow disease of the donor iliac artery can be treated by angioplasty and/or stenting prior to femoro-femoral crossover, but diffuse bilateral aorto-iliac disease in a fit patient is probably best treated by an aorto-bifemoral bypass, because of better long-term patency.

Axillo-bifemoral grafts have a lower patency rate and are rarely justified for claudication (see later). **Figure 3.7** outlines some typical options available for aorto-iliac disease. With the advent of percutaneous angioplasty and stenting, endarterectomy for localised aorto-iliac disease is rarely justified. For a claudicant with multilevel disease, it is usually better to assess the clinical benefit of an inflow procedure rather than embarking on an extensive combined suprainguinal and infrainguinal reconstruction.[84] Conventionally, the abdominal aorta is approached via a midline incision but a curved transverse upper abdominal incision provides better exposure and less postoperative pain. A unilateral transverse or oblique incision can be used for a retroperitoneal approach although exposure is more limited. Little evidence exists that the retroperitoneal or laparoscopically assisted approach offer any significant advantage.[85] The proximal anastomosis should be placed as high as possible on the infrarenal aorta as this is usually the site of least disease. The anastomosis can be either end-to-end or end-to-side. End-to-end anastomosis is indicated in patients with coexisting aneurysmal disease or complete aortic occlusion up to the renal arteries. Some surgeons claim that this configuration results in better long-term patency and less risk of an aorto-duodenal fistula, although there have been no randomised trials.[86,87] However, an end-to-side anastomosis seems easier to perform, with less risk of impotence. It can also preserve a patent inferior mesenteric or internal iliac arteries (**Fig. 3.8**).

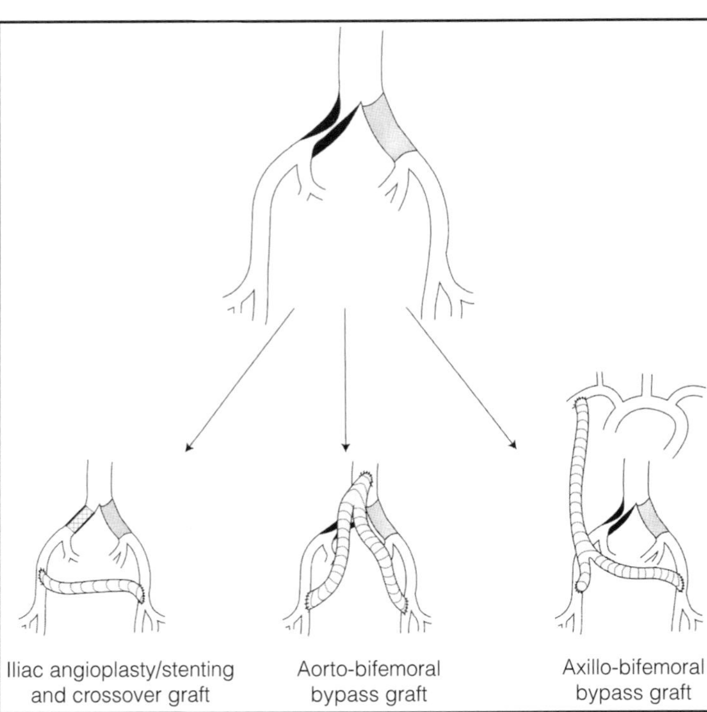

Figure 3.7 • Possible treatment options in a patient with aorto-iliac disease. Axillo-bifemoral bypass should be reserved for patients with critical ischaemia.

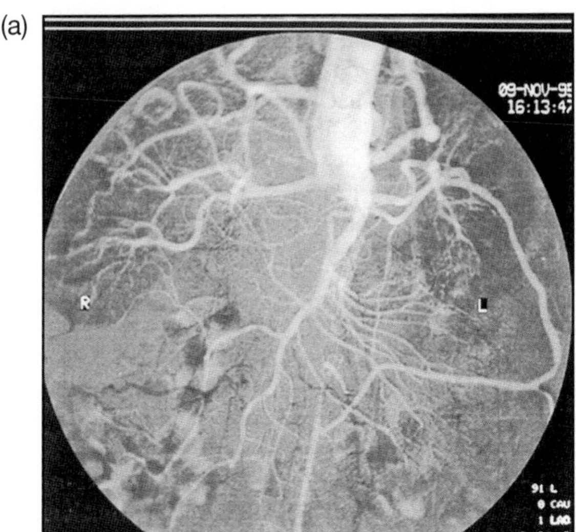

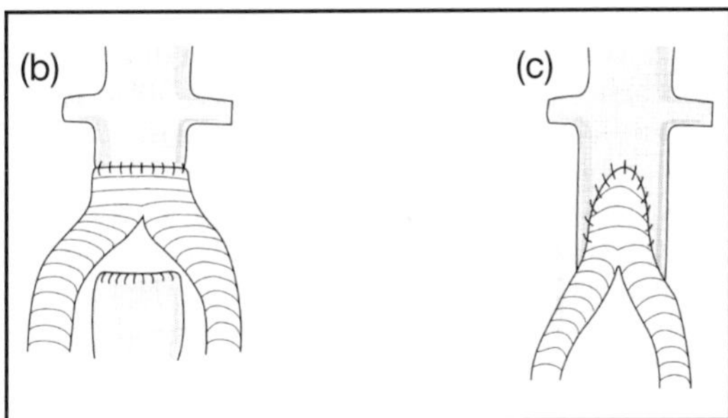

Figure 3.8 • **(a)** Aortogram showing occlusion of the aorta below the level of the renal arteries. In this case the proximal anastomosis of an aorto-bifemoral bypass should be end-to-end **(b)**. If there is continuity with the inferior mesenteric artery or internal iliac arteries, then an end-to-side anastomosis **(c)** may be preferable.

INFRAINGUINAL BYPASS

The results of above-knee femoro-popliteal bypass grafting are relatively good and in the first 2 years the patency of prosthetic grafts seems similar to vein (75–80%). Available prosthetic grafts include polytetrafluoroethylene (PTFE), polyester (Dacron) and various biological grafts (see Chapter 4). Using prosthetics in this position has the advantage that the vein is preserved for later use if necessary and they make the operation considerably quicker. However, the long-term results for prosthetics are less good. Occlusion may also result in CLI due to loss of the run-off caused by myointimal hyperplasia at the distal anastomosis.[88]

A large randomised trial comparing autologous saphenous vein with PTFE showed equivalent patency rates at 2 years for both above- and below-knee femoro-popliteal bypass grafts.[89] Thereafter the patency rates diverged. The 4-year patency rates for above-knee bypasses were 61% for vein (*N* = 85) and 38% for PTFE (*N* = 91), although this difference did not achieve significance. For below-knee bypasses the 4-year patency rates were significantly different at 76% for vein (*N* = 62) and 54% for PTFE (*N* = 80). Although large, this trial contained many methodological flaws, as have most others. The smaller, good-quality trial by Kumar et al.[90] compared the use of autologous vein, PTFE and Dacron for above-knee popliteal grafting. Primary patency rates were significantly better for saphenous vein (73%) compared with PTFE (54%) and Dacron (47%) at 4 years. Various claims have been made for other prosthetic grafts but there is little evidence that any do better than PTFE, and none seem as good as vein. A meta-analysis by Michaels[91] of approximately 40 femoro-popliteal graft studies concluded that saphenous vein was superior to prosthetic grafts. The average 5-year patency rate for above-knee prosthetic grafts was 43% compared with 62% for vein grafts. Below the knee the patency for prosthetics fell to 27% compared with 68% for vein.

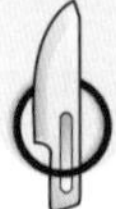

Bypass to below the knee is therefore harder to justify as the results are less good. Even though vein gives better results, there remains a 25–30% risk of further intervention for vein graft stenosis. Failure of a below-knee graft is often associated with worsening of the symptoms and occasionally limb loss, presumably due to damage to the geniculate collaterals. Use of a prosthetic graft in the femoro-popliteal position seems justified if the ipsilateral saphenous vein is unavailable or unsuitable. Ring-reinforced grafts should be used below the knee to reduce the risk of occlusion due to kinking. The use of a vein collar or patch will also improve patency. These adjuvant techniques together with vein graft preparation are discussed in Chapters 4 and 5.

The proximal anastomosis is usually to the common femoral artery, approached via a vertical groin incision. An oblique incision reduces the risk of wound breakdown but this can make proximal access to the external iliac artery or distal access to the profunda artery difficult. Use of the proximal superficial femoral artery (SFA) as an inflow site avoids the need for a groin incision but biplanar angiograms or a duplex scan are required to exclude a stenosis at its origin. For above-knee popliteal artery bypass, the distal incision is made medially in the thigh, posterior to adductor magnus and anterior to sartorius. Care should be taken to avoid injury to the saphenous vein lying posteriorly if a prosthetic graft is being used preferentially. A subsartorial tunnel should be used for both prosthetics and vein grafts, which should be reversed, as the in situ position does not sit well above the knee. The below-knee incision is made parallel to the posterior border of the tibia, again taking care to avoid damaging the long saphenous vein. The deep fascia is divided and the gastrocnemius muscle retracted posteriorly to enter the popliteal space. Prosthetic and reversed vein grafts are tunnelled between the head of gastrocnemius and then subsartorially. With the in situ vein technique, care must be taken to ensure that the vein is not compressed or kinked by the fascia or the semitendinosus and semi-membranosus tendons when the knee is extended. Divide these tendons if necessary. As graft patency is dependent on run-off, bypasses to an isolated popliteal artery or to a single calf vessel, though justified for limb salvage, are not indicated for claudication. **Figure 3.9** outlines some possible treatment options for a claudicant with femoro-popliteal disease.

Localised stenosis or occlusion of the common femoral artery can cause severe claudication because the profunda collaterals cannot develop (**Fig. 3.10**). This seems best treated by an endarterectomy and vein or prosthetic patch repair, extending down the profunda. Treatment of an isolated profunda stenosis rarely results in any significant benefit.[92] The operation can also be combined with suprainguinal or infrainguinal reconstruction, using the graft as the patch, which improves the run-off and long-term patency.[93] A bypass graft from the external iliac artery to the profunda or above-knee popliteal artery may better treat a long occlusion of the common femoral artery. Percutaneous angioplasty of the femoral bifurcation does not work well because of difficulties with access from the opposite groin and with the bulky calcified disease. Stents cannot be used at this level because the artery flexes with movements of the hip.

LUMBAR SYMPATHECTOMY

There is no objective evidence to support the use of lumbar sympathectomy in the treatment of IC. There is no increase in blood flow at rest or during exercise following the procedure.[28] It may have a role in the treatment of unreconstructable CLI as it interrupts cutaneous pain pathways to produce a degree of analgesia (see below).

Conclusion

IC is a common condition and although the diagnosis is usually straightforward, non-invasive assessment will confirm the diagnosis and give some idea of the haemodynamic severity of the disease. The most important aspects of the condition to

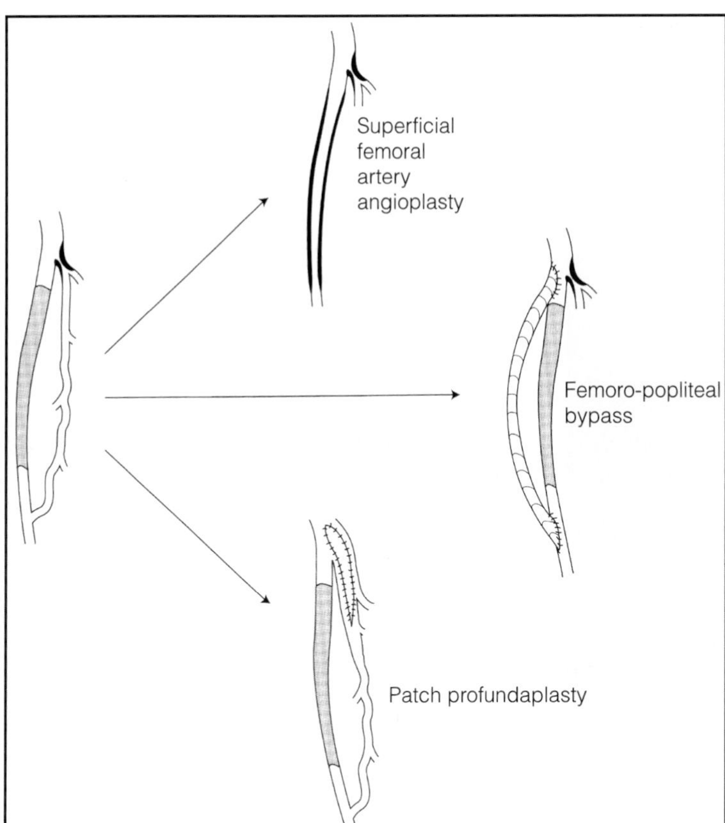

Figure 3.9 • Possible treatment options for a claudicant with femoro-popliteal disease. Angioplasty should be the first line of treatment for stenoses and occlusions less than 10 cm in length.

remember are the relatively benign prognosis for the local disease and the significant cardiovascular implications. Therefore, attention should be first directed at risk-factor modification. Several treatment options exist but there remains a lack of evidence for any of them, although the risks increase with the degree of intervention. Initially, it seems reasonable to adopt a non-interventional approach involving risk-factor modification and an exercise programme for all but the most severely affected patients. Reserve endovascular intervention for suitable lesions in those patients with severe symptoms or who fail to improve with risk-factor modification and exercise. The patient must be prepared to accept a small risk of worsening symptoms or even limb loss if the procedure fails. Surgical bypass may be indicated for those patients who seem unsuitable for endovascular treatment and in whom a simple femoro-popliteal bypass or inflow procedure appears possible. A history of significant cardiorespiratory disease would mitigate against intervention. The factors influencing the decision to intervene in claudication are outlined in **Box 3.1**.

Box 3.1 • Factors affecting the decision to intervene in claudication

For
Severe symptoms
Job affected
No improvement with exercise
Aortoiliac disease
Stenosis/short occlusion
Unilateral symptoms
Against
Short history
Still smoking
Other limiting conditions
Femoro-distal disease
Long occlusion
Multilevel disease

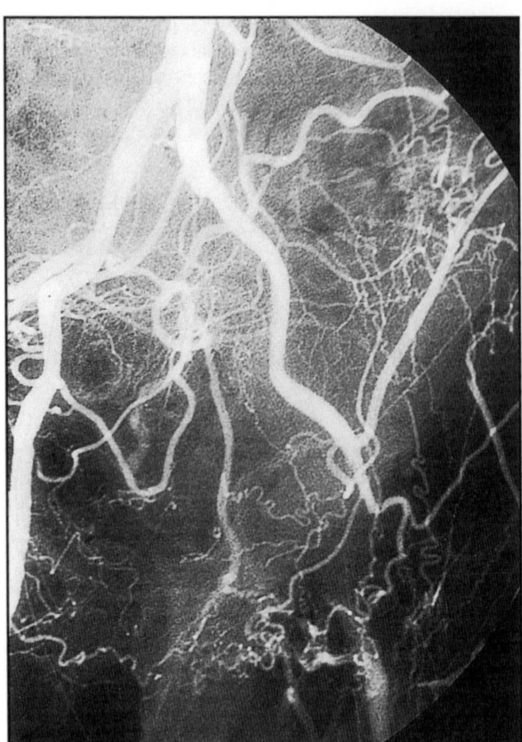

Figure 3.10 • Arteriogram of a claudicant showing a localised occlusion of the left common femoral artery, suitable for endarterectomy and patch repair.

TREATMENT OF CRITICAL LIMB ISCHAEMIA

There is little specific information on the incidence of CLI. Based on a national survey, the prevalence in the UK has been estimated at 20 000 cases per year, an annual incidence of 40 per 100 000 population.[94] This burden of disease will increase over the next decades due to the expanding elderly population. It will therefore generate a considerable workload for healthcare providers, especially with the increasing availability of therapeutic techniques. The majority of patients with CLI can now be offered a revascularisation procedure, mainly due to an increase in endovascular procedures.[95,96] The published results seem good in specialist centres, but intervention is often technically demanding and utilises significant hospital resources.[97] Furthermore, the prognosis for patients with CLI is poor, as about 25% will die within 1 year and 50% within 5 years, mainly from coronary and cerebral vascular disease (see Chapter 1). Many studies have shown that the presence of diabetes and renal failure result in worse outcomes in terms of limb salvage and mortality.[98–100] Therefore, treatment of CLI requires relatively short-term objectives, especially in patients with significant comorbidity.[97] There is some evidence that increased rates of vascular reconstruction are associated with a lower incidence of primary amputation (see Chapter 6).[28,95,101] A national survey by the Vascular Surgical Society of Great Britain and Ireland showed that 70% of patients with CLI underwent revascularisation, with a 75% chance of successful limb salvage.[94] Surgeons with a low throughput of patients performed more primary amputations than those who performed more than 30 infrainguinal reconstructions per year.

Economics, cost-effectiveness and quality of life

CLI creates a significant social and financial burden. A review of available statistics in 1994 estimated that £200 million was spent annually in the UK on this condition (30% on surgical procedures and 26% on amputations).[102] This figure can only increase with the rising prevalence of this condition and the expanding treatment options and will be compounded by escalating healthcare costs. With increasing demands on resources, it is important to select those patients who will gain the most from intervention, and avoid inappropriate procedures. The cost-effectiveness of any intervention therefore requires careful evaluation.[103] A retrospective analysis of CLI in elderly patients by Humphreys et al.[104] found that the operative cost of reconstruction was £10 222 compared with £6475 for amputation. However, if the community costs were added, the total costs rose to £13 546 and £33 095 respectively, partly because 66% of reconstructed patients were able to return home compared with only 33% of amputees. A more recent prospective study also found that amputation was more expensive than revascularisation at 1 year.[105] However, there was little difference between the cost of successful endovascular treatment compared with surgical reconstruction, because the length of inpatient stay was related more to the state of the foot than the treatment received.

A prospective study of 55 patients with CLI has shown that the overall quality of life improves after successful reconstruction.[106] Another prospective study from Sheffield of 150 patients with CLI found that activities of daily living improved significantly after successful reconstruction and primary amputation, as did pain scores.[107] Mobility was only improved by successful reconstruction. Thus the improvement in the overall quality of life of those undergoing successful reconstruction seems largely due to better mobility. Patients whose reconstruction fails leading to secondary amputation fare badly, in terms of both quality of life and cost, emphasising the need for a high success rate if undertaking this type of reconstruction.[106,107] This is especially true for infrainguinal bypass procedures. A prospective study by Panayiotopoulos et al.[108] showed that the median inpatient and rehabilitation cost of a successful distal bypass was £4320, a failed distal bypass leading to amputation £17 066, and a primary amputation in patients with non-reconstructable distal disease £12 730. The surgical ideal of an uncomplicated infrainguinal bypass operation, with rapid relief of pain, swift wound healing, a rapid return to premorbid function and no further intervention, was only achieved in 16 of 112 patients in a recent retrospective study.[109] Furthermore, failed reconstruction may result in a higher amputation level especially if an infected prosthetic graft requires removal.[110]

Patient selection

Most patients with CLI require some form of intervention. There are a few situations when this would be inappropriate and these patients should not undergo unnecessary investigation. If the general condition of the patient is poor and the chances of survival limited due to coexistent pathology, it seems reasonable to treat the patient with analgesia alone. However, if the patient has a reasonable quality of life and is likely to survive for more than a few months, it is probably better to attempt revascularisation whenever possible. No one wishes to see a patient spend the remaining few months of life struggling with an amputation as well as their primary disease.

Some patients present with such advanced ischaemia that there is little viable tissue left on the weight-bearing area of the foot. It is sometimes possible, with revascularisation and a customised forefoot amputation, to achieve a functional foot, but if this is not possible a primary amputation is the better option. In a few selected patients the foot can be salvaged with a free tissue transfer combined with revascularisation. This is technically demanding and is usually performed in conjunction with the plastic surgeon (**Fig. 3.11**). The chair- or bed-bound patient can provide a challenge when deciding on whether to intervene. Fixed flexion deformities and extensive tissue loss usually make amputation the best option. However, one should involve the rehabilitation team in this decision, as the patient's ability to transfer from a chair to the bed or toilet may depend on that limb, which should be preserved if possible. Unfortunately, the chances of long-term success after revascularisation in this situation are likely to be slim as patency after intervention depends upon flow, which is related to exercise.

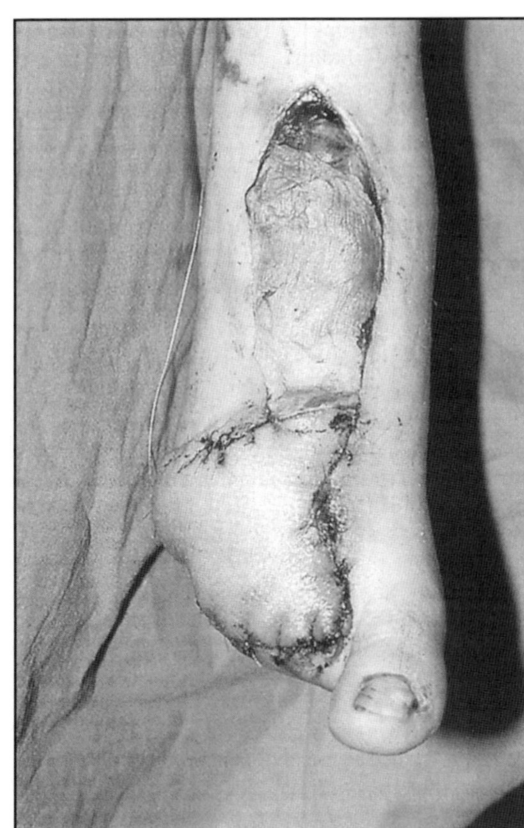

Figure 3.11 • Lateral arm free flap used to resurface the lateral aspect of the foot after femoro-distal bypass and ray amputation.

Preoperative independence and mobility have been shown to best predict postoperative independence and mobility after infrainguinal bypass for CLI.[111] Only 1 of 25 survivors who were not living independently before surgery achieved independent living 6 months postoperatively. Therefore, there seems little point in undertaking extensive revascularisation in the hope of achieving independence for a patient already requiring care in a nursing home.

Endovascular treatment

CLI is often due to multilevel, complex and diffuse arterial disease. More extensive disease is generally more difficult to treat using endovascular techniques, with reduced levels of long-term vessel patency.[28] Despite this and the fact that the haemodynamic durability of such endovascular intervention, particularly in infrainguinal disease, is not as prolonged as bypass surgery, the short-term effects may be sufficient to heal the threatened limb and re-occlusion does not necessarily result in clinical deterioration.[112] These patients often have significant comorbidity and have a very high short-term mortality of up to 25% at 6 months,[28] and are more likely to die than return for reintervention. Such patients are poor candidates for surgery because of the high rate of perioperative morbidity and mortality. For these reasons many institutions have now turned to a strategy of endovascular intervention in the first instance,[96] and such an approach is likely to be applicable in approximately 50–75% of cases.[113]

SUPRAINGUINAL INTERVENTION

With multilevel disease, as with claudication, aorto-iliac disease should be treated first, as it is likely to convert rest pain to claudication and optimises the inflow for any infrainguinal intervention. A detailed discussion of iliac angioplasty and stenting can be found in the section on the endovascular treatment of IC. When there is tissue loss, treatment of the inflow alone is probably less likely to result in limb salvage, and the aim then should be to achieve in-line flow to the foot. The infrainguinal disease can be managed by surgery or angioplasty or as a combined procedure, timed according to the clinical situation. When an occlusion of the ipsilateral iliac segment cannot be treated using endovascular techniques, then the contralateral side should be treated by angioplasty or stenting to facilitate a femoro-femoral crossover.[114] Endovascular intervention proximal to such a crossover graft does not interfere with the durability of the graft, and many would now advocate such an approach as significant inflow disease may jeopardise the graft.[115] Preoperative or peroperative angioplasty or stenting can improve graft inflow or run-off and reduce the length of the bypass. For example, angioplasty of an SFA stenosis may permit a short popliteal–pedal bypass rather than a full-length bypass from the femoral artery.

INFRAINGUINAL INTERVENTION

More extensive infrainguinal disease can be considered for endovascular intervention in patients with CLI compared with claudicants because a higher complication rate seems acceptable in the threatened limb. Despite the TASC recommendations that more complex type D lesions should be treated by bypass, the high risk of surgery in these patients and any lack of suitable vein for distal bypass make angioplasty invaluable as a treatment option. Advances in equipment and techniques mean that intervention includes angioplasty not only for occlusions of the superficial femoral and popliteal arteries but, in the context of limb salvage, also for stenoses and occlusions of the crural vessels (**Fig. 3.12**). Intentional subintimal angioplasty is an invaluable technique for treating long occlusions (**Fig. 3.13**). This permits any length of lesion to be treated, including flush occlusions of the SFA. Bolia and colleagues have reported a series of 200 subintimal angioplasties for long femoro-popliteal occlusions, with an initial success rate of 80%.[116] This technique is discussed in more detail in Chapter 5. Because the severity of disease and quality of run-off affects the success of angioplasty, published patency rates are considerably lower than the figures quoted for claudication. Results for vessel patency fall significantly with multilevel disease and poor run-off and may be as low as about 23% for long SFA occlusions in these circumstances.[28] However, it is important to focus on limb salvage, as long-term patency is not usually required to maintain a viable limb and limb salvage rates of 50–89% at 1 and 2 years have been reported.[112,113,117] Infrapopliteal angioplasty has also achieved limb salvage rates of 60–88% at 2 years, but if in-line flow to the foot cannot be achieved the results are considerably worse.[28,118–120] As for claudication there is little or no justification for primary stenting in femoro-popliteal disease. The preliminary results in CLI are probably even worse than those for claudicants, and stents cannot be deployed in the popliteal artery because of knee flexion.[28]

The complication rate from angioplasty in CLI is higher than that for claudication,[121] presumably because of the severity of comorbid disease and the tendency to treat more extensive lesions. Acute deterioration in the severity of ischaemia is usually due to distal embolisation or to dissection that removes collaterals or occludes flow. Embolisation should be managed by thrombo-aspiration in the first instance. If this fails, then surgical embolectomy or thrombolysis may be required. The administration of heparin during the procedure helps to limit thrombus formation. Spasm should be treated by the liberal use of antispasmodics, particularly in the tibial vessels. Clearly, these high-risk interventions should only be performed when surgical cover is available.

Occasionally, patients present with quite focal ischaemia of one or more toes with palpable pulses. Such a situation is referred to as the 'blue toe syndrome' and is usually due to a proximal, non-occlusive, ulcerating plaque causing distal platelet embolisation. It seems reasonable to treat these patients with antiplatelet drugs and angioplasty, which will convert the active lesion into something smooth and non-embologenic.

There is little in the way of randomised data comparing endovascular techniques with surgery in the management of chronic lower limb ischaemia. Holm et al.[122] randomised 102 patients, 66% of whom had CLI, and Wolf et al.[123] randomised 263 patients, 73% with claudication, to either angioplasty

(a)

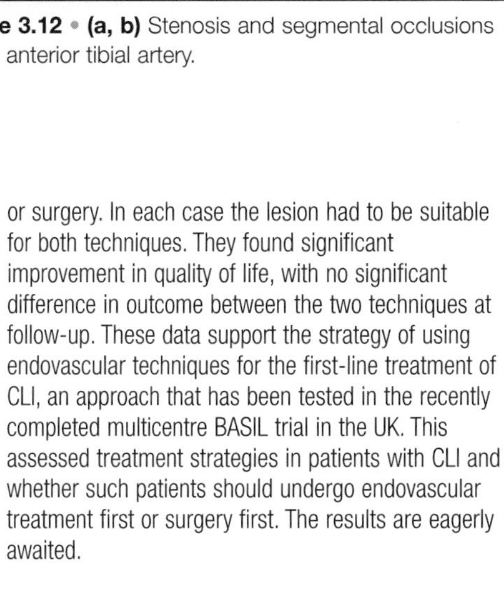

(b)

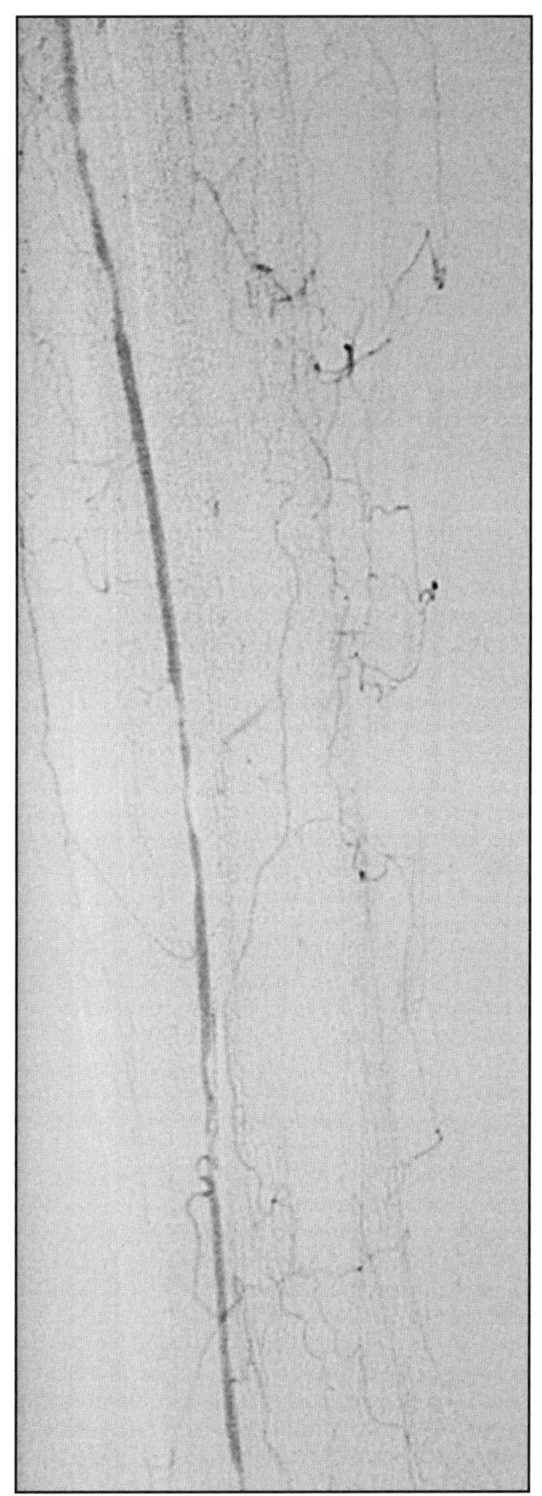

Figure 3.12 • **(a, b)** Stenosis and segmental occlusions of the anterior tibial artery.

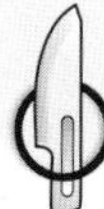

or surgery. In each case the lesion had to be suitable for both techniques. They found significant improvement in quality of life, with no significant difference in outcome between the two techniques at follow-up. These data support the strategy of using endovascular techniques for the first-line treatment of CLI, an approach that has been tested in the recently completed multicentre BASIL trial in the UK. This assessed treatment strategies in patients with CLI and whether such patients should undergo endovascular treatment first or surgery first. The results are eagerly awaited.

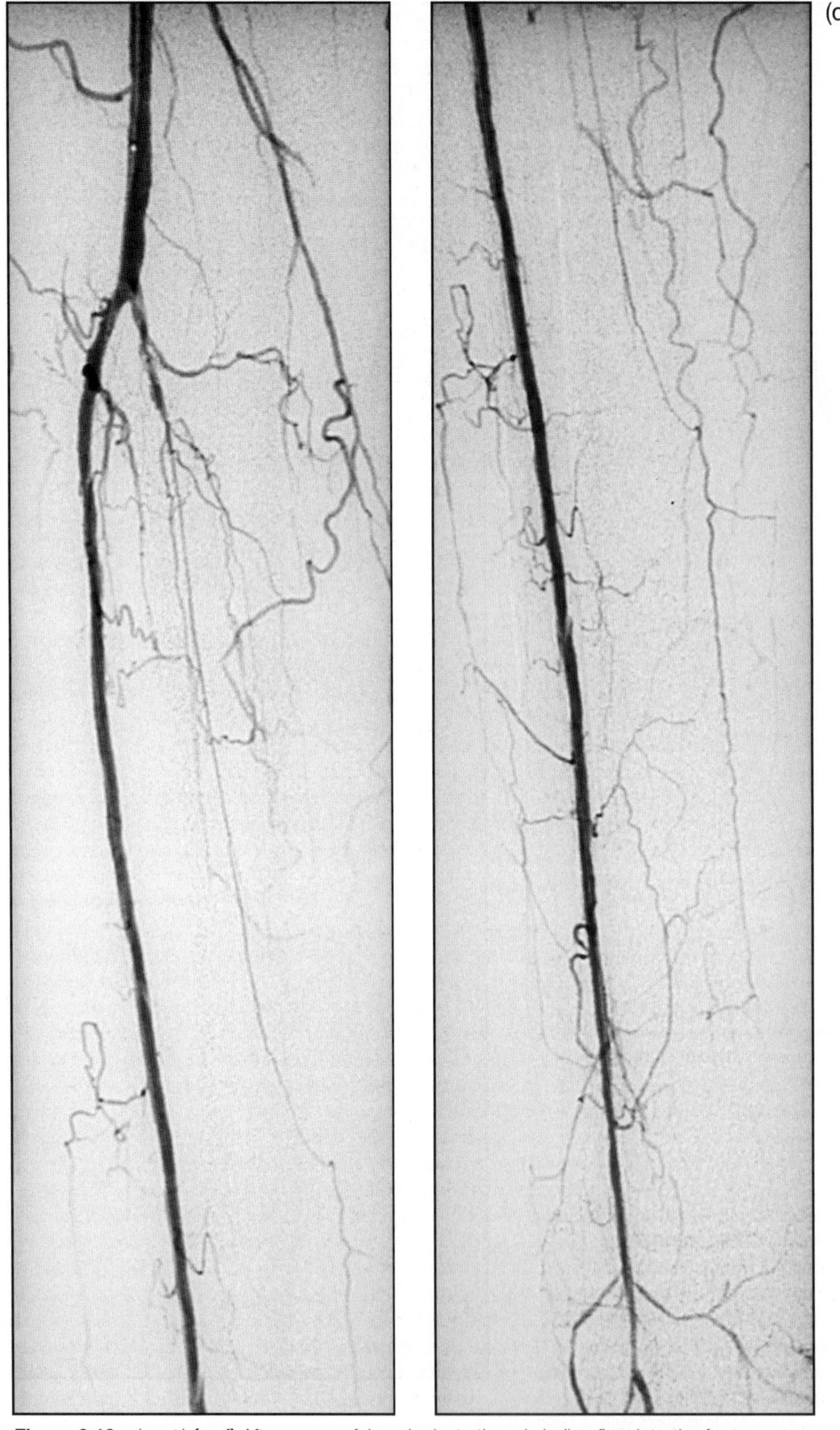

Figure 3.12 • (*cont.*) **(c–d)** After successful angioplasty there is in-line flow into the foot.

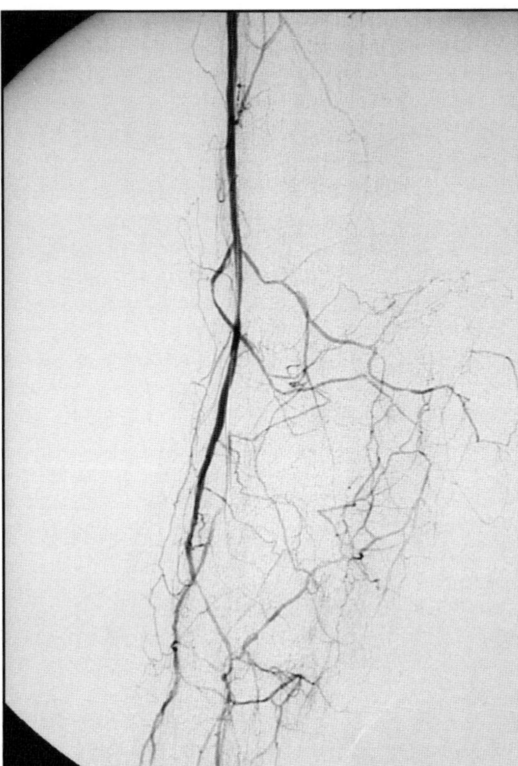

Figure 3.12 • *(cont.)* **(e)** After successful angioplasty there is in-line flow into the foot.

Surgical treatment

If the pattern of arterial disease is deemed unsuitable for endovascular treatment, surgical intervention will be required. The basic principles and techniques described for IC also apply to CLI. However, patients with aorto-iliac disease often require extra-anatomical bypass because they are unfit for aortic reconstruction. Infrainguinal reconstruction often requires femoro-distal bypass because of extensive disease.

SUPRAINGUINAL BYPASS

In patients without significant cardiac, respiratory or renal impairment, aorto-bifemoral bypass grafting gives excellent results in CLI. A meta-analysis by de Vries and Hunink[80] gave overall expected primary patencies of about 80% and 72% (patient based) at 5 and 10 years respectively. Operative mortality was reported as on average 3.3%, with systemic morbidity in 8%.

From a technical aspect, beware the heavily calcified aorta, which can make the proximal anastomosis hazardous. In those who are less fit, the options include femoro-femoral or ilio-femoral bypass for unilateral disease or axillo-bifemoral bypass for bilateral disease (see **Fig. 3.7**). The femoro-femoral bypass is conventionally performed from one common femoral artery to the other via vertical groin incisions. The graft (8 or 10 mm externally supported Dacron or PTFE) is tunnelled subcutaneously. Both the donor and recipient anastomoses face distally like an inverted 'C'. This is not an ideal haemodynamic configuration for the inflow. Anastomosis to the donor external iliac artery via a small oblique iliac fossa incision permits an S-shaped configuration. Other advantages are that the graft can then be tunnelled behind the rectus sheath and the groin preserved for radiological access if angioplasty of the donor iliac artery is subsequently required.

When performing an axillo-bifemoral bypass, brachial artery pressures should be measured on both sides and the supraclavicular fossae auscultated for bruits. If the pressures are equivalent, the right axillary artery should be chosen as the inflow vessel as it has a lower risk of proximal occlusive disease.[124] Axillo-bifemoral bypass has poorer patency than aorto-bifemoral bypass due to the long graft and lower flow, but better patency than axillo-unifemoral bypass, though the results are variable.[28] The donor arm is placed at right angles on an arm board and a mid-infraclavicular incision made. The axillary artery is exposed by splitting the fibres of pectoralis major and mobilising the axillary vein downwards. The tunneller is passed down under pectoralis major and minor and then subcutaneously to the groin. A long tunneller should be used to avoid staging incisions, thus eliminating a potential source of infection.[125] Improved results are obtained with supported grafts, and an 8 or 10 mm reinforced Dacron or PTFE graft should be used to prevent kinking or compression. Reported patency rates are 48–93% at 1 year and 19–79% at 5 years.[28] Review of these results does not reveal any significant differences between PTFE and Dacron, as the run-off is probably the main determinant of patency.

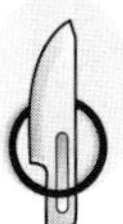

A randomised trial has shown that use of an axillo-bifemoral graft with a symmetrical 'flow splitter' bifurcation reduces the risk of the crossover limb occluding.[126]

Many of these patients will have associated distal disease and the main decision appears whether to undertake concomitant distal bypass. There seems no definitive answer but adding an infrainguinal bypass increases the operation time and risk to the patient. If the run-off, usually via the profunda artery, is good with little tissue loss in the foot, then it seems better simply to carry out the inflow

(a)

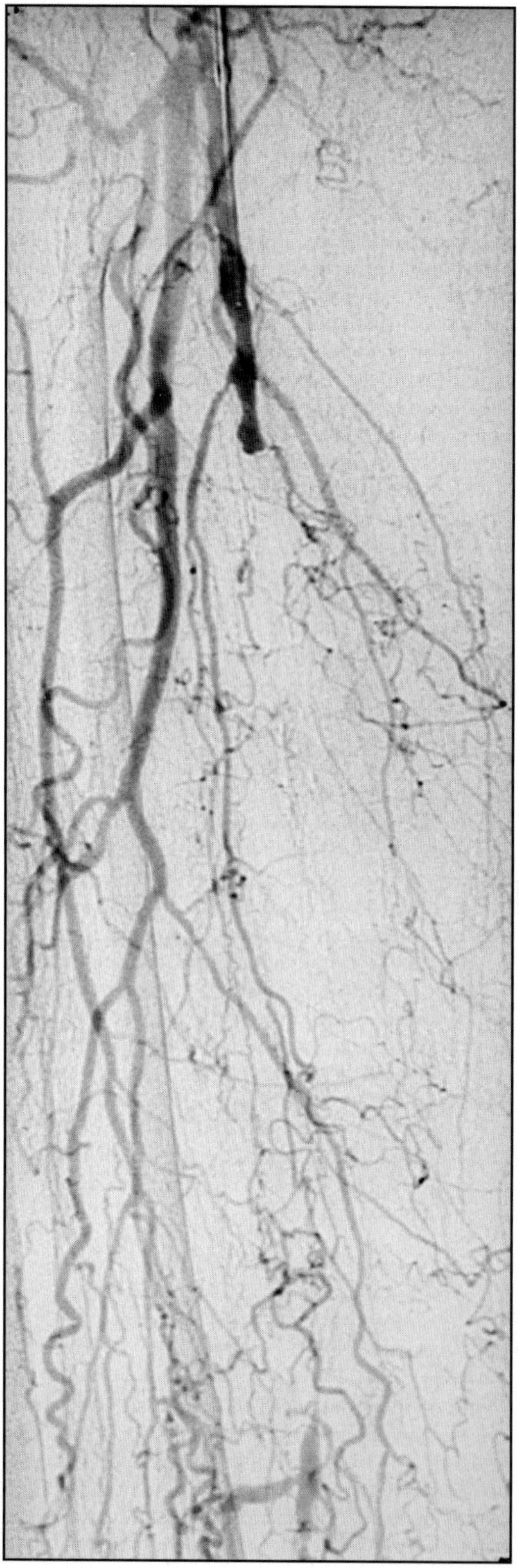

(b)

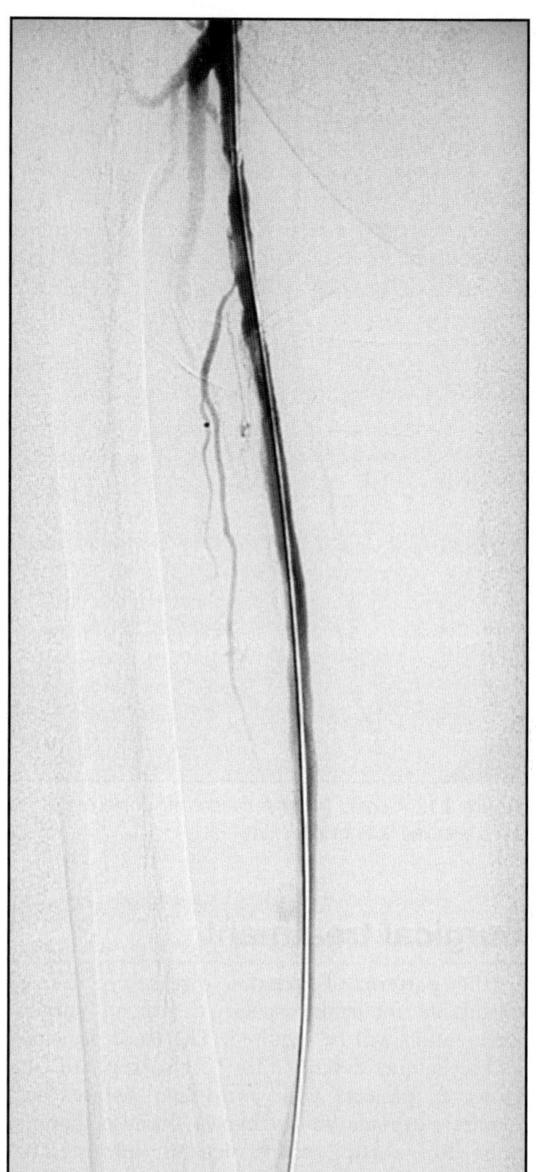

Figure 3.13 • **(a)** Long occlusion of the superficial femoral artery from just beyond its origin, successfully treated using subintimal angioplasty **(b–d)**.

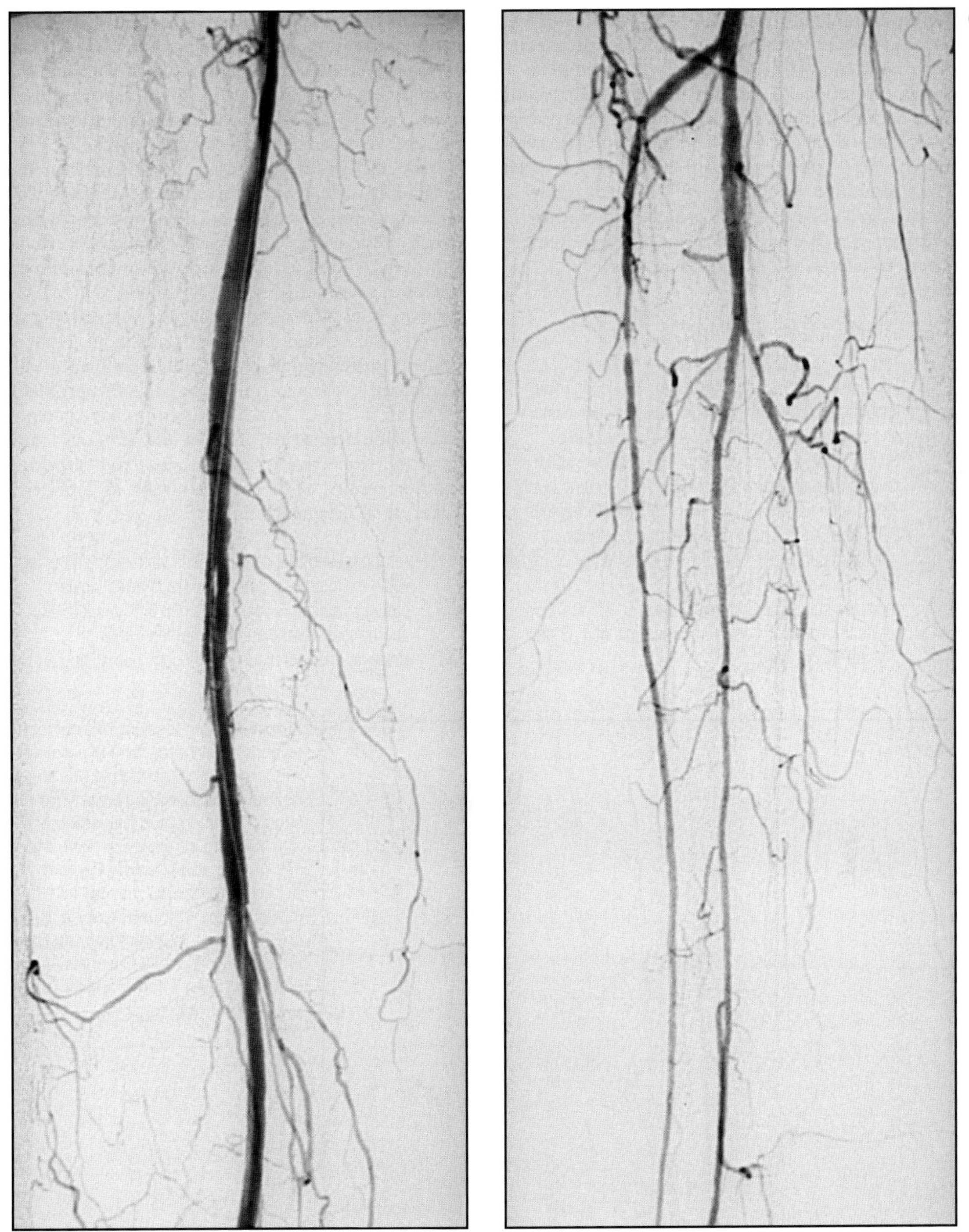

Figure 3.13 • (*cont.*) **(a)** Long occlusion of the superficial femoral artery from just beyond its origin, successfully treated using subintimal angioplasty **(b–d)**.

procedure, and only undertake a distal bypass if the inflow procedure proves to be insufficient. In patients with poor run-off or extensive pedal gangrene, it seems expeditious to combine the inflow correction with an infrainguinal bypass. Profundaplasty alone has a limited role in CLI. If there is no tissue loss, then it may relieve rest pain. However, it rarely heals ulceration or gangrene.[92] The best results of isolated profundaplasty are usually achieved in the presence of well-developed distal profunda femoris artery collaterals and patent tibial vessels.[127]

INFRAINGUINAL BYPASS

The majority of patients will require bypass to infrageniculate vessels (**Fig. 3.14**). Autologous vein should be used when possible, due to better patency and resistance to infection.[28] A meta-analysis by Hunink et al.[128] of femoro-popliteal bypass for CLI reveals primary patencies of 66% for vein (any level), 47% for above-knee PTFE and 33% for below-knee PTFE at 5 years. The pooled weighted data for primary patency rates for femoro-distal (tibial or pedal) bypass are reported in TASC as 85, 80 and 70% for femoro-distal bypass with vein and 70, 35 and 25% for femoro-distal bypass with prosthetic at 1, 3 and 5 years respectively.[28]

Most of the variation in outcomes is due to differences in case mix. The secondary patency and limb salvage rates are usually about 10% better than the primary rates. Vein graft patency depends upon many factors, including quality of the inflow, run-off, and vein quality, diameter and length.[129–131]

Preoperative duplex ultrasound mapping of the long saphenous vein facilitates harvesting, as well as identifying unsuitable small or diseased veins. When the long saphenous vein is unsuitable, veins can be harvested from the arm, the opposite long saphenous vein, the short saphenous vein or the deep leg veins. The disadvantage of using the contralateral long saphenous vein is that about 20% of patients subsequently require intervention for CLI in that leg.[132] Using arm veins avoids this problem. Holzenbein et al.[133] have reported primary patency rates using arm veins of 70% and 49% at 1 and 3 years respectively, but others have reported inferior results, with problems such as long-term aneurysmal degeneration.[134,135]

A randomised trial of saphenous vein versus deep leg veins for femoro-popliteal bypass showed similar patency rates at 3 years (60% vs. 64% respectively) and no long-term disability from leg swelling.[136] However, the technique seems quite demanding and

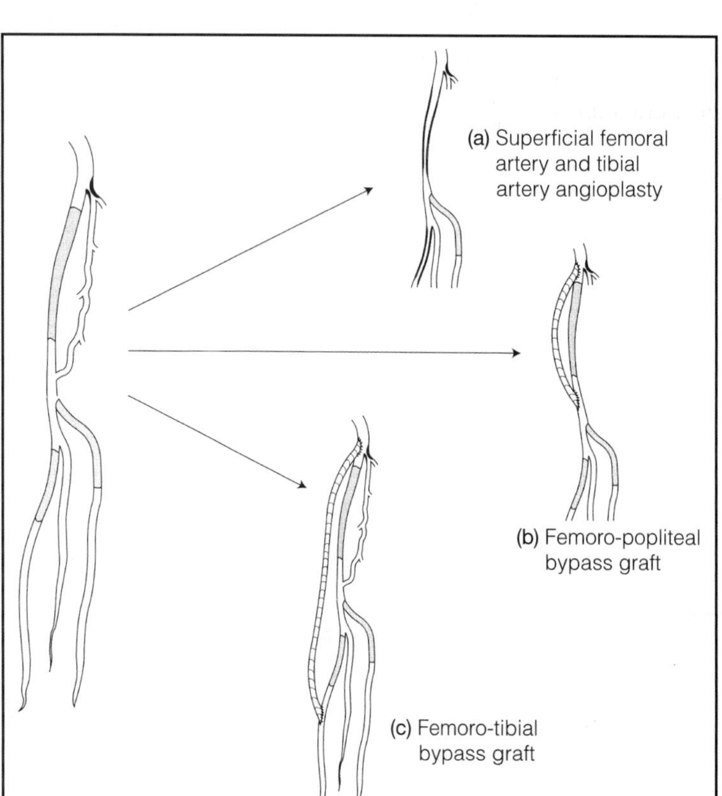

Figure 3.14 • Possible infrainguinal revascularisation options in a patient with critical limb ischaemia due to multilevel disease. Angioplasty **(a)** should be attempted if possible but may need to be extensive, with the risk of early re-occlusion. Femoro-popliteal bypass **(b)** may fail to reperfuse the foot unless at least one calf artery is patent into the foot. Extensive tissue loss or sepsis usually requires a femoro-tibial bypass graft **(c)**, especially in a diabetic.

only a short length of graft can be obtained. Proponents of the in situ technique claim that the taper of the vein gives better size matching between the graft and artery at both the proximal and distal anastomoses, which increases the proportion of veins that can be used for distal bypass, and initial good results led to claims for better long-term patency.[137] However, randomised trials of the in situ versus the reversed technique have shown no difference in utilisation or patency for femoro-popliteal or distal bypass.[138–140] Vein graft preparation, intraoperative monitoring and postoperative surveillance are discussed in Chapter 4.

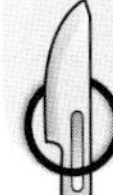

The common femoral artery appears the best site for the proximal anastomosis, but if the vein will not reach then the profunda is probably better than an endarterectomised segment of the SFA. The SFA or popliteal artery can be used as the inflow site providing there is no proximal disease. The distal anastomosis is usually selected from the pre-operative duplex scan or arteriogram. However, the artery chosen should always be inspected before harvesting the vein, as it is not uncommon to need a more distal site or different vessel. Femoro-popliteal grafts to isolated popliteal segments can be considered when no crural or pedal bypass is possible, but an adequate segment of popliteal artery with collateral outflow to the foot is required in order to have any hope of healing ulceration or gangrene and to ensure ongoing patency. With an isolated popliteal segment and a patent distal tibial vessel the best option would be a femoro-tibial bypass if there is enough vein or, if not, a femoro-popliteal prosthetic bypass with a vein extension to the tibial vessel.

The posterior tibial artery in the lower calf is easily reached by deepening the incision used to expose the long saphenous vein. The mid-portion of the peroneal artery is also accessible between the posterior tibial and soleus muscles. Access to the lower portion of the peroneal artery requires resection of a 6–8 cm segment of the fibula via a lateral incision (**Fig. 3.15**). The anterior tibial artery is reached by an incision 4 cm lateral to the anterior edge of the tibia. Vein grafts to the mid-portion of the anterior tibial artery need to be tunnelled through a window in the interosseous membrane. Grafts to the lower portion and the dorsalis pedis can be run across the front of the tibia. The calibre of the recipient tibial artery may be small and the artery and adjacent veins are easily damaged by manipulation. Fine Silastic slings or intraluminal occluders should be used rather than clamps. A long oblique end-to-side anastomosis should be performed with a double-ended monofilament 6-0 or 7-0 polypropylene (Prolene) suture, using magnifying loops.

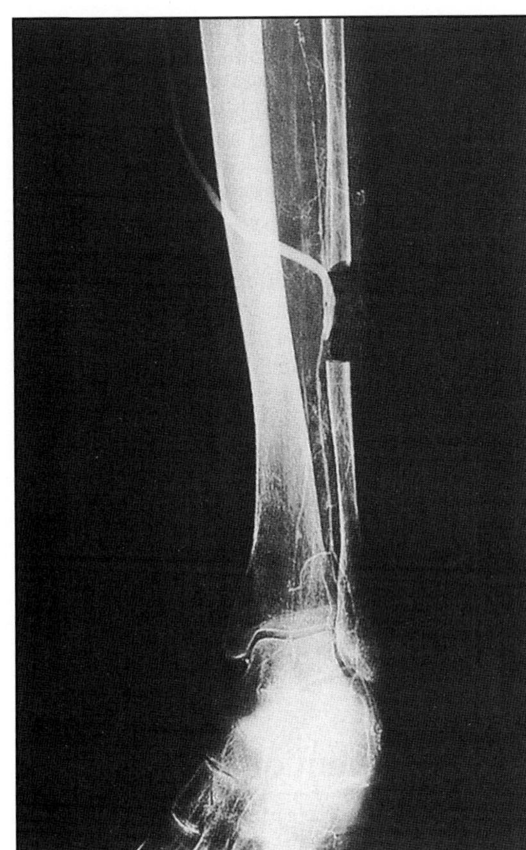

Figure 3.15 • Completion arteriogram of a femoro-peroneal vein bypass graft showing the fibulectomy required to access the peroneal artery from the lateral side of the leg.

In the absence of autologous vein, PTFE grafts to single calf vessels carry an unacceptable failure rate. Some have suggested that creation of an arteriovenous fistula to an adjacent vein at the distal anastomosis, using a common ostium technique, may improve patency due to increased blood flow.[141] Anecdotal reports of graft patency of 71% and limb salvage of 83% have been published.[142] However, a randomised trial of femoro-tibial prosthetic bypass with or without an adjuvant fistula found no significant difference in graft patency.[143] It seems that if used at all, this approach should be reserved for tibial or peroneal bypasses in those situations with poor run-off. Vein cuffs at the distal anastomosis have been described by a number of authors.[144,145] A multicentre randomised trial of femoro-popliteal prosthetic bypass with or without a vein cuff showed a significant improvement in patency rates for below-knee grafts with a vein cuff at 2 years (52% vs. 29%).[146] Grafts with a preformed prosthetic cuff are now available, for patients with no available vein to construct a cuff, and a recently published randomised comparison showed equivalence

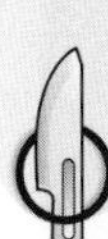

between these grafts and standard grafts with a vein cuff for infrageniculate bypass at 2 years, suggesting these are a reasonable alternative if a vein cuff cannot be fashioned.[147] There has been no randomised trial of vein cuffs at the tibial level, but given the significant improvement at the below-knee level it seems a sensible precaution. Chapter 4 covers the use of such adjuvant techniques in more detail.

Wolfe has estimated that about 14–20% of patients with CLI are unsuitable for distal arterial reconstruction because of occlusion of all the crural and pedal vessels. Many of these patients have diabetes and most require a major amputation (see Chapter 6). However, Taylor et al.[148] have recently described a bypass procedure in such patients from a patent inflow vessel proximal to the occlusion to the venous bed of the foot (dorsal venous arch or posterior tibial vein), after destruction of the venous valves. Of 18 grafts, three failed immediately, with a 1-year limb salvage rate of 75%. The bypass is technically exacting and causes substantial swelling due to venous hypertension, but this improves with time.

Non-interventional treatment

Several approaches have been tried as an alternative to amputation in patients with non-reconstructable disease (**Box 3.2**). Particular emphasis should also be targeted at risk-factor management and treatment of comorbid conditions such as coronary artery disease. Of pharmacological treatments, the most promising are the prostanoids. Prostacyclin (PGI_2) has antiplatelet, antileucocyte, vasodilatory and cytoprotective effects but a very short half-life. Iloprost (Schering), a stable prostacyclin analogue given by intravenous infusion, has a half-life of 30 minutes.

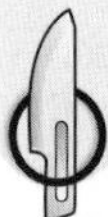

A meta-analysis of six randomised controlled studies of iloprost, involving more than 700 patients with CLI, suggests a significant reduction in death and amputation at 6 months (35% vs. 55%) for those patients receiving the drug.[149] However, the long-term benefit remains unclear for this expensive drug. Despite these impressive results, TASC recommendations are to only use prostanoids for CLI when revascularisation is not possible and the only other alternative is amputation.[28] However, iloprost does seem to have a definite role in the management of patients with ulceration due to severe vasospastic disorders, including scleroderma and Buerger's disease.[150]

Gene therapy aims to use recombinant formulations of angiogenic growth factors to produce therapeutic angiogenesis in order to expedite or augment collateral artery development. Using arterial gene transfer of vascular endothelial growth factor (VEGF) plasmid DNA, promising results have been reported in small numbers of patients.[151] More recently, intramuscular gene transfer has been reported to produce marked improvement in collateral vessel development in patients with CLI.[152] Though promising in the research environment, concerns with the safety of these approaches remain, predominantly the risk of development of malignant cells.

Box 3.2 • Non-surgical treatment options in critical limb ischaemia

Pressure care
Slow-release opiate analgesia
Prostacyclin analogues, e.g. iloprost
Gene therapy
Dorsal column stimulation
Chemical lumbar sympathectomy
Ambulation
Intermittent venous compression
Negative pressure application
Hyperbaric oxygen

Spinal cord stimulation has been used in some centres in Europe since the 1960s in patients with intractable pain from CLI as an alternative to amputation. The technique involves conduction of low-voltage electrical impulses from a subcutaneous pulse generator to electrodes positioned in the epidural space at the L3/4 level. Stimulation produces a sensation of paraesthesia and warmth.

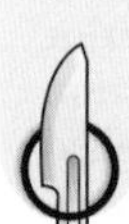

Two controlled studies of spinal cord stimulation have been published and although some benefits in terms of long-term pain control were found, ulcer healing, limb salvage and mortalilty rates were not significantly different in those treated with spinal cord stimulation.[153,154] Spinal cord stimulation also costs 26% more than best medical treatment.

Sympathetic denervation also has an analgesic effect by interrupting cutaneous pain pathways, and this is the basis for its use in CLI. Lumbar sympathectomy is a reasonable option in a patient with unreconstructable occlusive disease and rest pain or minimal tissue loss, as relief of pain is more likely than tissue healing. Published results are variable: some report long-term pain relief in 78% of cases, with 11% requiring amputation;[155] others report pain relief in only 6%, with 70% requiring early amputation.[156] Diabetics are unlikely to be helped because autonomic denervation invariably accompanies peripheral neuropathy.

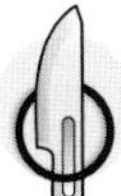

Controlled trials have clearly shown that there is no role for sympathectomy as an adjunct to lower limb revascularisation.[157,158]

Chemical sympathectomy[159] can produce results equal to a surgical lumbar approach,[160] which carries a significant mortality.

Exercise therapy and intermittent compression of the foot, calf or both have been shown to increase blood flow in limbs with PAOD. Limited walking was suggested in the Second European Consensus Document on CLI.[161] Similarly, there is some evidence that the application of external negative pressure to the leg increases blood flow in PAOD.[28] However, the role of these treatments has not been subject to assessment in any clinical trials for CLI.

There have been reports of the use of hyperbaric oxygen for treating early gangrene and the use of topical hyperbaric oxygen chambers for treating tissue loss or for stump healing problems, with encouraging results. However, there are no controlled trials to support its use and much of the improvement seen may have been due to other concomitant therapies. The treatment is also cumbersome and the equipment expensive. As a result these treatments cannot be recommended.[28]

Amputation

Amputation may become necessary despite the best efforts at revascularisation, or may be needed as a primary procedure. Primary amputation should only be considered in selected cases. Newer imaging techniques, such as MRI, and high-quality digital subtraction angiography can often detect patent distal vessels suitable for attempted revascularisation. That said, a complete lack of detectable distal vessels, especially with low ABPI values (<0.3), suggests that reconstruction is not possible and amputation then becomes inevitable. Other indications include necrosis of significant areas of weight-bearing parts of the foot and fixed unremediable flexion contracture of the leg. The goals of amputation are the relief of ischaemic pain, the complete removal of all diseased, infected and necrotic tissue, the achievement of complete healing and the construction of a stump suitable for ambulation. Many amputations follow previous attempts at revascularisation, and as such attempts at revascularisation do not predispose to a higher level of amputation, such an approach is reasonable.[162,163] When amputation is necessary, whether primary or not, selection of the appropriate level is important to try to avoid the need for revision or re-amputation. The lowest level of amputation that will heal is the ideal site for limb transection as this maintains mobility. Methods to help judge the level of amputation include measurements of Doppler pressure, transcutaneous oxygen levels and skin perfusion pressure, although there is little evidence that these methods are superior to clinical judgement.[28]

Conclusion

CLI has become a significant problem in the Western world. Many patients can be offered limb salvage but revascularisation is often technically demanding, time-consuming and costly.

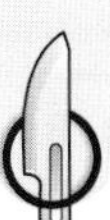

The Audit Committee of the Vascular Surgical Society of Great Britain and Ireland recommends that no patient with CLI should be treated without an expert vascular opinion.[164] Individual centres, surgeons and radiologists should maintain a careful audit of their results. The results of the BASIL trial may have a powerful influence on the way in which these cases are managed in the future.

Key points

- Chronic lower limb ischaemia is common and usually due to atherosclerotic arterial occlusion. With an ageing population the prevalence of disease is rising.
- All cases should have appropriate assessment of risk factors for vascular disease, and treatment should encompass secondary prevention for coronary and cerebrovascular events.
- Best medical treatment should include management of risk factors, including smoking cessation therapy and control of hyperlipidaemia, hypertension, diabetes and hyperhomocysteinaemia.
- Antiplatelet therapy and statins have established benefits in secondary prevention and are very important for all patients with PAOD.
- IC is a benign condition for the limb but is associated with a high risk to the patient, usually due to coronary or cerebrovascular events. Critical ischaemia is associated with a very high mortality, with 50% of patients dead in 5 years.
- Supervised exercise therapy is an effective management strategy for patients with IC, but lifestyle-limiting IC will often benefit more rapidly from angioplasty.
- Most patients with CLI can be offered some form of alternative to primary amputation.
- More diffuse and complex patterns of disease (TASC types C and D) will be more durably treated by surgery but if the risks of this are prohibitive, then angioplasty will often give excellent results, especially in the aortoiliac segment.
- Optimal management will often require a combination of open surgical and endovascular approaches.
- Angioplasty, including subintimal angioplasty, remains the mainstay of endovascular treatments for PAOD, although stents have a role, predominantly for suboptimal angioplasty results in the iliac arteries.
- The success of surgical bypass is most dependent on a good-quality vein and the run-off status.
- Autologous vein is the bypass material of choice for infrainguinal bypass.
- Pharmacotherapies and other non-interventional treatments, such as sympathectomy and gene therapy, for chronic limb ischaemia are generally disappointing, or their role is far from clear.
- All cases of chronic limb ischaemia should be assessed by an experienced team including surgeons and radiologists in order to provide the appropriate management for the individual, and to ensure there are mechanisms to audit the results of such a team approach.

REFERENCES

1. Maldini G, Teruya TH, Kamida C, Eklof B. Combined percutaneous endovascular and open surgical approach in the treatment of a persistent sciatic artery aneurysm presenting with acute limb-threatening ischemia: a case report and review of the literature. Vasc Endovasc Surg 2002; 36:403–8.
2. Brancaccio G, Falco E, Pera M et al. Symptomatic persistent sciatic artery. J Am Coll Surg 2004; 198:158.
3. Macfarlane R, Livesey SA, Pollard S, Dunn DC. Cystic adventitial arterial disease. Br J Surg 1987; 74:89–90.
4. Levien LJ, Veller MG. Popliteal artery entrapment syndrome: more common than previously recognized. J Vasc Surg 1999; 30:587–98.
5. Turnipseed WD. Popliteal entrapment syndrome. J Vasc Surg 2002; 35:910–15.
6. Levien LJ. Popliteal artery entrapment syndrome. Semin Vasc Surg 2003; 16:223–31.
7. Mills JL Sr. Buerger's disease in the 21st century: diagnosis, clinical features, and therapy. Semin Vasc Surg 2003; 16:179–89.
8. Doll R, Peto R, Wheatley K, Gray R, Sutherland I. Mortality in relation to smoking: 40 years' observations on male British doctors. Br Med J 1994; 309:901–11.
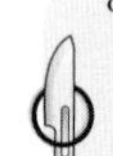
Publication from Doll's classic cohort study of British doctors, showing the hazards associated with long-term use of tobacco.
9. Cavender JB, Rogers WJ, Fisher LD et al. Effects of smoking on survival and morbidity in patients randomized to medical or surgical therapy in the Coronary Artery Surgery Study (CASS): 10-year follow-up. CASS Investigators. J Am Coll Cardiol 1992; 20:287–94.
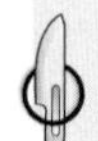
This study showed that among patients with documented coronary artery disease, continued cigarette smoking

may result in decreased survival, especially among those undergoing bypass surgery. Also, smokers had more angina, more unemployment, a greater limitation of physical activity and more hospital admissions.

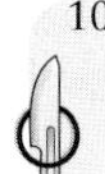
10. Silagy C, Lancaster T, Stead L, Mant D, Fowler G. Nicotine replacement therapy for smoking cessation. In: The Cochrane Library, issue 1. Chichester: John Wiley & Sons, 2005.

A systematic review of the evidence for the role of nicotine replacement therapy. It showed that all the commercially available forms of nicotine replacement therapy (gum, transdermal patch, nasal spray, inhaler and sublingual tablets/lozenges) are effective as part of a strategy to promote smoking cessation.

11. Murabito JM, D'Agostino RB, Silbershatz H, Wilson WF. Intermittent claudication. A risk profile from the Framingham Heart Study. Circulation 1997; 96:44–9.

12. Fowkes FG, Housley E, Riemersma RA et al. Smoking, lipids, glucose intolerance, and blood pressure as risk factors for peripheral atherosclerosis compared with ischemic heart disease in the Edinburgh Artery Study. Am J Epidemiol 1992; 135:331–40.

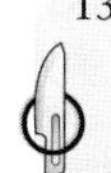
13. Leng GC, Price JF, Jepson RG. Lipid-lowering for lower limb atherosclerosis. In: The Cochrane Library, issue 1. Chichester: John Wiley & Sons, 2005.

The objective of this review was to assess the effects of lipid-lowering therapy in patients with lower limb atherosclerosis. It concluded that lipid-lowering therapy may be useful in preventing deterioration of underlying disease and in alleviating symptoms.

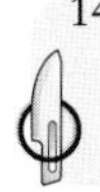
14. Scandinavian Simvastatin Survival Study (4S). Randomised trial of cholesterol lowering in 4444 patients with coronary heart disease. Lancet 1994; 344:1383–9.

This study shows that long-term treatment with simvastatin is safe and improves survival in patients with coronary heart disease.

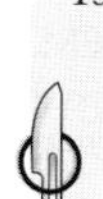
15. Sacks FM, Pfeffer MA, Moye LA et al. The effect of pravastatin on coronary events after myocardial infarction in patients with average cholesterol levels. Cholesterol and Recurrent Events Trial investigators. N Engl J Med 1996; 335:1001–9.

This trial demonstrates that the benefit of cholesterol-lowering therapy extends to the majority of patients with coronary disease who have average cholesterol levels.

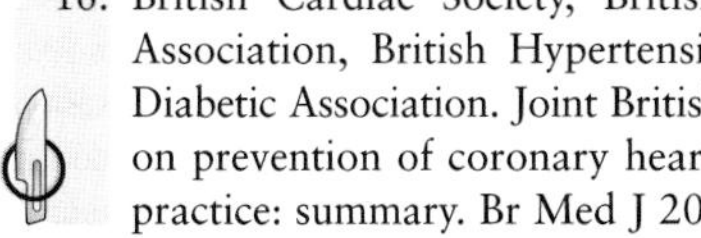
16. British Cardiac Society, British Hyperlipidaemia Association, British Hypertension Society, British Diabetic Association. Joint British recommendations on prevention of coronary heart disease in clinical practice: summary. Br Med J 2000; 320:705–8.

This paper summarises the aims of the joint societies, particularly in relation to cholesterol therapy, with target reductions of total cholesterol to less than 5 mmol/L or by 20–25%, of LDL cholesterol to less than 3 mmol/L or by 30%, and to achieve a triglyceride level of less than 1.7 mmol/L.

17. Jones P, Kafonek S, Laurora I, Hunninghake D. Comparative dose efficacy study of atorvastatin versus simvastatin, pravastatin, lovastatin, and fluvastatin in patients with hypercholesterolemia (the CURVES study). Am J Cardiol 1998; 81:582–7.

18. Neil HA, Fowler G, Patel H, Eminton Z, Maton S. An assessment of the efficacy of atorvastatin in achieving LDL cholesterol target levels in patients with coronary heart disease: a general practice study. Int J Clin Pract 1999; 53:422–6.

19. Kannel WB, McGhee DL. Update on some epidemiological features of intermittent claudication: the Framingham study. J Am Geriatr Soc 1985; 33:13–18.

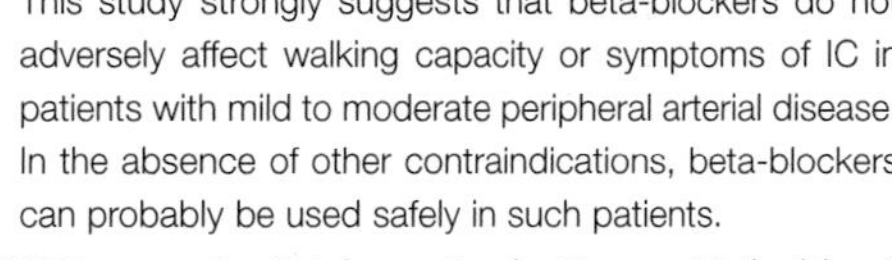
20. Radack K, Deck C. Beta-adrenergic blocker therapy does not worsen intermittent claudication in subjects with peripheral arterial disease. A meta-analysis of randomized controlled trials. Arch Intern Med 1991; 151:1769–76.

This study strongly suggests that beta-blockers do not adversely affect walking capacity or symptoms of IC in patients with mild to moderate peripheral arterial disease. In the absence of other contraindications, beta-blockers can probably be used safely in such patients.

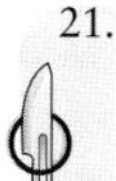
21. UK Prospective Diabetes Study Group. Tight blood pressure control and risk of macrovascular and microvascular complications in type 2 diabetes: UKPDS 38. Br Med J 1998; 317:703–13.

The results of this study show that tight blood pressure control in patients with hypertension and type 2 diabetes achieves a clinically important reduction in the risk of deaths related to diabetes, complications related to diabetes, progression of diabetic retinopathy and deterioration in visual acuity.

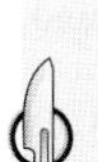
22. UK Prospective Diabetes Study (UKPDS) Group. Intensive blood-glucose control with sulphonylureas or insulin compared with conventional treatment and risk of complications in patients with type 2 diabetes (UKPDS 33). Lancet 1998; 352:837–53.

This study shows that intensive blood glucose control by either sulphonylureas or insulin substantially decreases the risk of microvascular complications, but not macrovascular disease, in patients with type 2 diabetes.

23. Cheng SW, Ting AC, Wong J. Fasting total plasma homocysteine and atherosclerotic peripheral vascular disease. Ann Vasc Surg 1997; 11:217–23.

24. Rauwerda JA, de Jong SC. Homocysteinaemia and vascular disease. Critical Ischaemia 1999; 9:53–7.

25. Hansrani M, Stansby G. Homocysteine lowering interventions for peripheral arterial disease and bypass grafts. In: The Cochrane Library, issue 1. Chichester: John Wiley & Sons, 2005.

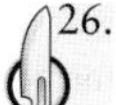
26. Kleijnen J, Mackerras D. Vitamin E for intermittent claudication. In: The Cochrane Library, issue 1. Chichester: John Wiley & Sons, 2005.

The authors of this study concluded that while vitamin E, which is inexpensive and has had no serious side effects reported with its use, may have beneficial effects, there is insufficient evidence to determine whether it is an effective treatment for IC.

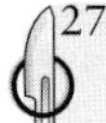
27. Ernst E. Chelation therapy for peripheral arterial occlusive disease: a systematic review. Circulation 1997; 96:1031–3.

This systematic review showed that chelation therapy for PAOD is not superior to placebo. It is associated with considerable risks and costs and should now be considered obsolete.

28. Trans-Atlantic Inter-Society Consensus (TASC) Working Group. Management of peripheral arterial disease (PAD). J Vasc Surg 2000; 31:S1–S296.

This overview summarises much of the available evidence for all aspects of the management of patients with PAOD, and is an invaluable reference.

29. Consensus statement. Antiplatelet therapy in peripheral arterial disease. Eur J Vasc Endovasc Surg 2003; 26:1–16.

A review and consensus statement of the evidence for the use of antiplatelet therapy in patients with PAOD.

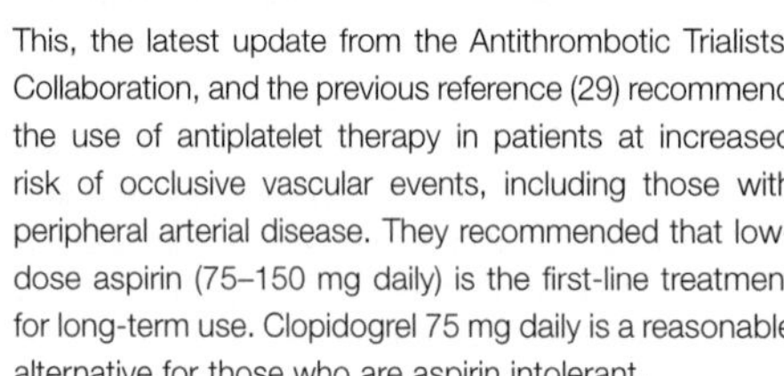
30. Antithrombotic Trialists' Collaboration. Collaborative meta-analysis of randomised trials of antiplatelet therapy for prevention of death, myocardial infarction, and stroke in high risk patients. Br Med J 2002; 324:71–86.

This, the latest update from the Antithrombotic Trialists' Collaboration, and the previous reference (29) recommend the use of antiplatelet therapy in patients at increased risk of occlusive vascular events, including those with peripheral arterial disease. They recommended that low-dose aspirin (75–150 mg daily) is the first-line treatment for long-term use. Clopidogrel 75 mg daily is a reasonable alternative for those who are aspirin intolerant.

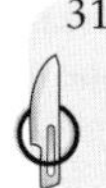
31. CAPRIE Steering Committee. A randomised, blinded, trial of clopidogrel versus aspirin in patients at risk of ischaemic events (CAPRIE). Lancet 1996; 348:1329–39.

This trial showed that long-term administration of clopidogrel to patients with atherosclerotic vascular disease was slightly more effective than aspirin in reducing the combined risk of ischaemic stroke, myocardial infarction or vascular death. The overall safety profile of clopidogrel was at least as good as that of medium-dose aspirin.

32. Breek JC, Hamming JF, De Vries J, Aquarius AE, van Berge Henegouwen DP. Quality of life in patients with intermittent claudication using the World Health Organisation (WHO) questionnaire. Eur J Vasc Endovasc Surg 2001; 21:118–22.

33. Muller-Buhl U, Engeser P, Klimm HD, Wiesemann A. Quality of life and objective disease criteria in patients with intermittent claudication in general practice. Fam Pract 2003; 20:36–40.

34. Rose GA. The diagnosis of ischaemic heart pain and intermittent claudication in field surveys. Bull WHO 1962; 27:645–58.

35. Leng GC, Fowkes FG. The Edinburgh Claudication Questionnaire: an improved version of the WHO/Rose Questionnaire for use in epidemiological surveys. J Clin Epidemiol 1992; 45:1101–9.

36. Housley E. Treating claudication in five words. Br Med J 1988; 296:1483–4.

37. Dormandy J, Mahir M, Ascady G et al. Fate of the patient with chronic leg ischaemia. A review article. J Cardiovasc Surg (Torino) 1989; 30:50–7.

38. Hughson WG, Mann JI, Tibbs DJ, Woods HF, Walton I. Intermittent claudication: factors determining outcome. Br Med J 1978; 1:1377–9.

39. Mathiesen FR, Larsen EE, Wulff M. Some factors influencing the spontaneous course of arterial vascular insufficiency. Acta Chir Scand 1970; 136:303–8.

40. Leng GC, Fowkes FG, Lee AJ et al. Use of ankle brachial pressure index to predict cardiovascular events and death: a cohort study. Br Med J 1996; 313:1440–4.

41. Bainton D, Sweetnam P, Baker I, Elwood P. Peripheral vascular disease: consequence for survival and association with risk factors in the Speedwell prospective heart disease study. Br Heart J 1994; 72:128–32.

42. McAllister FF. The fate of patients with intermittent claudication managed nonoperatively. Am J Surg 1976; 132:593–5.

43. Hiatt WR, Hoag S, Hamman RF. Effect of diagnostic criteria on the prevalence of peripheral arterial disease. The San Luis Valley Diabetes Study. Circulation 1995; 91:1472–9.

44. Hertzer NR, Beven EG, Young JR et al. Coronary artery disease in peripheral vascular patients. A classification of 1000 coronary angiograms and results of surgical management. Ann Surg 1984; 199:223–33.

45. Currie IC, Wilson YG, Baird RN, Lamont PM. Treatment of intermittent claudication: the impact on quality of life. Eur J Vasc Endovasc Surg 1995; 10:356–61.

46. Gardner AW, Poehlman ET. Exercise rehabilitation programs for the treatment of claudication pain. A meta-analysis. JAMA 1995; 274:975–80.

This study showed that the optimal exercise programme for improving claudication pain distances in patients with peripheral arterial disease uses intermittent walking to near-maximal pain for at least 6 months. Such a programme should be part of the standard medical care for patients with IC.

47. Leng GC, Fowler B, Ernst E. Exercise for intermittent claudication. In: The Cochrane Library, issue 1. Chichester: John Wiley & Sons, 2005.

The authors conclude that exercise is of significant benefit to patients with leg pain due to IC.

48. Perkins JM, Collin J, Creasy TS, Fletcher EW, Morris PJ. Exercise training versus angioplasty for stable claudication. Long and medium term results of a prospective, randomised trial. Eur J Vasc Endovasc Surg 1996; 11:409–13.

This study concluded that exercise training confers a greater improvement in claudication and maximum walking distance than percutaneous transluminal angioplasty, especially in patients with disease confined to the superficial femoral artery.

49. Whyman MR, Fowkes FG, Kerracher EM et al. Randomised controlled trial of percutaneous transluminal angioplasty for intermittent claudication. Eur J Vasc Endovasc Surg 1996; 12:167–72.

This study showed that patients treated with percutaneous transluminal angioplasty had a greater short-term improvement in walking and quality of life than with medical treatment alone, and that this was associated with less progression of disease.

50. Whyman MR, Fowkes FG, Kerracher EM et al. Is intermittent claudication improved by percutaneous transluminal angioplasty? A randomized controlled trial. J Vasc Surg 1997; 26:551–7.

The results at 2 years after percutaneous transluminal angioplasty showed that patients had less extensive disease than medically treated patients, but this did not translate into a significant advantage in terms of improved walking or quality of life.

51. Powell KE, Pratt M. Physical activity and health. Br Med J 1996; 313:126–7.

52. Lehert P, Comte S, Gamand S, Brown TM. Naftidrofuryl in intermittent claudication: a retrospective analysis. J Cardiovasc Pharmacol 1994; 23(suppl. 3):S48–S52.

This retrospective analysis based on a success/failure outcome was in favour of active treatment, as was an analysis of change in pain-free walking distance.

53. Barradell LB, Brogden RN. Oral naftidrofuryl. A review of its pharmacology and therapeutic use in the management of peripheral occlusive arterial disease. Drugs Aging 1996; 8:299–322.

54. Drug therapy for peripheral vascular disease. A National Clinical Guideline. Edinburgh: Scottish Intercollegiate Guidelines Network, 1998.

Oral naftidrofuryl improves the symptoms of IC in patients with POAD with minimal risk of adverse effects. It is recommended that in patients with Fontaine classification stage II POAD for whom lifestyle modifications and management of concomitant disease have provided insufficient benefit, naftidrofuryl is potentially useful.

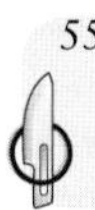

55. Beebe HG, Dawson DL, Cutler BS et al. A new pharmacological treatment for intermittent claudication: results of a randomized, multicenter trial. Arch Intern Med 1999; 159:2041–50.

This trial showed that compared with placebo, long-term use of cilostazol, 100 mg or 50 mg, twice a day significantly improves walking distances in patients with IC.

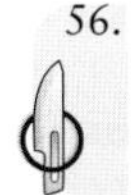

56. Dawson DL, Cutler BS, Hiatt WR et al. A comparison of cilostazol and pentoxifylline for treating intermittent claudication. Am J Med 2000; 109:523–30.

57. Dawson DL. Comparative effects of cilostazol and other therapies for intermittent claudication. Am J Cardiol 2001; 87(12A):19D–27D.

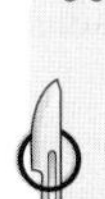

58. Dawson DL, Cutler BS, Meissner MH, Strandness DE Jr. Cilostazol has beneficial effects in treatment of intermittent claudication: results from a multicenter, randomized, prospective, double-blind trial. Circulation 1998; 98:678–86.

A collection of publications that show the potential benefit of cilostazol. It was significantly better than pentoxifylline or placebo for increasing walking distances in patients with IC, but was associated with a greater frequency of minor side effects.

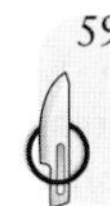

59. Money SR, Herd JA, Isaacsohn JL et al. Effect of cilostazol on walking distances in patients with intermittent claudication caused by peripheral vascular disease. J Vasc Surg 1998; 27:267–74.

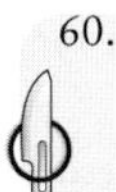

60. Reiter M, Bucek RA, Stumpflen A, Minar E. Prostanoids for intermittent claudication. In: The Cochrane Library, issue 1. Chichester: John Wiley & Sons, 2005.

It was not possible to pool results in this study, but based on the individual results of the published literature, patients with IC seem to benefit from administration (intravenous or intra-arterial) of PGE_1 by a significant improvement in their walking capacity.

61. Visser K, de Vries SO, Kitslaar PJ, van Engelshoven JM, Hunink MG. Cost-effectiveness of diagnostic imaging work-up and treatment for patients with intermittent claudication in The Netherlands. Eur J Vasc Endovasc Surg 2003; 25:213–23.

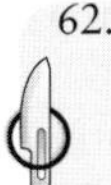

62. Chetter IC, Spark JI, Kent PJ et al. Percutaneous transluminal angioplasty for intermittent claudication: evidence on which to base the medicine. Eur J Vasc Endovasc Surg 1998; 16:477–84.

This study showed that unilateral claudicants undergoing percutaneous transluminal angioplasty to a solitary iliac lesion demonstrate the most marked quality-of-life benefits, and 12 months post-procedure report a quality of life approaching that of an age-matched population.

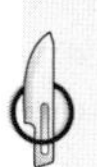

63. Bosch JL, van der Graaf Y, Hunink MG. Health-related quality of life after angioplasty and stent placement in patients with iliac artery occlusive disease: results of a randomized controlled clinical trial. The Dutch Iliac Stent Trial Study Group. Circulation 1999; 99:3155–60.

This group also showed that health-related quality of life improves following treatment of IC caused by iliac artery occlusive disease.

64. Hedeman Joosten PP, Ho GH, Breuking FA Jr, Overtoom TT, Moll FL. Percutaneous transluminal angioplasty of the infrarenal aorta: initial outcome and long-term clinical and angiographic results. Eur J Vasc Endovasc Surg 1996; 12:201–6.

65. Odurny A, Colapinto RF, Sniderman KW, Johnston KW. Percutaneous transluminal angioplasty of abdominal aortic stenoses. Cardiovasc Intervent Radiol 1989; 12:1–6.

66. McPherson SJ, Laing AD, Thomson KR et al. Treatment of infrarenal aortic stenosis by stent placement: a 6-year experience. Australas Radiol 1999; 43:185–91.

67. Sheeran SR, Hallisey MJ, Ferguson D. Percutaneous transluminal stent placement in the abdominal aorta. J Vasc Intervent Radiol 1997; 8:55–60.

68. Funovics MA, Lackner B, Cejna M et al. Predictors of long-term results after treatment of iliac artery obliteration by transluminal angioplasty and stent deployment. Cardiovasc Intervent Radiol 2002; 25:397–402.

69. Kamphuis AG, van Engelen AD, Tetteroo E, Hunink MG, Mali WP. Impact of different hemodynamic criteria for stent placement after suboptimal iliac angioplasty. Dutch Iliac Stent Trial Study Group. J Vasc Intervent Radiol 1999; 10:741–6.

70. Bosch JL, Hunink MG. Meta-analysis of the results of percutaneous transluminal angioplasty and stent placement for aortoiliac occlusive disease. Radiology 1997; 204:87–96.

This study showed that stent placement and percutaneous transluminal angioplasty yielded similar complication rates, but the technical success rate was higher after stent placement and the risk of long-term failure was reduced by 39%.

71. Richter G, Roeren T, Brado M et al. Further update of the randomised trial. Iliac stent versus PTA: morphology, clinical success rates and failure analysis (abstract). J Vasc Intervent Radiol 1993; 4:30–1.

72. Richter G, Roeren T, Noelge G. Prospective randomised trial: iliac stenting versus PTA (abstract). Angiology 1992; 43:268.

73. Tetteroo E, van der Graaf Y, Bosch JL et al. Randomised comparison of primary stent placement versus primary angioplasty followed by selective stent placement in patients with iliac-artery occlusive disease. Dutch Iliac Stent Trial Study Group. Lancet 1998; 351:1153–9.

This study showed that angioplasty followed by selective stent placement was as effective as primary stenting and less expensive, and should be the treatment of choice for lifestyle-limiting IC caused by iliac artery occlusive disease.

74. Leu AJ, Schneider E, Canova CR, Hoffmann U. Long-term results after recanalisation of chronic iliac artery occlusions by combined catheter therapy without stent placement. Eur J Vasc Endovasc Surg 1999; 18:499–505.

75. Muradin GS, Bosch JL, Stijnen T, Hunink MG. Balloon dilation and stent implantation for treatment of femoropopliteal arterial disease: meta-analysis. Radiology 2001; 221:137–45.

76. Duda SH, Pusich B, Richter G et al. Sirolimus-eluting stents for the treatment of obstructive superficial femoral artery disease: six-month results. Circulation 2002; 106:1505–9.

77. Becquemin JP, Favre JP, Marzelle J et al. Systematic versus selective stent placement after superficial femoral artery balloon angioplasty: a multicenter prospective randomized study. J Vasc Surg 2003; 37:487–94.

78. Saxon RR, Coffman JM, Gooding JM, Natuzzi E, Ponec DJ. Long-term results of ePTFE stent-graft versus angioplasty in the femoropopliteal artery: single center experience from a prospective, randomized trial. J Vasc Intervent Radiol 2003; 14:303–11.

79. Hansrani M, Overbeck K, Smout J, Stansby G. Intravascular brachytherapy for peripheral vascular disease. In: The Cochrane Library, issue 1. Chichester: John Wiley & Sons, 2005.

80. de Vries SO, Hunink MG. Results of aortic bifurcation grafts for aortoiliac occlusive disease: a meta-analysis. J Vasc Surg 1997; 26:558–69.

This study suggests that mortality and systemic morbidity rates of aortic bifurcation graft procedures have dropped since 1975, whereas patency rates seem to be fairly constant over the years. Expected primary patencies were 80% and 72% (patient based) at 5 and 10 years respectively.

81. Brewster DC. Current controversies in the management of aortoiliac occlusive disease. J Vasc Surg 1997; 25:365–79.

82. Berce M, Sayers RD, Miller JH. Femorofemoral crossover grafts for claudication: a safe and reliable procedure. Eur J Vasc Endovasc Surg 1996; 12:437–41.

83. Kalman PG, Hosang M, Johnston KW, Walker PM. Unilateral iliac disease: the role of iliofemoral bypass. J Vasc Surg 1987; 6:139–43.

84. Harris PL, Bigley DJ, McSweeney L. Aortofemoral bypass and the role of concomitant femorodistal reconstruction. Br J Surg 1985; 72:317–20.

85. Pierce GE, Turrentine M, Stringfield S et al. Evaluation of end-to-side v end-to-end proximal anastomosis in aortobifemoral bypass. Arch Surg 1982; 117:1580–8.

86. Dunn DA, Downs AR, Lye CR. Aortoiliac reconstruction for occlusive disease: comparison of end-to-end and end-to-side proximal anastomoses. Can J Surg 1982; 25:382–4.

87. Cambria RP, Brewster DC, Abbott WM et al. Transperitoneal versus retroperitoneal approach

for aortic reconstruction: a randomized prospective study. J Vasc Surg 1990; 11:314–24.

88. Sottiurai VS, Yao JS, Flinn WR, Batson RC. Intimal hyperplasia and neointima: an ultrastructural analysis of thrombosed grafts in humans. Surgery 1983; 93:809–17.

89. Veith FJ, Gupta SK, Ascer E et al. Six-year prospective multicenter randomized comparison of autologous saphenous vein and expanded polytetrafluoroethylene grafts in infrainguinal arterial reconstructions. J Vasc Surg 1986; 3:104–14.

This trial did not support the routine preferential use of PTFE grafts for either femoro-popliteal or more distal bypasses. However, it was felt that such grafts may be used preferentially in selected poor-risk patients for femoro-popliteal bypasses, particularly those that do not cross the knee. Although every effort should be made to use vein for infrapopliteal bypasses, a PTFE distal bypass is a better option than a primary major amputation.

90. Kumar KP, Crinnon JN, Ashley S, Gough MJ. Vein, PTFE or Dacron for above knee femoropoliteal bypass. Int Angiol 1995; 14:200–5.

This trial showed improved outcomes in terms of patency at 4 years for vein, with primary patency at 4 years of 73% for saphenous vein, 54% for PTFE and 47% for Dacron.

91. Michaels JA. Choice of material for above-knee femoropopliteal bypass graft. Br J Surg 1989; 76:7–14.

This paper used decision analysis to show that compared with vein the use of prosthesis for an initial graft will reduce the overall patency and substantially increase the requirement for reoperation for above-knee bypass.

92. Harward TR, Bergan JJ, Yao JS, Flinn WR, McCarthy WJ. The demise of primary profundaplasty. Am J Surg 1988; 156:126–9.

93. Prendiville EJ, Burke PE, Colgan MP et al. The profunda femoris: a durable outflow vessel in aortofemoral surgery. J Vasc Surg 1992; 16:23–9.

94. The Vascular Surgical Society of Great Britain and Ireland. Critical limb ischaemia: management and outcome. Report of a national survey. Eur J Vasc Endovasc Surg 1995; 10:108–13.

95. Pell JP, Whyman MR, Fowkes FG, Gillespie I, Ruckley CV. Trends in vascular surgery since the introduction of percutaneous transluminal angioplasty. Br J Surg 1994; 81:832–5.

96. Varty K, Nydahl S, Butterworth P et al. Changes in the management of critical limb ischaemia. Br J Surg 1996; 83:953–6.

97. Holdsworth RJ, McCollum PT. Results and resource implications of treating end-stage limb ischaemia. Eur J Vasc Endovasc Surg 1997; 13:164–73.

98. Fratezi AC, Albers M, De Luccia ND, Pereira CA. Outcome and quality of life of patients with severe chronic limb ischaemia: a cohort study on the influence of diabetes. Eur J Vasc Endovasc Surg 1995; 10:459–65.

99. Leers SA, Reifsnyder T, Delmonte R, Caron M. Realistic expectations for pedal bypass grafts in patients with end-stage renal disease. J Vasc Surg 1998; 28:976–80.

100. Hakaim AG, Gordon JK, Scott TE. Early outcome of in situ femorotibial reconstruction among patients with diabetes alone versus diabetes and end-stage renal failure: analysis of 83 limbs. J Vasc Surg 1998; 27:1049–54.

101. DHSS. Amputation statistics for England, Wales and Northern Ireland. London: Department of Health and Social Security, 1986.

102. Hart WM, Guest JF. Critical limb ischaemia: the burden of illness in the UK. Br J Med Econ 1995; 8:211–21.

103. Myhre H, Fosby B, Witsoe E, Groechenig E. Cost-effectiveness of therapeutic options for critical limb ischaemia. Critical Ischaemia 1996; 6:37–41.

104. Humphreys WV, Evans F, Watkin G, Williams T. Critical limb ischaemia in patients over 80 years of age: options in a district general hospital. Br J Surg 1995; 82:1361–3.

105. Singh S, Evans L, Datta D, Gaines P, Beard JD. The costs of managing lower limb-threatening ischaemia. Eur J Vasc Endovasc Surg 1996; 12:359–62.

106. Chetter IC, Spark JI, Scott DJ et al. Prospective analysis of quality of life in patients following infrainguinal reconstruction for chronic critical ischaemia. Br J Surg 1998; 85:951–5.

107. Johnson BF, Singh S, Evans L et al. A prospective study of the effect of limb-threatening ischaemia and its surgical treatment on the quality of life. Eur J Vasc Endovasc Surg 1997; 13:306–14.

108. Panayiotopoulos YP, Tyrrell MR, Owen SE, Reidy JF, Taylor PR. Outcome and cost analysis after femorocrural and femoropedal grafting for critical limb ischaemia. Br J Surg 1997; 84:207–12.

109. Nicoloff AD, Taylor LM Jr, McLafferty RB, Moneta GL, Porter JM. Patient recovery after infrainguinal bypass grafting for limb salvage. J Vasc Surg 1998; 27:256–63; discussion 264–6.

110. Panayiotopoulos YP, Reidy JF, Taylor PR. The concept of knee salvage: why does a failed femorocrural/pedal arterial bypass not affect the amputation level? Eur J Vasc Endovasc Surg 1997; 13:477–85.

111. Abou-Zamzam AM Jr, Lee RW, Moneta GL, Taylor LM Jr, Porter JM. Functional outcome after infrainguinal bypass for limb salvage. J Vasc Surg 1997; 25:287–95; discussion 295–7.

112. Ray SA, Minty I, Buckenham TM, Belli AM, Taylor RS, Dormandy JA. Clinical outcome and restenosis following percutaneous transluminal angioplasty for ischaemic rest pain or ulceration. Br J Surg 1995; 82:1217–21.

113. London NJ, Varty K, Sayers RD et al. Percutaneous transluminal angioplasty for lower-limb critical ischaemia. Br J Surg 1995; 82:1232–5.

114. Whitbread T, Cleveland TJ, Beard JD, Gaines PA. The treatment of aortoiliac occlusions by endovascular stenting with or without adjuvant femorofemoral crossover grafting. Eur J Vasc Endovasc Surg 1998; 15:169–74.

115. Perler BA, Williams GM. Does donor iliac artery percutaneous transluminal angioplasty or stent placement influence the results of femorofemoral bypass? Analysis of 70 consecutive cases with long-term follow-up. J Vasc Surg 1996; 24:363–9; discussion 369–70.

116. London NJ, Srinivasan R, Naylor AR et al. Subintimal angioplasty of femoropopliteal artery occlusions: the long-term results. Eur J Vasc Surg 1994; 8:148–55.

117. Greenfield AJ. Femoral, popliteal, and tibial arteries: percutaneous transluminal angioplasty. Am J Roentgenol 1980; 135:927–35.

118. Schwarten DE. Clinical and anatomical considerations for nonoperative therapy in tibial disease and the results of angioplasty. Circulation 1991; 83(2 suppl.):I86–I90.

119. Brown KT, Schoenberg NY, Moore ED, Saddekni S. Percutaneous transluminal angioplasty of infrapopliteal vessels: preliminary results and technical considerations. Radiology 1988; 169:75–8.

120. Tamura S, Sniderman KW, Beinart C, Sos TA. Percutaneous transluminal angioplasty of the popliteal artery and its branches. Radiology 1982; 143:645–8.

121. Belli AM, Cumberland DC, Knox AM, Procter AE, Welsh CL. The complication rate of percutaneous peripheral balloon angioplasty. Clin Radiol 1990; 41:380–3.

122. Holm J, Arfvidsson B, Jivegard L et al. Chronic lower limb ischaemia. A prospective randomised controlled study comparing the 1-year results of vascular surgery and percutaneous transluminal angioplasty (PTA). Eur J Vasc Surg 1991; 5:517–22.

The authors found that immediate and 1-year results showed similar success and complication rates for percutaneous transluminal angioplasty compared with surgery. However, there was a significantly shorter hospital stay for patients treated with percutaneous transluminal angioplasty.

123. Wolf GL, Wilson SE, Cross AP, Deupree RH, Stason WB. Surgery or balloon angioplasty for peripheral vascular disease: a randomized clinical trial. J Vasc Intervent Radiol 1993; 4:639–48.

This study found that patients in both treatment groups had prompt and sustained increases in haemodynamics and quality of life. There was no significant difference in outcomes during a median follow-up of 4 years.

124. Calligaro KD, Ascer E, Veith FJ et al. Unsuspected inflow disease in candidates for axillofemoral bypass operations: a prospective study. J Vasc Surg 1990; 11:832–7.

125. Taylor LM Jr, Park TC, Edwards JM et al. Acute disruption of polytetrafluoroethylene grafts adjacent to axillary anastomoses: a complication of axillofemoral grafting. J Vasc Surg 1994; 20:520–6.

126. Wittens CH, van Houtte HJ, van Urk H. Winner of the ESVS Prize 1991. European Prospective Randomised Multi-centre Axillo-bifemoral Trial. Eur J Vasc Surg 1992; 6:115–23.

The results showed that after 3 years, with a mean follow-up of 12 months (range 3–36 months), the prosthesis with a flow splitter had a significantly better patency rate after 2 years (84%) compared with the patency rate of the prosthesis with a 90° bifurcation (38%).

127. Kalman PG, Johnston KW, Walker PM. The current role of isolated profundaplasty. J Cardiovasc Surg (Torino) 1990; 31:107–11.

128. Hunink MG, Wong JB, Donaldson MC, Meyerovitz MF, Harrington DP. Patency results of percutaneous and surgical revascularization for femoropopliteal arterial disease. Med Decis Making 1994; 14:71–81.

The authors used a method based on the proportional-hazards model and the actuarial life-table approach. The results were adjusted for differences in case mix of the study populations. Adjusted 5-year primary patencies after surgery varied from 33 to 80%, the best results being for saphenous vein bypass performed for claudication.

129. Wengerter KR, Veith FJ, Gupta SK, Ascer E, Rivers SP. Influence of vein size (diameter) on infrapopliteal reversed vein graft patency. J Vasc Surg 1990; 11:525–31.

130. Panetta TF, Marin ML, Veith FJ et al. Unsuspected preexisting saphenous vein disease: an unrecognized cause of vein bypass failure. J Vasc Surg 1992; 15:102–10.

131. Davies AH, Magee TR, Baird RN, Sheffield E, Horrocks M. Pre-bypass morphological changes in vein grafts. Eur J Vasc Surg 1993; 7:642–7.

132. Tarry WC, Walsh DB, Birkmeyer NJ et al. Fate of the contralateral leg after infrainguinal bypass. J Vasc Surg 1998; 27:1039–47.

133. Holzenbein TJ, Pomposelli FB Jr, Miller A et al. Results of a policy with arm veins used as the first alternative to an unavailable ipsilateral greater saphenous vein for infrainguinal bypass. J Vasc Surg 1996; 23:130–40.

134. Schulman ML, Badhey MR. Late results and angiographic evaluation of arm veins as long bypass grafts. Surgery 1982; 92:1032–41.

135. Chang BB, Shah DM, Leather RP, Darling RC III. Finding autogenous veins for reoperative lower extremity bypasses: limitations of veins other than

the greater saphenous. Semin Vasc Surg 1994; 7:173–7.

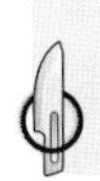
136. Schulman ML, Badhey MR, Yatco R. Superficial femoral–popliteal veins and reversed saphenous veins as primary femoropopliteal bypass grafts: a randomized comparative study. J Vasc Surg 1987; 6:1–10.

The study showed that the primary patency rates of randomized superficial femoral–popliteal veins (64% at 3 years) and reversed saphenous veins (60% at 3 years) were not significantly different. Similarly, there was no statistically significant difference in the secondary patency rates of 68% for superficial femoral–popliteal veins and 63% for reversed saphenous veins at 3 years.

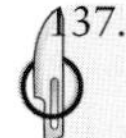
137. Leather RP, Shah DM, Chang BB, Kaufman JL. Resurrection of the in situ saphenous vein bypass. 1000 cases later. Ann Surg 1988; 208:435–42.

This was a retrospective analysis of 1000 in situ saphenous vein bypasses. The 30-day patency rate was 95%, and the cumulative patency rates, by life-table analysis at 1, 2, 3, 4 and 5 years, were 90, 86, 84, 80 and 76%, respectively.

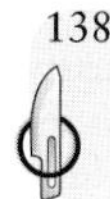
138. Wengerter KR, Veith FJ, Gupta SK et al. Prospective randomized multicenter comparison of in situ and reversed vein infrapopliteal bypasses. J Vasc Surg 1991; 13:189–97.

The trial results showed no significant difference in overall patency rates for the two types of vein grafts at 2.5 years.

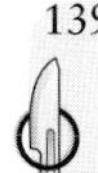
139. Watelet J, Soury P, Menard JF et al. Femoropopliteal bypass: in situ or reversed vein grafts? Ten-year results of a randomized prospective study. Ann Vasc Surg 1997; 11:510–19.

There was little difference between the two treated groups, with actuarial limb salvage at 10 years being 73.5% in the in situ graft group and 74.4% in the reversed graft group.

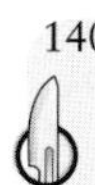
140. Moody AP, Edwards PR, Harris PL. In situ versus reversed femoropopliteal vein grafts: long-term follow-up of a prospective, randomized trial. Br J Surg 1992; 79:750–2.

This study showed that the in situ technique conferred neither short- nor long-term advantage over reversed vein grafting for femoropopliteal bypass.

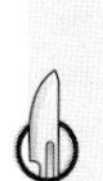
141. Ascer E, Gennaro M, Pollina RM et al. Complementary distal arteriovenous fistula and deep vein interposition: a five-year experience with a new technique to improve infrapopliteal prosthetic bypass patency. J Vasc Surg 1996; 24:134–43.

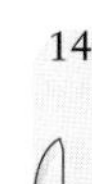
142. Jacobs MJ, Gregoric ID, Reul GJ. Prosthetic graft placement and creation of a distal arteriovenous fistula for secondary vascular reconstruction in patients with severe limb ischemia. J Vasc Surg 1992; 15:612–18.

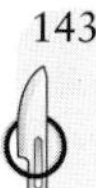
143. Hamsho A, Nott D, Harris PL. Prospective randomised trial of distal arteriovenous fistula as an adjunct to femoro-infrapopliteal PTFE bypass. Eur J Vasc Endovasc Surg 1999; 17:197–201.

This study showed that arteriovenous fistulas confer no additional significant clinical advantage over interposition vein cuff in patients having femoro-infrapopliteal bypass with ePTFE grafts for critical limb ischaemia.

144. Miller JH, Foreman RK, Ferguson L, Faris I. Interposition vein cuff for anastomosis of prosthesis to small artery. Aust NZ J Surg 1984; 54:283–5.

145. Tyrrell MR, Wolfe JH. New prosthetic venous collar anastomotic technique: combining the best of other procedures. Br J Surg 1991; 78:1016–17.

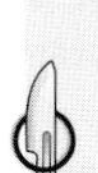
146. Stonebridge PA, Prescott RJ, Ruckley CV. Randomized trial comparing infrainguinal polytetrafluoroethylene bypass grafting with and without vein interposition cuff at the distal anastomosis. The Joint Vascular Research Group. J Vasc Surg 1997; 26:543–50.

In this study there was no improvement in the patency rate with the use of a distal anastomosis interposition vein cuff in above-knee femoro-popliteal PTFE bypass grafts, but there was a statistically significant advantage when PTFE bypass grafts were anastomosed to the popliteal artery below the knee.

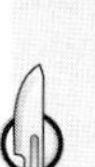
147. Panneton JM, Hollier LH, Hofer JM. Multicenter randomized prospective trial comparing a pre-cuffed polytetrafluoroethylene graft to a vein cuffed polytetrafluoroethylene graft for infragenicular arterial bypass. Ann Vasc Surg 2004; 18:199–206.

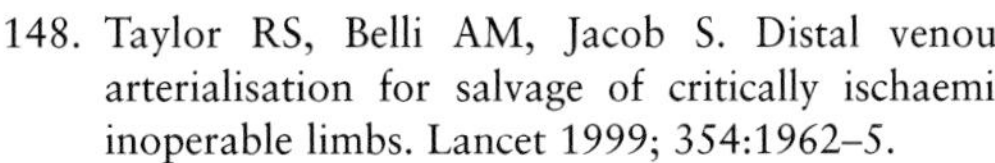
148. Taylor RS, Belli AM, Jacob S. Distal venous arterialisation for salvage of critically ischaemic inoperable limbs. Lancet 1999; 354:1962–5.

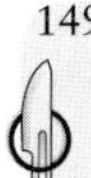
149. Loosemore TM, Chalmers TC, Dormandy JA. A meta-analysis of randomized placebo control trials in Fontaine stages III and IV peripheral occlusive arterial disease. Int Angiol 1994; 13:133–42.

This meta-analysis showed that for iloprost there was a significant beneficial effect over placebo on ulcer healing and pain relief. All other randomised controlled trials of pharmacotherapeutic agents in patients with Fontaine stage III and IV POAD showed no significant benefit over placebo for any of the endpoints reported.

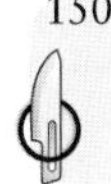
150. Fiessinger JN, Schafer M. Trial of iloprost versus aspirin treatment for critical limb ischaemia of thromboangiitis obliterans. The TAO Study. Lancet 1990; 335:555–7.

This study showed the benefits of iloprost in patients with Buerger's disease, with improved ulcer healing or pain relief compared with those treated with aspirin.

151. Isner JM, Walsh K, Symes J et al. Arterial gene therapy for therapeutic angiogenesis in patients with peripheral artery disease. Circulation 1995; 91:2687–92.

152. Baumgartner I, Pieczek A, Manor O et al. Constitutive expression of phVEGF165 after intramuscular gene transfer promotes collateral vessel development in patients with critical limb ischemia. Circulation 1998; 97:1114–23.

153. Jivegard LE, Augustinsson LE, Holm J, Risberg B, Ortenwall P. Effects of spinal cord stimulation (SCS) in patients with inoperable severe lower limb ischaemia: a prospective randomised controlled study. Eur J Vasc Endovasc Surg 1995; 9:421–5.

This controlled study showed that spinal cord stimulation provided long-term pain relief but did not significantly improve limb salvage at 18 months in this small study.

154. Klomp HM, Spincemaille GH, Steyerberg EW, Habbema JD, van Urk H. Spinal-cord stimulation in critical limb ischaemia: a randomised trial. ESES Study Group. Lancet 1999; 353:1040–4.

The results showed that spinal cord stimulation, in addition to best medical care, does not prevent amputation in patients with CLI.

155. Persson AV, Anderson LA, Padberg FT Jr. Selection of patients for lumbar sympathectomy. Surg Clin North Am 1985; 65:393–403.

156. Fulton RL, Blakeley WR. Lumbar sympathectomy: a procedure of questionable value in the treatment of arteriosclerosis obliterans of the legs. Am J Surg 1968; 116:735–44.

157. Barnes RW, Baker WH, Shanik G et al. Value of concomitant sympathectomy in aortoiliac reconstruction. Results of a prospective, randomized study. Arch Surg 1977; 112:1325–30.

In this randomised study the results showed that sympathectomy may improve pedal circulation, but does not appear to improve the results of aortoiliac reconstruction.

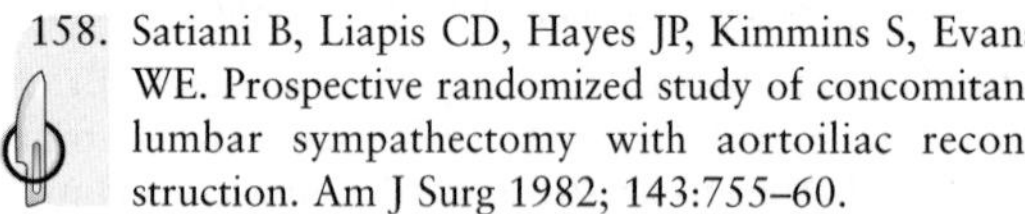

158. Satiani B, Liapis CD, Hayes JP, Kimmins S, Evans WE. Prospective randomized study of concomitant lumbar sympathectomy with aortoiliac reconstruction. Am J Surg 1982; 143:755–60.

In this randomised study, at a mean follow-up time of 11 months after aorto-femoral bypass, there was no significant difference in graft patency, need for subsequent distal bypass, or amputation rate between the sympathectomy and non-sympathectomy groups.

159. Walsh JA, Glynn CJ, Cousins MJ, Basedow RW. Blood flow, sympathetic activity and pain relief following lumbar sympathetic blockade or surgical sympathectomy. Anaesth Intensive Care 1985; 13:18–24.

160. Kim GE, Ibrahim IM, Imparato AM. Lumbar sympathectomy in end stage arterial occlusive disease. Ann Surg 1976; 183:157–60.

161. Second European Consensus Document on chronic critical leg ischemia. Eur J Vasc Surg 1992; 6(suppl. A):1–32.

162. Epstein SB, Worth MH Jr, el Ferzli G. Level of amputation following failed vascular reconstruction for lower limb ischemia. Curr Surg 1989; 46:185–92.

163. Bloom RJ, Stevick CA. Amputation level and distal bypass salvage of the limb. Surg Gynecol Obstet 1988; 166:1–5.

164. The Audit Committee of the Vascular Surgical Society of Great Britain and Ireland. Recommendations for the management of chronic critical lower limb ischaemia. Eur J Vasc Endovasc Surg 1996; 12:131–5.

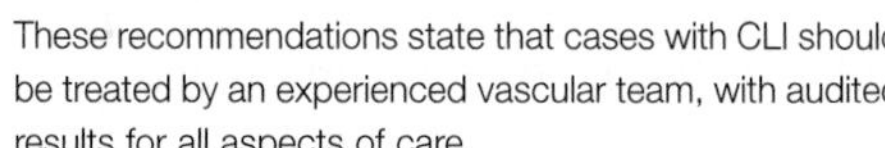

These recommendations state that cases with CLI should be treated by an experienced vascular team, with audited results for all aspects of care.

CHAPTER

Four

Vascular grafts, arterial sutures and anastomoses

Matthew Thompson

VASCULAR GRAFTS

The provision of materials used to replace diseased blood vessels has allowed vascular surgery to develop. The initial section of this chapter outlines the types of graft frequently used in peripheral vascular practice and reviews current developments in graft design and manufacture.

Vascular grafts can be classified into three broad groups: autogenous grafts, prosthetic grafts and biological prosthetic grafts (**Box 4.1**). Autogenous grafts are harvested from the same individual into which the graft is placed, and may be either arterial, venous or engineered. Prosthetic grafts are wholly manufactured. Biological prosthetic grafts can also be obtained from a human source (allografts) or from non-human species (heterografts).

Box 4.1 • Classification of vascular grafts

Autogenous grafts
Arterial
Venous
Tissue engineered grafts
Prosthetic grafts
Dacron
ePTFE
Polyurethane
Biological vascular grafts
Allografts (arterial and venous)
Xenografts

Autogenous grafts

ARTERIAL AUTOGRAFTS

Arterial autografts have many appealing features that make them ideal as arterial substitutes. They are resistant to degeneration, demonstrate proportional growth when used in children and exhibit normal flexibility at joints.

Arterial autografts can be harvested from various donor sites in the arterial system. They may be obtained from arteries that are dispensable, such as the internal mammary, radial and internal iliac arteries; these grafts can be harvested without the need for replacement. Other vessels, such as the external iliac and superficial femoral arteries, may also be harvested but require replacement by a prosthetic graft.

The use of arterial autografts has been most widespread in cardiac surgery, with the internal mammary, gastroepiploic and radial arteries being extensively used for coronary artery bypass. The internal mammary is commonly used for revascularisation of the left anterior descending artery, with patency rates superior to those of the saphenous vein.[1]

The use of arterial autografts is severely limited in peripheral vascular disease by lack of availability and relatively small diameter. However, renal artery revascularisation in children is best achieved by arterial autografting, usually employing the internal iliac artery as a free graft.[2] The use of saphenous veins in this context results in a high incidence of aneurysmal dilatation. Arterial autografts may be used to replace short arterial segments in contaminated or infected fields and may also be used preferentially in the repair of peripheral, visceral and mycotic aneurysms. The radial artery autograft has been successfully used for crural bypass in diabetic patients with high risk of infection.[3]

VENOUS AUTOGRAFTS

The commonest autogenous conduit in clinical use is vein. It is freely available, easily harvested, relatively resistant to infection, available in adequate length and adapts well to placement in the arterial circulation. The long saphenous vein is the first choice because of adequate calibre, being relatively thick-walled and the longest vein in the body. Alternative vein sources include the short saphenous vein, arm veins and deep veins such as the superficial femoral vein.

Most vascular surgeons will preferentially utilise vein grafts for infrainguinal reconstruction due to enhanced patency rates reported over prosthetic vascular grafts. Michaels[4] performed a meta-analysis of approximately 40 studies of femoropopliteal grafts and concluded that autogenous vein was superior to prosthetic grafts, with a mean 5-year patency rate of 62% versus 43% respectively for above-knee grafts and 68% versus 27% respectively for below-knee grafts. However, a recent Cochrane review suggested that only one of these trials was of adequate design and size, and that the advantages claimed in favour of vein grafts might be overestimated.[5]

Healing of vein grafts

Endothelial damage inevitably occurs during vein preparation for use as a bypass conduit. The amount of damage appears to be related to surgical technique and method of graft preparation.[6] Re-endothelialisation, often partial, occurs by proliferation of remaining endothelial cells, which demonstrate proliferation and migration for up to 6 months following bypass grafting.

As soon as the vein conduit is subject to arterial flow, focal loss of endothelial cells occurs, particularly at perianastomotic areas, together with fibrin deposition on the intima. Within 24 hours, subendothelial invasion of polymorphonuclear leucocytes occurs, and a patchy platelet clot forms on the subendothelial collagen surface where the endothelium has been lost. Over the next 4 days maturation of the clot on the intimal surface occurs, with cross-linking of fibrin and accumulation of red cells and leucocytes as well as platelets.

The underlying media shows oedema, cell necrosis and inflammatory reaction due to a combination of increased endothelial permeability and transmural flux, cellular and humoral factors, and damage caused by surgical manipulation and increased stretch. Vascular smooth muscle cells migrate from the media into the subendothelial intimal space, proliferate and later secrete extracellular matrix.[7] The adventitia becomes incorporated into the surrounding connective tissue by a process of periadventitial fibrosis, and revascularisation by the vasa vasorum commences from adjacent arterial vasa and connective tissue (**Fig. 4.1**). Eventually the vein graft shows long-term adaptive changes to arterial flow, with remodelling of the media and adventitia through cellular hyperplasia and secretion of extracellular matrix.[8]

Vein diameter and quality

The use of diseased saphenous veins as a bypass conduit adversely affects the patency rate of lower-extremity bypass grafting by up to 50%. Veins may be thick-walled, calcified, varicose or partially occluded.[9] Even in veins that appear macroscopically normal, approximately 20% demonstrate intimal and medial thickening, which may predispose to future vein graft stenosis (**Fig. 4.2**).[10]

(a)

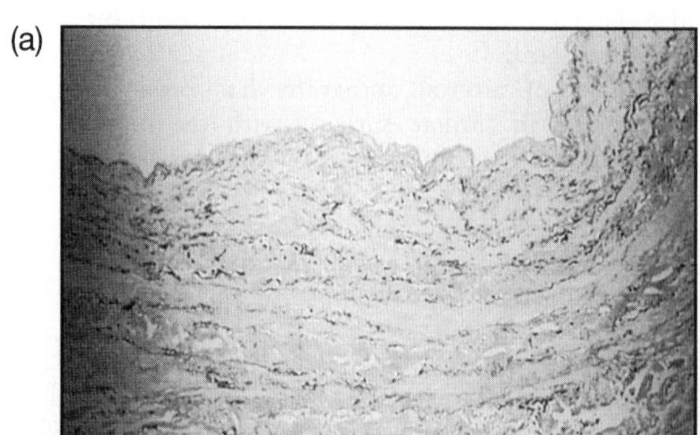

(b)

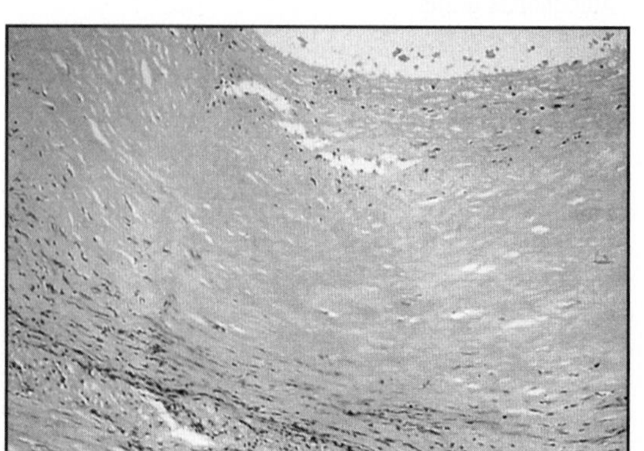

Figure 4.1 • 'Arterialisation' of vein graft after 1 year **(b)** demonstrating marked myointimal hyperplasia and loss of muscle architecture compared with vein graft prior to implantation **(a)**.

(a)

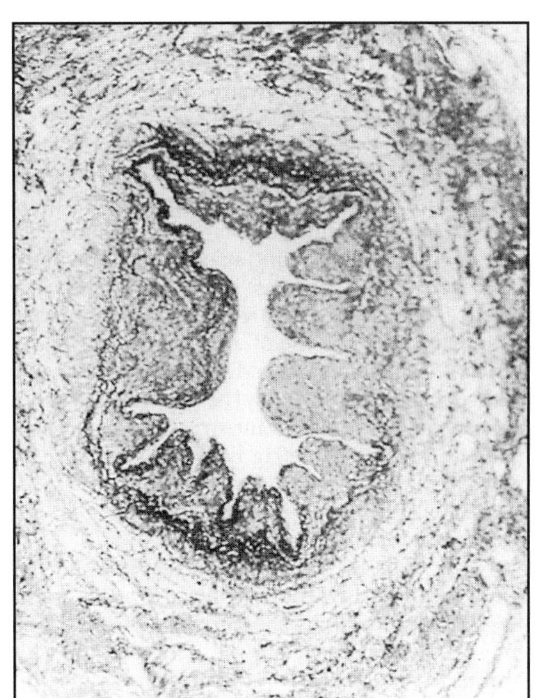

(b)

Figure 4.2 • Severe stenosis of harvested long saphenous vein **(b)** compared with relatively normal segment of same vein **(a)**. There is marked myointimal hyperplasia and longitudinal and circular muscle hypertrophy. Elastin Van Gieson stain ×50.

The optimum diameter for a bypass graft remains controversial, with the generally held concept that smaller grafts are at greater risk of failing. The poorer outcome of smaller grafts has been attributed to the greater likelihood of these veins having disease. There is no agreement as to the minimum vein diameter that is acceptable. Leather et al.[11] suggested 2.5 mm, whereas Towne et al.[12] suggested a diameter of 2 mm at maximal dilatation on preoperative evaluation. Stratification of vein graft diameter has failed to produce statistically significant data for early and long-term patency rates. Mills et al.[13] reported the same patency rates for infrapopliteal reversed vein grafts with diameters greater or less than 4 mm, but did not subdivide those with smaller diameters.

In situ versus reversed vein grafts

There are many advocates of the in situ and reversed techniques for infrainguinal bypass. Numerous advantages of the in situ technique have been proposed, including a better diameter match between the vein and the arteries, both at the proximal and distal anastomosis. Flow characteristics may therefore be improved and compliance mismatch reduced, with decreased turbulent flow leading to reduced incidence of graft thrombosis, anastomotic aneurysms and intimal hyperplasia. The vein is said to be better preserved if it is not removed from its bed and venous nutrition is not impaired.[14] The disadvantages of this technique include the need to lyse the valves with a valvulotome, leading to endothelial cell loss and smooth muscle damage, which might be expected to result in graft failure.[15] In addition, missed arterial tributaries necessitate repeat surgery or can lead to arteriovenous fistulas. These minor complications may be minimized by new minimally invasive vein preparation techniques, including angioscopically directed femoro-distal bypass.[16] Reversed vein grafts have the advantage of technically easier preparation and the ability to tunnel the grafts deep to sartorius to minimise the risk of graft infection.

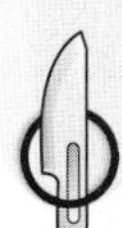

The debate between advocates of the two techniques is likely to continue for some time. Practically, different techniques should be applied to different situations as randomized trials have demonstrated no difference in haemodynamics,[17] compliance[18] or patency rates for both reversed and in situ techniques.[19,20]

Vein assessment, harvest and preparation

Duplex ultrasound seems the best method for the assessment of autologous vein as it can determine vein size, location, anatomical variation, patency and vein quality. Preoperative duplex ultrasound assessment of autologous vein has become invaluable in planning the surgical approach, selecting the best available vein and helping to diminish wound complications such as skin flap necrosis.[21]

Perioperative manipulation of veins before their insertion has been shown to produce cellular and molecular damage that may be important in future graft stenosis. Meticulous surgical technique is therefore important during vein harvest. Once the vein is harvested, several factors may influence future graft function: the pressure at which the vein is distended and the use of an appropriate physiological solution for storage. Distension pressures of over 600 mmHg can easily be generated using a syringe and cause significant structural damage. A pressure below 200 mmHg has been suggested for preventing vein injury.[22]

Superficial femoral vein

In recent years the use of superficial femoral veins for in situ reconstruction of infected aortic grafts has gained popularity. The superficial femoral vein may be harvested from the thigh to provide adequate vein length in order to reconstruct the aorto-iliac segment in bifurcated or unifemoral configuration. The vein is removed by division below the profunda femoris vein and may be harvested to the level of the knee joint without severe compromise of lower limb venous function. The vein is dissected on both sides of the sartorius muscle (**Fig. 4.3**, see also Plate 7, facing p. 116). Results from in situ venous reconstruction of infected prostheses have been encouraging and provide an alternative to extra-anatomic bypass or in situ prosthetic reconstruction.[23,24]

Mechanisms of vein graft failure

The causes of vein graft failure are listed in **Box 4.2**. Early graft occlusion refers to failure within 30 days of surgery and is usually due to technical errors or thrombotic problems. Most vein graft occlusions occur in the intermediate period up to 2 years, usually due to graft stenosis. Late occlusion after 2 years is usually due to progression of atherosclerosis in the inflow or outflow vessels or in the vein graft itself.

Box 4.2 • Causes of vein graft failure

Early (<30 days)
Inappropriate surgery
Technical error
Poor run-off
Small/diseased vein graft
Thrombophilia defect
Intermediate (<2 years)
Vein graft stenosis
Intimal hyperplasia
Late (>2 years)
Atherosclerosis
Aneurysmal degeneration

Graft stenosis Vein graft stenoses are caused by intimal hyperplasia within the vein graft. Haemodynamically significant stenoses develop in up to 30% of vein grafts and are equally distributed at the proximal and distal anastomoses and the main body of the vein graft.[25,26] Intimal hyperplasia is initiated by damage to the vein during the bypass procedure and as a response to arterial flow. Intimal hyperplasia is characterised by smooth muscle cell proliferation and migration from the arterial media to the intima. The intimal smooth muscle cells then

(a)
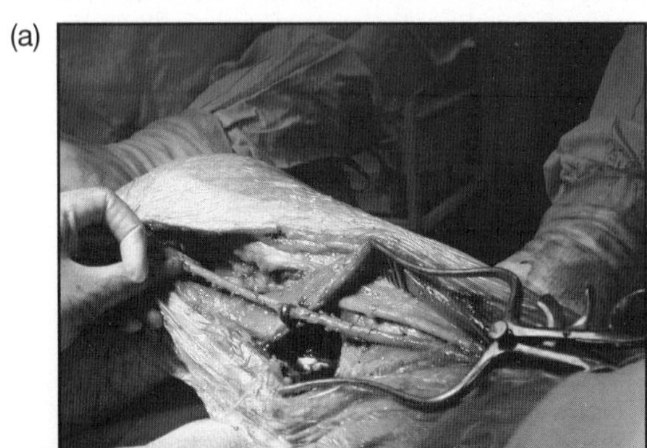

(b)
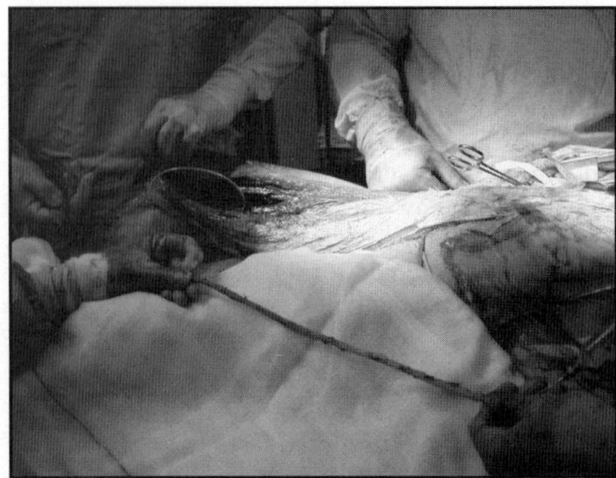

Figure 4.3 • Superficial femoral vein in situ **(a)** and following harvest **(b)**.

secrete large quantities of extracellular matrix, which results in development of a vein graft stenosis. Macroscopically, intimal hyperplastic lesions appear pale, smooth, firm and homogeneous; they are uniformly located between the endothelium and the medial smooth muscle cell layer of a vein graft.

There are a number of hypotheses that attempt to explain the development of intimal hyperplasia at specific sites within vein grafts. Low shear stress and low flow rates have been convincingly associated in experimental conditions. The sites of surgical trauma during bypass (valve cusps, valvulotomy trauma, tributaries and clamp sites) were not associated with location of intimal hyperplastic lesions.[27] Although the exact determinants of vein graft stenoses in individual patients remain undefined, the process is characterized by widespread secretion of inflammatory mediators and proteolytic enzymes.[28] In a population setting, age, sex, diabetes or concurrent medication are not risk factors for stenosis. Serum fibrinogen and continued cigarette smoking have been implicated, as has elevated serum lipoprotein (a).[29,30]

Venous atherosclerosis The venous system is generally resistant to atherosclerosis, but the same is not true of vein grafts implanted into the arterial system. These lesions have been termed 'accelerated atherosclerosis' in order to distinguish them from spontaneous atherosclerosis. Accelerated atherosclerotic lesions appear to be diffuse and more concentric and have a greater cellularity, with varying degrees of lipid accumulation and mononuclear cell infiltration. Vein graft atherosclerosis has been reported in 15% of femoro-popliteal vein grafts and in 7% of aorto-coronary vein grafts. These lesions characteristically occur 3–5 years after implantation.

Aneurysmal degeneration Aneurysmal degeneration is an infrequent cause of vein graft failure. The aetiology is uncertain but may be due to surgically induced ischaemia or a systemic predisposition to vascular dilatation in patients with aneurysmal disease.[31]

Prevention of vein graft failure

Early vein graft failure may be minimized by appropriate patient selection and rigorous quality control intraoperatively, with completion angiography, flow monitoring, duplex scanning or angioscopy. Therapeutic manipulations to improve early graft patency have been largely disappointing.

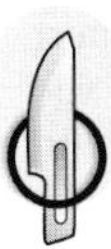

The prostacyclin analogue iloprost used as a single intraoperative intragraft injection or postoperative infusion appears to improve the outcome of prosthetic but not vein grafts.[32]

Early graft occlusion due to thrombosis is usually caused by platelet activation at the site of endothelial denudation.

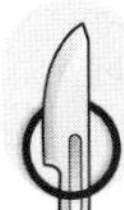

Several randomized trials have suggested that vein graft patency may be enhanced by antiplatelet medication,[33,34] although the optimum combination of agents has yet to be determined.[35]

Many vascular surgeons use formal anticoagulation in patients with vein grafts at high risk of thrombosis.

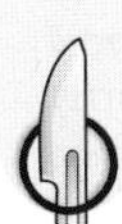

A randomized study by Arfvidsson et al.[36] failed to show any significant improvement in graft patency or limb salvage in patients given warfarin after vein or prosthetic bypass. However, a randomised trial has also reported significantly improved patency when aspirin was combined with warfarin in high-risk vein grafts (i.e. those with poor run-off, inferior vein quality or requiring revision).[37]

Until recently, drug therapy for intimal hyperplasia, although very effective in experimental models, had no clinical success. One randomised trial of low-molecular-weight heparin (once-daily injection) versus aspirin and dipyridamole found that heparin significantly improved 1-year patency following femoro-popliteal bypass in patients with critical limb ischaemia.[38] Recently, trials of immunosuppressive agents (rapamycin) bonded to coronary stents have revealed strikingly low rates of restenosis following coronary angioplasty. These trials have suggested that intimal hyperplasia may be effectively treated and a therapy for peripheral vascular use is likely to be available in the near future.[39,40]

Vein graft surveillance

In the absence of an effective pharmacological treatment, it appears reasonable to monitor vein grafts for the development of stenoses as 30% will develop a lesion. The results of treatment for occluded vein grafts are poor and so surgical or endovascular treatment of stenoses seems appropriate. As vein graft stenoses cannot be reliably detected by clinical examination,[41] routine surveillance of vein grafts with duplex scanning has become established.[42]

Most vascular surgeons agree that graft revision only seems justified for a stenosis with a diameter reduction of greater than 70% or a peak systolic velocity ratio exceeding 3.[43]

There have been two randomised controlled trials comparing vein graft patency using clinically based follow-up versus duplex surveillance. Ihlberg et al.[44] studied 185 infrainguinal vein grafts and found no significant difference in graft patency or limb salvage rates at 1 year, although there were problems with protocol violators and with the power of the study. However, a similar-sized study by Lundell et al.[45] did report a significant improvement in patency at 3 years (82% vs. 56%). The role of duplex surveillance of vein grafts is still questioned. The multicentre vein graft surveillance trial has recently been completed and data from this will allow formulation of protocols to minimize the risk of vein graft occlusion.

Prosthetic grafts

HEALING

Prosthetic grafts interact with the blood and with the surrounding tissues. Because of their inherent thrombogenicity, prosthetic vascular grafts become covered by fibrin and platelet thrombus shortly after implantation. This pannus persists and remains actively thrombogenic, although it may stabilize after 1 year. Healing of prosthetic grafts occurs by two mechanisms, endothelial cell migration along the graft and capillary ingrowth.

Endothelialisation of the graft may occur for variable distances around the anastomotic regions, as endothelial cells migrate from the host artery to the graft surface. Although this process may result in complete re-endothelialisation in animal models, human grafts do not develop an endothelial monolayer.[46] Capillary ingrowth occurs through the graft from surrounding tissues. The extent of perigraft incorporation is dependent on the porosity of the graft; the higher the porosity, the greater the extent of incorporation.

DACRON GRAFTS

Dacron yarn is a multifilament polyester yarn that is manufactured into grafts by weaving or knitting. Woven Dacron grafts are composed of threads interlaced in over and under patterns with two sets of yarns, the warp and the weft at right angles to each other (**Fig. 4.4**). Woven grafts are rigid and the cut ends of the graft are prone to fraying. These grafts have a low permeability (minimal bleeding during implantation) but have poor handling characteristics and very low compliance.

Knitted grafts have yarns inter-looped around each other oriented in a longitudinal (warp) or circumferential (weft) manner. Warp knitted grafts have more stability and the majority of commercially available grafts have this configuration. Knitted grafts have relatively high porosity and must therefore be pre-clotted to prevent bleeding. These grafts have a tendency to dilate with time, but encourage tissue ingrowth and have superior handling characteristics. In recent years most knitted grafts have been pre-impregnated with collagen,

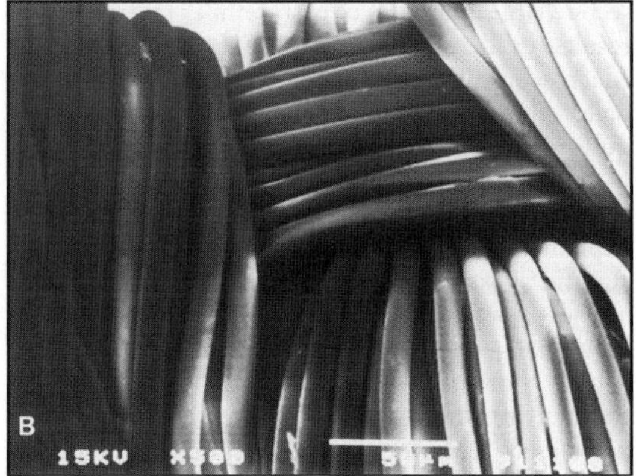

Figure 4.4 • Electron micrograph of a woven Dacron graft showing the multifilament yarn used for both the warp and the weft.

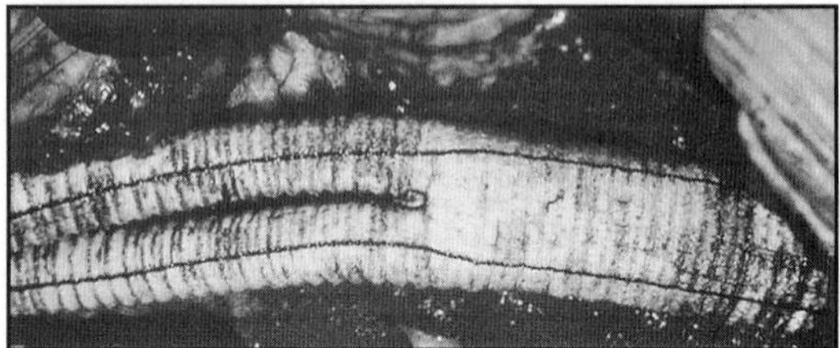

Figure 4.5 • Collagen-impregnated knitted Dacron (polyester) graft demonstrating almost zero porosity after implantation.

albumin or gelatin, which has abolished the need for pre-clotting (**Fig. 4.5**). Some evidence suggests that early thrombogenicity of the graft surface may be lessened by such graft coatings, with an expected improvement in graft patency. However, a randomised trial has shown no clinical evidence of reduced blood loss or improved patency.[47]

Knitted grafts may be made softer by adding yarns at right angles to the graft surface. The velour surface may allow the development of a stable neointima. Dacron grafts are usually crimped to impart flexibility, elasticity and shape retention.

EXPANDED POLYTETRAFLUOROETHYLENE

Expanded polytetrafluoroethylene (ePTFE) grafts are manufactured by extrusion of PTFE polymer, which produces a graft composed of solid nodes interconnected by fine fibrils (**Fig. 4.6**). The spaces between the individual fibrils are smaller than those between the fibres of a Dacron graft, producing a high-porosity low-permeability graft. PTFE is inert and has an electronegative charge that renders the graft hydrophobic. Some PTFE grafts have a thin outer wrap to increase wall strength and further

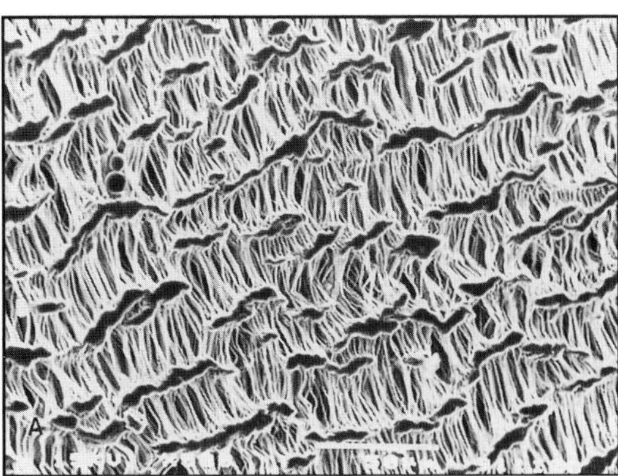

Figure 4.6 • Electron micrograph of an ePTFE graft demonstrating the solid nodes connected by fibrils.

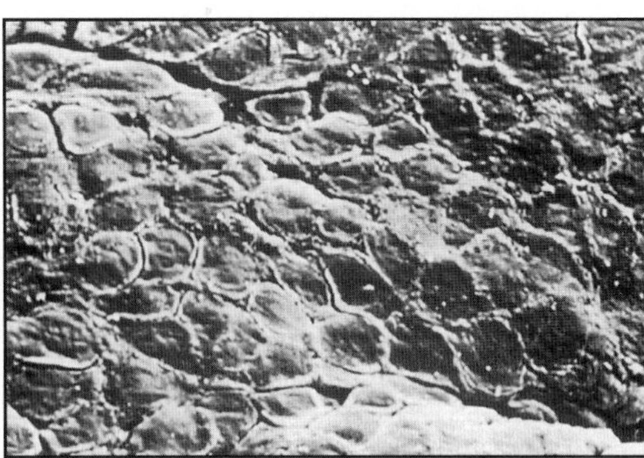

Figure 4.7 • Electron micrograph of confluent endothelial monolayer on a PTFE graft after endothelial seeding and incubation.

reduce permeability. PTFE grafts are now manufactured with thin walls to improve handling, and stretch grafts have longitudinal elasticity. These grafts may be externally supported to prevent kinking when placed across a joint, improving the chances of long-term patency. However, external support did not improve patency in a prospective randomised study.[48]

Some surgeons have used PTFE in preference to Dacron because of reports suggesting an improved resistance to infection and lower thrombogenicity in infrainguinal bypass.

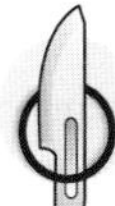

The only randomized comparison of Dacron and PTFE in aortic surgery suggested equivalent graft performance.[49]

Similarly, the preference for PTFE in lower limb revascularization has recently been assessed in a randomized trial, which showed comparable results in PTFE and Dacron grafts.[50,51]

MECHANISMS OF GRAFT FAILURE

Prosthetic vascular grafts have different mechanisms of failure compared with vein grafts. The dominant causes of prosthetic graft failure are luminal thrombogenicity, compliance mismatch and anastomotic intimal hyperplasia.

Luminal thrombogenicity, endothelial seeding and antithrombotic graft coatings

Prosthetic vascular grafts do not develop an endothelial monolayer in humans. The surface of the graft therefore remains inherently thrombogenic, with constant activation of platelets and the potential for thrombotic graft occlusion. The absence of the endothelial monolayer is considered to be a crucial factor in graft occlusion and thus lining the luminal surface of a graft with endothelial cells may produce a functioning biological graft, through a process termed 'endothelial cell seeding'.

Endothelial cell seeding involves attaching autologous endothelial cells to the graft surface. Endothelial cells may be harvested from vein, subcutaneous fat or omentum, and may be maintained in tissue culture. These cells can then be incubated with the luminal surface of a prosthetic graft to produce a stable endothelial monolayer (**Fig. 4.7**). Endothelial cell seeding may be a one-stage or two-stage procedure. Two-stage seeding involves the harvest of small numbers of endothelial cells from a peripheral vein, amplification of the cells in cell culture and subsequent attachment to a graft. This process usually takes up to 8 weeks. Single-stage seeding uses large numbers of microvascular endothelial cells harvested from omentum, which are then immediately attached to the luminal surface of a prosthetic graft.

Animal experimentation with endothelial-seeded grafts produced dramatic results, with increased graft patency and reduced thrombogenicity.[52,53] However, initial clinical results were disappointing, largely due to methodological difficulties. Recent studies have suggested that two-stage endothelial seeding is clinically possible and have revealed enhanced patency rates in infrainguinal and coronary artery bypass.[54,55] At present, endothelial seeding seems too technically demanding to warrant widespread use. However, future advances in cell culture and recombinant DNA technology may allow endothelial cells to be used as the vehicle for specifically targeted gene therapy aimed at reducing graft thrombogenicity and myointimal hyperplasia in both prosthetic and autologous vein grafts.[56,57]

Grafts have also been modified by attempts to produce a less thrombogenic luminal surface. Carbon coating of grafts imparts a negative charge on the intraluminal surface that may decrease thrombogenicity. Animal studies using carbon-coated ePTFE grafts have shown reduced platelet deposition,[58] although randomized studies have demonstrated no significant improvement in clinical patency.[58]

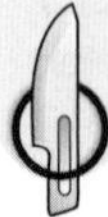

Heparin-bonded, small-calibre, collagen-sealed Dacron (HBD) grafts have also been developed. This reduces platelet aggregation in the short term but there is a small risk that platelet aggregation may be increased in sensitised individuals. A randomised trial of 209 patients undergoing femoro-popliteal bypass has shown a significantly better patency rate for HBD compared with ePTFE (55% vs. 42% at 3–4 years), but more importantly has demonstrated a significant improvement in limb salvage.[59]

A further commercially available graft incorporates a fluoropolymer that has been shown in experimental studies to cause less tissue reaction and to have reduced thrombogenicity.[60] There are no clinical data available to confirm any beneficial effect of this graft.

Compliance mismatch and anastomotic intimal hyperplasia

Compliance mismatch occurs when there is a difference in elasticity between a prosthetic graft and native artery. A compliant vessel acts as an elastic reservoir, storing energy in systole that is reduced during diastole. A rigid conduit diminishes this pulsatile energy by up to 60%. In prosthetic grafts, the compliance mismatch is particularly pronounced at the anastomoses. A paradoxical increase in compliance is observed a few millimetres each side of the suture line, the para-anastomotic hypercompliant zone. Anastomotic intimal hyperplasia preferentially develops in these zones.[61]

Compliance mismatch will lead to a region of excessive mechanical stress that may initiate proliferation of vascular smooth muscle cells and production of extracellular matrix. Changes in compliance are also known to affect flow and shear stress. Turbulent flow may cause low shear stress, which in turn can initiate the cellular changes leading to intimal hyperplasia. Experimentally, there is a correlation between graft compliance and patency rates.[62–65]

POLYURETHANE GRAFTS

Polyurethanes are segmented polymers with hard (urethane group) and soft (macromonomer) segments. Polyurethanes have superior viscoelastic properties compared with PTFE or Dacron and have excellent blood and tissue compatibility. In view of these characteristics, extensive efforts have been made to derive a polyurethane vascular graft for clinical use. Unfortunately, early clinical trials demonstrated poor patency rates and a tendency to degradation, which resulted in aneurysm formation.[66,67]

Recent developments have involved chemical modification to produce biologically stable polyurethane grafts that do not degenerate. Some of these grafts are now used in vascular access but none are yet used routinely in peripheral vascular surgery.

Biological vascular grafts

ALLOGRAFTS

Fresh or preserved arterial allografts were used as vascular substitutes in the 1940s and 1950s. Fresh allografts underwent rapid rejection and thrombosis. Allografts preserved by formalin, irradiation or freeze-drying fared better in the short term but subsequently underwent atheromatous degeneration and aneurysm formation.[68] The problems of unsatisfactory small-calibre synthetic grafts, revision surgery and graft infection have led to a renewed interest in allografts. Cryopreservation with liquid nitrogen and 15% dimethyl sulfoxide, an oxygen radical scavenger, decreases host immunological response and reduces the risk of viral transmission but late degeneration remains a problem. Allograft replacement following removal of an infected graft seems an attractive alternative to extra-anatomic reconstruction as it permits in situ reconstruction.[69]

The glutaraldehyde-tanned human umbilical vein graft was introduced in 1975. The human umbilical veins are placed on mandrils and tanned for extended periods in 1% glutaraldehyde solution. Cross-linking of the amino groups of the polypeptide collagen chains produces a non-antigenic conduit. Despite excellent results from some centres, there is little evidence that this graft has superior patency rates to small-calibre prosthetic grafts.[70] Aneurysmal dilatation occurs despite the use of a Dacron mesh wrap, which makes the anastomoses difficult. The manufacturing process was improved in 1989 but dilatation remains a long-term problem.[71]

HETEROGRAFTS

Arterial heterografts suffer from the same problem as allografts in that they are thrombogenic and prone to degeneration. Glutaraldehyde-treated bovine carotid artery and pericardium have been used clinically.

TISSUE-ENGINEERED GRAFTS

In the future, tissue engineering may be used to manufacture vascular grafts with lower thrombogenicity and tissue compatibility. Three approaches may be envisioned: addition of cells to synthetic polymers, biodegradable prostheses and synthesis of entire grafts in tissue culture. Addition of cells to synthetic polymers is a form of cell seeding, as has previously been described. The challenge in cell seeding is to derive an abundant source of cells that can be used immediately and that have antithrombotic properties. The advances in this field may lie in the mechanisms and methodology of cell harvesting.

The concept of biodegradable materials is that they provide initial vessel integrity but eventually allow the graft to be replaced by autogenous tissue. Both polydioxanone and polyglycolic acid have been used experimentally but clinical application seems some way off.[72] Tissue engineering has the potential to produce a vascular graft composed of autogenous smooth muscle, fibroblasts and endothelial cells. These cells can be cultured around a tissue support or can incorporate a prosthetic scaffold and may offer some promise in the future.[73]

MODIFICATIONS TO REDUCE INFECTION

Prosthetic vascular graft infection has become a serious problem, particularly if an aortic graft is involved. Most graft infections are due to implantation of bacteria at the time of operation. Despite optimum prophylactic antibiotic schedules, 1–3% of prosthetic grafts become infected.

The aim of bonding antibiotics to a graft is to prevent bacteria adhering at the time of surgery and for a few days thereafter. The antibiotic has to have an appropriate activity spectrum and adhere to the graft for long enough to be effective. Rifampicin, an antibiotic with good antistaphylococcal activity, has been shown to bind to the gelatin incorporated into some coated Dacron grafts by ionic bonding.[74] Rifampicin also bonds to albumin-coated grafts in vitro but no studies exist to confirm this bonding in grafts subjected to arterial blood flow. Active amounts of rifampicin can be shown to be present in gelatin-coated grafts in animal models 48–72 hours after implantation and reduce the risk of graft infection to a bacterial challenge.[75]

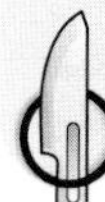

There have been two randomised controlled trials of rifampicin-bonded Dacron grafts with adequate follow-up. The first study from Italy involved 600 patients receiving aorto-femoral grafts.[76] The second from the UK involved 250 patients undergoing extra-anatomic bypass. Early wound infection rates were significantly reduced but at 2-year follow-up the reduction in graft infection rate was not significant.[77] Pragmatically, it seems appropriate to use rifampicin-bonded grafts in any situation where the risk of graft infection is raised.[78]

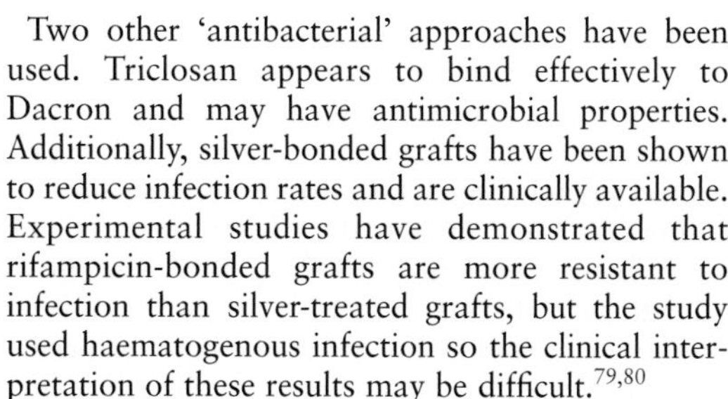

Two other 'antibacterial' approaches have been used. Triclosan appears to bind effectively to Dacron and may have antimicrobial properties. Additionally, silver-bonded grafts have been shown to reduce infection rates and are clinically available. Experimental studies have demonstrated that rifampicin-bonded grafts are more resistant to infection than silver-treated grafts, but the study used haematogenous infection so the clinical interpretation of these results may be difficult.[79,80]

ARTERIAL SUTURES

Alexis Carrel firmly established the basic principles and techniques of modern vascular anastomosis. In the recent past, surgeons continued to develop new techniques to improve arterial anastomosis. These techniques include adhesives and glues, staples, automated mechanical staplers, and laser welding. Nevertheless, suturing remains the basic technique in vascular surgery.

Suture size

The size of the suture should be as fine as possible in order to minimise the amount of material in contact with the endothelium but strong enough to support the anastomosis without risking disruption or aneurysm formation. As a reference, 2-0 or 3-0 is usually used for aortic anastomoses, 3-0 or 4-0 for the iliofemoral arteries, 5-0 or 6-0 for the popliteal arteries, and 6-0 or 7-0 for the tibial vessels.

Suture technique

Anastomotic techniques use interrupted, continuous or a combination suturing technique. A continuous suture line may be more likely to cause stenosis at the anastomosis than interrupted suturing, but has obvious advantages in terms of haemostasis and speed of surgery. Recent experimental studies have failed to prove significant haemodynamic differences or patency rates between both techniques,[81,82] although the use of interrupted sutures reduces compliance mismatch at vascular anastomoses.[83] The use of interrupted sutures is advocated by some authors for arterial and venous anastomoses in children, since theoretically they may permit the normal growth of the blood vessels between sutures.

Suture material

Monofilament polypropylene suture is now the most commonly used material for arterial and venous work. This suture has very good strength and durability and very little tissue reactivity, minimising the amount of scarring at the anastomosis. One important characteristic to remember when working with monofilament vascular sutures is that they are susceptible to fracture if handled inappropriately (**Fig. 4.8**). More recently, ePTFE suture has been advocated as better material for anastomosis involving ePTFE grafts. The main advantages of this material are its handling properties, as well as a better match between needle and suture size that minimises needle-hole bleeding (**Fig. 4.9**).

The ideal suture material for arterial anastomoses in children remains the object of experimental research since it is recognised that non-absorbable sutures are related to development of stenosis in the long term. There are no prospective randomised studies that prove any absorbable suture material to be advantageous over conventional non-absorbable sutures; however, monofilament polydioxanone seems to be a reasonable option.[84] Prosthetic grafts will probably always require non-absorbable sutures as these anastomoses never really heal.

Current vascular sutures are swaged onto fine, usually one-half to three-eighths circle, round needles with tapered or bevelled tips. Some of these needles have a tapered cutting edge on the side of the tip, which greatly facilitates penetration through atherosclerotic plaques and avoids bending the body of the needle in the process. The metallic composition of the needles has also been continuously improved, creating different stainless steel alloys (e.g. high-nickel alloys) that resist deforming even in the most delicate sizes. Haemostatic needles, which are slimmer than conventional vascular needles, are designed to reduce the mismatch between needle and suture diameter. However, these needles seem more delicate and bend easily if heavily calcified plaque is present.

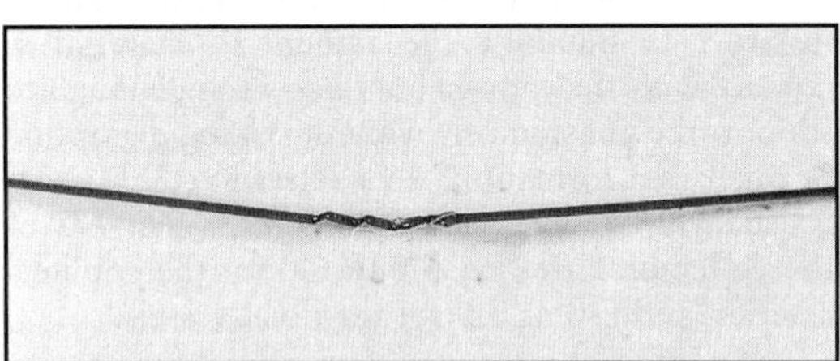

Figure 4.8 • Micrograph illustrating a 'fracture' on a polypropylene suture caused by handling with forceps.

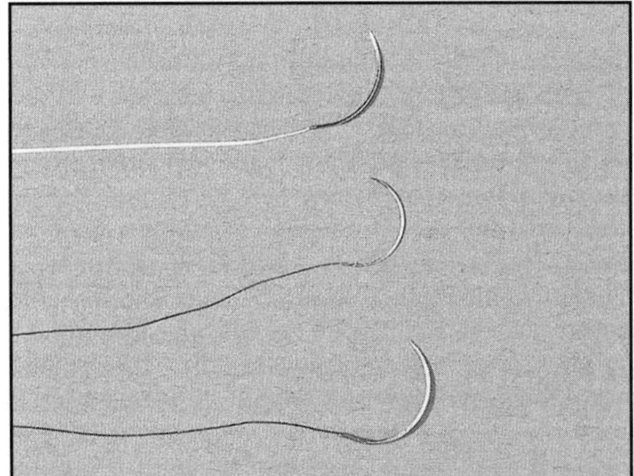

Figure 4.9 • Micrograph of modern vascular sutures: polypropylene suture with cutting needle (bottom); polypropylene suture with haemostatic needle (centre); ePTFE suture on haemostatic needle (top). Note the better match between needle and suture for the top two sutures.

Other materials and techniques

The standard technique for vascular reconstructions remains non-absorbable monofilament sutures but surgeons have continued to search for other alternatives. Adhesives and glues have been introduced but do not offer advantages or the security of standard suturing technique. They are currently being studied to aid in haemostasis of anastomoses involving prosthetic grafts[85] and to facilitate microvascular anastomosis in which four-quadrant interrupted sutures are used.[86]

A technique of anastomosis using laser energy for small vessels has been described. However, its clinical practice has been limited due to the risk of anastomotic failure due to weakness associated with laser welding. These problems may be overcome by the addition of a chromophore.[87,88]

More recently, non-penetrating arcuate-legged clips have been used for vascular anastomoses. The technique has already been used in clinical practice, mainly in haemodialysis access procedures, some femoro-popliteal bypass reconstructions, carotid endarterectomies, plastic surgery microvascular procedures[89] and coronary anastomoses. The results of some clinical reports are encouraging; however, with the exception of trials in haemodialysis access, there are no prospective randomised studies with long-term follow-up. Therefore, its applicability in current vascular practice remains to be defined. One potential advantage of clips is that the vessel wall is not penetrated and so damage to the endothelium may be minimized with potential reduction in myointimal hyperplasia.[90,91]

Future developments are likely to include laparoscopic stapling devices for use in aortic surgery.

ARTERIAL ANASTOMOSES

There are three basic anastomotic configurations: end-to-end, end-to-side and side-to-side. Each of these methods can be tailored according to the experience of the surgeon to suit the specific requirements of the reconstructive procedure in which it is used. Small modifications to the different types of anastomosis can also be introduced depending on the circumstances in which the procedure is being performed.

End-to-end anastomosis

End-to-end anastomoses require mobilisation of the two vessel ends to ensure appropriate placement of the sutures. This anastomotic configuration has a tendency to be constrictive, which risks significant stenosis. In most practices, end-to-end anastomoses are used when the vessels involved are of large calibre (e.g. aorta and iliac arteries).

When a small-calibre end-to-end anastomosis is required, the two vessel ends are spatulated and an oblique anastomosis is performed. This type of anastomosis is particularly useful for grafts composed of two segments of vein joined together or for composite grafts of vein and prosthetic material. Modifying the angle of the anastomosis means that diameter mismatches between the vessels can be easily accommodated without altering significantly the haemodynamics across the suture line.[92]

End-to-side anastomosis

The end-to-side anastomosis is the most common configuration used in arterial reconstructive surgery and constitutes the basis for most bypass grafting procedures, although haemodynamically this anastomotic technique may be at a slight disadvantage compared with the end-to-end technique.[93]

The length and the angle of the end-to-side anastomosis have been the object of in vitro and in vivo studies.[94] With some slight variations, it is accepted that the ideal length of the anastomosis should be close to twice the diameter of the native vessel. The angle at which the graft approaches the native vessel seems to be a critical factor when considering that low shear forces along the areas at the 'heel' and 'toe' of the anastomosis have been related with increased development of intimal hyperplasia. In vitro studies have demonstrated that for small native vessels (e.g. infrapopliteal vessels) an acute angle is recommended. It is accepted that an anastomotic angle of about 30° produces good results for infrapopliteal bypass.[95,96] For larger vessels, which can more easily accommodate the changes related with intimal hyperplasia, less acute angles are acceptable. Anatomical considerations mean that certain anastomoses require much wider angles (e.g. axillo-femoral bypass, and subclavian to carotid artery transposition). These types of anastomoses are often performed at angles of 75–90° without significant haemodynamic compromise or patency differences.

Side-to-side anastomosis

This is the least common type of vascular anastomosis. The better-known examples of this technique are arteriovenous fistulas for haemodialysis access, and sequential bypasses at the infrapopliteal level. In most instances, the technique for this type of anastomosis resembles the technique and principles used for the end-to-side anastomosis.

Adjuvant techniques

ARTERIOVENOUS FISTULAS

The patency of prosthetic grafts depends on luminal blood flow velocity, as thrombosis rapidly occurs below the threshold thrombotic velocity. This velocity varies but all prosthetic materials have a much higher threshold than autogenous vein. The velocity in low-flow infrainguinal grafts can be increased by reducing the graft diameter, but prosthetic grafts less than 6 mm tend to occlude due to the resistance caused by the small calibre of the graft itself.[97] One solution is to increase blood flow velocity by the creation of an adjuvant venous fistula at, or close to, the distal anastomosis.

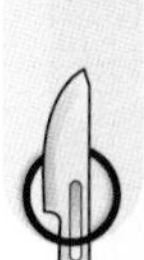

Although blood flow ought to be increased by this technique, a recent randomised trial comparing graft patency and limb salvage rates after femoro-tibial prosthetic bypass with and without adjuvant arteriovenous fistula failed to prove a significant difference.[98]

VENOUS PATCHES AND CUFFS

Interposition vein patches or cuffs between the prosthetic graft and the recipient small-calibre artery at the distal anastomosis were originally developed to facilitate a technically demanding anastomosis. The technique was first described in 1970 and a number of vein configurations have been described, including the Miller collar, Taylor patch, St Mary's boot, Linton patch and Karacagil cuff (**Fig. 4.10**).[64]

The venous cuff reduces compliance mismatch at the prosthetic–arterial anastomosis, stimulates biphasic arterial flow and alters the haemodynamics of the anastomosis.[99] Additionally, the cuff acts as a 'reservoir' of endothelium at the vascular anastomosis and may stimulate endothelial migration along the prosthetic graft. It has been demonstrated that the strip of vein used to make the Miller cuff is more compliant in its longitudinal than its transverse axis.[100] Bench studies of

(a)

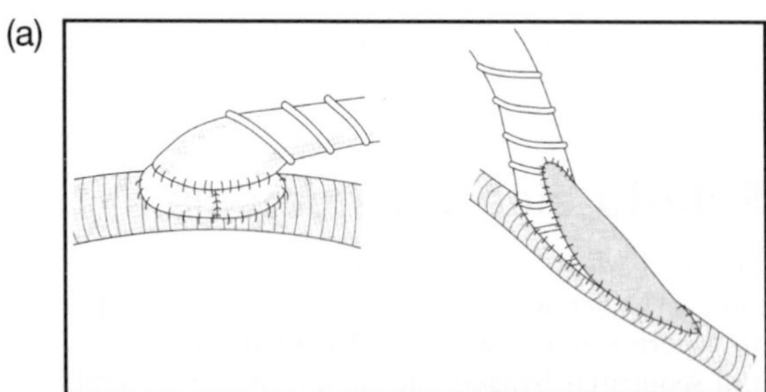

(b)

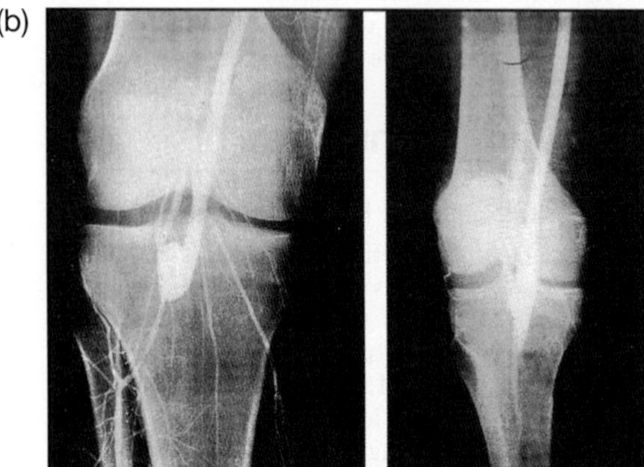

Figure 4.10 • **(a)** Venous cuff described by Miller (left) and venous patch described by Taylor (right); **(b)** corresponding completion angiograms of below-knee popliteal anastomoses.

anastomotic haemodynamics using cineangiography have shown that vein cuffs induce a large vortex that forms just after peak systole. This vortex is highly cohesive and persists until late diastole.[101] Blood flow through a conventional end-to-side anastomosis is essentially laminar (**Fig. 4.11**). However, areas of flow separation near the 'toe', 'heel' and floor of the anastomosis cause constant areas of low wall shear stress that may explain myointimal hyperplasia at these sites.[102] In the cuffed anastomosis, the regions of low wall shear stress are located within the cuff, away from the artery. Furthermore, the repeated formation and dissipation of the vortex means that no single area is constantly exposed to low wall shear stress. This may inhibit the development of myointimal hyperplasia.

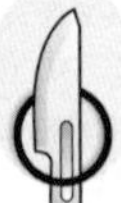

Clinically, venous cuffs improve patency and limb salvage of prosthetic vascular grafts in infragenicular anastomoses but not in the larger above-knee vessels.[103]

Recently, it has been suggested that prosthetic grafts with a 'cuffed' configuration at the distal anastomtic region have similar patency rates to those of vein collars, but these data were uncontrolled and should be interpreted with caution.[104]

(a)

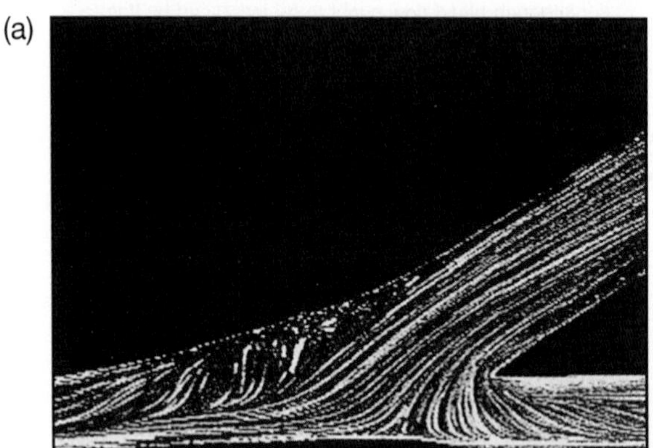

(b)

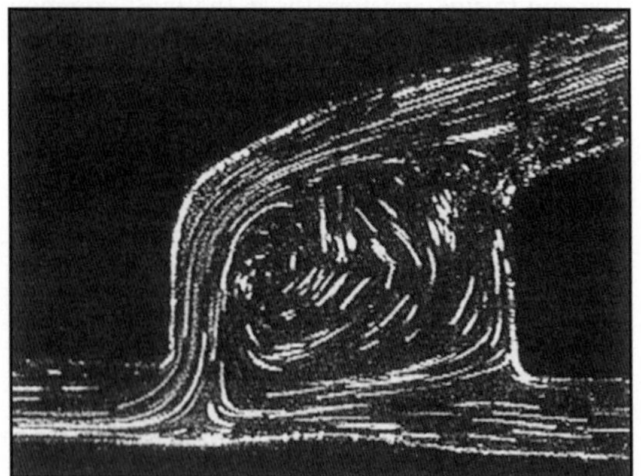

Figure 4.11 • Laminar flow pattern at the end of systole in a conventional end-to-side anastomosis **(a)** compared with the large vortex in a Miller cuff **(b)**. Reproduced with kind permission of Mr P.L. Harris.

Key points

- Venous autografts are the preferred choice for infrainguinal bypass. There appears to be no difference in patency rates for the reversed or in situ techniques.
- Evidence suggests that intensive vein graft surveillance may improve graft patency rates, although results from a randomized trial are awaited.
- Superficial femoral vein has become an essential tool in treating aortic graft infection
- Dacron and PTFE grafts perform similarly in femoro-popliteal bypass. There is some evidence to support the use of HBD in lower limb bypass.
- There is little evidence to support rifampicin bonding of grafts to reduce graft infection. However, most authors support the use of a bonded graft in high-risk cases.
- Vein cuffs improve patency of below-knee grafts.

REFERENCES

1. Boylan MJ, Lytle BW, Loop FD et al. Surgical treatment of isolated left anterior descending coronary stenosis. Comparison of left internal mammary artery and venous autograft at 18 to 20 years of follow-up. J Thorac Cardiovasc Surg 1994; 107:657–62.
2. Novick AC, Stewart BH, Straffon RA. Autogenous arterial grafts in the treatment of renal artery stenosis. J Urol 1977; 118:919–22.
3. Fearn SJ, Parkinson E, Nott DM. Radial artery as a conduit for diabetic crural bypass. Br J Surg 2003; 90:57–8.
4. Michaels JA. Choice of material for above-knee femoropopliteal bypass graft. Br J Surg 1989; 76:7–14.
5. Mamode N, Scott RN. Graft type for femoro-popliteal bypass surgery. Cochrane Database Syst Rev 2000; CD001487.
6. Dilley RJ, McGeachie JK, Prendergast FJ. A review of the histologic changes in vein-to-artery grafts, with particular reference to intimal hyperplasia. Arch Surg 1988; 123:691–6.
7. Lemson MS, Tordoir JH, Daemen MJ, Kitslaar PJ. Intimal hyperplasia in vascular grafts. Eur J Vasc Endovasc Surg 2000; 19:336–50.
8. Dashwood MR, Gibbins R, Mehta D et al. Neural reorganisation in porcine vein grafts: a potential role for endothelin-1. Atherosclerosis 2000; 150:43–53.
9. Milroy CM, Scott DJ, Beard JD, Horrocks M, Bradfield JW. Histological appearances of the long saphenous vein. J Pathol 1989; 159:311–16.
10. Davies AH, Magee TR, Baird RN, Sheffield E, Horrocks M. Vein compliance: a preoperative indicator of vein morphology and of veins at risk of vascular graft stenosis. Br J Surg 1992; 79:1019–21.
11. Leather RP, Shah DM, Chang BB, Kaufman JL. Resurrection of the in situ saphenous vein bypass: 1000 cases later. Ann Surg 1988; 208:435–42.
12. Towne JB, Schmitt DD, Seabrook GR, Bandyk DF. The effect of vein diameter on patency of in situ grafts. J Cardiovasc Surg (Torino) 1991; 32:192–6.
13. Mills JL, Fujitani RM, Taylor SM. The characteristics and anatomic distribution of lesions that cause reversed vein graft failure: a five-year prospective study. J Vasc Surg 1993; 17:195–204.
14. Corson JD, Leather RP, Balko A et al. Relationship between vasa vasorum and blood flow to vein bypass endothelial morphology. Arch Surg 1985; 120:386–8.
15. Sayers RD, Watt PA, Muller S, Bell PR, Thurston H. Endothelial cell injury secondary to surgical preparation of reversed and in situ saphenous vein bypass grafts. Eur J Vasc Surg 1992; 6:354–61.
16. Rosenthal D. Angioscopy in vascular surgery. Cardiovasc Surg 1997; 5:245–55.
17. Gannon MX, Simms MH, Goldman M. Does the in situ technique improve flow characteristics in femoropopliteal bypass? J Vasc Surg 1986; 4:595–9.
18. Beard JD, Lee RE, Aldoori MI, Baird RN, Horrocks M. Does the in situ technique for autologous vein femoropopliteal bypass offer any hemodynamic advantage? J Vasc Surg 1986; 4:588–94.
19. Harris PL, Veith FJ, Shanik GD et al. Prospective randomized comparison of in situ and reversed infrapopliteal vein grafts. Br J Surg 1993; 80:173–6.

   Multicentre trial demonstrating no difference in patency between in situ and reversed vein grafts.

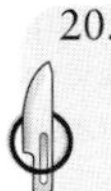

20. Watelet J, Soury P, Menard JF et al. Femoro-popliteal bypass: in situ or reversed vein grafts? Ten-year results of a randomized prospective study. Ann Vasc Surg 1997; 11:510–19.

Randomised trial of in situ versus reversed vein grafts. Actuarial patency rates were higher in the reversed group. Veins with larger diameters demonstrated improved patency.

21. Davies AH, Magee TR, Jones DR et al. The value of duplex scanning with venous occlusion in the preoperative prediction of femoro-distal vein bypass graft diameter. Eur J Vasc Surg 1991; 5:633–6.

22. Ramos JR, Berger K, Mansfield PB, Sauvage LR. Histologic fate and endothelial changes of distended and nondistended vein grafts. Ann Surg 1976; 183:205–28.

23. Gibbons CP, Ferguson CJ, Edwards K, Roberts DE, Osman H. Use of superficial femoropopliteal vein for suprainguinal arterial reconstruction in the presence of infection. Br J Surg 2000; 87:771–6.

24. Gibbons CP, Ferguson CJ, Fligelstone LJ, Edwards K. Experience with femoro-popliteal vein as a conduit for vascular reconstruction in infected fields. Eur J Vasc Endovasc Surg 2003; 25:424–31.

25. Szilagyi DE, Elliott JP, Hageman JH, Smith RF, Dall'olmo CA. Biologic fate of autogenous vein implants as arterial substitutes: clinical, angiographic and histopathologic observations in femoro-popliteal operations for atherosclerosis. Ann Surg 1973; 178:232–46.

26. Varty K, Porter K, Bell PR, London NJ. Vein morphology and bypass graft stenosis. Br J Surg 1996; 83:1375–9.

27. Moody AP, Edwards PR, Harris PL. The aetiology of vein graft strictures: a prospective marker study. Eur J Vasc Surg 1992; 6:509–11.

Prospective study to determine the relationship between vein manipulation and development of vein graft stenoses. It was concluded that there was no correlation between valve sites, tributaries, clamp sites or residual valve cusps and the development of vein graft strictures.

28. Clowes AW, Reidy MA. Prevention of stenosis after vascular reconstruction: pharmacologic control of intimal hyperplasia. A review. J Vasc Surg 1991; 13:885–91.

29. Hicks RC, Ellis M, Mir-Hasseine R et al. The influence of fibrinogen concentration on the development of vein graft stenoses. Eur J Vasc Endovasc Surg 1995; 9:415–20.

30. Cheshire NJ, Wolfe JH, Barradas MA, Chambler AW, Mikhailidis DP. Smoking and plasma fibrinogen, lipoprotein (a) and serotonin are markers for postoperative infrainguinal graft stenosis. Eur J Vasc Endovasc Surg 1996; 11:479–86.

31. Loftus IM, McCarthy MJ, Lloyd A et al. Prevalence of true vein graft aneurysms: implications for aneurysm pathogenesis. J Vasc Surg 1999; 29:403–8.

32. The Iloprost Bypass International Study Group. Effects of perioperative iloprost on patency of femorodistal bypass grafts. Eur J Vasc Endovasc Surg 1996; 12:363–71.

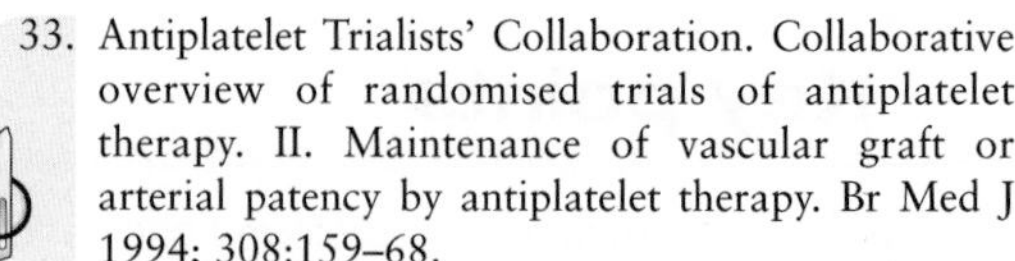

33. Antiplatelet Trialists' Collaboration. Collaborative overview of randomised trials of antiplatelet therapy. II. Maintenance of vascular graft or arterial patency by antiplatelet therapy. Br Med J 1994; 308:159–68.

Overview of antiplatelet therapy in bypass graft and native arterial stenoses.

34. Watson HR, Belcher G, Horrocks M. Adjuvant medical therapy in peripheral bypass surgery. Br J Surg 1999; 86:981–91.

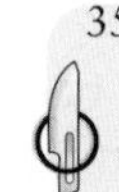

35. Smout JD, Mikhailidis DP, Shenton BK, Stansby G. Combination antiplatelet therapy in patients with peripheral vascular bypass grafts. Clin Appl Thromb Hemost 2004; 10:9–18.

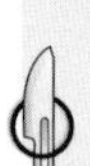

36. Arfvidsson B, Lundgren F, Drott C, Schersten T, Lundholm K. Influence of coumarin treatment on patency and limb salvage after peripheral arterial reconstructive surgery. Am J Surg 1990; 159:556–60.

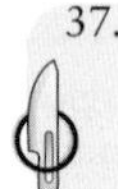

37. Sarac TP, Huber TS, Back MR et al. Warfarin improves the outcome of infrainguinal vein bypass grafting at high risk for failure. J Vasc Surg 1998; 28:446–57.

Randomised prospective trial in 56 patients at high risk of graft occlusion. Addition of warfarin to standard aspirin therapy increased limb salvage and graft patency rates.

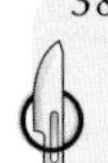

38. Edmondson RA, Cohen AT, Das SK, Wagner MB, Kakkar VV. Low-molecular-weight heparin versus aspirin and dipyridamole after femoropopliteal bypass grafting. Lancet 1994; 344:914–18.

Randomised trial demonstrating that 3 months of low-molecular-weight heparin (compared with aspirin and dipyridamole) improved graft patency in patients undergoing surgery for limb salvage.

39. Lemos PA, Saia F, Ligthart JM et al. Coronary restenosis after sirolimus-eluting stent implantation: morphological description and mechanistic analysis from a consecutive series of cases. Circulation 2003; 108:257–60.

40. Moses JW, Leon MB, Popma JJ et al. Sirolimus-eluting stents versus standard stents in patients with stenosis in a native coronary artery. N Engl J Med 2003; 349:1315–23.

Drug-eluting stents demonstrate significantly reduced intimal hyperplasia.

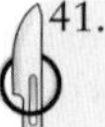

41. Moody P, Gould DA, Harris PL. Vein graft surveillance improves patency in femoro-popliteal bypass. Eur J Vasc Surg 1990; 4:117–21.

Observational study revealing that a programme of vein graft surveillance improved graft patency when compared with historical controls.

42. McCarthy MJ, Olojugba D, Loftus IM et al. Lower limb surveillance following autologous vein bypass should be life long. Br J Surg 1998; 85:1369–72.

43. Olojugba DH, McCarthy MJ, Naylor AR, Bell PR, London NJ. At what peak velocity ratio value

should duplex-detected infrainguinal vein graft stenoses be revised? Eur J Vasc Endovasc Surg 1998; 15:258–60.

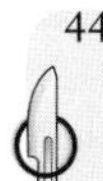

44. Ihlberg L, Luther M, Tierala E, Lepantalo M. The utility of duplex scanning in infrainguinal vein graft surveillance: results from a randomised controlled study. Eur J Vasc Endovasc Surg 1998; 16:19–27.

Study comparing ankle–brachial pressure index with duplex scanning in vein graft surveillance. There was no benefit to duplex scanning.

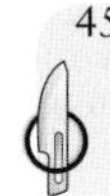

45. Lundell A, Lindblad B, Bergqvist D, Hansen F. Femoropopliteal–crural graft patency is improved by an intensive surveillance program: a prospective randomized study. J Vasc Surg 1995; 21:26–33.

Randomised trial demonstrating that intensive vein graft surveillance programmes lead to improved graft patency.

46. Wu MH, Shi Q, Wechezak AR et al. Definitive proof of endothelialization of a Dacron arterial prosthesis in a human being. J Vasc Surg 1995; 21:862–7.

47. Chakfe N, Kretz JG, Petit H et al. Albumin-impregnated polyester vascular prosthesis for abdominal aortic surgery: an improvement? Eur J Vasc Endovasc Surg 1996; 12:346–53.

48. Gupta SK, Veith FJ, Kram HB, Wengerter KR. Prospective, randomized comparison of ringed and nonringed polytetrafluoroethylene femoropopliteal bypass grafts: a preliminary report. J Vasc Surg 1991; 13:163–72.

Data from this study failed to support the recommendation that ringed PTFE grafts be used preferentially over conventional PTFE grafts in patients who require femoropopliteal bypass with a synthetic graft.

49. Polterauer P, Prager M, Holzenbein T et al. Dacron versus polytetrafluoroethylene for Y-aortic bifurcation grafts: a six-year prospective, randomized trial. Surgery 1992; 111:626–33.

Long-term patency for Dacron and PTFE was equivalent in aortic surgery.

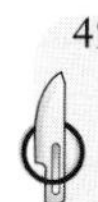

50. Abbott WM, Green RM, Matsumoto T et al. Prosthetic above-knee femoropopliteal bypass grafting: results of a multicenter randomized prospective trial. Above-Knee Femoropopliteal Study Group. J Vasc Surg 1997; 25:19–28.

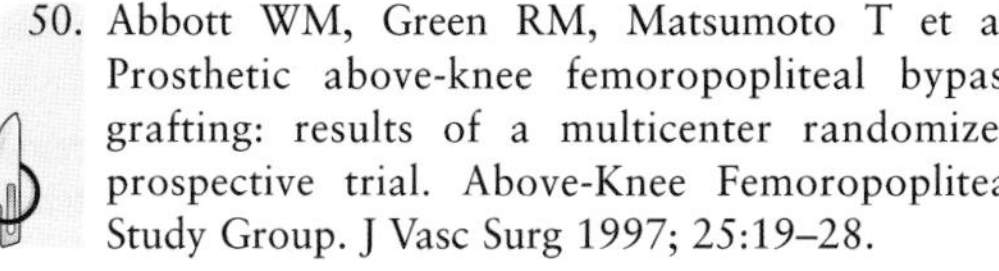

Prospective, randomized, multicentre trial of Dacron and PTFE in above-knee popliteal bypass. Equivalent outcomes with both prosthetic materials.

51. Robinson BI, Fletcher JP, Tomlinson P et al. A prospective randomized multicentre comparison of expanded polytetrafluoroethylene and gelatin-sealed knitted Dacron grafts for femoropopliteal bypass. Cardiovasc Surg 1999; 7:214–18.

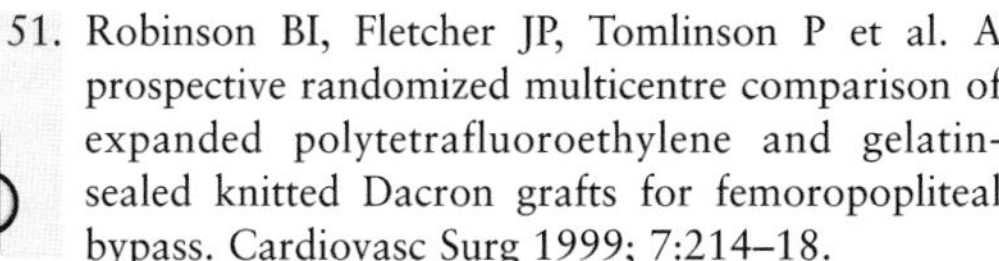

Prospective, randomized, multicentre trial of Dacron and PTFE in above-knee and below-knee femoro-popliteal bypass. Equivalent outcomes with both prosthetic materials.

52. Budd JS, Allen KE, Hartley G, Bell PR. The effect of preformed confluent endothelial cell monolayers on the patency and thrombogenicity of small calibre vascular grafts. Eur J Vasc Surg 1991; 5:397–405.

53. Budd JS, Allen K, Hartley J et al. Prostacyclin production from seeded prosthetic vascular grafts. Br J Surg 1992; 79:1151–3.

54. Deutsch M, Meinhart J, Fischlein T, Preiss P, Zilla P. Clinical autologous in vitro endothelialization of infrainguinal ePTFE grafts in 100 patients: a 9-year experience. Surgery 1999; 126:847–55.

55. Laube HR, Duwe J, Rutsch W, Konertz W. Clinical experience with autologous endothelial cell-seeded polytetrafluoroethylene coronary artery bypass grafts. J Thorac Cardiovasc Surg 2000; 120:134–41.

56. Wilson JM, Birinyi LK, Salomon RN et al. Genetically modified endothelial cells in the treatment of human diseases. Trans Assoc Am Physicians 1989; 102:139–47.

57. Wilson JM, Birinyi LK, Salomon RN et al. Implantation of vascular grafts lined with genetically modified endothelial cells. Science 1989; 244:1344–6.

58. Tsuchida H, Cameron BL, Marcus CS, Wilson SE. Modified polytetrafluoroethylene: indium 111-labeled platelet deposition on carbon-lined and high-porosity polytetrafluoroethylene grafts. J Vasc Surg 1992; 16:643–9.

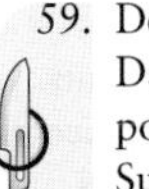

59. Devine C, Hons B, McCollum C. Heparin-bonded Dacron or polytetrafluoroethylene for femoropopliteal bypass grafting: a multicenter trial. J Vasc Surg 2001; 33:533–9.

Randomised multicentre trial of HBD and PTFE for femoro-popliteal bypass. HBD achieved better patency than PTFE, which carried a high risk of subsequent amputation.

60. Rhee RY, Gloviczki P, Cambria RA, Miller VM. Experimental evaluation of bleeding complications, thrombogenicity and neointimal characteristics of prosthetic patch materials used for carotid angioplasty. Cardiovasc Surg 1996; 4:746–52.

61. Abbott WM, Megerman J, Hasson JE, L'Italien G, Warnock DF. Effect of compliance mismatch on vascular graft patency. J Vasc Surg 1987; 5:376–82.

62. Salacinski HJ, Goldner S, Giudiceandrea A et al. The mechanical behavior of vascular grafts: a review. J Biomater Appl 2001; 15:241–78.

63. Tai NR, Salacinski HJ, Edwards A, Hamilton G, Seifalian AM. Compliance properties of conduits used in vascular reconstruction. Br J Surg 2000; 87:1516–24.

64. Tiwari A, Cheng KS, Salacinski H, Hamilton G, Seifalian AM. Improving the patency of vascular bypass grafts: the role of suture materials and surgical techniques on reducing anastomotic compliance mismatch. Eur J Vasc Endovasc Surg 2003; 25:287–95.

65. Tiwari A, Salacinski H, Seifalian AM, Hamilton G. New prostheses for use in bypass grafts with special emphasis on polyurethanes. Cardiovasc Surg 2002; 10:191–7.

66. Bull PG, Denck H, Guidoin R, Gruber H. Preliminary clinical experience with polyurethane vascular prostheses in femoro-popliteal reconstruction. Eur J Vasc Surg 1992; 6:217–24.

67. Dereume JP, van Romphey A, Vincent G, Engelmann E. Femoropopliteal bypass with a compliant, composite polyurethane/Dacron graft: short-term results of a multicentre trial. Cardiovasc Surg 1993; 1:499–503.

68. Callow AD. Arterial homografts. Eur J Vasc Endovasc Surg 1996; 12:272–81.

69. Ruotolo C, Plissonnier D, Bahnini A, Koskas F, Kieffer E. In situ arterial allografts: a new treatment for aortic prosthetic infection. Eur J Vasc Endovasc Surg 1997; 14(suppl. A):102–7.

70. Dardik H, Miller N, Dardik A et al. A decade of experience with the glutaraldehyde-tanned human umbilical cord vein graft for revascularization of the lower limb. J Vasc Surg 1988; 7:336–46.

71. Strobel R, Boontje AH, Van Den Dungen JJ. Aneurysm formation in modified human umbilical vein grafts. Eur J Vasc Endovasc Surg 1996; 11:417–20.

72. Mikucki SA, Greisler HP. Understanding and manipulating the biological response to vascular implants. Semin Vasc Surg 1999; 12:18–26.

73. L'Heureux N, Paquet S, Labbe R, Germain L, Auger FA. A completely biological tissue-engineered human blood vessel. FASEB J 1998; 12:47–56.

74. Gahtan V, Esses GE, Bandyk DF et al. Antistaphylococcal activity of rifampin-bonded gelatin-impregnated Dacron grafts. J Surg Res 1995; 58:105–10.

75. Lachapelle K, Graham AM, Symes JF. Antibacterial activity, antibiotic retention, and infection resistance of a rifampin-impregnated gelatin-sealed Dacron graft. J Vasc Surg 1994; 19:675–82.

76. D'Addato M, Curti T, Freyrie A. Prophylaxis of graft infection with rifampicin-bonded Gelseal graft: 2-year follow-up of a prospective clinical trial. Italian Investigators Group. Cardiovasc Surg 1996; 4:200–4.

No difference in graft infection rates in 600 patients randomized to rifampicin-bonded or non-bonded Dacron grafts.

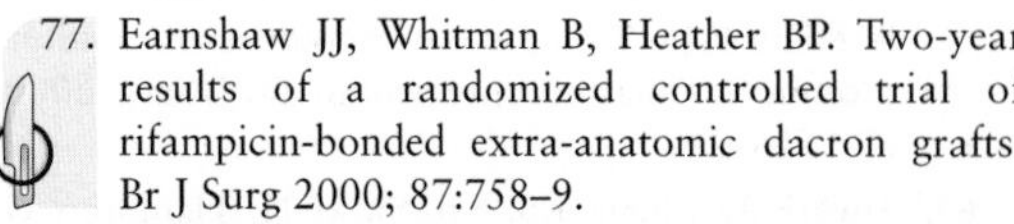
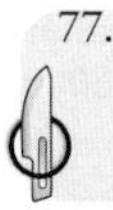

77. Earnshaw JJ, Whitman B, Heather BP. Two-year results of a randomized controlled trial of rifampicin-bonded extra-anatomic dacron grafts. Br J Surg 2000; 87:758–9.

Randomised trial of rifampicin bonding in extra-anatomic graft failed to show any difference in graft infection rates.

78. Earnshaw JJ. The current role of rifampicin-impregnated grafts: pragmatism versus science. Eur J Vasc Endovasc Surg 2000; 20:409–12.

79. Hernandez-Richter T, Schardey HM, Wittmann F et al. Rifampin and triclosan but not silver is effective in preventing bacterial infection of vascular dacron graft material. Eur J Vasc Endovasc Surg 2003; 26:550–7.

80. Goeau-Brissonniere OA, Fabre D, Leflon-Guibout V et al. Comparison of the resistance to infection of rifampin-bonded gelatin-sealed and silver/collagen-coated polyester prostheses. J Vasc Surg 2002; 35:1260–3.

81. Dobrin PB, Mirande R, Kang S, Dong QS, Mrkvicka R. Mechanics of end-to-end artery-to-PTFE graft anastomoses. Ann Vasc Surg 1998; 12:317–23.

82. Baumgartner N, Dobrin PB, Morasch M, Dong QS, Mrkvicka R. Influence of suture technique and suture material selection on the mechanics of end-to-end and end-to-side anastomoses. J Thorac Cardiovasc Surg 1996; 111:1063–72.

83. Hasson JE, Megerman J, Abbott WM. Suture technique and para-anastomotic compliance. J Vasc Surg 1986; 3:591–8.

84. Wang ZG, Pu LQ, Li GD, Du W, Symes JF. Polydioxanone absorbable sutures in vascular anastomoses: experimental and preliminary clinical studies. Cardiovasc Surg 1994; 2:508–13.

85. Milne AA, Murphy WG, Reading SJ, Ruckley CV. Fibrin sealant reduces suture line bleeding during carotid endarterectomy: a randomised trial. Eur J Vasc Endovasc Surg 1995; 10:91–4.

Fibrin sealant reduced suture line bleeding in 17 patients undergoing carotid endarterectomy.

86. Detweiler MB, Detweiler JG, Fenton J. Sutureless and reduced suture anastomosis of hollow vessels with fibrin glue: a review. J Invest Surg 1999; 12:245–62.

87. Oz MC, Williams MR, Souza JE et al. Laser-assisted fibrinogen bonding of umbilical vein grafts. J Clin Laser Med Surg 1993; 11:123–6.

88. McCarthy WJ, LoCicero J, Hartz RS, Yao JS. Patency of laser-assisted anastomoses in small vessels: one-year follow-up. Surgery 1987; 102:319–26.

89. Shenoy S, Miller A, Petersen F et al. A multicenter study of permanent hemodialysis access patency: beneficial effect of clipped vascular anastomotic technique. J Vasc Surg 2003; 38:229–35.

90. Dal Ponte DB, Berman SS, Patula VB, Kleinert LB, Williams SK. Anastomotic tissue response associated with expanded polytetrafluoroethylene access grafts constructed by using nonpenetrating clips. J Vasc Surg 1999; 30:325–33.

91. Berman SS, Kirsch WM, Zhu YH, Anton L, Chai Y. Impact of nonpenetrating clips on intimal hyperplasia of vascular anastomoses. Cardiovasc Surg 2001; 9:540–7.

92. Weston MW, Rhee K, Tarbell JM. Compliance and diameter mismatch affect the wall shear rate

distribution near an end-to-end anastomosis. J Biomech 1996; 29:187–98.

93. Ojha M, Ethier CR, Johnston KW, Cobbold RS. Steady and pulsatile flow fields in an end-to-side arterial anastomosis model. J Vasc Surg 1990; 12:747–53.

94. Keynton RS, Rittgers SE, Shu MC. The effect of angle and flow rate upon hemodynamics in distal vascular graft anastomoses: an in vitro model study. J Biomech Eng 1991; 113:458–63.

95. Staalsen NH, Ulrich M, Winther J et al. The anastomosis angle does change the flow fields at vascular end-to-side anastomoses in vivo. J Vasc Surg 1995; 21:460–71.

96. Ulrich M, Staalsen N, Djurhuus CB et al. In vivo analysis of dynamic tensile stresses at arterial end-to-end anastomoses. Influence of suture-line and graft on anastomotic biomechanics. Eur J Vasc Endovasc Surg 1999; 18:515–22.

97. Jones DN, Rutherford RB, Ikezawa T et al. Factors affecting the patency of small-caliber prostheses: observations in a suitable canine model. J Vasc Surg 1991; 14:441–8.

98. Hamsho A, Nott D, Harris PL. Prospective randomised trial of distal arteriovenous fistula as an adjunct to femoro-infrapopliteal PTFE bypass. Eur J Vasc Endovasc Surg 1999; 17:197–201.

Randomised trial demonstrating that an adjunctive arteriovenous fistula confers no additional significant clinical advantage over interposition vein cuff in patients having femoro-infrapopliteal bypass with ePTFE grafts for critical limb ischaemia.

99. How TV, Rowe CS, Gilling-Smith GL, Harris PL. Interposition vein cuff anastomosis alters wall shear stress distribution in the recipient artery. J Vasc Surg 2000; 31:1008–17.

100. Tyrrell MR, Chester JF, Vipond MN et al. Experimental evidence to support the use of interposition vein collars/patches in distal PTFE anastomoses. Eur J Vasc Surg 1990; 4:95–101.

101. da Silva AF, Carpenter T, How TV, Harris PL. Stable vortices within vein cuffs inhibit anastomotic myointimal hyperplasia? Eur J Vasc Endovasc Surg 1997; 14:157–63.

102. Sottiurai VS, Yao JS, Batson RC et al. Distal anastomotic intimal hyperplasia: histopathologic character and biogenesis. Ann Vasc Surg 1989; 3:26–33.

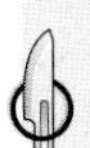

103. Stonebridge PA, Prescott RJ, Ruckley CV. Randomized trial comparing infrainguinal polytetrafluoroethylene bypass grafting with and without vein interposition cuff at the distal anastomosis. The Joint Vascular Research Group. J Vasc Surg 1997; 26:543–50.

Multicentre randomised trial demonstrating that there was no improvement in the patency rate with the use of a distal anastomosis interposition vein cuff in femoropopliteal PTFE bypass grafts above the knee, but there was a statistically significant advantage when PTFE bypass grafts were anastomosed to the popliteal artery below the knee.

104. Fisher RK, Kirkpatrick UJ, How TV et al. The distaflo graft: a valid alternative to interposition vein? Eur J Vasc Endovasc Surg 2003; 25:235–9.

CHAPTER

Five

Angioplasty and stents

Duncan F. Ettles

INTRODUCTION

This chapter considers the principles and current practice of angioplasty and stenting in the peripheral and visceral circulation. While many of these procedures share similarities, technique varies between individual operators. Local practice and experience will determine the approach to specific clinical problems.

REFERRAL, SELECTION AND INFORMED CONSENT

The scope and complexity of lesions referred for endovascular treatment continues to increase. With a growing body of experience and technological improvements, virtually all arterial lesions are accessible and amenable to treatment. However, appropriate selection of cases for intervention is the key to good practice and is based on many factors other than technical feasibility alone.

In most UK vascular units, referral of patients for intervention follows a combination of clinical examination, non-invasive assessment and angiographic investigation. Investigation by duplex ultrasound and magnetic resonance angiography allows intervention to be planned without invasive investigation in the majority of cases of aortoiliac and femoro-popliteal occlusive disease. Best practice is exemplified by the discussion of all potential cases at a vascular multidisciplinary team meeting, before the patient goes forward to treatment. As well as symptomatology and the presence of comorbid disease, any particular technical factors can be considered that may determine whether patients should be treated by endovascular or conventional surgical approaches. While published data from controlled trials offer guidance as to the efficacy and durability of treatment in particular conditions, each individual case must still be considered on its own merits. For instance, while attempted angioplasty of a long femoro-popliteal occlusion is unlikely to offer good long-term patency, it may be the most appropriate treatment for a patient with critical limb ischaemia who is at high risk from general anaesthesia and reconstructive surgery. In contrast, while endovascular techniques manage the majority of patients with aortoiliac disease, there are cases better managed by the vascular surgeon. Despite the plethora of publications relating to angioplasty, there are many grey areas in the selection process, where no sufficient evidence base yet exists to offer definitive guidelines. For this reason, regular audit of outcome data on patients treated by angioplasty and stenting remains of great importance in any unit undertaking such procedures.

The practice of informed consent has undergone considerable scrutiny and revision over the past few years. Once the decision to offer endovascular treatment has been made, careful discussion of the proposed intervention between the interventional radiologist and patient is required well before the planned procedure date. It is increasingly common for interventionists to run outpatient clinics specifically for this purpose. A clear description of risks and benefits is needed in a way the patient can understand. This demands considerable time and can be helped by providing patients with information leaflets.

PRETREATMENT ASSESSMENT AND INVESTIGATION

Pretreatment evaluation aims to identify and correct risk factors, minimise potential risks and maximise the potential benefits of endovascular treatment. Clinical examination should be supported by biochemical investigation to detect and treat hyperlipidaemia and hypertension, correct anaemia and exclude diabetes. Smoking should be strongly discouraged. For day-case intervention, assessment of the patient's home circumstances is important.

Abnormal renal function is not uncommonly found in this elderly population, many of whom are diabetics. It is important that this is recognised since iodinated contrast agents may cause significant deterioration in renal function. Such patients with a creatinine above 150 µmol/L before the procedure should have anti-inflammatory drugs and metformin withdrawn and intravenous fluids provided.

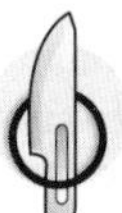

Consideration should be given to the elective administration of acetylcysteine[1] or one of the new iso-osmolar contrast agents.[2]

The potential dangers of lactic acidosis induced by contrast media in patients taking metformin, particularly in those patients with abnormal renal function, have been widely published.[3] Nevertheless, in an emergency, contrast administration may be unavoidable, requiring careful postprocedural monitoring of renal function. Routine coagulation screening and crossmatching are unnecessary because the incidence of significant postprocedural bleeding is negligible.

In patients taking long-term anticoagulation for atrial fibrillation or previous pulmonary embolism, cessation of warfarin 3 days prior to a planned procedure is usually sufficient to bring the international normalised ratio (INR) below 1.5, but this should always be checked prior to intervention except in emergency. For those patients taking anticoagulants for a prosthetic heart valve, significantly reducing the level of anticoagulation may be hazardous even for a short while and therefore patients are admitted for conversion to heparin prior to the procedure.

Antiplatelet therapy is advocated in all patients with peripheral vascular disease and reduces the risk of stroke and fatal and non-fatal myocardial infarction.[4] Preprocedural ankle–brachial pressure indices should be recorded as a baseline for comparison at follow-up, as well as an assessment of walking distance by treadmill testing if possible. Although there is evidence to suggest that exercise programmes may be of considerable benefit in the claudicant,[5] resource limitations mean that many centres are unable to offer supervised exercise programmes.

CARE OF THE ANGIOPLASTY PATIENT

Such are the demonstrable efficacy and low complication rates of angioplasty and stenting that endovascular treatment is often viewed as a routine procedure. This can, in turn, foster a false sense of security among junior medical and nursing staff about the safety of such procedures. Puncture site complications, discussed later, remain an important cause of morbidity and, occasionally, even death. The complexity of most endovascular procedures is poorly understood even by referring clinicians and continued education of ancillary staff is therefore vitally important to maintaining high standards of patient care.

The problems of coexisting coronary, carotid and renovascular disease in patients with peripheral vascular disease are widely recognised.[6] All patients undergoing endovascular treatment should have continuous blood pressure, ECG and pulse oximetry monitoring, and adequate venous access should be established.

The great majority of procedure-related complications are likely to occur during, or in the first few hours following, intervention. Supervision by dedicated staff experienced in vascular intervention in a day-case or vascular ward is optimal. In patients returning to wards less familiar with endovascular procedures, close liaison between the radiology and ward staff is essential to minimise complication rates.

Because of the availability of low-profile balloon/stent systems and low intrinsic complication rates, many procedures can now be performed on a day-case basis. However, in patients with important comorbidity, the elderly and poorly supported, hospital admission is still advisable.

EQUIPMENT FOR ANGIOPLASTY AND STENTING

Equipment availability and selection in interventional suites reflects the range of procedures being carried out as well as the operator's experience and training. Although standard approaches to many procedures are established and predictable, more complex cases require a flexible approach to treatment and therefore a wide range of guidewires, balloons and stents must be stocked. Additional devices, such as atherectomy devices, snares and covered stents, should also be available as well as arterial closure devices.

Guidewires and catheters

A range of guidewires is required for arterial access, negotiation of the access vessels and the target lesion. Standard PTFE-coated 0.035-inch wires are used for arterial access and sheath placement. They are often double-ended, with straight and J-configured tips. In the presence of simple stenotic disease, a standard wire may be all that is needed to successfully cross a lesion and allow angioplasty. Wires with a hydrophilic coating are very valuable in negotiating tortuous vessels and in crossing complex stenoses. In less experienced hands they may cause vessel dissection and they cannot be passed through puncture needles as this causes damage and stripping of the hydrophilic coating.

Low-profile balloon systems use 0.018-inch wires but these cannot be used routinely for arterial access. Specialised wires with graduated gauge from proximal to distal (e.g. TAD wire, Mallincrodt, Hennef/Sieg, Germany) are useful in renal and visceral intervention, and stiff wires (e.g. Amplatz wire, Boston Scientific, Miami, USA) can be used to aid catheter and balloon stability in tortuous vessels. Exchange wires are long-length (180 or 260 cm) wires used to maintain access across a lesion while exchanging balloon catheters or introducing stents.

Angiographic catheters with a variety of predetermined curves are used in conjunction with a guidewire to negotiate vessel stenoses and occlusions. The challenge of complex angioplasty usually lies in the geometry of the lesion being treated and familiarity with a wide range of catheters is therefore essential. Catheters designed for use in cardiac angiography, which can be particularly useful in the supra-aortic and crural vessels, augment the wide range of catheters manufactured for peripheral intervention.

Access sheaths

The great majority of angioplasty and stenting procedures are performed through 11-cm long 5 Fr or 6 Fr sheaths. After antegrade or retrograde puncture, the sheath is positioned using a standard 0.035-inch guidewire to allow introduction of catheters, balloons and stents through the haemostatic valve. The side arm of the sheath permits contrast to be injected for angiographic monitoring of the procedure and is used to administer anticoagulants and other drugs. Longer sheaths may be needed to provide additional stability if the angioplasty site is remote from the puncture site. In my unit, an increasing number of iliac and femoropopliteal lesions are treated using contralateral femoral access and newer flexible braided sheath designs (e.g. Arrow Sheath, Arrow International, Reading, USA) allow very good support and directional control across the aortic bifurcation, avoiding the need for antegrade access or a second retrograde puncture.

Many commercially available stents of up to 10 mm diameter can be placed through a 6 Fr sheath but larger-gauge sheaths are required for some types of self-expanding and balloon-mounted stents.

Angioplasty balloons

Manufacturers offer a large range of angioplasty balloons, with those 3–10 mm in diameter generally available for use through 5 Fr or 6 Fr sheaths and using 0.035-inch guidewires. Angioplasty balloons are available on standard or long shafts and in varying balloon lengths. For ipsilateral work, shaft lengths of around 90 cm are best; for contralateral angioplasty or when using brachial access, longer shaft lengths of up to 130 cm are used. For femoropopliteal lesions, balloons of 4–6 mm diameter are most useful in 4- and 10-cm lengths. Iliac lesions require larger balloon diameters of 6–10 mm. Where possible, the length of the balloon should allow coverage of the entire length of the lesion in order to reduce procedure time and the number of manipulations required within the target vessel. Most balloons used for peripheral angioplasty are non-compliant in type and once their predetermined size has been reached, further pressure increase causes no further expansion. A smaller number of semicompliant balloons are available that allow the balloon to be used over a small range of sizes. Many operators tend to favour one particular manufacturer's products as familiarity with the balloon's tolerance and behaviour is important.

For smaller vessels such as the tibial arteries, balloons of 2–3 mm diameter based on an 0.018-inch or smaller guidewire are available. These balloons are more expensive but can be used through a 4 Fr sheath.

The precise selection of balloon diameters and lengths is not well understood or reported. Some operators prefer to deliberately undersize the balloon with respect to the reference vessel diameter, while others exactly size or oversize the balloon to the vessel. In heavily calcified or resistant lesions, high-pressure balloons made of thicker material, with rated burst pressures of around 2020 kPa, may be used.

The inflation times of balloon dilatation is very variable. Most units inflate the balloon for 1–3 minutes but in the carotid artery the inflation time is necessarily short, and when tacking back dissections long inflation times (3–5 minutes) are used.

Metallic stents

Metallic stents have been routinely used in the treatment of peripheral arterial disease since the 1990s, although Dotter[7] introduced a prototype design almost 20 years before. An increasing number of stent designs made from various materials are available and these are being constantly refined. The radial force exerted by the stent on the vessel wall maintains the lumen and allows remodelling of the intima while minimising elastic recoil and restenosis. Initially, stents were deployed following suboptimal balloon angioplasty or in cases of restenosis after angioplasty. With increased experience, the concept of primary stenting has evolved and may be applicable for certain lesion types and territories.

The ideal stent should be flexible enough to be tracked to its deployment site using a small-gauge delivery system and be easily visible to allow accurate deployment. It should be able to adapt to the contour of the vessel but exert sufficient force on the vessel wall to resist recoil. Its surface characteristics should minimise thrombus formation but allow rapid re-endothelialisation with minimal neointimal hyperplasia. In practice, however, such a stent does not yet exist and several factors need to be considered in choosing a specific stent for use in any given lesion.[8]

The deployed stent is effectively a focus of trauma to the vessel wall and produces strain across the vessel wall. Deployment is followed by the deposition of surface thrombus, with subsequent cellular ingrowth and neointima formation.[9,10] The response of the vessel to stenting is therefore not passive and as yet incompletely understood mechanisms must ultimately influence the tendency to restenosis or occlusion.

DESIGN AND CONSTRUCTION

Arterial stents are broadly divided into self-expanding and balloon-expandable types. The inherent characteristics of the different stent types largely relate to the materials from which they are constructed and these influence their clinical applications.

The most commonly used metals for stent manufacture are stainless steel 316L (e.g. Palmaz stent, Cordis, Miami, USA), nitinol (e.g. SMART stent, Cordis, Miami, USA) and a cobalt–chromium-based alloy used in the Wallstent (Boston Scientific, Natick, USA). Nitinol is a nickel–titanium alloy that has thermal memory and also demonstrates the property of superelasticity. During manufacture, the nitinol is heated and maintained in the desired shape for around 30 minutes. When it is cooled, it can then be deformed into a shape that allows it to be loaded into its delivery system. Upon release at body temperature, the nitinol stent again resumes its predetermined shape. This property of superelasticity may have particular advantages in tortuous pulsatile vessels such as the iliac arteries.

Numerous stent designs have been introduced but there are three basic types. The stent can be produced from a single tube of stainless steel, which is then laser cut to allow it to be compressed around a balloon and subsequently re-expanded. This was the design of the original Palmaz stent, which allowed high radial strength at the expense of flexibility. By linking several short stents or stainless steel hoops with welded junctions, complex balloon-expandable designs with greater flexibility are produced. Nitinol stents can similarly be produced from a slotted tube of the material or by using nitinol wires wound into a zigzag configuration to produce a tube or coil. The Wallstent differs from these designs and is constructed from 24 braided wires to produce a woven mesh design whose strength relates to the crossing angles of the wires.

Both the surface charge of an implanted stent and its surface characteristics influence the tendency to thrombosis and neointimal hyperplasia.[11] The intimal surface of arteries carries a weakly negative charge that is resistant to thrombus formation. Both nitinol and stainless steel are electropositive in saline solution, which may be advantageous as it is associated with less neointima formation. Increased thromboresistance is afforded by a smoother stent surface and is achieved by electropolishing.

STENT SELECTION IN SPECIFIC TERRITORIES

Balloon-expandable stents are usually supplied premounted on a balloon dilatation catheter, but some can be purchased separately and mounted onto a catheter by the operator. In general terms, they offer the advantage of greater radial strength than self-expanding stents at the expense of flexibility. They are therefore particularly suited to the treatment of relatively short arterial lesions in non-tortuous vessels and are preferred in the renal and brachiocephalic artery origins. Placement tends to be more accurate than with self-expanding stents but there is less potential for the stent to conform to vessel curvature or variation in vessel calibre.

Self-expanding stents have a much greater ability to conform to the shape and diameter of the target vessel. This avoids distortion of the vessel, which can occur with balloon-expandable stents. Adequate oversizing of stents relative to the target vessel (usually 1 or 2 mm) is necessary to ensure adequate stent–vessel apposition and prevent migration.

In practice, most departments will carry one self-expanding and one balloon-expandable design to cope with the great majority of lesions being treated. Lower-profile systems are becoming increasingly popular for renal arterial stenting and may be advantageous for day-case work. No particular stent design or manufacturer can be recommended based on our current evidence base, as randomised comparative trials of different stent types have never been documented. The fact that broadly similar outcomes are reported for different stent types in similar territories suggests that patient selection and lesion characteristics may have more influence on outcome than stent design, material or construction.

Covered stents (such as the Wallgraft) are more expensive and often ordered specifically for planned cases, but one or two of these should be kept in stock by all departments undertaking angioplasty to deal with the occasional but potentially disastrous complication of vessel rupture. This is most common in the iliac arteries and therefore covered stents to treat vessels of 6–8 mm in diameter and 8–10 cm in length are most useful.

DRUG-ELUTING STENTS

Restenosis after arterial intervention remains the greatest single challenge in endovascular therapy. Restenosis is related to elastic recoil following angioplasty, late vessel remodelling and neointimal hyperplasia.[12,13] While stent implantation minimises recoil and prevents remodelling, intimal hyperplasia within stents remains an important cause of stent restenosis and failure. Adjuvant therapy in the form of brachytherapy or balloon-administered antiproliferative agents has been evaluated as a potential solution to this problem, but the use of the stent itself to deliver high-concentration site-specific drug therapy seems to offer an attractive alternative. Drug-eluting stents are coated with a polymer matrix, which incorporates and controls the release of the active pharmacological agent. A variety of antithrombotic agents have been evaluated in this way but of most interest are the potential applications of cytotoxic and immunosuppressive drugs. Sirolimus (rapamycin) has been quite extensively investigated within the coronary arteries and has demonstrated very impressive results both in terms of almost complete abolition of restenosis and high event-free survival rates.[14,15]

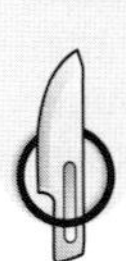

The question of whether these results could be reduplicated in the peripheral circulation using sirolimus-eluting stents was the subject of the SIROCCO trial using the Cordis Cypher SMART stent, which compared the use of eluting and non-eluting stents in femoral lesions. In the group with the sirolimus-eluting stent, the binary restenosis rate at 6 months was 0%; surprisingly, restenosis in the group with the bare stent was only 23.5% ($P = 0.1$).[16]

While several other agents have been trialled within the coronary circulation, the use of coated stents in the peripheral circulation is in its early stages. Ongoing research into optimal agents and stent delivery is likely to have a profound effect on current strategies for the management of peripheral vascular disease.[17]

BRACHYTHERAPY AND IRRADIATED STENTS

Endovascular irradiation (brachytherapy) at the site of angioplasty to prevent restenosis offers an alternative strategy to drug-eluting stents. Irradiation of the target site is usually achieved by insertion of a radioactive wire into a prepositioned catheter or by means of radioactive fluid injected into a balloon. A further method involves the implantation of radioactive metallic stents.[18,19] There seems no doubt that local irradiation using doses of 6–30 Gy is safe and effectively suppresses neointimal hyperplasia and possibly the progression of atherosclerotic disease. The major drawbacks of brachytherapy relate to the logistics of using highly radioactive sources (such as iridium-192 and phosphorus-32) while maintaining operator and staff safety. Automated delivery systems are efficient but occasional complications are reported. In addition irradiated stents exhibit the so-called 'candy-wrapper' effect, whereby neointimal hyperplasia appears to be accelerated at the edges of the irradiated segment, and late stent thrombosis. Recently published data have confirmed that brachytherapy in the femoro-popliteal segments can significantly reduce restenosis rates,[20,21] but it is likely that in the face of improved stent technology, eluting stents and better pharmacotherapy, brachytherapy will prove to be a less valuable clinical tool.

Arterial closure devices

The use of arterial closure devices has been most widely described in cardiological practice but has increased in peripheral intervention. There are two main types, the first using some form of suture delivered into the vessel via a sheath (e.g. Perclose device) and the second purified bovine collagen to seal the arterial puncture (e.g. Vasoseal and Angioseal devices). They provide rapid haemostasis with effectively no need for manual compression. However, their introduction has not led to a reduction in complication rates and, worryingly, recognised sequelae include puncture site infection and distal embolisation of components of the closure device.[22] Significant advantages include early mobilisation, which allows increased day-case work, and the ability to perform angioplasty and stenting in patients who require continuing anticoagulation. Operator convenience does not justify the use of these devices as an alternative to careful manual compression in the great majority of cases.

Other devices

A small number of other devices are of considerable help in peripheral procedures. Snare catheters use a prefashioned loop or lasso, which is introduced through a 5 Fr catheter and can be used to retrieve and reposition stents, catheters and guidewires. Atherectomy and thrombectomy devices can be used to remove or debulk atheroma or thrombus from within native vessels, vascular grafts and stents. However, they are expensive and generally unnecessary in routine practice.

GENERAL PRINCIPLES OF ANGIOPLASTY AND STENTING

Arterial access

The great majority of peripheral and visceral interventions are performed via the common femoral arteries using either retrograde or antegrade puncture. I prefer to use a single-part needle for both approaches with single wall puncture, but two-part Seldinger needles are favoured by other operators and can be helpful in difficult antegrade access. While the usual relationship between the femoral artery, vein and nerve makes femoral access a generally straightforward procedure, the recognition and understanding of anatomical variants is important. High bifurcation of the common femoral artery and venous tributaries crossing anterior to the common femoral artery are not uncommon. When the femoral pulse is diminished or even absent, the use of a hand-held Doppler probe in a sterile cover (such as a rubber glove) can be used to locate the artery and guide puncture. Even better is the use of duplex ultrasound to identify the course and site of the vessel. Following puncture, the J-tip end of a guidewire is passed into the vessel and an access sheath can then be placed. A J-tip is preferable because it is less likely to cause intimal damage or to track beneath arterial plaque. In patients who have undergone previous intervention or vascular surgery, transfemoral access can be very difficult because of perivascular fibrosis and in such cases the use of stiff guidewires may be necessary.

Antegrade puncture of the common femoral artery is a more difficult technique than retrograde puncture and the operator must ensure that the puncture site is below the level of the inguinal ligament to avoid retroperitoneal haemorrhage. Fluoroscopic screening of the position of the femoral head may be helpful in indicating the position of the common femoral artery, but careful palpation of the position of the inguinal ligament is vital to avoid inadvertently high puncture. Again, duplex ultrasound can be of value in locating the common femoral artery. Not uncommonly after antegrade puncture, the guidewire may preferentially select the profunda branch, and several techniques, including the use of curved catheters and additional guidewires, may be needed to cannulate the superficial femoral artery.

Retrograde puncture of the popliteal artery is occasionally required for the treatment of femoropopliteal disease. The patient is placed prone and, because of the close relationship of vein and artery, ultrasound-guided puncture is preferred.

Transbrachial and transaxillary arterial access is less commonly used, but may be necessary in the approach to anatomically unfavourable or angulated renal and visceral arteries. The use of antispasmodics, such as papaverine or glyceryl trinitrate (GTN), is advocated although in my experience attention to careful technique is probably more important in avoiding vessel spasm.

Antiplatelet and anticoagulant therapy

Unless specifically contraindicated, antiplatelet therapy should be commenced at least 72 hours prior to any planned intervention and continued indefinitely following treatment. Apart from the carotid territory any added benefit of combining aspirin with clopidogrel has not yet been demonstrated. Oral anticoagulant therapy may occasionally be of value, for instance in the patient with multilevel disease and low cardiac output.

Heparin should be administered during all angioplasty and stenting procedures and should be given as soon as arterial access has been achieved. Practice is variable, but adequate anticoagulation is achieved for 30 minutes with 3000 units and for 45 minutes with 5000 units.[23] In complex cases or when angiographic patency is suboptimal after treatment, conversion to intravenous or therapeutic subcutaneous heparinisation may be useful with the aim of maintaining the activated partial thromboplastin time at between two and three times control. The use of platelet glycoprotein receptor (GPIIb-IIIAa) inhibitors such as abciximab has been widely described in the coronary literature and there is growing interest in the use of these agents for peripheral intervention, despite the attendant increase in bleeding complications.[24]

Catheter technique and contrast dose

As a general principle, the number of manipulations and guidewire and catheter changes should be kept to a minimum during any angioplasty or stenting procedure. This reduces the incidence of puncture site complications and minimises the risk of cholesterol embolisation. The administered dose and strength of contrast media should be kept as low as possible. Allergic and idiosyncratic reactions to injected contrast are rare, but transient renal impairment is common.

Transluminal and subintimal angioplasty techniques

In the presence of arterial stenoses, the lesion can usually be negotiated using a combination of an angled wire-tip and suitably shaped catheter. The treatment of occluded arterial segments is more technically demanding and passage of the guidewire–catheter combination through the occluded lumen may be impossible. The alternative technique of subintimal angioplasty, first described by Bolia, provides an important alternative and widely adopted technique in the recanalisation of occluded vessels at many sites in the peripheral circulation.[25,26] The basic technique involves the use of a shaped catheter and guidewire to deliberately initiate intimal dissection at the proximal end of the vessel occlusion (**Fig. 5.1**). Looping the guidewire and passing it forward then produces a subintimal channel. Distal to the occlusion, where the intima is less firmly adherent, the guidewire loop tends naturally to re-enter the vessel lumen and, once this is achieved, balloon angioplasty can then be performed in the conventional manner (**Fig. 5.2**). Problems using the subintimal technique may be encountered in the presence of significant vessel wall calcification, when re-entry of the guidewire into the vessel lumen may prove difficult. Vessel perforation may also occur more frequently in these circumstances. The presence and position of major collaterals around an occlusion is an important

(a)

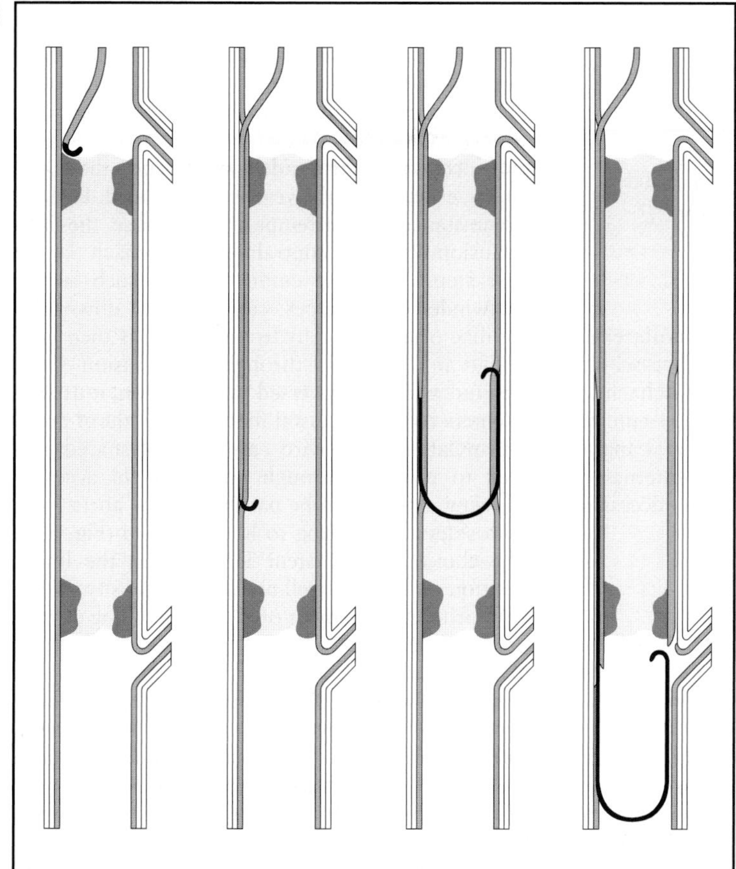

Figure 5.1 • **(a)** The occlusion is approached with a catheter/wire combination, the tip of which is pointing away from any important collaterals. Advancing the catheter/wire in this direction initiates a dissection without difficulty. The catheter/wire is traversed through the length of the occlusion. When most of the length of the occlusion has been crossed, the wire is manipulated to form a wide loop, which allows re-entry into the lumen to be achieved in the majority of cases.

(b)

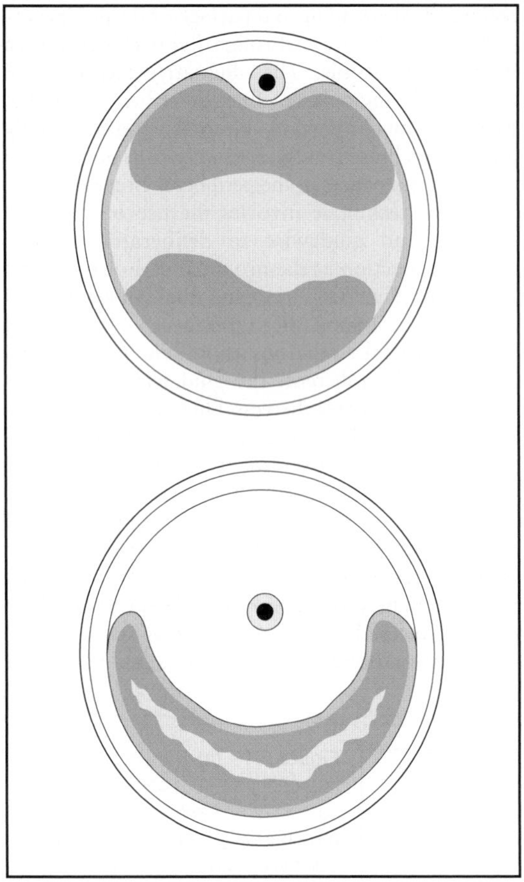

Figure 5.1 • (*cont.*) **(b)** Cross-section showing the catheter position and following dilatation: the occluding material is displaced to one side, leaving a smooth disease-free lumen in the recanalised segment.

consideration because stripping of collaterals coupled with failure to re-enter the distal vessel has the potential to render the limb acutely ischaemic. In my experience, if the lumen cannot be re-entered distally, then a further attempt at subintimal angioplasty 2–3 weeks later often allows an alternative subintimal tract to be established, with successful recanalisation and angioplasty.

ANGIOPLASTY AND STENTING IN SPECIFIC TERRITORIES

Aortoiliac disease

Stenotic and occlusive iliac lesions are usually approached using ipsilateral common femoral access. When the lesion lies in the distal external iliac artery, contralateral access may be preferable as it avoids puncture too close to the angioplasty site. Bilateral access is required for simultaneous iliac origin stent placement and for the treatment of some cases of iliac occlusion, as described below. The primary treatment of iliac artery stenoses is by simple balloon angioplasty. Balloon diameters range from 7–10 mm in the common iliac arteries to 5–7 mm in the external iliac arteries. The stenotic lesion is crossed using a standard or hydrophilic guidewire and a shaped end-hole catheter such as the Van Schie or Cobra type. The challenge in crossing such lesions is one of geometry rather than force and for this reason angled catheters are useful. Once the lesion has been crossed, a balloon of appropriate diameter and suitable length to cover the lesion is inflated. Angiographic assessment is followed by pressure measurement across the angioplasty site. This is best done using an end-hole catheter (such as the Van Andel catheter) through which a 0.018-inch (0.46-mm) safety wire can be passed to ensure that wire access across the lesion is maintained until completion of the procedure. Pressure measurements should be performed after administration of 40 mg papaverine or other vasodilator to simulate the vessel bed dilatation that accompanies exercise. A residual pressure gradient of 10 mmHg systolic or greater equates to angioplasty failure and the further options (repeat balloon dilatation or stent placement) must then be considered (**Fig. 5.3**).

Iliac occlusions often involve the common iliac artery origins and it can prove challenging to cross these occlusions retrogradely and re-enter the aortic lumen, especially if the vessels are calcified. In these circumstances, an attempt to recanalise the iliac occlusion using a contralateral approach is the next step. A reverse curve catheter, such as the Sidewinder or Sos types, can be pulled down into the iliac origin and a hydrophilic wire is then used to find an initial tract through the occlusion. Once the guidewire has traversed the occlusion, it usually re-enters the patent distal iliac vessel without much manipulation. The wire can then be snared and used to provide 'through and through' access,[27] allowing catheters to be passed into the aorta from both sides and stenting to be performed (**Fig. 5.4**). The choice of iliac stent is based on the lesion position and site as well as vessel tortuosity. In my unit, primary placement of a self-expanding stent is preferred in iliac occlusion followed by balloon dilatation if necessary to bring the stent to its nominal diameter. For shorter lesions, balloon-expandable stents may be preferable. As a general rule, the strategy used in stenting should aim to keep the number of stents deployed to a minimum.

Iliac rupture during angioplasty and stenting is rare, but is commoner in the external iliac artery, calcified vessels and in patients taking long-term

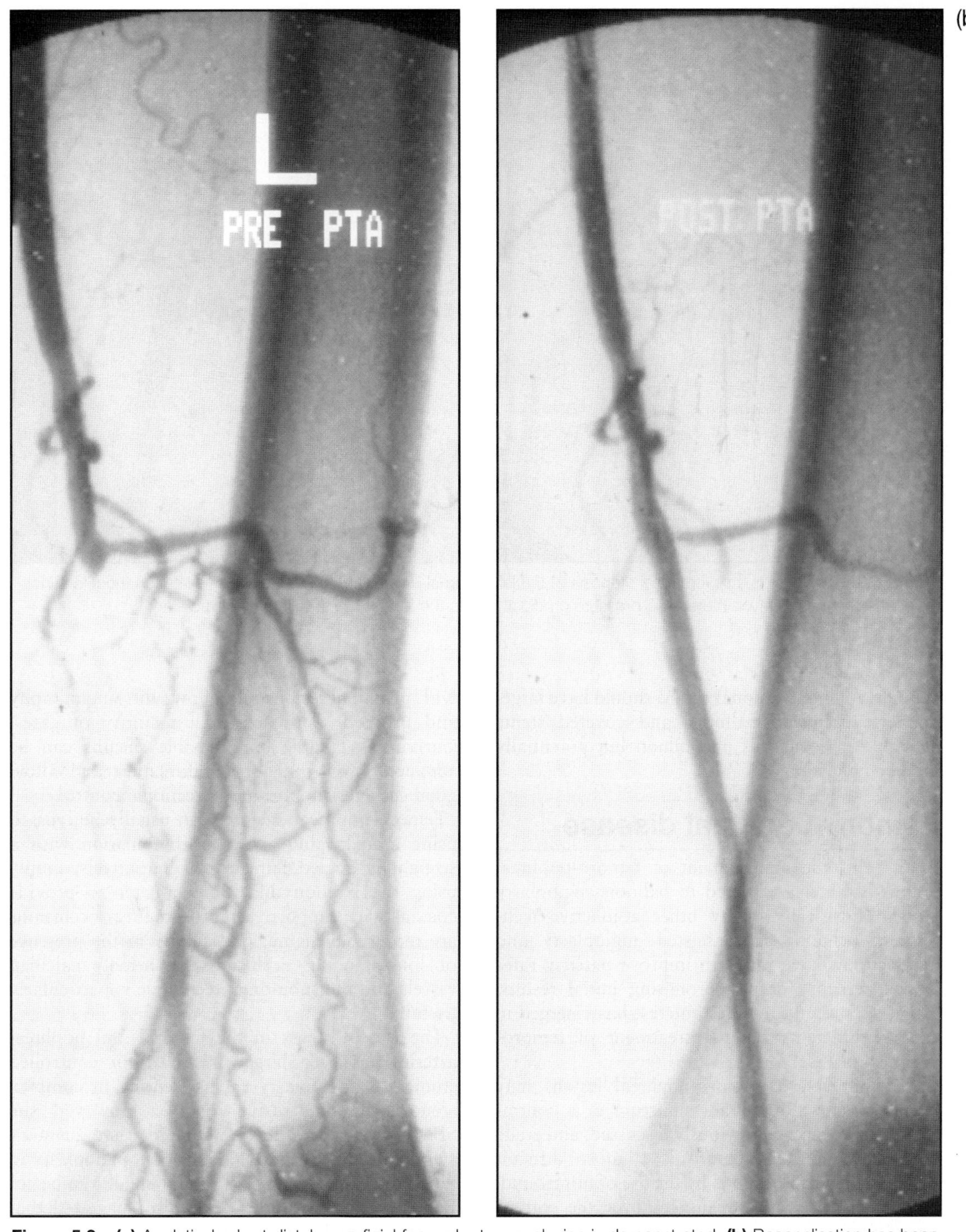

Figure 5.2 • **(a)** A relatively short distal superficial femoral artery occlusion is demonstrated. **(b)** Recanalisation has been performed using the subintimal technique. The major collateral has been preserved.

(a) (b)

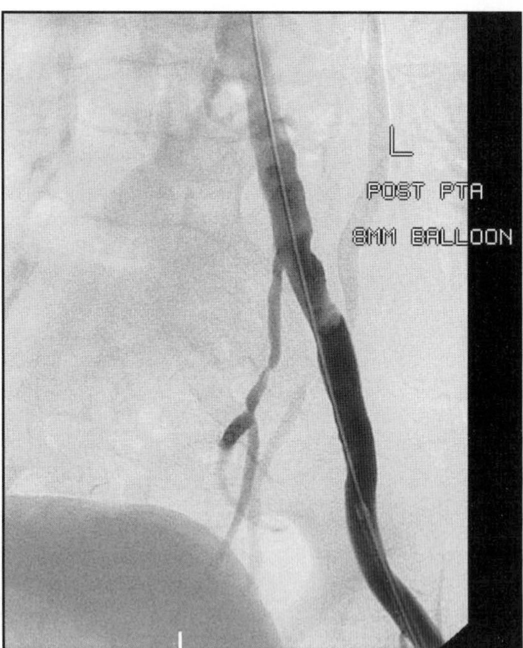

Figure 5.3 • **(a)** There is a severe focal stenosis of the left external iliac artery. **(b)** After balloon dilatation there is minor residual stenosis. However, there is no pressure gradient across the lesion and stenting is not required.

steroids. All interventional rooms should have large-diameter occlusion balloons and covered stents available to cover this uncommon but potentially fatal complication.

Femoro-popliteal disease

In the UK, the management of femoro-popliteal lesions is largely restricted to balloon angioplasty alone. Historically, many other adjunctive techniques, including laser-assisted angioplasty and atherectomy, have failed to improve patency rates in this territory despite promising initial results. However, recently renewed interest has emerged in the use of stents for the treatment of femoro-popliteal disease.[16]

The approach to femoro-popliteal lesions may be via ipsilateral antegrade puncture or a contralateral approach. As previously discussed, antegrade common femoral puncture is a more difficult technique but can be aided by the use of ultrasound. It does have certain advantages over the contralateral approach, in particular the closer proximity of the lesion to the operator's hands and the ease with which occlusions and difficult tibial anatomy are negotiated. In addition, it is easier to perform bale-out techniques, e.g. thrombus aspiration or stent placement. Puncture above the inguinal ligament must be avoided. The contralateral approach to femoral lesions is particularly helpful in dealing with proximal lesions and allows the 'angiography and proceed' approach in a majority of cases. Currently available long flexible sheaths can be advanced over the aortic bifurcation and allow good catheter support and directional control.

Femoro-popliteal stenoses can usually be crossed using a hydrophilic wire in combination with a straight or angled catheter or, alternatively, simply using the balloon dilatation catheter to provide coaxial wire support. Femoro-popliteal occlusions are more challenging, particularly in the presence of long-standing occlusions or heavily calcified vessels and the subintimal technique is particularly useful.[25]

The use of stents in the femoral and popliteal arteries has been largely reserved for controlled studies of angioplasty versus stenting in complex stenotic and occlusive disease. However, the SIROCCO study has suggested that primary stenting may be superior to balloon angioplasty in terms of primary patency[16] and a small number of European cohort studies have also suggested that stenting may be preferable in this territory. This is likely to be the subject of further randomised controlled studies and, for the time being, primary stenting for femoro-popliteal disease should be largely confined to clinical studies. However, in the context of critical ischaemia and acute closure of an angioplasty site following intervention, stenting has an important role as a bale-out technique.

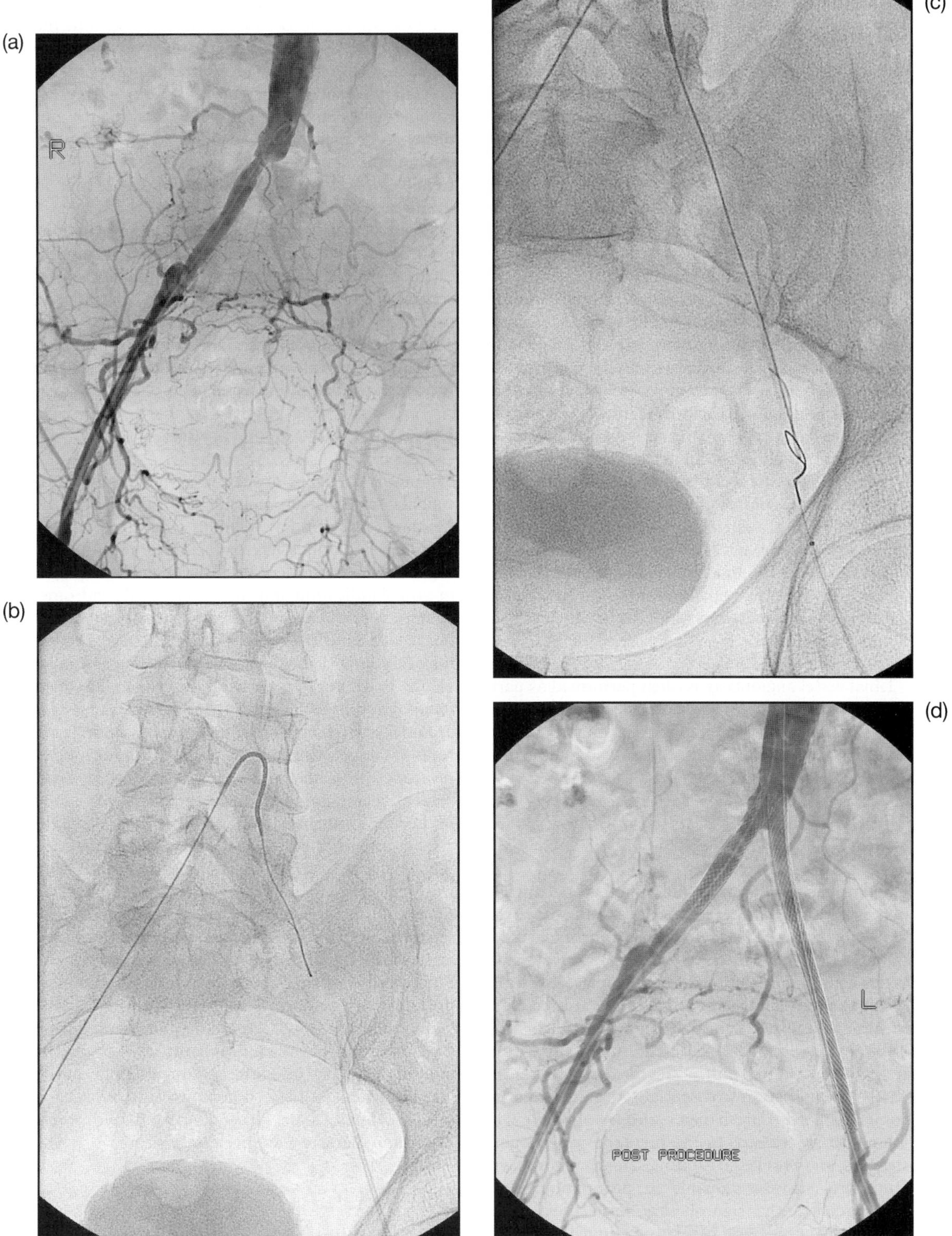

Figure 5.4 • **(a)** Attempts to cross the long left iliac occlusion retrogradely were unsuccessful. **(b)** Using a Sos catheter and hydrophilic wire, a channel has been created through the iliac occlusion. **(c)** The guidewire has re-entered the true lumen of the left external iliac artery. It has been snared and can now be pulled out through the femoral sheath . 'Through and through' access has now been achieved. **(d)** With bilateral access, stents have now been placed to complete the recanalisation procedure.

Crural and limb salvage angioplasty

In patients with rest pain, tissue loss and ulceration, angioplasty is now commonly regarded as the first line of therapy if possible before proceeding to distal reconstruction. Many such patients have significant comorbid disease and are at high risk from general anaesthesia. Crural angioplasty can be performed without compromise to potential distal graft anastomoses and has a very low associated morbidity and mortality.[28,29]

The objective of below-knee limb salvage angioplasty is to restore 'in-line' flow to the foot arches if possible. Using conventional 5 Fr systems, vessels down to 3 mm diameter can be treated. The availability of low-profile balloons based on a 0.018-inch (0.46-mm) guidewire allows balloon dilatation of vessels as small as 2 mm in diameter. The same techniques of transluminal and subintimal angioplasty[30] are employed in the crural vessels as elsewhere and ipsilateral antegrade access allows the best directional control in these technically difficult cases. The crural vessels are more prone to spasm than more proximal vessels and thus vasodilator drugs such as GTN and isosorbide are preferred by many interventionists. Balloon inflation times and guidewire manipulations should be kept to a minimum to reduce the risk of vessel spasm and acute closure.

Tibial vessel angioplasty is often performed as part of a multilevel angioplasty procedure and severe proximal lesions may need to be treated first to allow access to the more distal crural lesions (**Fig. 5.5**).

Visceral and renal angioplasty

Standard access for renal and mesenteric angioplasty is via the femoral arteries but in the presence of steeply angulated vessel origins, transbrachial or radial access may offer a simpler approach and better control during intervention. Available systems for angioplasty and stenting are based around 5 Fr sheaths with 0.018-inch (0.46-mm) guidewires and 6 Fr sheaths with 0.035-inch (0.89-mm) guidewires. Renal ostial lesions offer the greatest technical challenge but the use of specialised guidewires in conjunction with preshaped catheters allows most lesions to be crossed. In the presence of 'pinhole' stenoses, low-profile 0.014-inch (0.36-mm) coronary guidewires can be valuable in negotiating such lesions. Once the stenosis has been crossed, a larger-gauge guidewire can be positioned to allow subsequent predilatation of the lesion and stent placement. While simple balloon angioplasty is preferred for non-ostial renal artery stenosis, primary stenting is currently believed to offer the best approach to ostial lesions.[31,32] Ideally, the chosen stent should be long enough to cover the lesion and protrude 2–3 mm into the aortic lumen. If bilateral renal artery stenting is performed, great care is needed to ensure that the first stent is not distorted or even dislodged by subsequent catheter manipulations in the contralateral vessel. Typically, stents of 5–7 mm in diameter and 15–25 mm in length are required.

Angioplasty and stenting of coeliac and superior mesenteric artery origins is less commonly undertaken. Lateral (cross-table) angiography is the best technique for identifying and negotiating the proximal portions of these vessels and allows accurate stent placement. The balloons and stents employed in renal artery intervention are suitable for use in the visceral arteries.

Upper limb angioplasty

Symptomatic lesions of the subclavian and brachiocephalic arteries are considered here, while the treatment of carotid arterial disease is dealt with in Chapter 16. Patients with subclavian and brachiocephalic disease present with the typical symptoms of arm claudication and subclavian steal syndrome. Stenotic lesions can be treated by angioplasty alone but most authorities prefer primary stent placement for occlusions. The approach to such lesions can be via the brachial artery or from the groin. Combined femoral and brachial access can be very useful as it provides better control angiography during the recanalisation of occlusions. If a sufficient 'nipple' protrudes into the vessel from the aortic arch, recanalisation, angioplasty and stenting may all be performed through a femoral approach (**Fig. 5.6**). This is often not the case as the vessel is occluded 'flush' with the aorta and retrograde catheterisation from the ipsilateral arm is then preferable. The potential problem encountered using this technique relates to failure of the guidewire to re-enter the aortic arch and this is more common if the arch is calcified. Embolisation to the hindbrain is rare because most proximal lesions are associated with retrograde vertebral artery flow. Cerebral embolisation during the treatment of brachiocephalic lesions can be minimised by carotid artery compression during manipulation. As these lesions usually involve the vessel origins, short balloon-expandable stents (7–10 mm diameter) are preferred.

COMPLICATIONS AND THEIR MANAGEMENT

A comprehensive review of the complications of angioplasty and stenting is outwith the scope of this

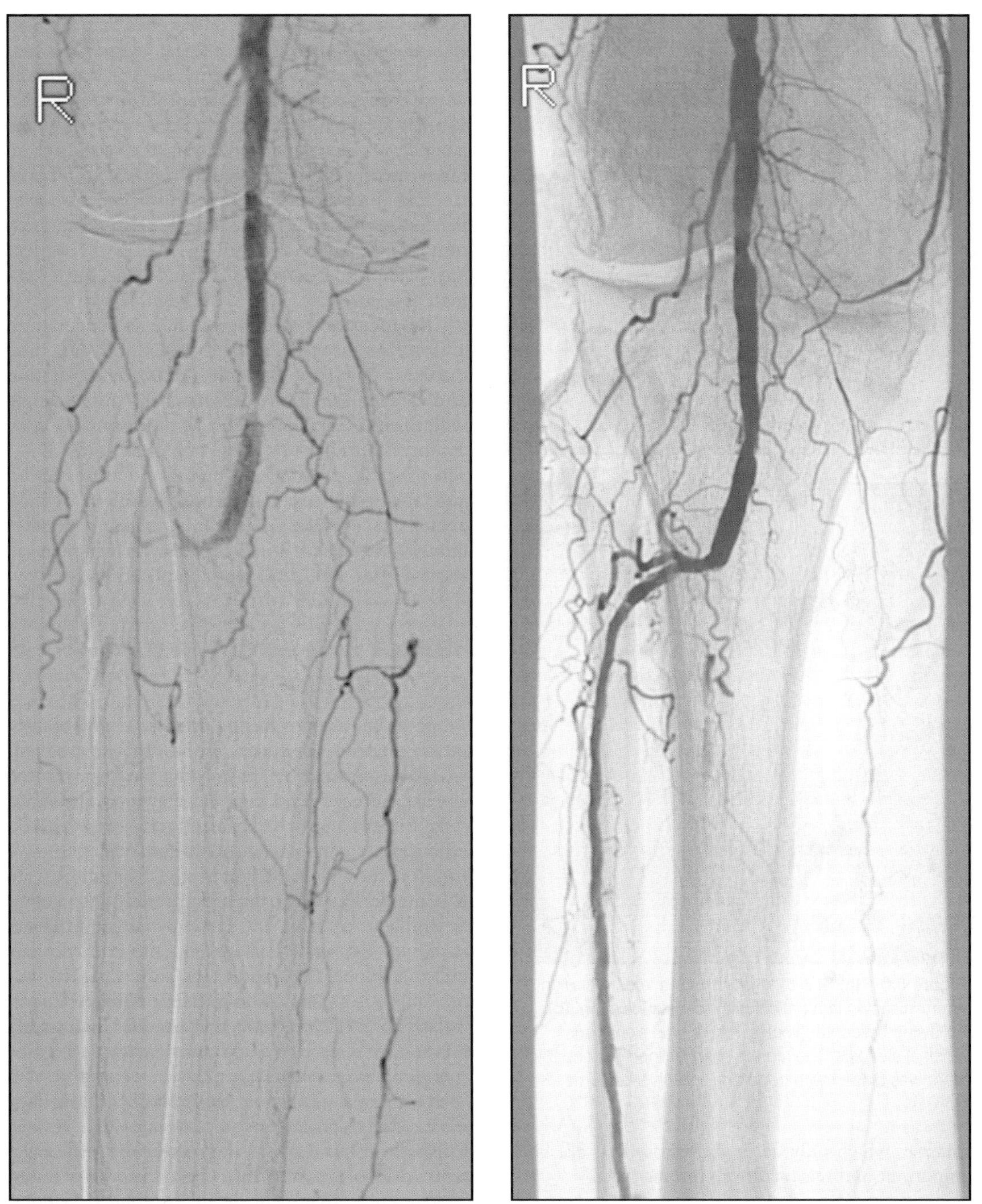

Figure 5.5 • **(a)** Proximal occlusion of all the crural vessels is demonstrated in an elderly patient with critical limb ischaemia. **(b)** Using a 4 Fr system, recanalisation of the anterior tibial artery has been performed allowing in-line flow to the foot and immediate relief of symptoms.

(a)

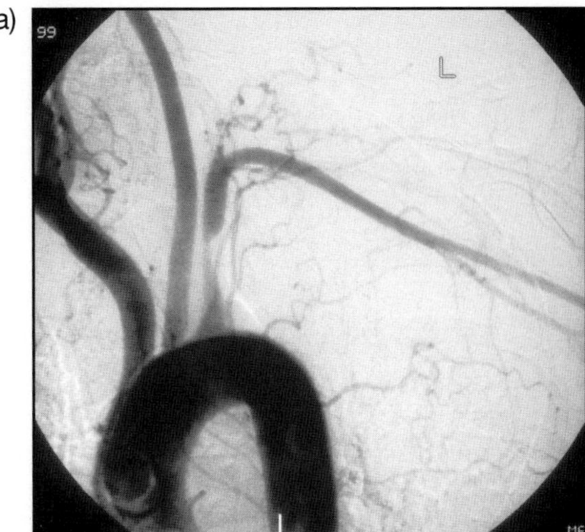

(b)

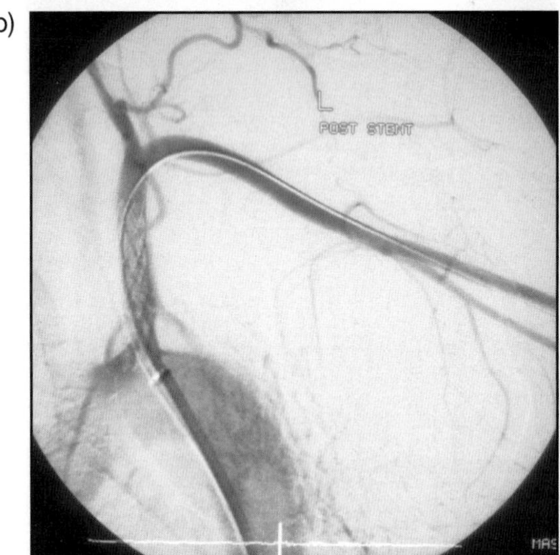

Figure 5.6 • **(a)** Severe stenosis of the left subclavian artery is shown in a patient with arm claudication. **(b)** Following balloon angioplasty there was significant residual stenosis. Therefore a short balloon-expandable stent was placed with good angiographic outcome.

chapter, which only deals with those that are both important and reasonably common.

Puncture site complications

These remain the most frequent complications, with reported incidence varying between 2 and 6%.[33,34] Postprocedure bleeding and haematoma formation relate to several variables including puncture site, operator experience, device size and the use of anticoagulation. Patient characteristics, such as restlessness, confusion, obesity and hypertension, increase the risk of bleeding complications. In most cases, manual compression and conservative management is sufficient, but, rarely, surgical evacuation and blood transfusion may be required. The potentially lethal complication of retroperitoneal haematoma formation may occur as an extension of groin haematoma but is more likely in the setting of an inadvertently high antegrade femoral puncture. If clinical observations raise suspicion of retroperitoneal bleeding, then urgent pelvic computed tomography should be arranged after the patient has been resuscitated and blood sent for cross-matching.

False aneurysms at the groin are not uncommon and are predisposed to by low femoral puncture, the use of aggressive periprocedural anticoagulation and careless attention to haemostasis. While some will thrombose spontaneously, ultrasound-guided compression offers a success rate of around 75%.[35] The procedure is time-consuming and often painful and, increasingly, percutaneous treatment of false aneurysms by direct injection of thrombin under ultrasound guidance is undertaken, with high reported success rates and infrequent complications.[36,37]

Target site and distant complications

Acute vessel closure during attempted angioplasty or stenting can occur as a result of local dissection, vessel thrombosis or spasm and these may often coexist. In most cases, treatment by local thrombolysis, antispasmodic drugs and additional balloon inflations or stent placement are sufficient to restore patency. Intimal dissection at the angioplasty site is common but while limited retrograde dissection is unlikely to lead to haemodynamic sequelae, antegrade dissection may extend and limit flow as pulsatile blood flow enters the false channel and maintains its patency. Additional prolonged balloon inflations (5–10 minutes) will usually successfully tamponade dissection tracts but stents have a major role in bale-out when vessel closure persists.

Arterial rupture is very uncommon but has been most often reported in the external iliac vessels. Clinically, this is recognised by severe and prolonged pain in association with a vagal response. Initial endovascular treatment is by prolonged balloon tamponade at the angioplasty site but if this fails then a covered stent should be placed (**Fig. 5.7**).[38,39]

Certain device-specific complications may be encountered at the target site. In current practice, these are perhaps most often associated with the use of metallic stents, where device migration and failure of deployment can occur. A variety of techniques can be used to reposition or recover maldeployed stents but sometimes the only option is deployment at a site other than the target lesion.

(a)

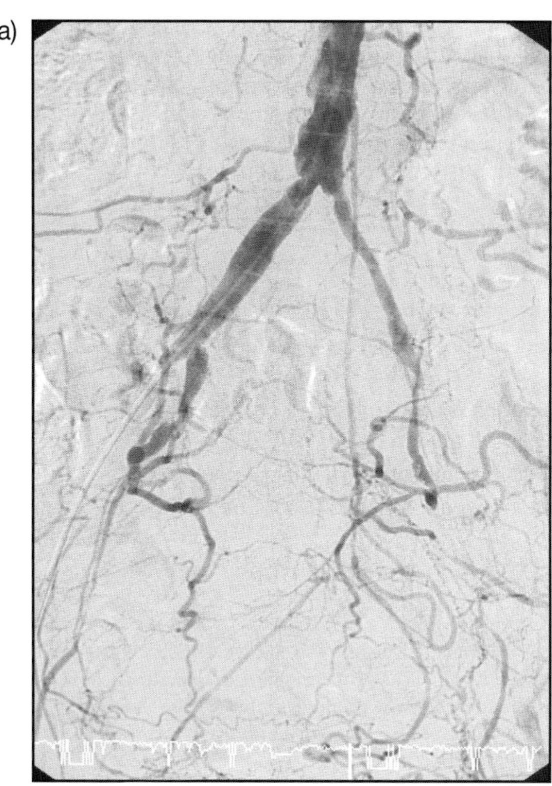

(b)

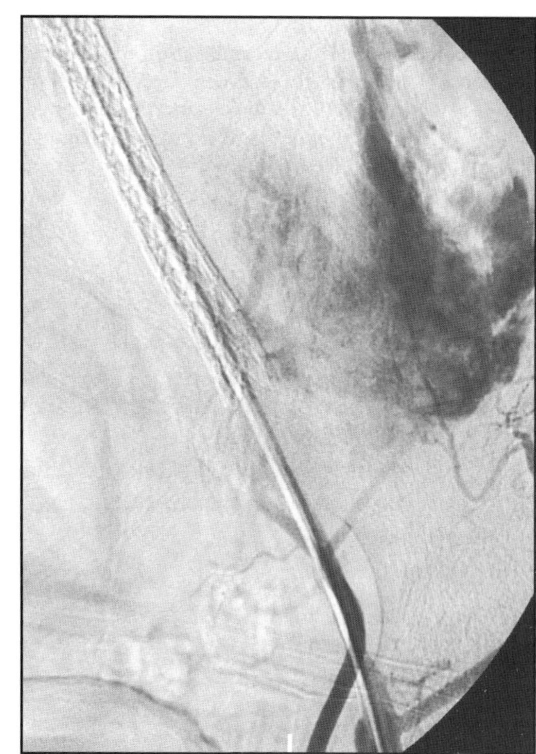

(c)

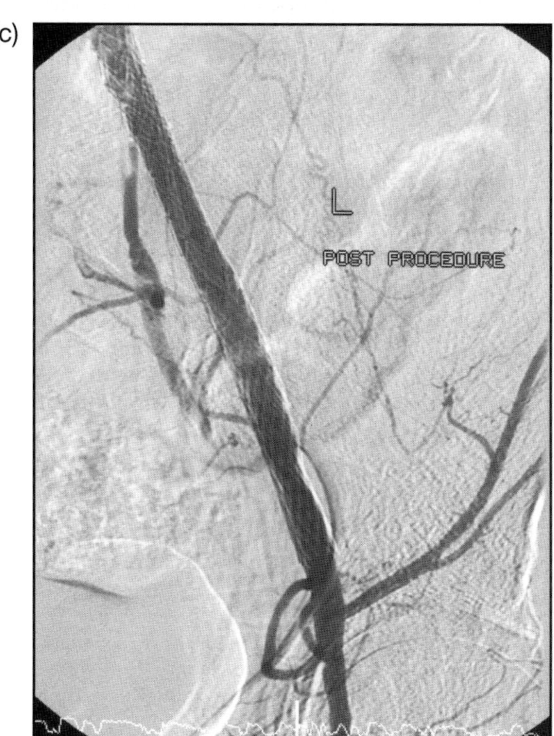

Figure 5.7 • **(a)** There is left external iliac occlusion and severe disease of the right external iliac artery, which is occluded by the diagnostic catheter. **(b)** Initial balloon dilatation causes iliac rupture. A covered stent has been placed but there is still considerable contrast extravasation. **(c)** A second overlapping covered stent has been placed and extravasation has now ceased.

Distal embolisation occurs in up to 5% of cases and is commoner during recanalisation of occluded segments.[40] Most of these events are unlikely to have any adverse clinical sequelae and go unnoticed, while larger emboli may result in acute ischaemia. Patients with single-vessel below-knee run-off are at the greatest potential risk and this should be considered in case selection and planning of the intervention. Small emboli can be managed using a combination of suction embolectomy and local thrombolysis,[41] but occasionally surgical intervention is required.

Key points

- Angioplasty and stenting have become first-line therapy in most cases and are unlikely to compromise future surgical treatment.
- Subintimal angioplasty offers an important alternative in the management of long occlusions, although long-term results are unknown.
- Further developments of drug-eluting stents are likely to reduce restenosis rates significantly.
- Serious complications of angioplasty and stenting are infrequent and can usually be managed without surgical intervention.

REFERENCES

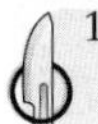

1. Birck R, Krzossok S, Markowetz F et al. Acetylcysteine for prevention of contrast nephrotoxicity: meta-analysis. Lancet 2003; 362:598–603.

   Review of seven trials including 805 patients demonstrated a 56% reduction in contrast nephropathy if patients are pretreated with acetylcysteine.

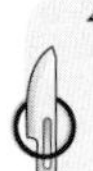

2. Aspelin P, Aubrey P, Fransson S-V et al. for the NEPHRIC study investigators. Nephrotoxic effects in high-risk patients undergoing angiography. N Engl J Med 2003; 348:491–9.

   A study of 129 diabetic patients with known renal impairment randomised to an iso-osmolar dimeric or low-osmolar monomeric contrast agent. The iso-osmolar agent demonstrated significantly less deterioration in renal function.

3. Nawaz S, Cleveland TJ, Gaines PA, Chan P. Clinical risk associated with contrast angiography in metformin-treated patients: a clinical series. Clin Radiol 1998; 53:342–4.
4. Antiplatelet Trialists' Collaboration. Secondary prevention of vascular disease by prolonged antiplatelet treatment. Br Med J 1988; 296:320–31.
5. Hiatt WR, Regensteiner JG, Hargarten ME, Wolfel EE, Brass EP. Benefit of exercise conditioning for patients with peripheral arterial disease. Circulation 1990; 81:602–9.
6. Dormandy J, Mahir M, Ascady G et al. Fate of the patient with chronic leg ischaemia. J Cardiovasc Surg 1989; 30:50–7.
7. Dotter CT. Transluminally-placed coilspring endarterial tube grafts. Long term patency in the canine popliteal artery. Invest Radiol 1969; 4:329–32.
8. Dyet JF, Watts WG, Ettles DF, Nicholson AA. Mechanical properties of metallic stents: how do these specific properties influence the choice of stent for specific lesions? Cardiovasc Intervent Radiol 2000; 23:47–6.
9. Palmaz JC. Intravascular stents: tissue–stent interactions and design considerations. Am J Roentgenol 1993; 160:613–18.
10. Schatz RA, Palmaz JC, Tio FO, Garcia FJ, Reuter SR. Balloon-expandable intracoronary stents in the adult dog. Circulation 1987; 76:450–7.
11. Palmaz JC, Tio FO, Schatz RA et al. Early endothelialisation of balloon expandable stents: experimental observations. J Intervent Radiol 1988; 3:119–24.
12. Fischman DL, Leon MB, Baim DS et al. A randomised comparison of coronary stent placement and balloon angioplasty in the treatment of coronary artery disease. Stent Restenosis Study Investigators. N Engl J Med 1994; 331:496–501.
13. Grimm J, Muller-Hulsbeck S, Jahnke T et al. Randomised study to compare PTA alone versus PTA with Palmaz stent placement for femoropopliteal lesions. J Vasc Intervent Radiol 2001; 12:935–42.
14. Serryus PW, Regar E, Carter AJ. Rapamycin eluting stent: the onset of a new era in interventional cardiology. Heart 2002; 87:305–7.
15. Morice MC, Serryus PW, Sousa JE. A randomised comparison of a sirolimus-eluting stent with a standard stent for coronary revascularisation. N Engl J Med 2002; 346:1773–80.

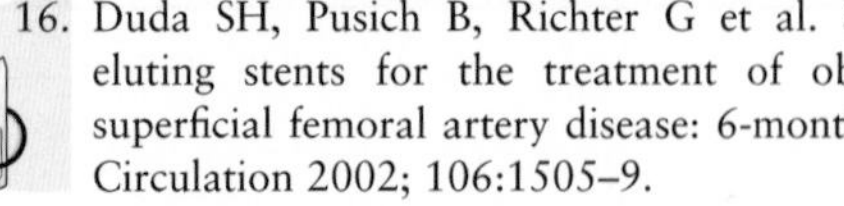

16. Duda SH, Pusich B, Richter G et al. Sirolimus eluting stents for the treatment of obstructive superficial femoral artery disease: 6-month results. Circulation 2002; 106:1505–9.

This is the first randomised trial of a sirolimus-eluting versus conventional self-expanding stent in the superficial femoral artery. The 6-month data are unimpressive, with no significant difference in restenosis. Longer-term data are awaited.

17. Duda SH, Poerner TC, Wiesinger B et al. Drug-eluting stents: potential applications for peripheral arterial occlusive disease. J Vasc Intervent Radiol 2003; 14:291–301.
18. Moura A, Yamada A, Hauer D et al. Salmarium-153 for intravascular irradiation therapy with liquid-filled balloons to prevent restenosis: acute and long-term results in a hypercholesterolemic rabbit restenosis model. Cardiovasc Radiat Med 2001; 2:69–74.
19. Albierio R, Adamian M, Kobayashi N et al. Short and intermediate-term results of P-32 radioactive beta-emitting stent implantation in patients with coronary artery disease: the Milan dose–response study. Circulation 2000; 10:18–26.
20. Waksman R, Laird JR, Jurkovitz CT et al. Intravascular radiation therapy after balloon angioplasty of narrowed femoropopliteal arteries to prevent restenosis: results of the PARIS feasibility clinical trial. J Vasc Intervent Radiol 2001; 12:915–21.
21. Krueger K, Landwehr P, Bendel M et al. Endovascular gamma irradiation of femoropopliteal de novo stenoses immediately after PTA: interim results of prospective randomised controlled trials. Radiology 2002; 224:519–28.
22. Hoffer EK, Bloch RD. Percutaneous arterial closure devices. J Vasc Intervent Radiol 2003; 14:865–85.
23. Zaman SM, de Vroos Meiring P, Gandhi MR, Gaines PA. The pharmacokinetics and UK usage of heparin in vascular intervention. Clin Radiol 1996; 51:113–16.
24. Stavropoulos SW, Solomon JA, Soulen MC et al. Use of abciximab during infrainguinal peripheral vascular interventions: initial experience. Radiology 2003; 227:657–61.
25. Bolia A, Miles K, Brennan J, Bell P. Percutaneous transluminal angioplasty of occlusions of the femoral and popliteal arteries by subintimal dissection. Cardiovasc Intervent Radiol 1990; 13:357–63.
26. Reekers J, Kroumhout J, Jacobs M. Percutaneous intentional extraluminal recanalisation of the femoropopliteal artery. Eur J Vasc Surg 1994; 8:723–38.
27. Gaines PA, Cumberland DC. 'Wire-loop' technique for the angioplasty of total iliac occlusions. Radiology 1989; 168:275–6.
28. London NJM, Varty K, Sayers RD et al. Percutaneous transluminal angioplasty for lower-limb critical ischaemia. Br J Surg 1995; 82:1232–5.
29. Wolf GL, Wilson SE, Cross AP et al. Surgery or balloon angioplasty for peripheral vascular disease: a randomised trial. J Vasc Intervent Radiol 1993; 4:639–48.
30. Bolia A, Sayers R, Thompson M, Bell P. Subintimal and intraluminal recanalisation of occluded crural arteries by percutaneous balloon angioplasty. Eur J Vasc Surg 1994; 8:214–19.
31. Blum U, Krumme B, Flugel P et al. Treatment of ostial renal-artery stenosis with vascular endoprostheses after unsuccessful balloon angioplasty. N Engl J Med 1997; 336:459–65.
32. Van de Ven PJG, Kaatee R, Beutler JJ et al. Arterial stenting and balloon angioplasty in ostial atherosclerotic renovascular disease: a randomised trial. Lancet 1999; 353:282–6.
33. Gardiner GA, Meyerovitz MF, Stokes KR et al. Complications of transluminal angioplasty. Radiology 1986; 159:201–8.
34. Belli AM, Cumberland DC, Knox AM et al. Complications of transluminal angioplasty. Clin Radiol 1990; 41:380–3.
35. Fellmeth BD, Roberts AC, Bookstein JJ et al. Postangiographic femoral artery injuries: nonsurgical repair with US-guided compression. Radiology 1991; 178:671–5.
36. Liau C-S, Ho F-M, Chen M-F et al. Treatment of iatrogenic femoral artery pseudoaneurysms with percutaneous thrombin injection. J Vasc Surg 1997; 26:18–23.
37. Kang SS, Labropoulos N, Mansour M et al. Percutaneous guided thrombin injection: a new method for treating postcatheterisation femoral pseudoaneurysms. J Vasc Surg 1998; 27:1032–8.
38. Lois JF, Takiff H, Schechter MS et al. Vessel rupture by balloon catheters complicating chronic steroid therapy. Am J Roentgenol 1985; 144:276–9.
39. Joseph N, Levy E, Lipman S. Angioplasty related iliac artery rupture: treatment by temporary balloon occlusion. Cardiovasc Intervent Radiol 1987; 10:276–9.
40. Sniderman K, Bodner L, Saddekni S, Srur M, Sos T. Percutaneous embolectomy by transcatheter aspiration. Radiology 1984; 150:357–61.
41. Cleveland TJ, Cumberland DC, Gaines PA. Percutaneous aspiration thromboembolectomy to manage the embolic complications of angioplasty and as an adjunct to thrombolysis. Clin Radiol 1994; 49:549–52.

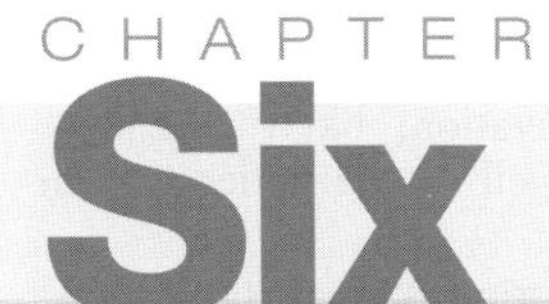

Amputation, rehabilitation and prosthetic developments

Dipak Datta and
Gillian Atkinson

INTRODUCTION

In some patients with lower limb ischaemia, amputation seems the best option. This may be because revascularisation appears impracticable or unjustified, or because it has not succeeded. Amputation should not be regarded as 'failure' of treatment but should be seen by patients as well as clinicians as a positive procedure. Amputation should achieve relief of symptoms, remove dead or severely ischaemic or infected tissue, as well as restore function and quality of life. This is true even for the patients who may not be able to return to functional walking with prostheses.

The planning and process of rehabilitation of amputees should start prior to amputation and continue into the community. Expert and holistic assessment of the patient leading to careful selection of the level of amputation, good surgical technique and optimal postoperative management are all vital in the initial stage of amputee rehabilitation. The process then dovetails into postamputation early rehabilitation, e.g. use of early walking aids, wheelchair and home assessments, prosthetic rehabilitation where appropriate, and continuing follow-up and support to patients and their families in the community.

This chapter concentrates on the rehabilitation of patients undergoing amputation because of lower limb ischaemia, although the principles involved are similar to amputations due to other causes.

EPIDEMIOLOGY

Peripheral arterial occlusive disease accounts for the vast majority of lower limb amputations in westernised societies. More than 80% of all amputations carried out in the UK are said to be due to vascular causes, of which 20–30% are due to diabetes mellitus.[1] The overall risk of amputation is six times higher in insulin-dependent diabetics compared with non-insulin-dependent diabetics. A global study group reported a marked difference in the incidence of amputation between ten centres in six different countries. Rates were highest in the North American and northern European centre and lowest in Spain, Taiwan and Japan. In the Navajo population, a very high prevalence of diabetes was thought to be the explanation for their high amputation rates.[2]

The National Amputee Statistical Data Base for the UK reported that in 70% of cases of lower limb amputees referred to the prosthetic services centre in 2001/2002, dysvascularity was the stated cause.[3] The prevalence of limb loss and incidence of amputation are difficult to estimate in the UK as data collection is incomplete. It is estimated that in the UK approximately 10 000 amputations are performed per annum.[4] The annual incidence of critical limb ischaemia is 500–1000 per million population and up to one-quarter of these patients undergo major amputations.[5]

There is some evidence that the impact of modern vascular surgery may reduce the incidence of amputation.[6] The Danish National Amputation Register has demonstrated a 27% fall in the number of major amputations due to peripheral vascular disease in the decade 1980–90. This decline was attributed to the increased use of (distal) bypass operations.[7] A paper from Finland also reported that it was possible to reduce amputation rates with an aggressive reconstruction policy in critical limb ischaemia.[8] However, the West Coast Vascular Surgeons Study Group in Sweden failed to demonstrate a negative correlation between amputation and revascularisation rates.[9]

It has been quoted that 30% of vascular amputees may be expected to lose the opposite leg within 2 years and 50% to die within 5 years.[10,11] In a more recent study in Scotland, the overall survival of patients who had an amputation as a result of peripheral vascular disease was found to be 4 years. Survival was significantly lower in patients with diabetes mellitus (3 years 8 months) than in those without diabetes (4 years 2 months). In this study, analysis of two 10-year cohorts of amputees indicates that survival is improving.[12]

INDICATIONS FOR AMPUTATION

The decision to perform amputation seems straightforward where there is extensive tissue loss or no reasonable prospect of revascularisation. However, the precise role of amputation in the management of critical limb ischaemia remains controversial. If it is predicted that vascular reconstruction is likely to be unsuccessful, then primary amputation perhaps offers the best outcome in terms of quality of life and cost–benefit.[13] (Chapter 3 discusses the treatment of chronic lower limb ischaemia and covers these issues of economics and quality of life in more detail.) Where patients with critical limb ischaemia also have coexisting disabilities or other medical conditions that would render them unable to make use of a salvageable limb, then primary amputation and appropriate rehabilitation offers the best option. Examples of such patients include those with severe dementia, dense hemiplegia or spinal paralysis, severe arthritis and severe cardiorespiratory disease.

LEVEL SELECTION

Selection of the ideal level of amputation depends on the healing potential, rehabilitation potential and prosthetic considerations. The potential for rehabilitation and likely goals can only be set by a full holistic assessment of the patient by the specialist amputee rehabilitation team. This assessment should include other illnesses and disabilities, cognitive state and motivation, likely discharge destination, lifestyle, as well as the patient's own aspirations and wishes.

In general terms, the more proximal the level of amputation, the more difficult it will be for the patient to achieve independent walking. Therefore the more distal the amputation site, the better the rehabilitation potential for walking, as this provides longer stump length and preserves more joints and hence more control of the prosthesis. **Figure 6.1** is an algorithm dealing with level selection.

Except in diabetics with good foot pulses (see Chapter 7), amputation of single or multiple toes generally does not heal unless the foot can be revascularised. Transmetatarsal or ray amputation, if technically feasible, produces excellent functional results. Chopart's mid-tarsal amputation and Symes' through-ankle amputation are rare in chronic limb ischaemia and are not recommended because of the risks of developing equinus deformity (in Chopart's), movement of the distal flap (in Symes'), poor long-term flap viability and considerable technical difficulties in prosthetic fitting. Thus, the commonest major levels of amputation in limb ischaemia are transtibial, knee disarticulation, Gritti–Stokes and transfemoral. Hip disarticulation and hindquarter amputation are rare and in 2001–02 accounted for just over 1% of all cases of lower limb amputations referred to the prosthetic centres in the UK. Dysvascularity was given as the cause for these levels of amputation in only 18% of cases.[3]

Preservation of the knee joint has enormous advantages in terms of mobility. In one study, 80% of transtibial amputees achieved unlimited household mobility or better compared with 40% of above-knee amputees.[14] In a Sheffield study, only 26% of transfemoral vascular amputees achieved community ambulation compared with 50% of transtibial vascular amputees at 1-year follow-up of a group of amputees who underwent prosthetic rehabilitation. In this study group, the figures for household mobility were 48% and 63% respectively for transfemoral and transtibial vascular amputees at 1-year follow-up.[15]

Transcutaneous oximetry ($tcPO_2$),[16] photoplethysmography,[17] laser Doppler velocimetry,[18] thermography[19] and isotope clearance rates[20] have all been shown to correlate with subsequent stump healing. However, while all these methods seem superior to Doppler ankle pressures,[21] a review concluded that sensitivities and specificities were inadequate to recommend their clinical use.[22]

The energy cost of walking with prostheses for vascular amputees is increased by 63% and 117% respectively in unilateral transtibial and transfemoral amputees compared with non-amputees. In bilateral transfemoral amputees, it is calculated that

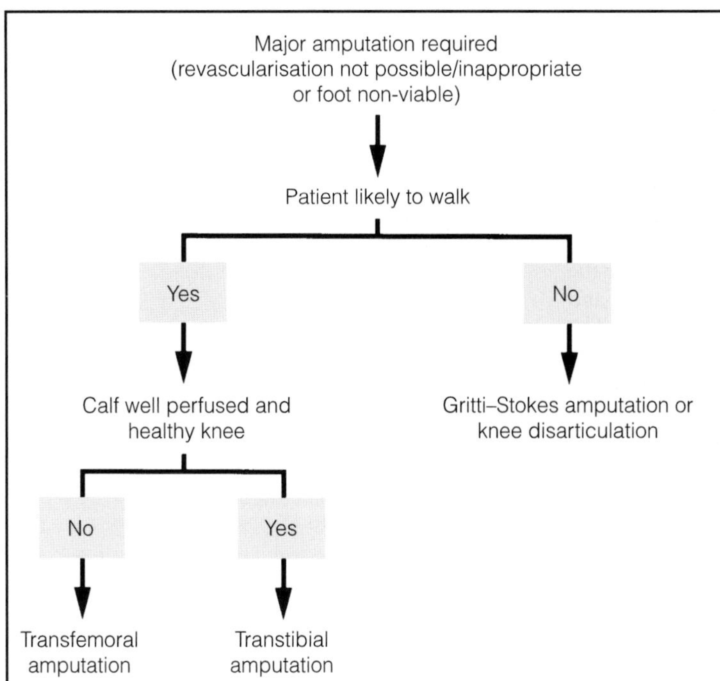

Figure 6.1 • Algorithm for the selection of amputation level.

energy cost is 280% higher.[23] Therefore, it should not seem surprising that even in a selected group of bilateral transfemoral amputees who were successfully trained to walk with prostheses in an inpatient rehabilitation facility, the majority of them abandoned walking when they returned home and preferred to be wheelchair-dependent.[24]

Thus, for patients in whom major lower limb amputations are necessary, the following points should be remembered.

- Preserve the knee joint whenever possible if it is anticipated that the patient has the potential to achieve prosthetic walking or has the potential to use a prosthetic limb for assisting transfers from chair, bed, etc.
- In patients likely to remain chair- or bed-bound following amputation, a transtibial amputation risks non-healing and may become a hindrance to transfers if flexion contractures of the knee and hip joints develop. In such patients, knee disarticulation or Gritti–Stokes amputation seems a better option.
- Where there is a fixed knee flexion deformity of 35° or more, satisfactory fitting of a prosthesis is not possible. In such cases, a more proximal amputation should be undertaken.
- For patients likely to remain wheelchair- or bed-bound, including bilateral amputees, knee disarticulation or Gritti–Stokes amputation is preferable to transfemoral or transtibial as longer lever lengths and larger surface area are more conducive to transferring and provide a much better seating balance.
- In patients where a transtibial amputation is not possible but the patient has the potential to walk, most amputee rehabilitation units prefer a transfemoral rather than knee disarticulation or Gritti–Stokes amputation. This is because of problems of prosthetic fitting compromising cosmetic appearance and function.

SURGICAL CONSIDERATIONS

All amputations should be carried out by surgeons experienced in the procedure and should not be delegated to unsupervised and inexperienced junior staff. The following important general principles should be followed.

- Tissues must be handled with care.
- Flaps should be oversized initially and then shaped and trimmed as required.
- Good-quality sensate skin coverage of stump without tension.
- Bone edges should be smoothed off and bevelled.

- Skin and muscle flaps should be trimmed and shaped to prevent dog ears, redundant tissue or a bulbous stump.
- Creating the correct shape of the stump is the responsibility of the surgeon at the time of surgery.

Transfemoral amputation

Ensure adequate muscle (myoplastic) cover over the cut end of femur to prevent pain and discomfort and allow balanced action of flexors and extensors.[25] The technique of myodesis, where drill holes are made in the bone to fix muscles, may not be applicable in ischaemic limbs due to poor tissue quality. However, this minimises the risk of the muscles slipping off the end of the femur. The myoplasty and myodesis need to be performed with the hip joint in the neutral and naturally adducted position.

Allow at least 12 cm of clearance from distal end of stump to knee joint level in order to allow space for incorporating a prosthetic knee joint. The exact level of bone section will depend on thickness of the myoplasty and subcutaneous tissue. This will prevent the unacceptable cosmetic and functional disability of a lowered knee centre in the prosthetic limb.

Gritti–Stokes and through-knee amputation

These seem useful options for patients in whom transtibial amputation will not heal and who are deemed incapable of walking.[26] The longer stump assists transfers and sitting balance and maintains muscle attachment and proprioception. Limitations in prosthetic fitting due to a lowered knee centre, and limited availability of stance and swing phase control mechanism in the prosthetic knee joint at this level, make these procedures unpopular with prosthetists, although good ambulation can be achieved.[27]

In the Gritti–Stokes amputation, the femoral condyles are removed to avoid a bulbous stump. Adequate fixation of patella is vital as a mobile and non-united patella prevents end bearing. In the modified Gritti–Stokes amputation there is a long anterior semicircular flap, which transects the patellar tendon to enter the knee joint. The patella is then retracted and the femur divided just above the condyles at a 30° backward angle. This makes the patella lock over the end of the femur once the articular surface has been removed (**Fig. 6.2**).

In the through-knee amputation, mediolateral flaps should be devised to allow the scar to retract into the condylar notch away from the end-bearing area. The bulbous end of the stump may make fitting and cosmesis of a prosthesis unacceptable.

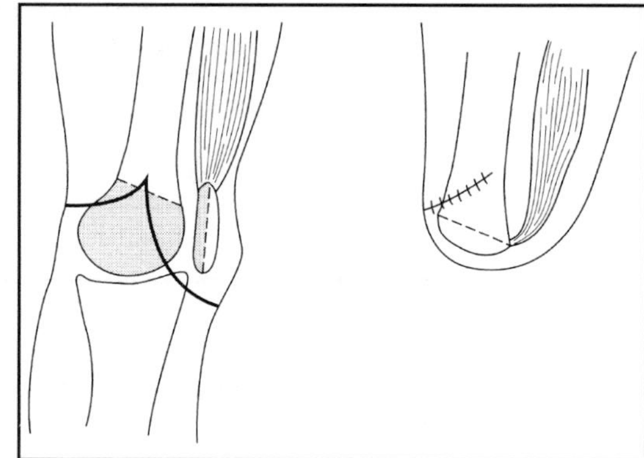

Figure 6.2 • Transection of the femur with a backward angle results in a more stable attachment of the patella in the modified Gritti–Stokes amputation.

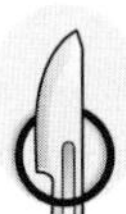

A randomised study of through-knee versus Gritti–Stokes amputation has reported poorer healing rates with the former as a result of synovial fluid leakage.[28]

Transtibial amputation

Many surgeons favour the skew flap technique[29] rather than the traditional Burgess long posterior flap.[30] In the skew flap technique, the flaps are based on the arteries that run with the long and short saphenous veins, which provide the main blood supply to the skin. In a small study of posterior flap and skew flap techniques, evaluation of flap hypoxia demonstrated that the posterior flap was associated with greater and more persistent reduction in tc$P\text{O}_2$.[31]

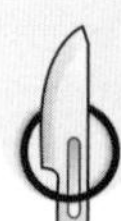

Randomised trials have shown no difference in healing between the skew flap and traditional Burgess long posterior flap.[32] However, the time to limb-fitting and early mobility was shorter in the skew flap group due to a less bulbous stump (**Fig. 6.3**).

The Burgess amputation still seems useful when skew flaps might be compromised by the medial skin incision of a failed femoro-distal bypass graft or following fasciotomies.

A tibial section at about 15 cm is considered ideal. The fibula should be divided around 1.5 cm proximal to the level of the tibial section. A short bevel and rounding off the sharp corners of the tibia must be undertaken. Much shorter transtibial stumps (up to 8 cm), though not ideal, can be fitted with supracondylar or ICEROSS sockets. Avoidance of a bulbous distal end of stump is vital for this level of amputation.

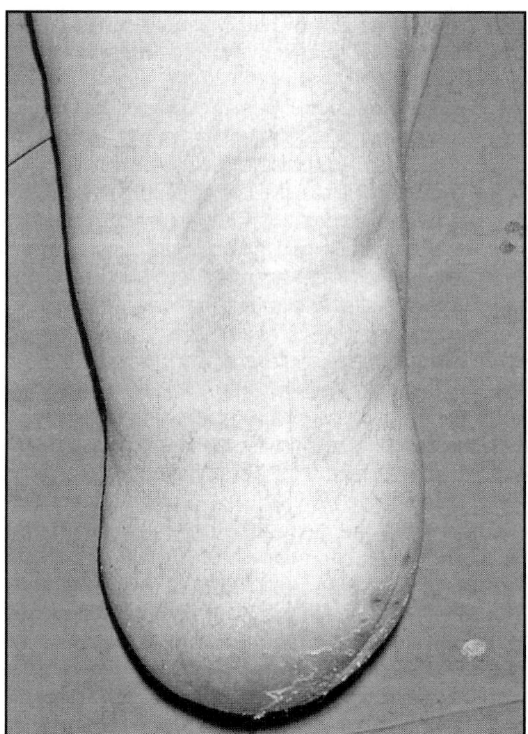

Figure 6.3 • Skew flap transtibial amputation at 1 week showing a nicely shaped stump suitable for early limb-fitting.

Foot amputation

Digital amputation is most commonly performed in diabetics because of their susceptibility to infection. In general, a digital amputation will only heal if foot pulses are present or can be restored. Therefore it is better to leave toes with partial dry gangrene alone. Amputation is best performed through the base of the proximal phalanx, leaving the wound open to heal by secondary intention. When infection extends beyond the proximal phalanx, a 'ray amputation' is indicated, especially in diabetics. After excision of the relevant toes, the line of excision is carried back through the infected tissue until healthy tissue is reached. The underlying metatarsal head is excised and the wound left open like a 'fish mouth'.

Infection of the first or fifth metatarsophalangeal joint requires a 'tennis-racquet' incision; the handle of the racquet can usually be closed after excision of the metatarsal head. A transmetatarsal amputation can be useful when all the toes are gangrenous but when the plantar skin is still viable. A dorsal skin incision is made at mid-metatarsal level with a long plantar flap and bone transection through the metatarsal bases. As much soft tissue as possible should be preserved and the flaps left open with delayed closure, as infection and gangrene of the flaps may occur if primary closure is attempted. Vacuum-assisted closure systems may facilitate the healing of such open foot amputations.

REHABILITATION

The process of rehabilitation for vascular amputees, who are usually elderly and often have a number of other concurrent disabilities and illnesses, can pose a considerable challenge. A 'team approach' in amputee rehabilitation is gaining popularity and has been shown to be cost-effective.[33] The core members of the team should include a vascular surgeon, a specialist in rehabilitation medicine, specialist physiotherapist and occupational therapist, and a prosthetist. Ready availability of a social worker, a community nurse, a clinical psychologist and a chiropodist is invaluable. Other multidisciplinary team members include wheelchair personnel, housing and adaptation officers, social services and orthotists. Close liaison and cooperation between all members of the team are vital. Counsellors and amputee volunteers, if available, can be extremely valuable. The British Society of Rehabilitation Medicine has recently updated and published standards and guidelines in amputee and prosthetic rehabilitation based on national consensus.[34]

In smaller district general hospitals where fewer amputations are carried out, it is not practical to develop such a multidisciplinary team. In such situations an experienced senior physiotherapist specialising in amputee rehabilitation should be given the coordinating role with the surgical team, liaising closely with the nearest regional or sub-regional amputee rehabilitation centre.

Planning

A pre-amputation consultation by specialists in rehabilitation medicine and their team is ideal but impractical for every patient for whom an amputation is planned. However, a member of the amputee rehabilitation team (usually a therapist) should see all patients prior to amputation in order to make an initial assessment and prepare the patient for the likely programme to be implemented, instil realistic expectations and resolve any specific questions or anxieties. Other members of the multidisciplinary team may be involved at this stage if specially required. In our unit, specialist physiotherapists cover the boundary between the vascular and rehabilitation units and we find that this works extremely effectively. In cases where amputation is a treatment option rather than a necessity, and in situations where there is some uncertainty regarding level selection, we recommend that the surgical team obtain advice from an appropriate consultant in rehabilitation medicine.

Stump management

Tight or elasticated stump bandaging should not be used in vascular amputees as it can generate unacceptable pressures and cause tissue breakdown.[35] Rigid dressings of plaster of Paris are not generally used for vascular amputees in the UK, although some studies have suggested that they reduce the knee contracture rate following transtibial amputation. Adhesive clear-plastic film dressing applied postoperatively can be very useful as this allows easier and regular wound inspection. This type of dressing makes life easier for the physiotherapist when inspecting wounds before and after application of early walking aids. Where a more conventional dressing for the wound is required, an elasticated tubular bandage (e.g. Tubifast) is usually placed on the stump to hold these dressings in place. If the wound is healed or healing satisfactorily, then elasticated and graduated pressure stump shrinker socks (e.g. Juzo) are applied to the stump about 2–3 weeks postoperatively to control postoperative oedema. Appropriate stump supports are fitted to the wheelchair so that the patients can keep their below-knee stumps elevated. Sometimes appropriate stump supports may also be necessary for long transfemoral or knee disarticulation stumps. Appropriate and specialist footwear to protect the other leg from damage by the wheelchair may be an important consideration. In our centre we find pressure-relieving ankle foot orthoses effective for this purpose and also relieve pressure on the heel whilst lying down.

Pain management

Controlling stump and phantom pains is vital for the patient to participate successfully in a rehabilitation programme. Houghton et al.[36] found a significant relationship between pre-amputation pain and phantom pain in the first 2 years after amputation in vascular amputees. Nikolajsen et al.[37] in a study of mostly vascular amputees found a relationship between preoperative pain and incidents of phantom pain at 1 week and 3 months after amputation, but not after 6 months. Early involvement of the 'pain team' in appropriate cases is most beneficial. Numerous medical interventions have been proposed over the years but tricyclic antidepressants and sodium channel blockers are currently considered to be the drugs of choice for neuropathic pain.[38] The anticonvulsant carbamazepine, a non-specific sodium channel blocker, has been reported to be effective in phantom pain.[39,40]

In a randomised, double-blind, placebo-controlled, crossover study of 19 patients, gabapentin monotherapy was better than placebo in relieving postamputation phantom limb pain.[41] In a randomized study of 25 patients undergoing amputation, Bach et al. established that incidents of phantom pain were reduced 6 months after amputation but not after 1 week or after 12 months in the group receiving epidural analgesia for 72 hours prior to amputation compared with a controlled group.[42] In a blinded and placebo-controlled trial of 60 patients who received epidural analgesia for 1 day before amputation, it was concluded that it is not possible to prevent phantom pain by an epidural block of short duration.[43]

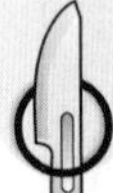

In addition to the medical treatment of stump and phantom pains, various non-invasive treatments such as transcutaneous electrical nerve stimulation, vibration therapy, acupuncture, hypnosis and biofeedback can prove useful, although evidence of efficacy is limited.

Early rehabilitation

The occupational therapist and physiotherapist should work closely together to ensure an effective and timely rehabilitation programme. Following amputation the physiotherapist usually sees the amputee on the first postoperative day and will begin a programme of bed mobility, joint movements, transferring and wheelchair mobility, depending on the patient's general condition and pain control. Stump exercises, exercises for the remaining limb and upper limbs, muscle strengthening, maintaining range of movements of the proximal joints, sitting balance and improvement of general cardiovascular fitness will all be incorporated into the programme. Each amputee will be assessed for an appropriate wheelchair and cushion as early as possible to facilitate discharge. The amputee will be taught the skills necessary for independent use of the wheelchair. By around the 1-week assessment, the therapist is usually reasonably sure of a patient's potential ability to use a prosthesis or not; however, some amputees are too unwell at the early postoperative stage but later may recover sufficiently to benefit from prosthetic rehabilitation. Therefore appropriate follow-up assessment may need to be arranged for this group of amputees.

Extreme frailty, severe dementia, severe cardiorespiratory disease, gross fixed flexion contractures and severe arthritis are contraindications to prosthetic rehabilitation. It is generally the practice in our unit to guide elderly bilateral vascular transfemoral amputees away from prosthetic rehabilitation.

Assessing the home environment and adaptations, advice regarding driving, hobbies and employment also need addressing as an integral part of the rehabilitation.

Primary prosthetic rehabilitation

All amputees who receive a prosthesis should undergo prosthetic rehabilitation to achieve the best prosthetic outcome. The physiotherapist will play a key role in this. Prosthetic rehabilitation should aim to establish an energy-efficient gait based on normal physiological walking patterns. The physiotherapist should teach efficient control of the prosthesis through postural control, weight transference, use of proprioception, and specific muscle strengthening and stretching exercises to prevent and correct gait deviations. Prosthetic rehabilitation will work towards the individual's own realistic goals, and should include functional activities relevant to that person and his or her lifestyle. All encouragement should be given to enable the individual to resume hobbies, sports, social activities, driving and return to work. The British Association of Chartered Physiotherapists in Amputee Rehabilitation have published useful evidence-based clinical guidelines for the physiotherapy of adults with lower limb prostheses.[44]

PROSTHESES

There are three main types of early walking aids used in the UK (**Figs 6.4** and **6.5**). The best known is the pneumatic post-amputation mobility aid (PPAM Aid). The PPAM Aid is widely used and can be used for transtibial, through-knee and transfemoral levels of amputation. The amputee mobility aid (AMA) is designed for transtibial amputation only, and allows amputees to flex and extend their knee during the gait cycle. It also has a foot rather than a rocker end, allowing a more natural gait. The Femurette is an excellent early walking aid for transfemoral amputees; it mimics a definitive transfemoral prosthesis in terms of ischial tuberosity-bearing socket configuration and knee joint and it also has a foot.[45] The early walking aids are excellent morale boosters and are also used as assessment tools to estimate an amputee's potential for walking. They allow stump desensitisation, assist in reduction of stump oedema and may promote wound healing, and allow re-education of postural reflexes, balance and gait. The early walking aids should be considered around 1 week after

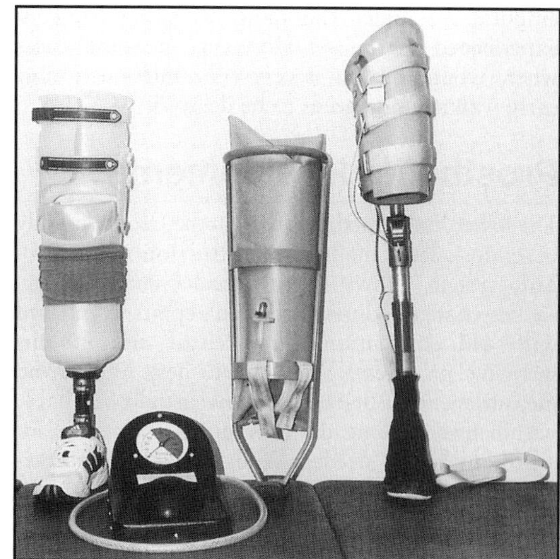

Figure 6.4 • A selection of early walking aids. From left to right: amputee mobility aid (AMA); pneumatic post-amputation mobility aid (PPAM Aid); Femurette. A foot pump to inflate the AMA and PPAM Aid is also shown.

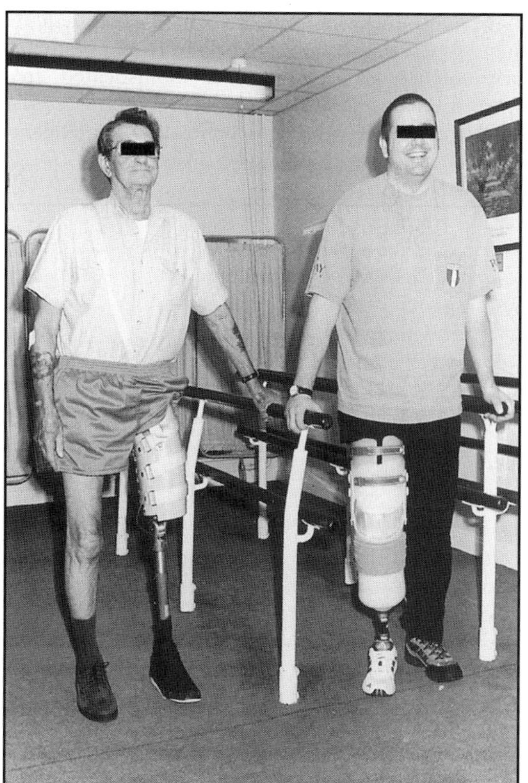

Figure 6.5 • A patient wearing Femurette (left) and a patient wearing AMA (right).

amputation, under the judicious supervision of experienced therapists. However, in some cases where wound healing is very poor, introduction of early walking aids needs to be delayed.

Prosthetic developments

The lower limb prostheses used in the UK are mainly of endoskeletal modular construction (**Fig. 6.6**). This system allows much speedier manufacture, socket change, adjustments and repairs compared with old conventional exoskeletal and labour-intensive prostheses. A complete new limb, from measurement to delivery, is now usually available within five working days for primary patients, or even quicker if needed. The modern prostheses usually incorporate thermoplastic materials like polypropylene or laminated plastics as socket materials and carbon fibre or lightweight alloy for fabrication of the weight-bearing structures.

Usually, vascular amputees are measured for their first prosthesis at about 6–8 weeks from amputation, although earlier fitting can take place subject to wound healing status and the general condition of the stump. It is not imperative that the stump be completely healed before a prosthesis can be provided.

Younger vascular transfemoral amputees may have good musculature of the stump and adequate hand function and agility to benefit from prostheses with suction socket fitting and sophisticated 'free knee' mechanisms like pneumatic or hydraulic swing phase controls. Microchip-controlled 'intelligent' knee joints providing improved swing phase control are used to some benefit for transfemoral amputees, but experience so far has been generally limited to younger and more active amputees.[46] In the UK, most elderly and dysvascular transfemoral amputees, if they are accepted for a prosthetic rehabilitation programme, are provided with non-suction prostheses with some form of waist-belt suspension and a 'locked' knee (bends only to sit down).

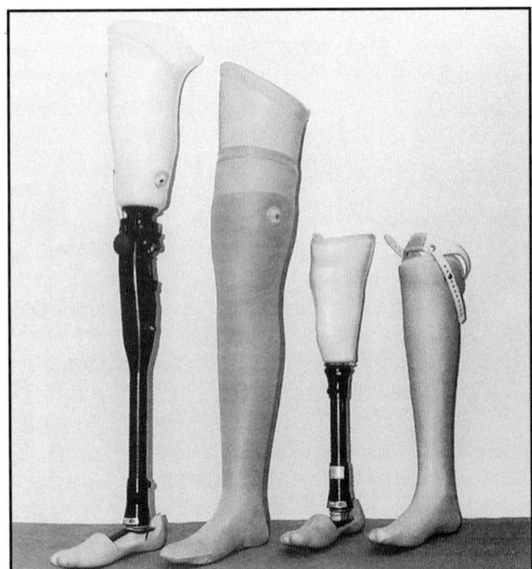

Figure 6.6 • Modular endoskeletal prostheses for transfemoral and transtibial amputation, with and without cosmetic covers.

For knee disarticulation, Gritti–Stokes or long transfemoral amputees, prosthetic options are limited. Use of polycentric knee joints like four-bar linkage knee mechanisms have eased some of the difficulties, though prostheses at these levels still create cosmetic as well as functional difficulties.

For transtibial amputees the introduction of the ICEROSS prosthesis has found favour with some patients as it provides much improved suspension as well as reducing friction and shear forces at the stump–socket interface[47] (**Fig. 6.7**). This type of prosthesis uses a silicone sleeve directly on the stump, which is then locked into the prosthetic socket. Much shorter transtibial amputation stumps can now be fitted successfully, which was not possible previously with the traditional patellar tendon-bearing prosthesis.

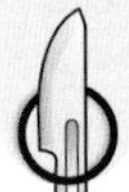

Direct casting of socket on the amputation stump using the pressure-casting method of ICECAST has been available more recently. This type of socket and prostheses for transtibial amputation can be made much more speedily but it is considerably more expensive and has shown not to improve gait and only minor comfort preference in a randomized controlled study.[48]

Computer-aided socket design and manufacture are also being used more frequently in the UK, eliminating the need for plaster models.

Energy-saving prosthetic feet, e.g. Dynamic Response Foot (Blatchford), Flex Foot, Seattle Foot, are generally provided to younger active amputees (**Fig. 6.8**). They are more expensive than the usual uniaxial or multiaxial ankle joints and moulded foot provided for the vast majority of lower limb amputees. A patient-adjustable heel height device is available when shoes with different heel height are to be worn. Special components are also available and may be of benefit in appropriate cases, such as a torsion device and vertical shock absorber in the shin of a prosthesis that absorbs vertical forces and rotational torque, turntables that allow sitting cross-legged on the floor, or individually created highly life-like silicone cosmetic cover, swimming or shower legs. Selection of the prostheses and components will be determined by the amputee's wishes, realistic goals, progress in rehabilitation and ability to benefit from a prescribed device.

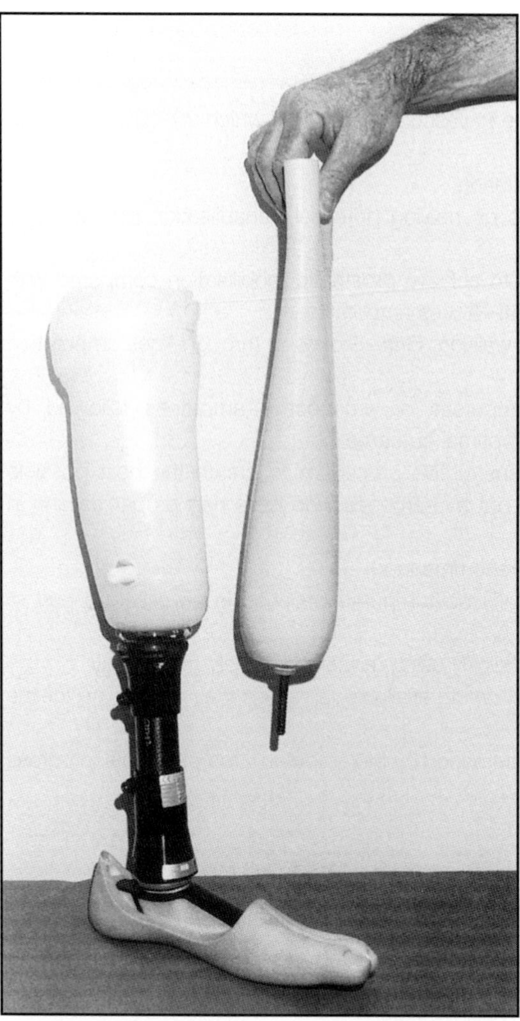

Figure 6.7 • ICEROSS below-knee prosthesis. The hand is holding the silicone liner, which is applied by rolling over the stump and then locked into the plastic socket.

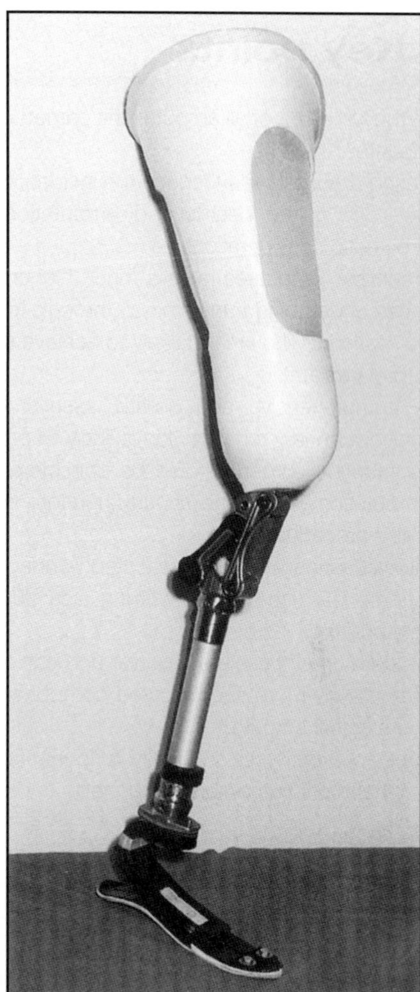

Figure 6.8 • A knee disarticulation prosthesis incorporating a four-bar linkage knee joint and a Flex Foot.

Key points

- In the UK, 80% of all amputations carried out are due to vascular disease, of which 20–30% are due to diabetes.
- Vascular surgery may reduce the incidence of amputation.
- Selection of the ideal level of amputation depends on healing potential, rehabilitation potential and prosthetic considerations.
- Transtibial amputees have a much higher potential to achieve prosthetic mobilisation compared with those undergoing transfemoral, through-knee or Gritti–Stokes amputation.
- For patients who are not likely to achieve prosthetic walking, Gritti–Stokes or through-knee amputation is preferable.
- A comprehensive and holistic assessment of amputees or prospective amputees followed by multidisciplinary rehabilitation is likely to provide the optimal outcome.
- Amputation surgery should be considered as a constructive procedure to create the best possible amputation stump and should therefore be carried out by surgeons who have had proper training in these procedures.
- Stump bandaging with elasticated bandages is not recommended.
- Appropriate use of early walking aids during the early postamputation period is an essential part of rehabilitation.
- Modern prostheses are modular and can be made quickly using modern materials technology.
- Increasingly more sophisticated components are becoming available, although they tend to be for the more active amputee.
- Types of prostheses and their components will be determined by the amputee's realistic goals, progress in rehabilitation and ability to benefit.

REFERENCES

1. Fyfe NCM. Amputation and rehabilitation. In: Davies AH, Beard JD, Wyatt MG (eds) Essential vascular surgery. London: WB Saunders, 1999; pp. 243–51.
2. The Global Lower Extremity Amputation Study Group. Epidemiology of lower extremity amputation in centres in Europe, North America and East Asia. Br J Surg 2000; 87:328–37.
3. Amputee Statistical Database for the United Kingdom 2001–02: Information and Statistic Division. Edinburgh: National Health Service Scotland, 2003.
4. Dormandy JA, Thomas PRS. What is the natural history of a critical ischaemic patient with and without his leg? In: Greenhalgh R, Jamieson CW, Nicolaides AN (eds) Limb salvage and amputation for vascular disease? Philadelphia: WB Saunders, 1988; pp. 11–26.
5. Price JF, Fowkes FGR. Epidemiology of peripheral vascular disease. In: Davies AH, Beard JD, Wyatt MG (eds) Essential vascular surgery. London: WB Saunders, 1999; pp. 18–30.
6. Gutteridge W, Torrie P, Galland R. Trends in arterial reconstruction, angioplasty and amputation. Health Trends 1994; 26:88–91.
7. Ebskov LB, Scroeder TV, Holstein PE. Epidemiology of leg amputation: the influence of vascular surgery. Br J Surg 1994; 81:1600–3.
8. Luther M. The influence of arterial reconstruction surgery on the outcome of critical leg ischaemia. Eur J Vasc Surg 1994; 8:682–9.
9. The West Coast Vascular Surgeons Study Group. Variations of rates of vascular surgical procedures for chronic critical limb ischaemia and lower limb amputation rates in Western Swedish counties. Eur J Vasc Endovasc Surg 1997; 14:310–14.
10. English AWG, Dean AAG. The Artificial Limb Service. Health Trends 1980; 12:77–82.
11. Couch NP, David JK, Tilney NL, Crane L. Natural history of the leg amputee. Am J Surg 1977; 133:469–73.
12. Stewart CPU, Jain AS, Ogden SA. Lower limb amputee survival. Prosthet Orthot Int 1992; 16:11–18.
13. Johnson B, Evans L, Datta D, Morris-Jones W, Beard JD. Surgery for limb threatening ischaemia. A reappraisal of costs and benefits. Eur J Vasc Endovasc Surg 1995; 9:181–8.
14. Houghton AD, Taylor PR, Thurlow S, Rootes E, McColl I. Success rates for rehabilitation of vascular amputees: implications for preoperative

assessment and amputation level. Br J Surg 1992; 79:753–5.

15. Davies B, Datta D. Mobility outcome following unilateral lower limb amputation. Prosthet Orthot Int 2003; 27:186–190.

16. Ratcliffe DA, Clyne CAC, Chant ADB, Webster JHH. Prediction of amputation wound healing: the role of transcutaneous pO_2 assessment. Br J Surg 1984; 71:219–22.

17. Van Den Broek TAA, Dwars BJ, Rauwerda JA, Bakker FC. Photoplethysmographic selection of amputation level in peripheral vascular disease. J Vasc Surg 1988; 8:10–13.

18. Karanfilian RG, Lynch TG, Zinsl VT et al. The value of laser Doppler velocimetry and transcutaneous oxygen tension determination in predicting healing of ischaemic forefoot ulcerations and amputations in diabetic and non-diabetic patients. J Vasc Surg 1986; 4:511–16.

19. Stoner HB, Taylor L, Marcuson RW. The value of skin temperature measurements in forecasting the healing of below-knee amputation for end-stage ischaemia of the leg in peripheral vascular disease. Eur J Vasc Surg 1989; 3:355–61.

20. Moore WS, Henry RE, Malone JM et al. Prospective use of xenon Xe-133 clearance for amputation level selection. Arch Surg 1981; 166:86–8.

21. Welch GH, Leiberman DP, Pollock JG, Angerson W. Failure of Doppler ankle pressure to predict healing of conservative forefoot amputations. Br J Surg 1985; 72:888–91.

22. Savin S, Sharni S, Shields DA, Scurr JH, Coleridge-Smith PD. Selection of amputation level: a review. Eur J Vasc Surg 1991; 5:611–20.

The authors reviewed the evidence for many tests (Doppler indices, segmental pressures, skin blood flow, skin perfusion pressure, $tcPo_2$, thermography) to predict the likelihood of successful healing of an amputation stump. They concluded that the foremost requirement to raise the below-knee/above-knee ratio is to promote awareness among surgeons of the value of medical management and encourage the use of routinely available tests such as ankle–brachial pressure index and Doppler segmental pressures. The value of more specialised tests remains to be established.

23. Huang CT, Jackson JR, Moore NB et al. Amputation: energy cost of ambulation. Arch Phys Med Rehabil 1979; 60:18–24.

24. Datta D, Nair PN, Payne J. Outcome of prosthetic management of bilateral lower limb amputees. Disability Rehab 1992; 14:98–102.

25. Chadwick SJD, Lewis JD. Above-knee amputation. Ann R Coll Surg Engl 1991; 73:152–4.

26. Dovan J, Hopkinson BE, Makin GS. The Gritti–Stokes amputation in ischaemia: a review of 134 cases. Br J Surg 1978; 65:135–6.

27. Houghton A, Allen A, Luff R, McColl I. Rehabilitation after lower limb amputation: a comparative study of above-knee and Gritti–Stokes amputations. Br J Surg 1989; 76:622–4.

28. Campbell WB, Morris PJ. A prospective, randomised comparison of healing in Gritti–Stokes and through-knee amputations. Ann R Coll Surg Engl 1986; 69:1–4.

In this study, 22 patients with a median age of 79 years had 24 amputations about knee joint level. The patients were randomised to undergo either Gritti–Stokes or through-knee amputation; 12 (75%) Gritti–Stokes amputations underwent uncomplicated primary healing compared with only 2 of 12 (17%) through-knee procedures (P = 0.04). Two through-knee amputations required revision to above the knee (17%), whereas all Gritti–Stokes amputations healed.

29. Robinson KP, Hoile R, Coddington T. Skew flap myoplastic below knee amputation: a preliminary report. Br J Surg 1992; 69:554–7.

30. Burgess EM. The below knee amputation. Bull Prosth Res 1968; 10:19–25.

31. Johnson WC, Watkins MT, Hamilton J, Baldwin D. Transcutaneous partial oxygen pressure changes following skew flap and Burgess-type below knee amputations. Arch Surg 1997; 132:261–3.

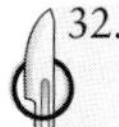

32. Ruckley CV, Stonebridge PA, Prescott RJ. Skewflap versus long posterior flap in below-knee amputations: multicenter trial. J Vasc Surg 1991; 13:423–7.

A multicentre trial of 191 patients with end-stage occlusive vascular disease needing transtibial amputation were randomised to skew flap technique in 98 and long posterior flap technique in 93 patients. The two groups were well matched: 30-day mortality rate, date of wound at 1 week and need for surgical revision at same or higher level were not statistically significant between the groups. Follow-up information at 6 months showed 64 (84%) of skew flaps and 50 (77%) of long posterior flaps were fitted with prostheses. Walking, alone or with support, was achieved in 59 (78%) and 46 (71%), respectively. None of these differences reached statistical significance.

33. Ham RO, Thornberry DJ, Regan JF et al. Rehabilitation of the vascular amputee: one method evaluated. Physiother Pract 1985; 1:6–13.

34. British Society of Rehabilitation Medicine. Amputee and prosthetic rehabilitation standards and guidelines, 2nd edn. Report of the Working Party (chair Hanspal, RS). London: British Society of Rehabilitation Medicine, 2003.

35. Isherwood PA, Robertson JC, Rossi A. Pressure measurements beneath below-knee stump bandages. Elastic bandaging, the Puddifoot dressing and a pneumatic bandaging technique compared. Br J Surg 1975; 62:982–6.

36. Houghton AD, Nicholls G, Houghton AL, Saadah E, McColl L. Phantom pain: natural history and association with rehabilitation. Ann R Coll Surg Engl 1994; 76:22–5.

37. Nikolajsen L, Ilkjaer S, Kroner K, Christensen JH, Jensen TS. The influence of preamputation pain on postamputation stump and phantom pain. Pain 1997; 72:393–405.

38. Nikolajsen L, Jensen TS. Phantom limb pain. Br J Anaesth 2001; 87:107–16.

39. Elliott F, Little A, Milbrandt W. Carbamazepine for phantom limb phenomena. N Engl J Med 1976; 295:678.

40. Patterson JF. Carbamazepine in the treatment of phantom limb pain. South Med J 1988; 81:1101–2.

41. Bone M, Critchley P, Buggy DJ. Gabapentin in postamputation phantom limb pain: a randomised, double-blind, placebo-controlled, cross-over study. Reg Anesth Pain Med 2002; 27:481–6.

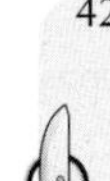

In this study, 17 patients attending a multidisciplinary pain clinic with phantom limb pain were randomised to a double-blind, placebo-controlled, crossover study. A daily dose of gabapentin was administered in increments of 300 mg to 2400 mg or the maximum tolerated dose. Fifteen patients completed both arms of the study. It was concluded that after 6 weeks, gabapentin monotherapy was better than placebo in relieving postamputation phantom pain. There were no significant differences in mood, sleep interference and activities of daily living.

42. Bach S, Norenz MF, Tjellden NU. Phantom limb pain in amputees during the first twelve months following limb amputation after pre-operative lumbar epidural seventy-two hours pre-operation. Pain 1988; 33:297–301.

The aim of this study was to investigate if it was possible to reduce postoperative phantom limb pain by lumbar epidural blockade (LEB) with bupivacaine and morphine for 72 hours prior to the operation. Twenty-five patients were interviewed about their limb pain before limb amputation and about their phantom limb pains 7 days, 6 months and 1 year after limb loss. Seven patients received LEB, so that they were pain-free 3 days prior to operation. The control group of 14 patients all had preoperative limb pain. After 6 months, all patients in the LEB group were pain-free, whereas five patients in the control group had pain ($P < 0.05$).

43. Nikolajsen L, Ilkjaer S, Kroner K, Christensen JH, Jensen TS. Randomized trial of epidural bupivacaine and morphine in prevention of neuropathic pain following amputation. Lancet 1997; 350:1353–7.

In a randomised double-blind trial, 60 patients scheduled for lower limb amputation were randomly assigned to epidural (bupivacaine and morphine) 18 hours before and during the operation (29 patients) or epidural saline and oral or intramuscular morphine (31 patients). All patients had general anaesthesia for the amputation and were asked about stump and phantom pain after 1 week and then at 3, 6 and 12 months. The authors concluded that perioperative epidural blockade did not prevent phantom or stump pain.

44. Broomhead P, Dawes D, Hale C et al. Evidence based clinical guidelines for physiotherapy management of adults with lower limb prostheses. London: Chartered Society of Physiotherapy, 2003.

45. Ramsay EM. A clinical evaluation of the LIC Femurette as an early training device for the primary above knee amputee. Physiotherapy 1988; 74:598–601.

46. Datta D, Howitt J. Conventional versus microchip controlled pneumatic swing-phase control for trans-femoral amputees. Prosthet Orthot Int 1998; 22:129–35.

47. Datta D, Vaidya S, Howitt J, Gopalan L. Outcome of fitting of ICEROSS prosthesis: views of trans-tibial amputees. Prosthet Orthot Int 1996; 20:111–15.

48. Datta D, Harris I, Heller B, Howitt J, Martin R. Gait cost and time implications for changing from PTB to ICEX® sockets. Prosthet Orthot Int 2004; 28:115–20.

In this study, 27 established transtibial amputees were randomised to be fitted with either a conventional patella tendon bearing socket by conventional plaster-casting methods (control) or were fitted with a new ICEX socket created directly on the patients' amputation stump by using air pressure (experimental). Twenty-one subjects completed the trial. No significant difference was found in the gait parameters in the two groups. ICEX prostheses were considerably more expensive, although they could be manufactured more quickly. Patients showed only minor comfort preference for ICEX prostheses.

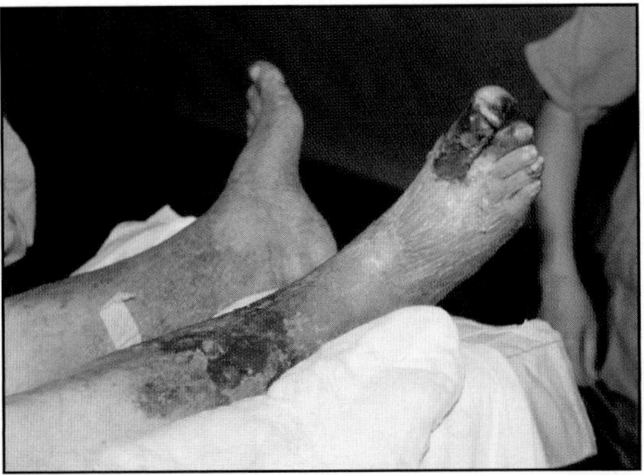

Plate 1 • Severe ischaemia over 3 months has resulted in gangrene of the great toe and ulceration of the venous type above the ankle as this man has been sleeping overnight in a chair.

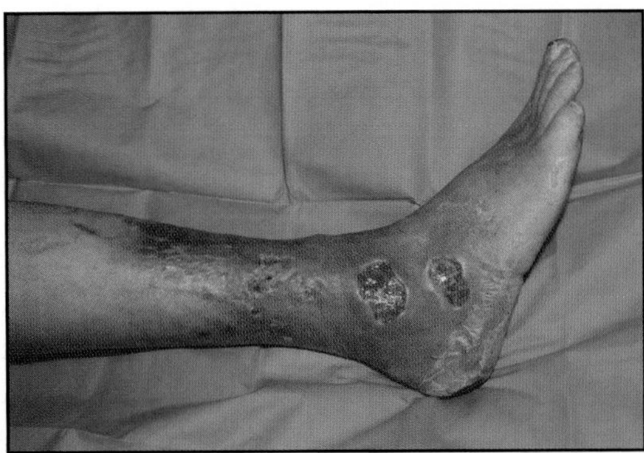

Plate 3 • Typical features of venous ulceration are apparent with pigmentation and lipodermatosclerosis. However, these atypical ulcers on the lateral aspect suggest mixed arterial and venous ulceration with an ankle pressure in this patient of only 65 mmHg (ABPI 0.4).

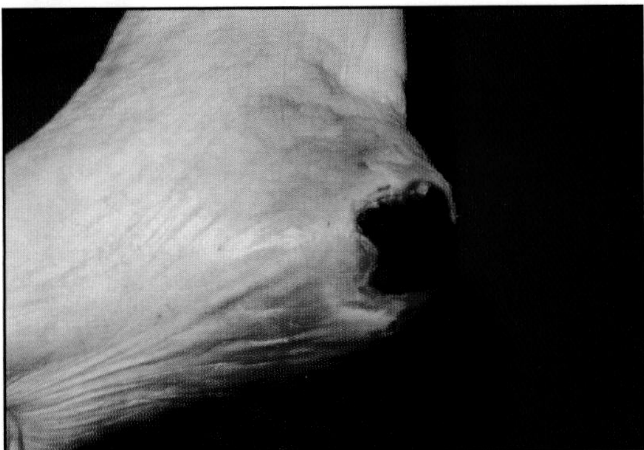

Plate 2 • Pressure necrosis of the type illustrated over this heel occurs easily in rest ischaemia of the foot, as tissue perfusion pressures are low and easily overwhelmed by compression within a shoe or against the mattress at night.

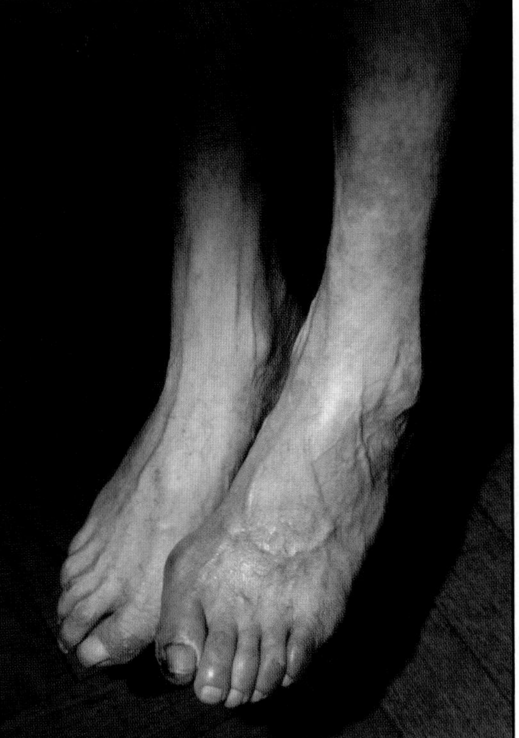

Plate 4 • There is profound vasodilatation of the toes and forefoot on the left typical of severe ischaemia. The appearances may be red or even cyanosed in dependency but on elevation this foot would become pale with venous guttering.

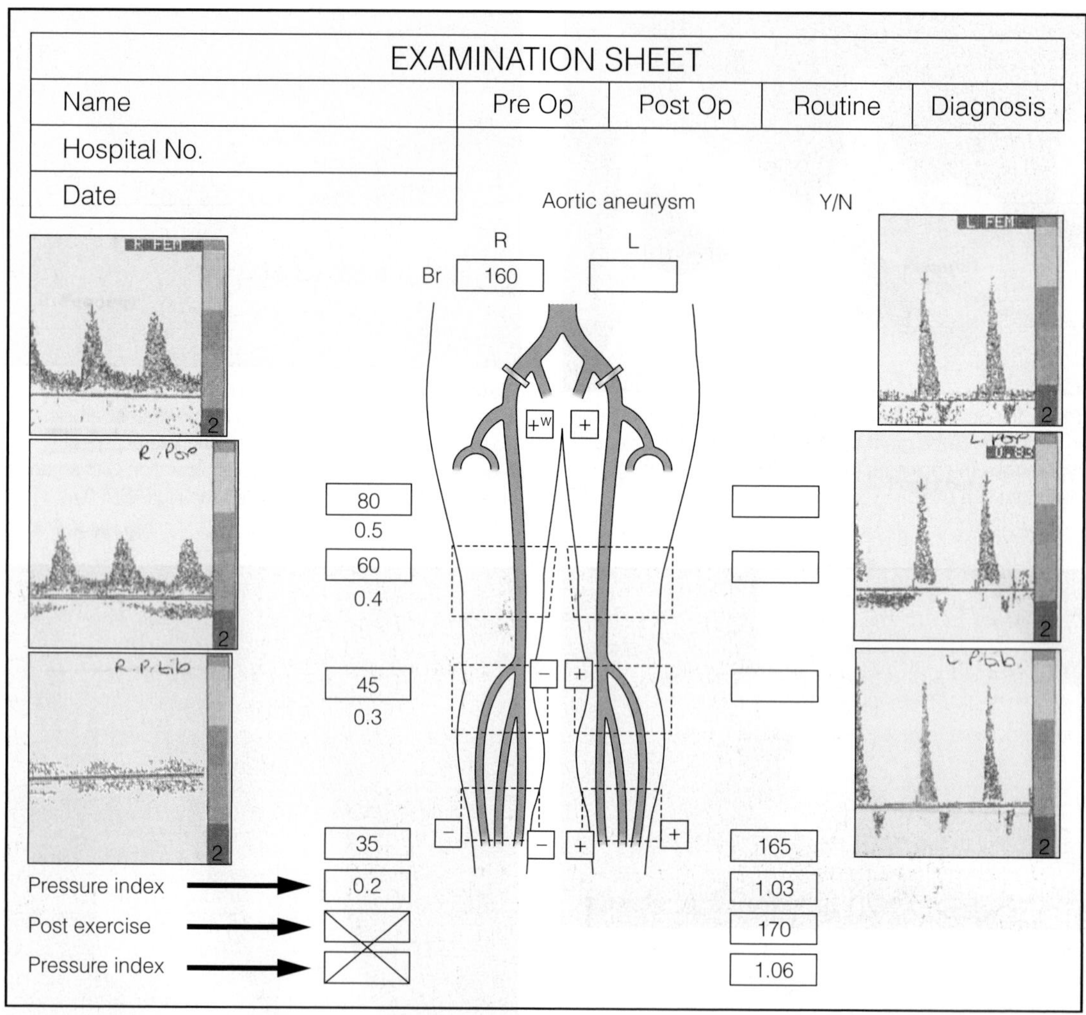

Plate 5 • Segmental arterial waveforms may help discriminate the functional significance of multisegment disease, such as the right iliac and superficial femoral occlusions in this patient. Theoretically, correcting the high thigh pressure to normal will approximately double the ankle arterial pressure to a level that should relieve ischaemic rest pain.

(a)

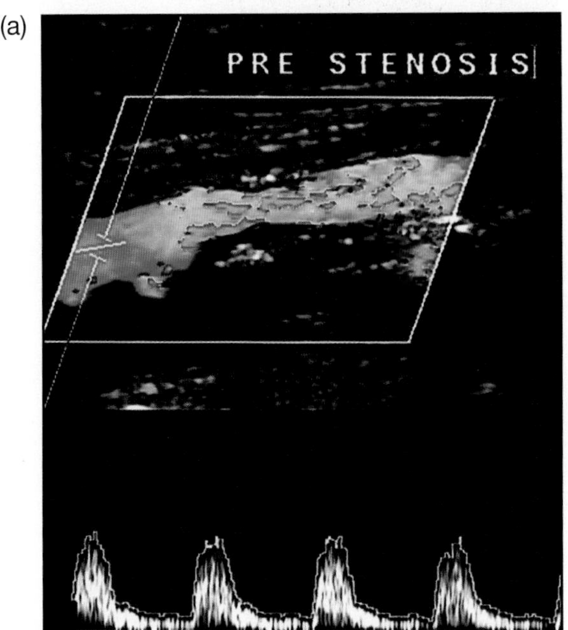

(b)

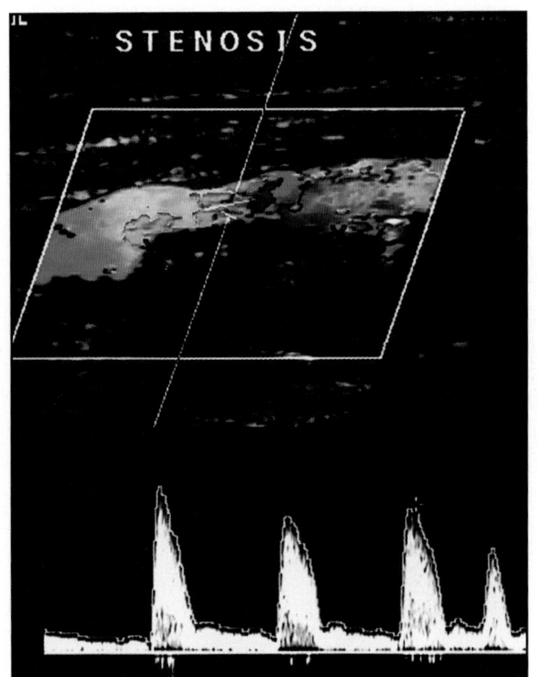

Plate 6 • Duplex imaging demonstrating the measurement of peak flow velocities **(a)** above and **(b)** within a stenosis allows the ratio of peak flow velocity to be calculated as an indication of the severity of stenosis.

(a)

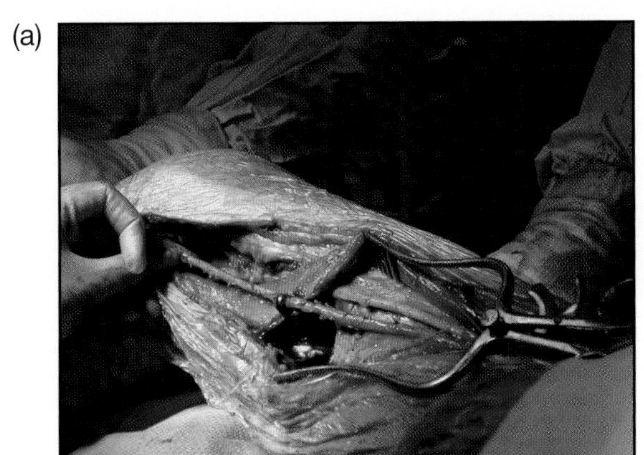

(b)

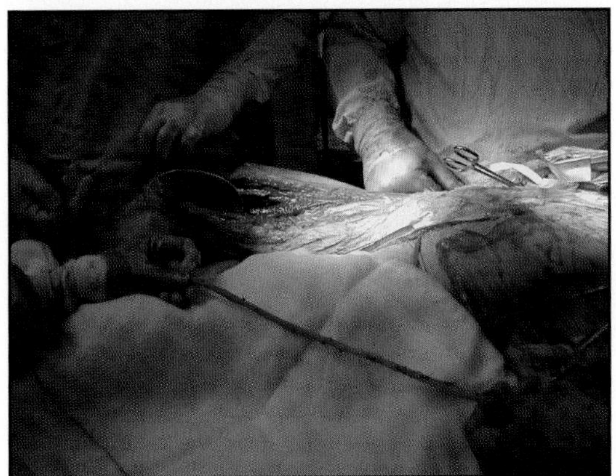

Plate 7 • Superficial femoral vein in situ **(a)** and following harvest **(b)**.

(a)

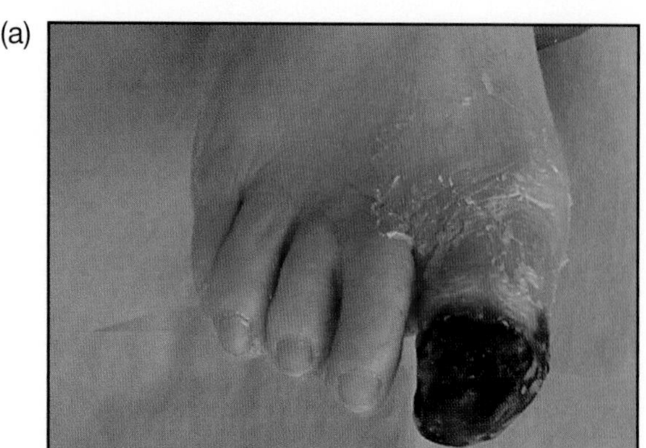

(b)

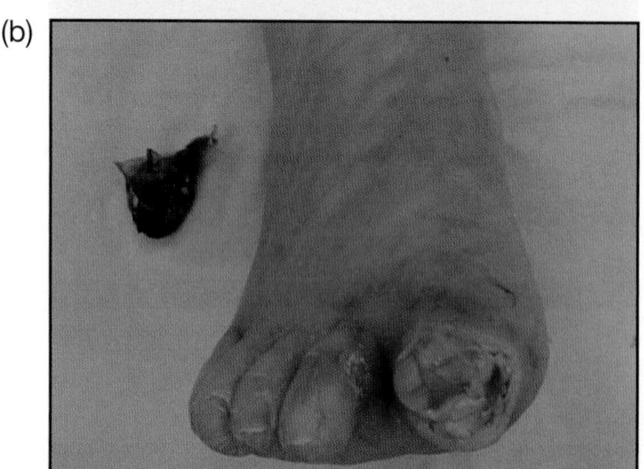

(c)

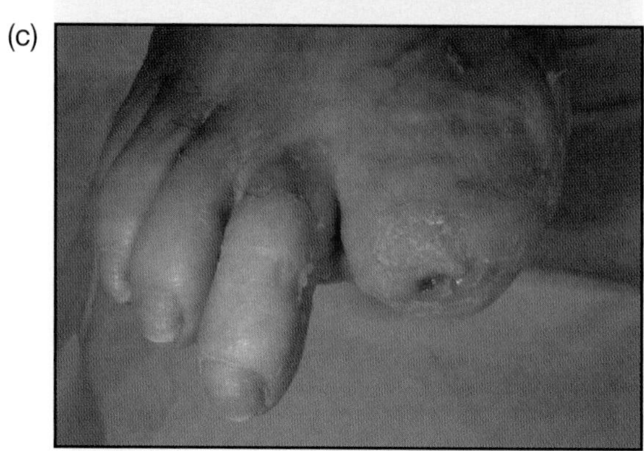

Plate 8 • Patient with digital gangrene **(a)** resulting in autoamputation **(b)** and healing of the wound **(c)**.

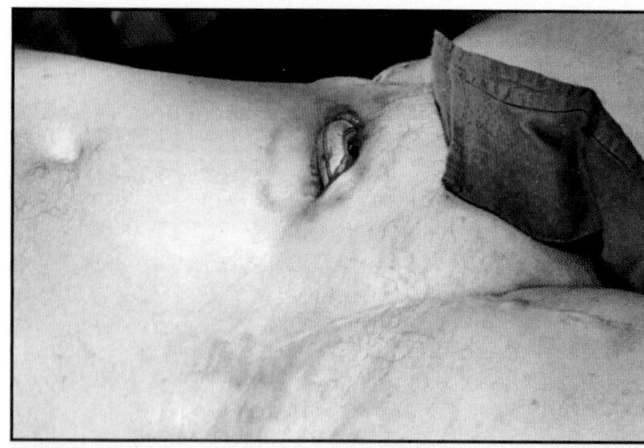

Plate 9 • A chronically exposed femoro-femoral bypass graft.

(a)

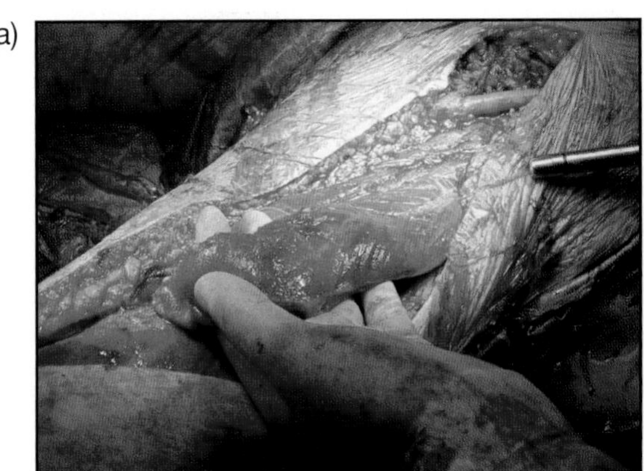

(b)

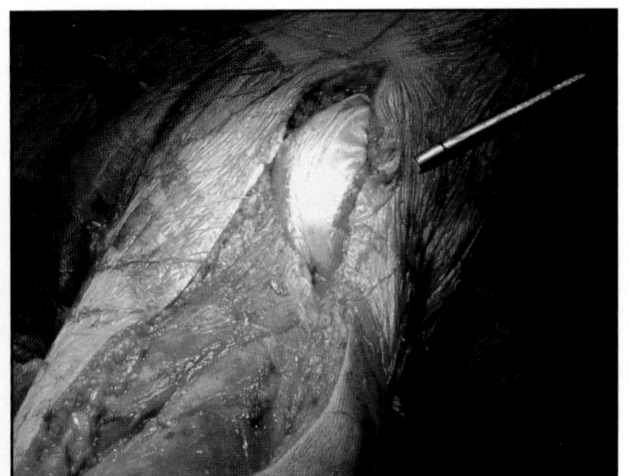

Plate 10 • Use of a rectus femoris flap to cover a femoral anastomsosis: **(a)** after mobilisation of the flap; **(b)** with the flap in position over the anastomosis.

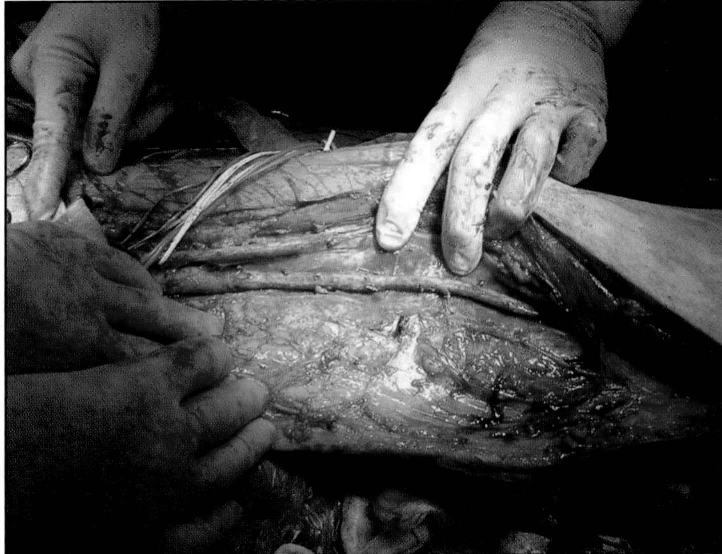

Plate 11 • Exposure of the femoral vein.

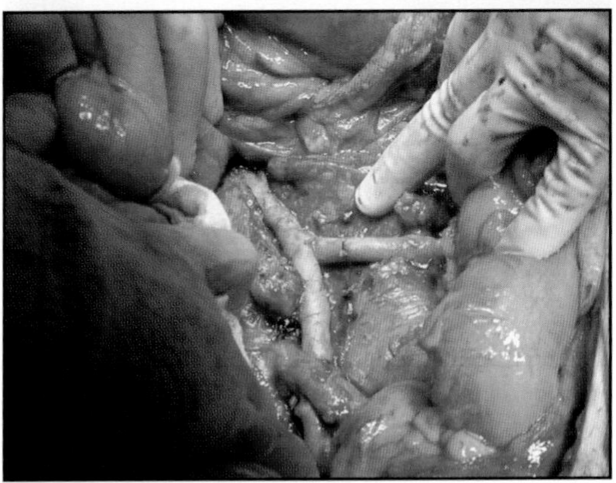

Plate 12 • Aortic reconstruction using femoral vein after excision of an infected aortic graft.

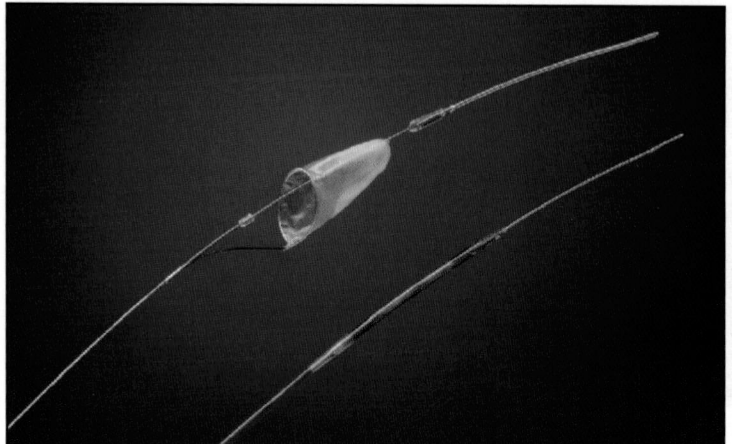

Plate 13 • Cerebral protection device incorporating a filter (Filterwire EZ, Boston Scientific Corporation).

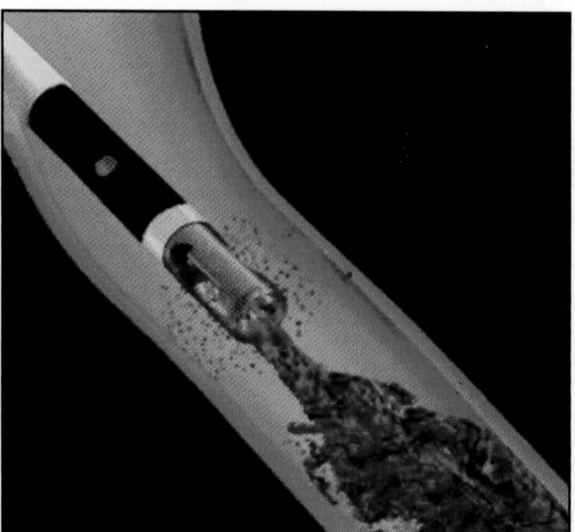

Plate 14 • Amplatz rotational thrombectomy device.

(a)

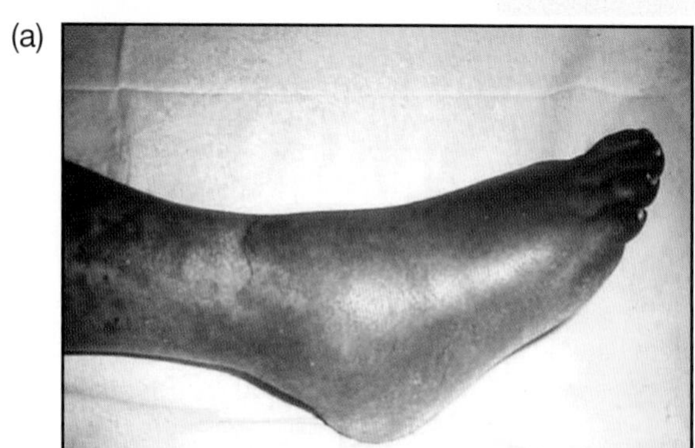

(b)

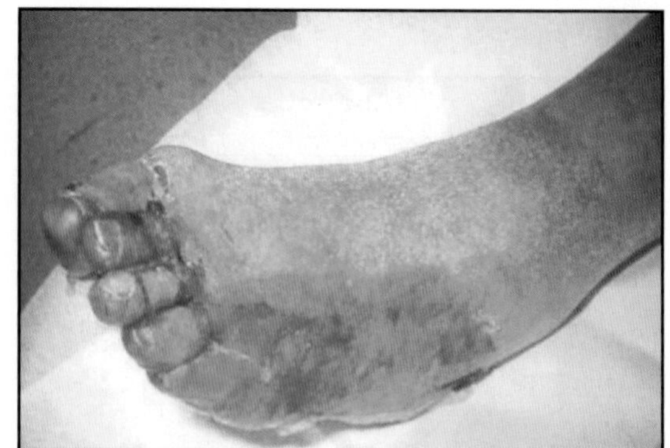

Plate 15 • **(a)** Acutely swollen cyanotic limb of phlegmasia caerulea dolens before treatment in a patient with carcinoma of the colon. **(b)** Limb salvage has been achieved at 3 days.

CHAPTER

Seven

The diabetic foot

Edward B. Jude and
Andrew J.M. Boulton

INTRODUCTION

Diabetes mellitus is increasing by epidemic proportions, presenting a major burden of healthcare as a result of end-organ damage caused by long-term hyperglycaemia.[1] Foot ulceration is the commonest major endpoint among diabetic complications. Diabetic neuropathy and peripheral vascular disease are the main aetiological factors in foot ulceration and may act alone, together or in combination with other factors such as microvascular disease, biomechanical abnormalities, limited joint mobility and increased susceptibility to infection. Foot problems in diabetic patients account for more hospital admissions than any other long-term complication of diabetes and also result in increasing morbidity and high mortality.[2–4] The 'diabetic foot syndrome' encompasses a number of pathologies, including diabetic neuropathy, peripheral vascular disease, Charcot neuroarthropathy, foot ulceration, osteomyelitis and the potentially preventable endpoint amputation.[5] Patients with the diabetic foot can also have multiple diabetic complications and because caring for such patients may require attention to many different areas, a multidisciplinary approach is usually necessary. Among the many aspects of the diabetic foot, this review concentrates on the aetiology and management of foot ulceration.

EPIDEMIOLOGY

Prevalence and incidence studies of foot ulceration have looked at a number of different community-based populations. Kumar et al.[6] found a history of current or previous ulceration in 5.3% of patients with type 2 diabetes; a study from Oxford found foot ulceration in 7% of diabetic patients over the age of 60 years;[7] and Borssen et al.[8] reported a history of ulceration in 3% of type 1 diabetic patients aged 15–50 years. In a recent study in the north-west of England, the annual incidence of foot ulceration was reported to be 2.2% among 10 000 community-based diabetic individuals with type 2 diabetes,[9] and in the Wisconsin study the 4-year incidence of ulcers in diabetic patients with type 1 and type 2 diabetes was 9.5% and 10.5%.[10] In another study from the USA, 5.8% of 8905 patients followed up over a 3-year period developed a foot ulcer, or in other words nearly 2% per year.[11]

With regard to the aetiology of foot ulceration, 45–60% are purely neuropathic, about 10% purely ischaemic and 25–45% of mixed neuroischaemic origin. In a more recent study we found a slight increase in the incidence of neuroischaemic (52.3%) and ischaemic (11.7%) foot ulcers, with a reduction in neuropathic ulcers (36%).[12] This changing pattern in the presentation of diabetic foot ulcers may be an indication of the greater awareness created by the initiation of multidisciplinary foot clinics as well as the importance placed on the education of patients who are 'at risk' of foot ulceration.

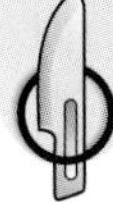

Lower limb amputation is performed 15 times more frequently in diabetic than non-diabetic patients;[13] after unilateral amputation, rates for both mortality and contralateral amputation are depressingly high. Like neuropathy and peripheral vascular disease, both amputation and ulceration are more common in males. Racial differences exist, with the amputation rate in Asian subjects being only one-quarter that in Caucasians.[14]

AETIOLOGY OF FOOT ULCERATION

Diabetic neuropathy

The numerous manifestations of diabetic neuropathy affect up to 50% of patients, but despite much intensive research the pathophysiology remains unclear and opinion is divided between microvascular disease leading to nerve hypoxia, and the direct effects of hyperglycaemia on neuronal metabolism. Recently, attempts to unite these two hypotheses have demonstrated abnormalities in nitric oxide metabolism, resulting in perineural vasoconstriction and nerve damage.

There are a number of manifestations of diabetic neuropathy, including mononeuropathies and polyneuropathies. As far as the diabetic foot is concerned, distal sensory polyneuropathy is the most important type. However, the motor and autonomic fibres may also be involved. It is not uncommon for a patient to have more than one type of neuropathy. The development of neuropathy is linked to poor glycaemic control over many years and thus increases in frequency with both age and duration of diabetes. Estimates of the prevalence of neuropathy vary because of different diagnostic criteria and populations. A number of studies have indicated a prevalence of neuropathy of approximately 30% among diabetic patients attending hospital,[15] with lower rates closer to 20% seen in population-based samples.[9,16] Among the elderly, the prevalence may be as high as 50%.

Symptoms of neuropathy do not occur in every patient and a significant number of patients are completely unaware of their marked sensory loss, which can therefore only be detected by regular and annual screening of the asymptomatic diabetic patient. Over time, as the neuropathy evolves, patients will experience symptoms, although these may simply be 'negative' and might comprise 'numbness' or 'deadness' in the lower limbs. Positive symptoms most commonly include burning pain, altered and uncomfortable temperature perception, paraesthesiae, shooting, stabbing and lancinating pain, hyperaesthesiae and allodynia. Many patients find the symptoms difficult to describe, but most report them to be extremely uncomfortable, distressing and prone to nocturnal exacerbation. The feet and lower legs are most commonly affected, although some patients with long-standing neuropathy may experience similar though less severe symptoms in the upper limbs. About an equal number of patients report no symptoms and distal symmetrical polyneuropathy cannot be excluded without a careful neurological examination. These can be differentiated from intermittent claudication most easily by the nocturnal exacerbations, the lack of relationship to exercise and the location of symptoms mainly in the foot rather than the calf (**Table 7.1**). Although no drugs have been demonstrated to improve the underlying neuropathy, painful symptoms are often well controlled by tricyclic antidepressants or anticonvulsants, such as gabapentin and carbamazepine.[17,18] Topical creams containing capsaicin may also provide relief, especially at night.[19]

Autonomic neuropathy reduces sweating in the skin and opens arteriovenous shunts, leading to increased blood flow to the leg.[20] Thus, the neuropathic foot is typically warm with bounding pulses and has dry, sometimes cracked, skin. Motor neuropathy mainly affects the intrinsic muscles of the foot (as they are the most distal) and can lead to wasting (guttering between the metatarsals) and an altered foot shape, with clawed toes and prominent metatarsal heads. It can be seen therefore that the insensitive neuropathic foot is at risk from unperceived external trauma (e.g. ill-fitting shoes), repetitive painless injury to high-pressure areas

Table 7.1 • Comparison of signs and symptoms of neuropathic and ischaemic pain

	Neuropathic pain	Intermittent claudication	Ischaemic rest pain
Site	Foot/shin	Calf/thigh	Foot/calf
Nature	Tingling/burning/shooting	Cramping	Aching
Exacerbating factors	Night time	Exercise	Elevation
Relieving factors	Exercise	Rest	Dependency of foot
Clinical signs in the foot	Warm, bounding pulses	Weak/absent pulses	Cold/pulseless

under the metatarsal heads during walking, and easy access to infection through dry cracked skin. Although vascular disease and infection were once thought to be the main causes of foot ulceration, prospective studies have now clearly demonstrated the important role of neuropathy.[21,22] Neuropathy is responsible for a high proportion of foot ulcers,[23,24] and leads to a sevenfold to tenfold increase in the risk of ulceration.

The diagnosis of neuropathy is usually simple and can be made by clinical examination, which reveals a 'stocking' distribution of sensory loss to one or more of pain, temperature and vibration modalities with absent ankle reflexes. If present, neuropathic symptoms and the typical appearance (described above) are useful. Quantitative sensory testing (of vibration, pressure and temperature perception thresholds) may provide a useful adjunct, and of the different tests available, measurement of the pressure perception threshold is the simplest. Using a nylon monofilament pressed against the skin until it buckles, a load of 10 g can be accurately applied. Patients unable to feel this on the sole of the foot are at high risk of ulceration. Simple bedside tests are all that is required to identify the foot at risk of neuropathic ulceration, and nerve conduction studies are rarely needed in clinical practice. For more details on the epidemiology, diagnosis and management of neuropathy, readers are directed to a recent extensive review.[25]

Peripheral vascular disease

Atherosclerotic vascular disease is probably present (at least in subclinical form) in all patients with long-duration diabetes. Vascular disease is responsible for up to 70% of deaths in type 2 diabetes, the premenopausal protection from vascular disease is lost in female diabetic patients, and peripheral vascular disease may be 20 times more common in diabetes.[26] The basic pathophysiology of atherosclerosis is probably no different in diabetes and is characterised by endothelial damage followed by platelet aggregation, lipid deposition and smooth muscle proliferation with plaque formation. The same risk factors also operate and include smoking, hypertension, dyslipidaemia, abnormal fibrinolysis and altered platelet function. Although some of these risk factors are much more prevalent in the diabetic population, a full explanation of the excess of vascular disease in diabetes remains elusive.

The distribution of vascular disease in the lower limb is thought to be different in diabetes, with more frequent involvement of vessels below the knee (**Fig. 7.1a**). Surprisingly, however, there are few good studies available to support this widely held belief, although Strandness et al.[27] reported that two-thirds of diabetic patients with peripheral vascular disease had infrapopliteal disease, and King et al.[28] found that involvement of the profunda femoris was increased in diabetes (**Fig. 7.1b**). In our random study of patients referred for angiography, no difference was seen in proximal disease (iliac, femoro-popliteal vessels) but distal disease (calf vessel) was twice as high in diabetic compared with non-diabetic patients.[29] The difficulties posed by the distribution may be further complicated by a reduced ability to develop a contralateral supply, but despite these problems revascularisation procedures are frequently successful, although a more distal anastomosis may be required. Indeed comparative studies have shown similar long-term outcomes of revascularisation for patients with and without diabetes,[30] and a number of centres have reported reduced amputation rates due to an increase in the number of bypass procedures.

Diabetic patients with peripheral vascular disease may develop intermittent claudication, but often this seems absent and the first clinical presentation may be ischaemic foot ulceration. Typically, this is at the ends of the toes, and in the absence of neuropathy is painful. The foot is usually cool with absent pulses, but do not be reassured by warmth in a neuroischaemic foot; swelling suggests deep infection. The most helpful non-invasive investigation is measurement of the ankle–brachial pressure index (ABPI).[31] When below 0.9 this is clearly indicative of ischaemia, but often it may be falsely elevated due to medial calcification of vessel walls, a phenomenon frequently seen in diabetic neuropathy (**Fig. 7.2**). In this situation, the Doppler waveform seems useful, as loss of the normal triphasic waveform indicates vascular disease. Measurement of toe pressures provides additional information, as the digital arteries are less frequently affected by calcification (see Chapter 2). Elevation of the leg using the pole-test[32] improves the reliability of both ankle and toe pressure measurements as it remains unaffected by calcification. Finally, transcutaneous oxygen tension (measured by an electrode placed on the foot) accurately reflects skin oxygenation and can be used to determine the severity of ischaemia, the likelihood that an ulcer will heal, and an appropriate level for amputation.[33] Despite advances in non-invasive investigations, arteriography (which must include pedal arteries) remains the gold standard for both diagnosis and planning of treatment. However, care is needed with contrast media in patients with renal impairment, since they can precipitate an acute deterioration in renal function. If the serum creatinine is greater than 200 μmol/L, a nephrologist should be consulted prior to contrast arteriography (see Chapter 2).

(a)

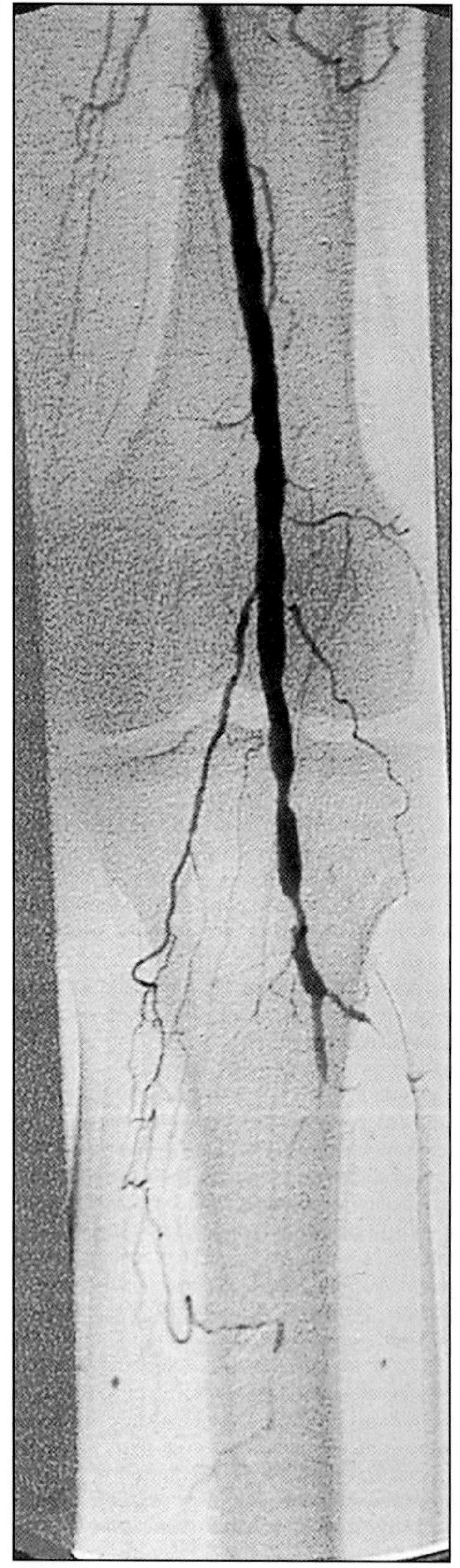

(b)

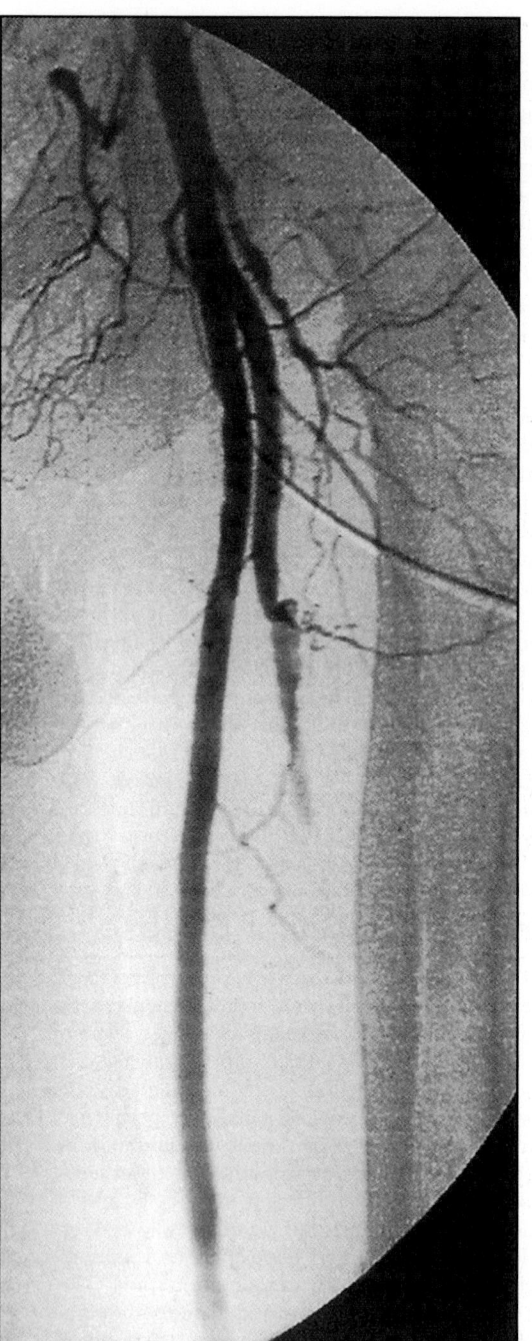

Figure 7.1 • Typical distribution of atherosclerosis affecting the popliteal trifurcation and tibial arteries **(a)**. The distal profunda is also often affected **(b)**, which reduces the ability for collaterals to develop around a superficial femoral occlusion.

(a)

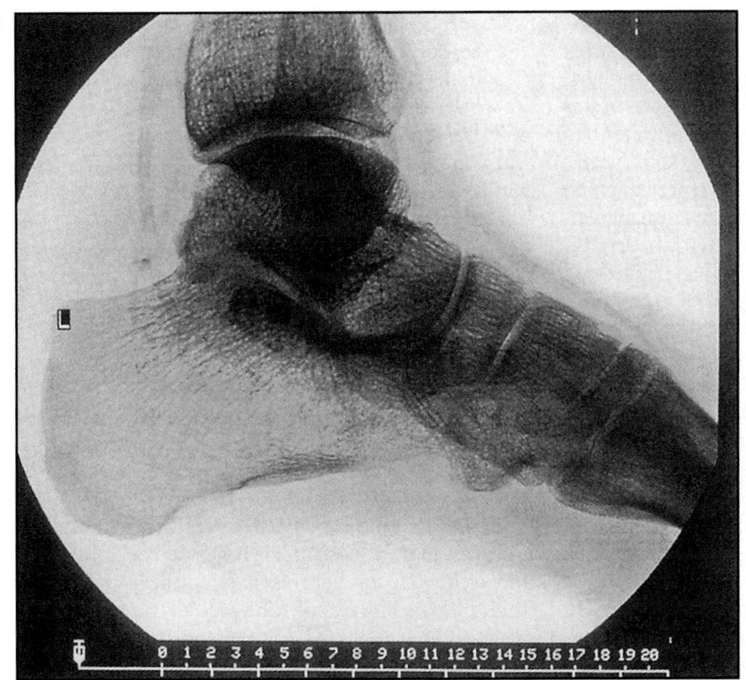

(b)

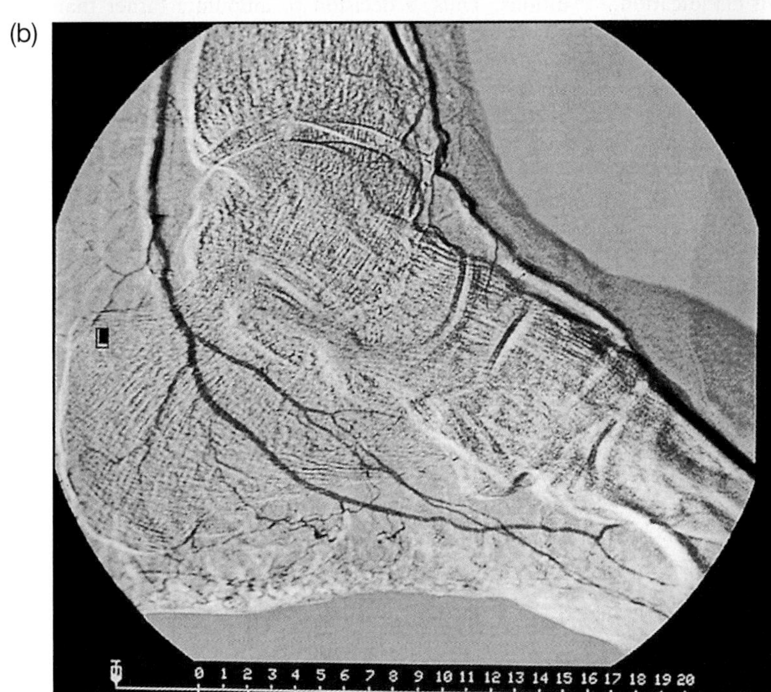

Figure 7.2 • **(a)** Calcification of the posterior tibial, anterior tibial and dorsalis pedis arteries in diabetes. The calcification is in the media and may falsely elevate Doppler pressures and make pulses difficult to palpate. However, good arterial flow may still be present **(b)**.

An antiplatelet agent such as aspirin, dipyridamole or clopidogrel will lower the risk of thrombotic vascular events, and has been shown to reduce vascular death in patients with intermittent claudication by about 25%.[36] Hypertension should be treated to target (130/80 mmHg for patients with diabetes),[37] with an angiotensin-converting enzyme (ACE) inhibitor probably being the treatment of choice. The HOPE study showed that the ACE inhibitor ramipril reduces cardiovascular morbidity and mortality in patients with peripheral arterial disease by around 25%.[38] Patients with hyperlipidaemia should have their cholesterol levels lowered to target. The Heart Protection Study showed that lowering total and LDL-cholesterol by 25% with a statin reduces cardiovascular mortality and morbidity in patients with peripheral arterial disease by around one-quarter.[39]

Three indicated therapies are available to improve walking distance. Two of these (naftidrofuryl, pentoxifylline) are considered to be less suitable for prescribing.[40] The third, and newest, therapy is cilostazol (Pletal), which has been shown to significantly improve maximal and pain-free walking distance in patients with intermittent claudication, both in patients with diabetes and in those without diabetes.

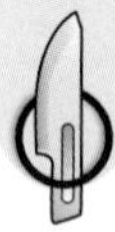

Regular exercise has been shown to be beneficial in diabetic patients with intermittent claudication, where it more than doubled the symptom-free walking distance.[34] Based on current evidence, the most effective exercise regimen consists of walking sessions approximately 1 hour long three times a week during which the patient walks to near maximal pain (preferably on a treadmill during supervised therapy), stops until the pain is relieved, and then resumes walking to near maximal pain again.[35] Exercise training in patients with intermittent claudication can produce a significant improvement in walking distance in those patients who adhere to the programme. Unfortunately, compliance in such patients is often poor and only a minority are able to attend supervised exercise classes.

Cilostazol, a selective phosphodiesterase III inhibitor, has vasodilating, antithrombotic and antiplatelet properties but its exact mechanism of action in patients with intermittent claudication is unknown.[41] A pooled analysis of the results of eight phase III controlled clinical trials of 436 patients with intermittent claudication who also had diabetes showed that the 216 patients who received cilostazol (100 mg b.d.) increased their maximal walking distances, initial claudication distance and absolute claudication distance significantly more than the 220 patients who received placebo.[42,43] Patients with diabetes showed no significant differences from those without diabetes who had taken cilostazol with respect to improvements in walking distances and response rates. Mean percentage change in maximal walking distance from baseline was 53% for patients with diabetes versus 60% for patients without diabetes. However, increases in maximal walking distance were slightly lower in patients with diabetes, as these patients had a lower baseline walking distance and a higher incidence of concomitant cardiovascular disease. Safety data in the patients with diabetes were in line with those seen in patients without diabetes. Cilostazol is contraindicated in several subpopulations of patients, particularly those with congestive heart failure and severe hepatic or renal impairment. However, current data would appear to support the use of cilostazol as a promising therapy for patients with intermittent claudication and diabetes, among the limited options available for these patients.

The indications for invasive treatment of peripheral vascular disease are progressive claudication and ischaemic or neuroischaemic ulceration. Suitability of an individual for vascular reconstruction needs to be considered and depends on appropriate anatomy and the presence of other medical conditions. Thus, a decision to amputate rather than revascularise in a patient with renal failure and ischaemic heart disease may be based on their substantial perioperative risk from a prolonged distal bypass, rather than the availability of a vessel to graft onto. However, an aggressive approach to revascularisation is known to save limbs, and other conditions may need treating or controlling before vascular surgery. Finally, when severe foot infection is present, this needs treating promptly with incision, drainage and débridement. Only when the infection has been controlled can revascularisation be performed.

Biomechanical aspects

The most important cause of foot ulceration is loss of protective pain sensation, permitting 'painless' repetitive trauma and tissue injury. However, vertical pressure applied to the plantar surface of the feet during walking and standing predisposes to ulceration. Plantar pressures can be measured by various methods, dynamic and static. Dynamic measurements are made using optical pedobarograph, Podotrack,[44] in-shoe or in-sole pressure transducers and static measurements using a Harris mat or a polytechnic-modified force plate. Patients with peripheral neuropathy and particularly ulcer patients have high plantar pressures,[45] although high pressures alone in the absence of insensitivity do not lead to ulceration.[46] Using an optical pedobarograph, Van Schie et al.[44] showed that plantar ulcers developed in one-third of patients with foot pressures greater than 12.3 kg/cm^2, whereas no ulcers developed in patients with pressures below 12.3 kg/cm^2. However, Frykberg et al.,[47] using an F-scan mat system, identified patients at risk of ulceration with foot pressures greater than 6 kg/cm^2. Using the Pedar in-shoe pressure analysis system, Stacpoole-Shea et al.[48] demonstrated its ability to predict sites of potential foot ulceration, with a sensitivity of 83% and a specificity of 69%. Additionally, neuropathy with altered proprioception and small muscle wasting leads to alteration in foot shape, clawing of the toes, prominent metatarsal heads and a high arch, all of which result in changes in foot pressures.[49] Patients with previous amputations have higher foot pressures and greater risk of foot ulceration.[50] The more severe deformity of the Charcot foot, with joint dislocation and bony deformities, can also result in increased foot pressures and foot ulceration.

Limited joint mobility is a further contributing factor to elevated plantar pressures. Chronic hyperglycaemia results in glycosylation of proteins and when collagen is involved the collagen bundles become thickened and cross-linked. This results in thick, tight, waxy skin and restriction of joint movement. Limited joint mobility of the subtalar joint alters the mechanics of walking and is strongly associated with high plantar pressure.[51]

Neuropathy alone does not lead to spontaneous ulceration. It is only the combination of trauma and insensitivity that results in tissue damage. The trauma sometimes takes the form of a single event, such as standing on a nail, but more frequently occurs as repeated minor trauma, such as unperceived shoe rubbing to the toes or increased pressure beneath the metatarsal heads during walking. It is now possible to measure dynamic vertical plantar pressure accurately, and a number of studies have clearly demonstrated that this is elevated in diabetic neuropathy and especially in patients with a history of plantar ulceration.[52,53] More importantly, a prospective study has shown that elevated plantar pressures are predictive of plantar ulceration, with 28% of neuropathic feet with high foot pressures ulcerating during a 30-month follow-up period.[45] Plantar ulcers only occurred in those who had both neuropathy and high foot pressures. The presence of callus (produced in response to pressure) may exacerbate the problem both by acting as a foreign body and by increasing plantar pressures.[54] Thus, removal of callus significantly reduces foot pressures.[55] Increased plantar tissue thickness has also been demonstrated in the neuropathic foot thus making these patients at higher risk for foot ulceration.[56]

The main cause of increased pressure is thought to be the alteration in foot shape (described earlier) resulting in prominent metatarsal heads. Neuropathy causes atrophy of the intrinsic muscles of the foot (predominantly plantar flexors of the toes), altering the flexor/extensor balance at the metatarsophalangeal joints. This results in clawing of the toes and may be associated with subluxation at the metatarsophalangeal joints. There is also anterior displacement of the submetatarsal fat pads and indeed reduced subcutaneous tissue thickness at the metatarsal heads has been confirmed in diabetic neuropathy.[57]

The accurate measurement of foot pressures requires sophisticated and expensive systems, which are currently available only in specialised centres. However, clinical examination that both inspects foot shape and identifies the presence of callus provides very valuable information, which can be used to select patients in need of pressure relief (see below). Indeed, the presence of callus may in some ways be superior to pressure measurement, as it results not only from vertical pressure but also from shear forces, which cannot currently be measured. Furthermore, the presence of haemorrhage into callus should be seen as a pre-ulcerative phenomenon and requires urgent attention.

Abnormalities of the microcirculation

Thickening of capillary basement membranes seems central to the development of diabetic retinopathy and nephropathy, and is closely linked with neuropathy. Similar changes can be found in most tissues and although microvascular disease alone does not cause foot ulceration, it is almost certainly a contributory factor. Evidence of a functional microvascular disorder can be found in uncomplicated diabetes, diabetic neuropathy and macrovascular disease. The key abnormalities are increased resting microvascular flow, impaired postural vasoconstriction and a reduced hyperaemic response to nociceptive stimulation. In the neuropathic foot, much of the excessive resting flow is through arteriovenous shunt vessels[58] and although there is also evidence of increased flow through nutritive skin capillaries, this may not be enough to compensate for the increased metabolic requirements resulting from the warmth of the neuropathic foot.

Intact autoregulatory mechanisms maintain constant flow at varying perfusion pressures and induce vasoconstriction in the foot when the leg is dependent. When this postural vasoconstriction is lost, capillary flow and pressure increase on standing[59] and oedema may occur. This oedema, which is seen in both neuropathy and ulceration, impairs wound healing. Nociceptive stimulation, either iontophoretically applied acetylcholine or a needle prick, normally results in a flare response that may last for 24 hours. The loss of this response, particularly marked in neuropathy,[60] impairs the ability of the tissue to respond appropriately to trauma.

Other risk factors

A number of inherent immunological abnormalities have been documented in diabetes. Neutrophil function is impaired, with abnormalities of adherence, chemotaxis, phagocytosis and killing ability,[61] and these may be partly due to ascorbic acid transport defects.[62] Several studies have shown an increased infection rate in postoperative wounds.[63] Thus although no study has specifically examined reduced immunity in the context of diabetic foot ulceration, it seems likely that this forms part of the explanation of the common clinical problem of infection in the diabetic foot.

Advancing age is frequently accompanied by impaired vision and immobility, both of which make foot inspection more difficult and delay the time when help is sought for an ulcer. The prevalence of neuropathy and peripheral vascular disease is also high among the elderly. Thus, lower limb amputation is more common among older diabetic patients.[13]

Diabetic nephropathy and renal failure are usually associated with numerous other problems, including diabetic retinopathy, neuropathy, macrovascular disease, reduced resistance to infection and peripheral oedema, all of which place such patients at very high risk of ulceration.

THE PATHWAY TO ULCERATION

As evidenced by the number of different risk factors (**Box 7.1**), the pathway to ulceration and amputation is often complex, and two or more elements are nearly always required. Ulceration of the insensitive foot only occurs when it is subjected to trauma, and the addition of peripheral vascular disease reduces the external pressure required to cause local ischaemia and tissue breakdown. Conversely, in patients with elevated plantar pressures due to rheumatoid arthritis, ulceration does not occur because sensation is intact and pain protects the feet from repeated injury.

Box 7.1 • Risk factors for diabetic foot ulceration

Previous ulceration
Neuropathy
Peripheral vascular disease
Altered foot shape
High foot pressures
Increasing age
Visual impairment
Living alone

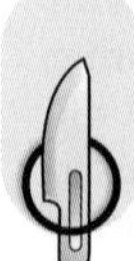

A two-centre prospective study confirmed that the commonest factors leading to foot ulceration were neuropathy, deformity (e.g. claw toes, prominent metatarsal heads) and trauma (e.g. ill-fitting shoes).[24]

The corollary of this multifactorial aetiology is that the pathways can be interrupted at any point. Tight glycaemic control in the first 10–20 years of diabetes will prevent the development of neuropathy and other complications, but the provision of good education about foot care to patients with high-risk feet may be equally successful at preventing ulceration.

MANAGEMENT

The management of diabetic foot problems requires input from a number of different healthcare professionals and the evidence strongly suggests that specialised diabetic foot clinics can significantly reduce ulceration and amputation rates.[64] Such a clinic requires a doctor with an interest in diabetes, a nurse, a podiatrist and orthotist, as well as rapid access to the services of vascular and orthopaedic surgeons. Before considering the details of the management of foot ulcers it is essential to recognise the crucial role of prevention, which initially involves identification of the 'at-risk' foot.

The 'at-risk' foot

The identification of patients at risk of foot ulceration is most easily done on an annual basis and must be performed on all patients with diabetes. Screening does not involve expensive equipment or testing and can be done in an ordinary clinic setting. Sadly, foot examination is frequently overlooked,[65] perhaps because doctors are reassured by the patient not reporting any symptoms. However, as discussed earlier, neuropathy, vascular disease and even ulceration are frequently asymptomatic but can be easily diagnosed by simple clinical examination. Peripheral neuropathy can be recognised with standard clinical tools by finding reduced or absent vibration, pin-prick or thermal (cold tuning fork) sensation in the foot, usually accompanied by the loss of the ankle reflex. As described earlier, quantitative sensory testing is a useful adjunct. Dry and cracked skin on the feet usually signifies autonomic neuropathy, and neuropathic symptoms (burning, paraesthesiae, etc.) should be sought. The peripheral vascular status is usually indicated by palpation of peripheral pulses and it should be remembered that absent foot pulses may be due to arterial wall calcification not absent flow. The ABPI should be measured whenever there is any doubt, but further investigations will be dictated by individual clinical requirements. If a patient is at risk by virtue of having either neuropathy or peripheral vascular disease, then a more detailed assessment of additional risk factors is required. Foot inspection may reveal deformities of foot shape and areas of callus that indicate sites exposed to high pressure or friction. Immobility and social circumstances may influence a patient's ability to understand and carry out appropriate foot care. Finally, a history of previous ulceration should be sought, as this is probably the strongest single predictor of ulceration.

As most of the risk factors (apart from vascular disease) are not directly modifiable by treatment, the most important element of the management of at-risk patients is the provision of good education on foot care.

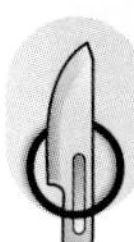

Even a simple approach can have considerable success, as demonstrated by Malone et al.,[66] who reported a two-thirds reduction in amputation and ulceration as a result of a 1-hour educational session.

A number of different educational approaches have been used and options include group sessions, printed material, videos and opportunistic education. Areas covered by education need to include both the correction of patient misconceptions[67] (does the patient know what a foot ulcer is and how it might be prevented?) and advice on foot care. With regard to the latter, it is important to concentrate on positive recommendations rather than prohibitions. The basic elements of foot care advice are shown in **Box 7.2**. Patients also need to know how to gain rapid access to advice and treatment from the foot-care team.

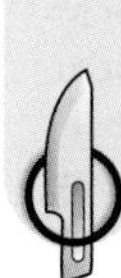

Areas of high pressure need to be accommodated in appropriate footwear and the evidence suggests that when high-risk patients wear the footwear provided, ulceration rates are reduced.[68] A small randomised study showed that injecting liquid silicone under areas of callus and high pressure resulted in reduced ulceration at these sites.[69]

Extra-depth shoes provide enough room for clawed toes, and cushioned insoles reduce plantar pressures. It is not clear whether flat insoles provide greater pressure relief than custom-moulded insoles. Padded hosiery may further reduce pressure and also protect the dorsum of the toes.[70] Most patients can be fitted with 'off the shelf' extra-depth shoes, with custom-made shoes being reserved for patients with major foot deformity. Further shoe modifications are possible, for example a rigid rocker bottom sole can be added. With the rocker axis posterior to the metatarsal heads, metatarsal head pressure can be reduced by up to 40%.[71] Regular podiatry is required for most at-risk patients. Callus needs to be débrided regularly because although it develops in response to pressure and friction, its removal reduces pressure.[55] Furthermore, callus can sometimes hide ulceration, which will only be revealed when the callus is removed. Without its removal, infection and abscess formation are encouraged, but it is important to explain to the patient that the podiatrist has not caused the ulcer. The presence of callus should always prompt a search for its cause, and shoe modification may be necessary.

The surgical correction of specific foot deformities is sometimes necessary to prevent ulceration. However, this should only be done after confirming that there is a good peripheral circulation and it is important to bear in mind that the correction of a hallux valgus may leave a rigid hallux with high plantar pressures. Metatarsal head resection (through a dorsal incision) is sometimes used to

Box 7.2 • Principles of foot care education

1. Target the level of information to the needs of the patient. Those not at risk require only general advice about foot hygiene and footwear
2. Make positive rather than negative recommendations

   DO inspect the feet daily

   DO report any problems, even if painless

   DO buy shoes with a square toe box and laces

   DO inspect the inside of shoes for foreign objects every day before putting them on

   DO attend a fully trained podiatrist regularly

   DO cut your nails straight across and not rounded

   DO keep your feet away from heat (fires, radiators, hot water bottles) and check the bath water with your hand or elbow

   DO always wear something on your feet to protect them and never walk barefoot
3. Repeat the advice at regular intervals and check for compliance
4. Disseminate the advice to other family members and other healthcare professionals involved in the care of the patient

reduce pressures; the only study that has examined the results of this procedure showed a 40–70% fall in pressure, with no evidence of transfer of pressure to other metatarsal heads.[72] However, the follow-up period was short and our own observations suggest that, after a few months, pressures may start to increase again. Correction of deformity is usually only performed in patients with a history of ulceration, rather than for primary prevention.

Ulcer management

A number of different classifications of diabetic foot ulcers have been devised. The Wagner classification[73] is probably the most widely used in the literature and grades ulcers on the depth of penetration and extent of tissue necrosis. However, it makes no reference to aetiology and, for clinical practice, a more helpful classification is to divide ulcers into neuropathic, neuroischaemic and purely ischaemic, combined with an assessment of the presence and severity of infection. All diabetic patients presenting with foot ulcers need at the very least a clinical examination of peripheral sensation and circulation (supplemented with measurement of ABPI if there is any doubt at all about the circulation) in order to classify the ulcer. Radiography of the foot should also be carried out if the ulcer is deep or resistant to therapy to exclude underlying osteomyelitis (**Fig. 7.3**). Any type of ulcer can be infected and the management of infection will be considered separately.

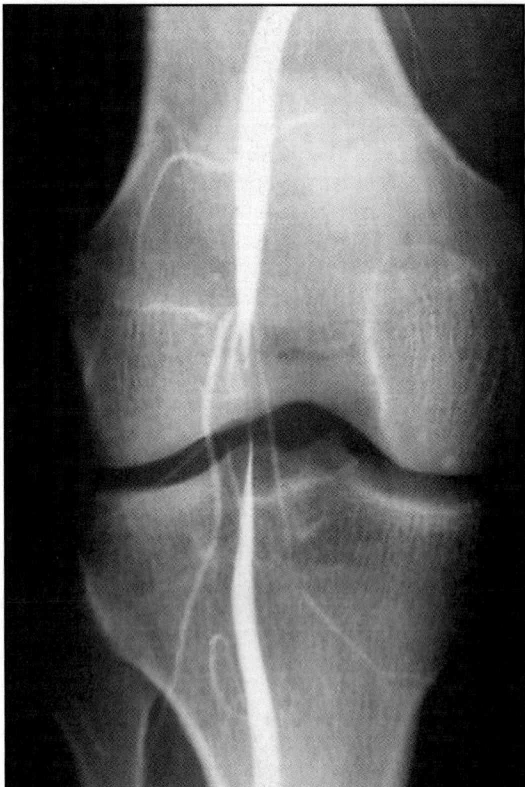

Figure 7.3 • Osteomyelitis of the first interphalangeal joint causing bony destruction. Calcification of the digital artery between the first and second metatarsals can also be seen.

A second commonly used classification is the University of Texas Wound Classification system. This assesses ulcer depth, the presence of wound infection and the presence of clinical signs of lower-extremity ischaemia.[74] The system uses a matrix of grade on the horizontal axis and stage on the vertical axis. Grade 0 is a pre- or post-ulcerative site that has healed; Grade 1 a superficial wound not involving tendon, capsule or bone; Grade 2 a wound penetrating to tendon or capsule; and Grade 3 a wound penetrating bone or joint. Within each wound grade there are four stages: clean wounds (A), non-ischaemic infected wounds (B), ischaemic non-infected wounds (C) and ischaemic infected wounds (D). This classification system has recently been shown to be a better predictor of outcome in terms of healing and amputations compared with the Wagner system.[75]

NEUROPATHIC ULCERS

Typically, the foot is warm and well perfused with bounding pulses and distended veins. The ulcer is usually at the site of repetitive trauma and most commonly due to a shoe rub on the dorsum of the toes or a high-pressure area under the metatarsal heads. The ulcer may be hidden under callus and only revealed when this is removed by a podiatrist. Occasionally, a foreign body causes ulceration: either a nail penetrates the sole of the shoe and the skin, or a stone or other object gets into the shoe. Neuropathic patients may walk on a foreign body for hours or even days without being aware of it.

The key to management is pressure relief. With shoe-induced ulcers, appropriate footwear must be provided, irrespective of patients' protestations that their own shoes (which caused the ulcer) are comfortable. However, merely providing shoes may not be enough, as many patients do not wear prescribed shoes on a regular basis. Failure to wear the provided shoes may be because of their appearance or the belief (common in the elderly) that they are only for outdoors and that slippers are suitable footwear in the home.

In order to relieve pressure from a plantar ulcer, a more aggressive approach is required. Bed rest is simple and attractive, but is expensive in hospital and difficult to enforce in a patient who feels well and is free of pain. Therefore, several ambulatory methods have been designed.

(a)

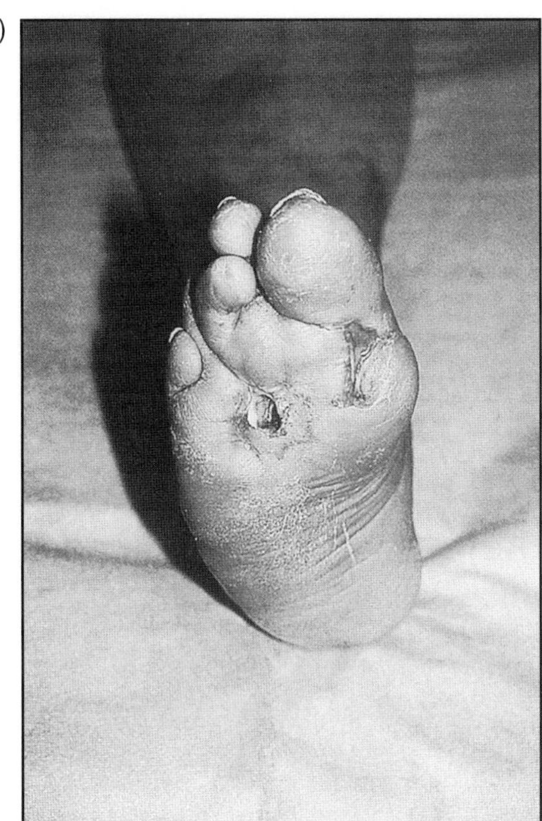

(b)

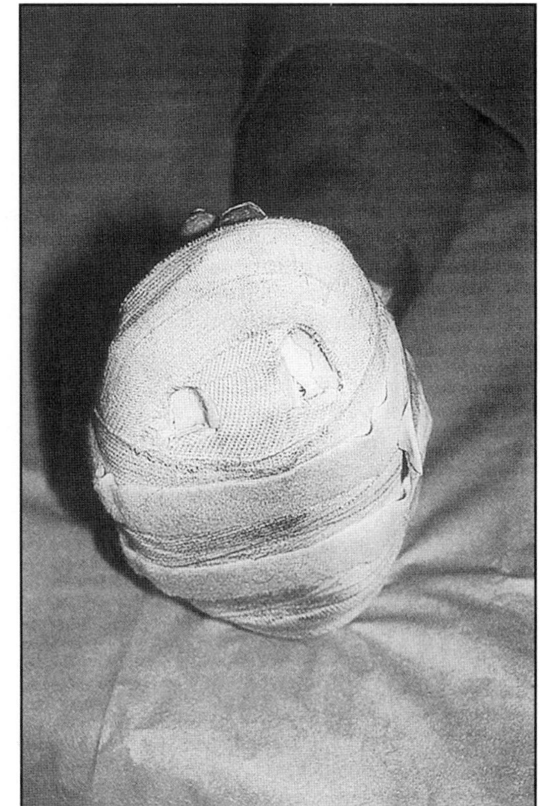

(c)

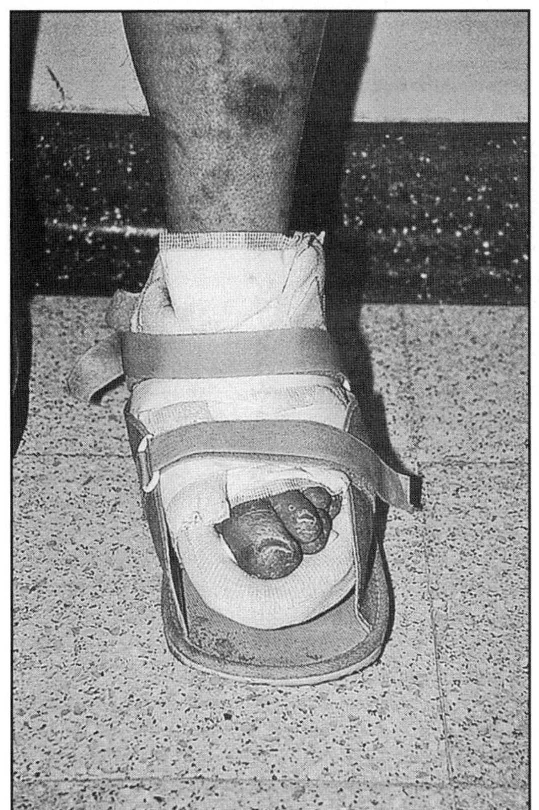

Figure 7.4 • Plantar ulcers due to diabetic neuropathy **(a)** treated by a windowed Scotch cast boot **(b)** to relieve pressure on the metatarsophalangeal joints when walking **(c)**.

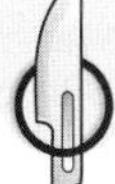

The total contact cast was originally used for patients with neuropathic ulcers due to leprosy and was modified by Paul Brand for use in diabetic neuropathy. The cast extends from below the knee and encases the whole foot. Only minimal padding is used, except in the forefoot. Excellent healing rates have been reported and in a randomised controlled trial total contact cast was associated with faster healing compared with other removable devices.[76]

The cast works by transferring load from the forefoot to the heel and directly to the leg via the cast walls,[77] as well as by reducing oedema and shear forces. Its main disadvantages are that it is labour intensive, as it may need frequent changes, and signs of wound infection or ulceration secondary to the cast may not be seen. An alternative is the Scotch cast boot.[78] This is a removable fibreglass boot that is moulded to the contours of the plantar surface of the foot and a window cut out at the site of the ulcer (**Fig. 7.4**). A number of commercially produced pressure-relieving boots are now available and although their capacity to reduce pressure has been demonstrated, only the total contact cast has been tested in trials of ulcer healing.

The second important element of management of neuropathic ulcers is débridement of callus. Wounds heal from the margins and callus prevents the migration of epidermal cells from the wound margin, and encourages wound infection. Débridement of callus and necrotic tissue is usually required on a weekly basis and the continued presence of callus should prompt a review of the pressure relief being employed.

ISCHAEMIC AND NEUROISCHAEMIC ULCERS

The purely ischaemic ulcer is relatively rare and most are in fact neuroischaemic. Typical sites include the toes, heel and medial aspect of the first metatarsal head. Callus is usually absent and the ulcer is often surrounded by a rim of erythema and may have a necrotic centre. The presence of pain depends on the degree of neuropathy. Ulceration is often precipitated by minor trauma and the most common culprit is ill-fitting shoes. Prompt vascular assessment is crucial and angiography is often required. Revascularisation should be performed whenever possible, both for ulcer healing (ischaemic and neuroischaemic ulcers only rarely heal without improvements in blood flow) and to prevent future ulceration. As described earlier, this may involve a distal bypass, although the outcome of vascular surgery is just as good in patients with and without diabetes.[30]

Gangrene and amputation are among the most feared complications of diabetes. Although gangrene may complicate neuropathic ulceration (microorganisms in infected digital ulcers may produce necrotising toxins, which lead to thrombotic occlusion of digital arteries and subsequent gangrene), it usually only occurs when significant vascular disease is present. Gangrenous tissue must be removed, and when it involves a dry digit with a clear demarcation line this will usually occur spontaneously, leaving a healed stump (**Fig. 7.5**, see also Plate 8, facing p. 116). However, when these conditions are not met, local amputation is mandatory. Local amputation includes simple removal of a toe, ray amputation (of a toe and metatarsal), or a transmetatarsal amputation. The general rule is to remove all necrotic tissue, ensuring that no bone is left exposed, while leaving part of the wound open to allow drainage. If arterial reconstruction is possible, then this can be combined with amputation to enable the healing of the amputation site. This is not possible when major sepsis is present, and in such circumstances revascularisation should be done at a second procedure when infection has been controlled by débridement and antibiotics. The amputation site is determined by both the extent of tissue involvement and the level at which the circulation will support wound healing. With regard to the latter, the transcutaneous oxygen tension provides useful information; in a large study, values under 40 mmHg were strongly associated with failure of healing at the amputation site.[32]

(a)

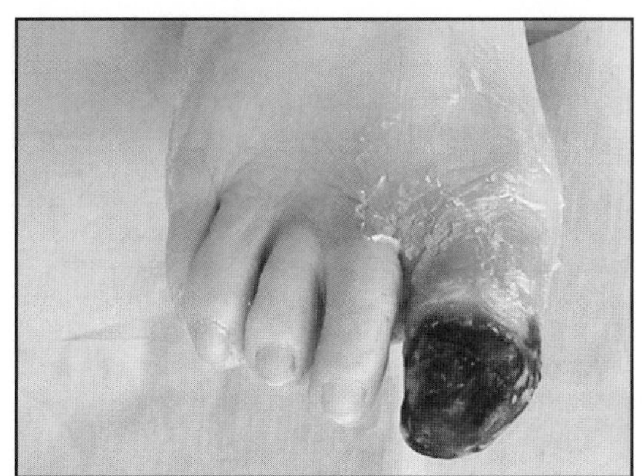

(b)

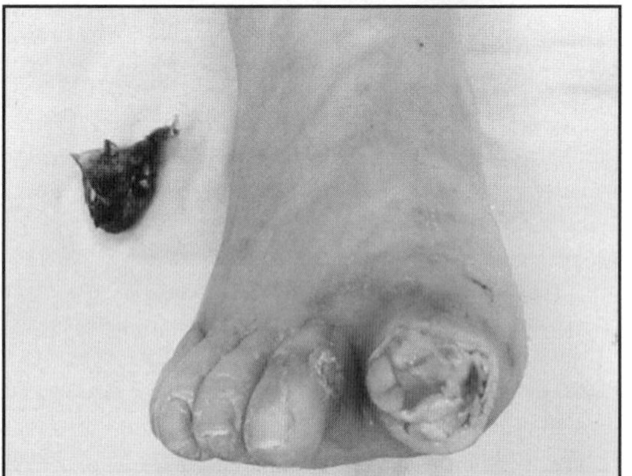

(c)

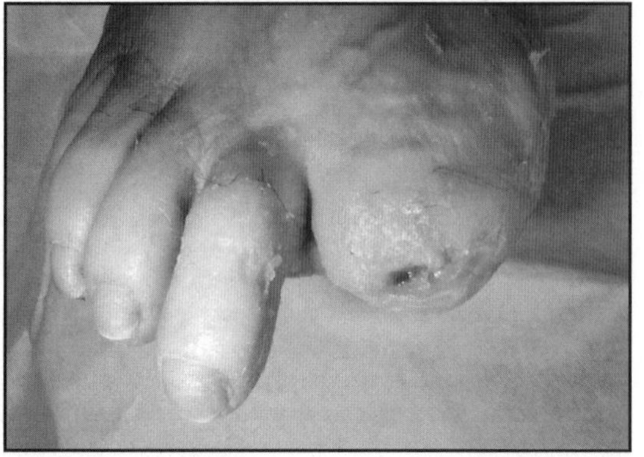

Figure 7.5 • Patient with digital gangrene **(a)** resulting in autoamputation **(b)** and healing of the wound **(c)**.

INFECTION

An infected diabetic foot ulcer can lead to limb loss in a matter of days, but by no means are all ulcers infected, although bacterial colonisation seems universal. The distinction between colonisation and infection can be difficult and is not aided by microbiological investigations. Clinical signs are the most reliable indicators of infection. Evidence of systemic upset (e.g. fever, leucocytosis) is frequently absent, and signs of local inflammation, swelling and the presence of pus are usually used to dictate the need for antibiotics. With severe infection, there may be crepitus due to gas formation and fluctuance indicating the presence of an abscess. Infections are usually polymicrobial, with typically three to six organisms isolated per ulcer.[79,80] The most commonly found organisms include staphylococci, streptococci, Gram-negative species such as *Proteus* and *Pseudomonas* and anaerobes such as *Bacteroides*, and synergy between organisms may increase pathogenicity. Recently, methicillin-resistant *Staphylococcus aureus* (MRSA) has posed an increasing problem, and was found to be present in over 20% of ulcers in a specialised diabetic foot clinic and increasing in prevalence.[81,82] In non-limb-threatening infections, microbiological investigation is not essential, but when swabs are taken the method is important. Superficial swabs are likely to isolate colonising rather than pathogenic bacteria[79] and the deeper the sample, the more reliable the results are. Ideally, curettings from the ulcer base should be transported and cultured aerobically and anaerobically.

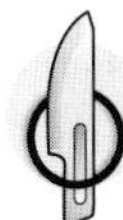

Osteomyelitis should be suspected in any deep ulcer, if a sinus tract is present or if an ulcer fails to heal despite adequate pressure relief.

Osteomyelitis is an important predisposing factor for amputation. Though sometimes obvious from plain radiographs, the sensitivity and specificity of radiography in diagnosing osteomyelitis are only about 70%.[83,84] This may be improved with serial radiographs taken at 2-weekly intervals or by using isotope scans. Three-phase bone scans and indium-labelled white cell scans improve the sensitivity but not necessarily the specificity.[83,84] However, a recent report has indicated that by combining bone and white cell scan images, sensitivity is over 90% and specificity greater than 80%.[85] Magnetic resonance imaging is now also proving useful by showing marrow oedema before cortical bone loss occurs, and is particularly valuable in differentiating infection from Charcot neuroarthropathy. Interestingly, a simple clinical test (the ability to probe to bone with a blunt instrument at the base of an ulcer) has proved to be a useful test for osteomyelitis,[86] with a sensitivity of 66% and positive predictive value of 89% (i.e. bone can be probed in 66% of all cases of osteomyelitis, and in all ulcers where bone can be probed 89% have osteomyelitis). Simple laboratory markers, such as erythrocyte sedimentation rate and C-reactive protein, may assist in the diagnosis.

The threshold for initiating antibiotic treatment should be low, and the agents used should have a broad spectrum of activity to include the known common pathogenic organisms.[87] There is limited evidence on which to base the choice of antibiotic regimen, although it has been demonstrated that antibiotic treatment is not required in neuropathic ulcers that are not clinically infected.[88]

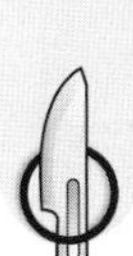

In limb-threatening diabetic foot infections, amoxicillin or ampicillin combined with a β-lactamase inhibitor (clavulanic acid or sulbactam) are effective and give very similar results to those achieved with either ofloxacin used alone[89] or imipenem combined with cilastatin.[90]

Clindamycin or the combination of amoxicillin with flucloxacillin are also suitable outpatient treatments and cover most of the required spectrum, although they do not have trial data to support their use. Preferably the antibiotic of choice should be against common organisms causing infection in the diabetic foot and the most frequent organism found is *S. aureus*. Caution should be exercised in patients with pencillin hypersensitivity and clindamycin can be the first choice in these patients.

Organisms that are commonly isolated are shown in **Box 7.3**. MRSA is also being seen increasingly, causing a major problem in antibiotic choices. A new class of antimicrobial agents has been identified, represented by linezolid, an oxazolidinone, which acts against bacteria by inhibiting the initiation of protein synthesis at the ribosomal subunit.[91] Linezolid has excellent activity against staphylococci, including MRSA, streptococci and other Gram-positive organisms.[92] It can also be used in patients with penicillin allergy. It has recently been approved for use in skin and soft tissue infection but is not currently licensed for the treatment of osteomyelitis. However, pharmacological data, supported by case reports, suggest that linezolid may be a useful option in the treatment of bone infection due to resistant Gram-positive bacteria.[93] Furthermore, linezolid has excellent oral absorption, giving the potential for oral therapy of deep-seated infections. However, it can be used intravenously in the initial period and then converted to oral dosage when the patient is less toxic or able to take medications by mouth. Regular monitoring of blood counts is required for patients on this antibiotic.

However, antibiotics should be used with care. Aminoglycosides are potentially nephrotoxic, and clindamycin (as well as other agents) can cause

Box 7.3 • Organisms isolated from diabetic foot ulcers in a specialised diabetic foot clinic

Gram-positive aerobes	59 (56.7%)
Staphylococcus aureus	30 (28.8%)
Coagulase-negative *Staphylococcus*	5 (4.8%)
Streptococcus spp.	11 (10.6%)
Gram-negative aerobic bacilli	31 (29.8%)
Enterobacter species	22 (21.1%)
Pseudomonas species	4 (3.8%)
Anaerobic species	14 (13.5%)
Cases with mixed skin flora	12 (17.9%)
Results by category	
Aerobes only	53 (79.1%)
Anaerobes only	3 (4.5%)
Aerobes and anaerobes	11 (16.4%)
Monomicrobial infection	35 (52.2%)
Methicillin-resistant *Staphylococcus aureus*	12 (15.2%)

From Tentolouris N, Jude EB, Smirnof I et al. Methicillin-resistant *Staphylococcus aureus*: an increasing problem in a diabetic foot clinic. Diabet Med 1999; 16:767–71, with permission.

Clostridium difficile diarrhoea. Quinolones (such as ofloxacin) sometimes have limited potency against Gram-positive cocci. Serious limb-threatening infections often demand multiple drug regimens, which should be administered carefully with monitoring for adverse effects, and in consultation with a microbiology department. Infected and necrotic tissue must be aggressively débrided, and when osteomyelitis is present infected bone nearly always needs resecting, although prolonged antibiotic courses may successfully eradicate the bone infection. Limb-threatening infections require urgent hospitalisation, bed rest, surgical débridement and broad-spectrum antibiotics.

The choice of dressings remains controversial due to the lack of large well-controlled comparative studies. When slough is present, desloughing agents are often effective (although more expensive than a scalpel) and hydrocolloid dressings are useful in cleaner ulcers. Interest has recently focused on actively influencing the complex environment that exists within chronic wounds. Growth factors are central to this process, and are responsible for triggering and controlling the events that finally result in healing and skin closure. Silver-containing dressings have also been found to have antibacterial activity and may be used in certain foot ulcers where antibiotics may not be necessary or in conjunction with antibiotics.

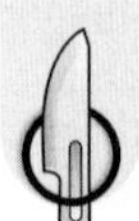

Various newer topical therapies have been researched recently and have been shown to be of some benefit in the healing of chronic diabetic foot ulcers. These include platelet-derived growth factor (becaplermin), living dermal equivalent (Dermagraft) and living human skin equivalents (Graftskin). However, they are not appropriate for all patients and should be used judiciously with good wound care being paramount.

Becaplermin, a formulation of platelet-derived growth factor that is applied directly to the ulcer, has recently been shown to improve healing times for neuropathic diabetic foot ulcers,[94] and studies of other growth factors are currently underway. Living dermal replacements can now be manufactured from neonatal fibroblasts, which are cultured in vitro onto a bioabsorbable mesh. The product is applied as a dressing to the wound, and the fibroblasts within it are metabolically active, producing a full array of growth factors. Evidence is now available that this skin substitute may also improve healing,[95] although some uncertainty remains about the validity of the data. Hyperbaric oxygen therapy has been used for a variety of conditions including wound healing. It improves tissue oxygenation, enhances the killing capacity of neutrophils, and directly inhibits the growth of anaerobic organisms. A controlled trial of this treatment modality in limb-threatening diabetic foot ulcers indicated its efficacy, especially when ischaemia was a major problem.[96]

The recent development of living human skin equivalents, produced by tissue engineering techniques, offers new opportunities for wound healing in chronic ulcers caused by venous disease and diabetic neuropathy. Graftskin is a bilayered cultured skin equivalent, consisting of human epidermis and a collagenous dermal layer containing human fibroblasts. A prospective, randomised, controlled trial has demonstrated the efficacy of Graftskin in the management of chronic neuropathic diabetic foot ulcers.[97] Graftskin or a standard treatment (saline moisturized gauze) was applied to more than 200 patients who also received standardized foot care for their foot ulcers, which comprised sharp débridement and offloading. After 12 weeks of treatment, 56% of Graftskin-treated patients achieved complete healing compared with 38% of the controls.

It appears therefore that treatments such as Graftskin and possibly Dermagraft might be useful adjuncts in the treatment of diabetic neuropathic foot ulcers. These new treatments offer a variety of exciting options, but are expensive and are limited in their indications (e.g. growth factors and skin substitutes should only be used in non-infected ulcers). Their availability should not obscure the fact that most ulcers respond to simple care, comprising pressure relief, débridement and control of infection, and must not be seen as a replacement but as an addition to good wound care.

Granulocyte colony-stimulating factor

Neutrophil superoxide generation, a crucial part of neutrophil bactericidal activity, is impaired in diabetes. Granulocyte colony-stimulating factor (G-CSF) increases the release of neutrophils from the bone marrow and improves neutrophil function. In a placebo-controlled trial, G-CSF (filgrastim) treatment was associated with improved clinical outcome of foot infection in diabetic patients. This improvement may be related to an increase in neutrophil superoxide production.[98]

Larva débridement therapy

Larva débridement therapy (the use of maggots to cleanse wounds) is hardly new. Indeed, an early reference to larval therapy was made during the Napoleonic wars when it was observed that those wounds accidentally infected by maggots did not become infected and appeared to heal better.

In recent years the use of sterile larvae (of the greenbottle fly, *Lucilia sericata*) has been investigated with encouraging results, and is becoming increasingly popular as therapy for infected and necrotic wounds.[99,100] It is thought that maggots remove necrotic tissue by secreting powerful enzymes that break down dead tissue into a liquid form, which is then ingested.[101] The mechanisms by which larvae prevent or combat infection are also complex but there is anecdotal evidence that they may also help in combating antibiotic-resistant strains of bacteria. There is a growing body of clinical experience with the use of larval therapy that suggests that it is useful in the management of patients with necrotic, sloughing and often neuro-ischaemic ulcers. The use of this therapy is now quite widespread in foot care for infected diabetic ulcers.

MEDICAL PROBLEMS ON THE SURGICAL WARD

By the time that a diabetic patient reaches the vascular surgeon, numerous complications will often have developed. Apart from somatic neuropathy and peripheral vascular disease, coronary artery disease, diabetic nephropathy (with or without renal failure) and cardiac autonomic neuropathy are frequently present in this population and may play a major role in determining the overall outcome. Thus patients need careful screening to identify potential problems. All patients with a significant degree of renal impairment should ideally be reviewed by a renal physician prior to any procedures.

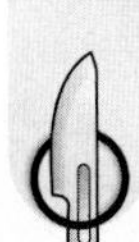

Angiography with contrast media carries a risk of worsening renal function, which may be as high as 50% among patients with diabetic nephropathy.[102] However, it has been shown that hydration with normal saline alone provided better protection than when diuretics were added.[103]

Metformin must also be stopped for 48 hours before elective angiography because of the risk of lactic acidosis, which carries a high mortality (see Chapter 2). Coronary artery disease and cardiac autonomic neuropathy increase the risk of perioperative cardiac events. Invasive monitoring (e.g. Swan–Ganz catheterisation) and regional anaesthetic techniques help to reduce this risk. The hormonal and metabolic changes associated with surgery present a particular problem in diabetes. Intravenous insulin (plus dextrose and potassium) is usually needed for the perioperative period, unless the duration of anaesthesia is short (<45 minutes) and the patient is not on insulin. It is mostly simply administered as part of a 'GKI' regimen,[104] in which 15 units of soluble insulin and 10 mmol of potassium chloride are added to 500 mL of 10% dextrose, the solution being infused at 100 mL/hour. Despite its simplicity, this regimen provides remarkably stable glycaemic control, although many centres prefer the insulin to be administered separately, allowing adjustment of the rate according to capillary glucose measurements, using a sliding scale.

Patients with neuropathy are at great risk of developing posterior heel ulcers when lying in bed immobile for several days. These can be very difficult to heal, are entirely preventable and medico-legally indefensible. The simple provision of foam leg troughs is all that is needed to relieve the pressure on the heels while the patient is in bed. This should be done routinely in patients at risk. Pressure-relieving boots (**Fig. 7.6**) seem useful for wheelchair-bound patients.

CHARCOT NEUROARTHROPATHY

Charcot neuroarthropathy is characterised by bone and joint destruction, fragmentation and remodelling. It can be one of the most devastating foot complications of diabetes, and was first described as a complication of tabes dorsalis. It can develop in any joint and has been reported in most sensory

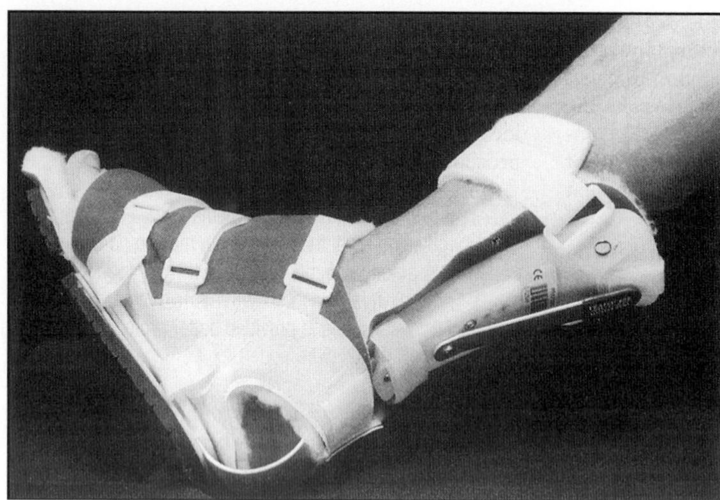

Figure 7.6 • Routine use of pressure-relieving boots reduces the risk of pressure ulcers in bed- or chair-bound patients.

neuropathies, but diabetes is now the commonest cause of the Charcot foot. Although once thought to be very rare, it is now known to affect nearly 10% of patients with neuropathy and over 16% of those with a history of neuropathic ulceration.[105] The exact mechanism remains unclear. Unperceived trauma, followed by weight-bearing on an injured limb, is thought by some to account for the fractures and joint destruction; however, there is evidence that increased blood flow to bone, resulting from autonomic neuropathy, activates osteoclasts and leads to localised osteoporosis,[106,107] perhaps allowing fractures to occur with minimal trauma. The matter is further complicated by the observation that fractures may not develop until several weeks after the foot becomes swollen. We have noted that periarticular erosions are common around affected joints and sometimes precede fractures and fragmentation, suggesting that an inflammatory arthropathy (possibly secondary to trauma) is the first stage of the process and that continued weight-bearing prolongs this phase, allowing periarticular bone resorption and fractures. Typically, patients present with a warm swollen foot. Although most textbooks describe it as a painless condition, there is frequently discomfort but not enough to prevent walking. The presentation is often several weeks after the onset of symptoms and, because of the lack of significant pain, simple radiographs may unfortunately not be performed. However, plain radiography is usually adequate to make the diagnosis, but isotope scans and magnetic resonance imaging are sometimes necessary to exclude osteomyelitis. The natural history is such that after a matter of months, during which bone resorption continues, the swelling and warmth begin to resolve. Treatment is aimed at shortening this time in order to minimise bone and joint destruction. The midfoot is a common site of Charcot neuroarthropathy and when affected can result in midfoot collapse, with a plantar bony prominence and 'rocker' foot, which has a very high risk of ulceration (**Fig. 7.7**). The mainstay of treatment is rest and immobilisation usually in a total contact cast, which may need to be continued for many months until disease activity has subsided. Disease activity is usually judged by measuring the temperature of the overlying skin with an infrared thermometer; when this is 2°C warmer than the other foot, an inflammatory response is still present. The only treatment directed at the excessive osteoclastic activity is with the intravenous bisphosphonate pamidronate. In an open study, pamidronate led to a rapid clinical improvement, together with a decrease in foot temperature and alkaline phosphatase.[108] In a randomised trial a single infusion of pamidronate resulted in a significant reduction in symptoms and an additional improvement in disease activity, as well as a reduction in bone turnover markers compared with standard care.[109]

Surgery to the foot is contraindicated in the early stages, due to the gross hyperaemia of involved bone and the risk that it (like trauma) will trigger bone resorption. However, corrective surgery may be useful at a later stage in order to remove bony prominences. At this stage, appropriate (usually custom-made) footwear is required, and great care should be taken of the other foot as there is a high risk of contralateral Charcot changes.

(a)

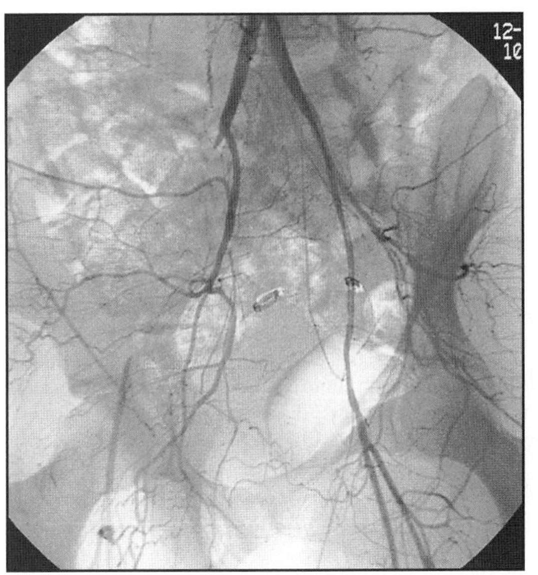

(b)

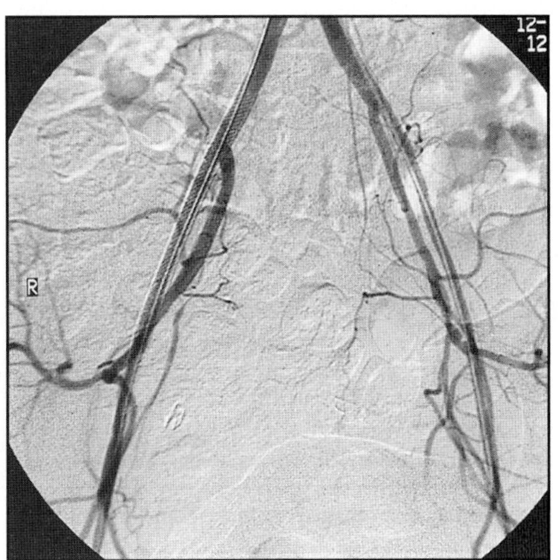

Figure 7.7 • Charcot neuroarthropathy resulting in midfoot collapse **(a)** with a plantar bony prominence and ulceration **(b)**.

Key points

- The management of the diabetic foot is challenging and requires a multidisciplinary approach, ideally coordinated by a specialised clinic.
- Identification of high-risk patients requires screening that must be both comprehensive and regular, and patient education should be part of this process.
- Once ulceration has developed, aggressive management can achieve excellent results with a significant reduction of both amputation and re-ulceration rates.
- Future research may ultimately enable the prevention of foot ulcers and the predisposing factors that lead to ulceration and may demonstrate superior ways of healing ulcers. However, the dissemination of current 'best practice' is already starting to have a major impact on the outlook for this condition.

REFERENCES

1. Wild S, Roglie G, Green A, King H. Global prevalence of diabetes: estimates for 2000 and projections for 2030. Diabetes Care 2004; 27:1047–53.
2. Boyko EJ, Ahroni JH, Smith DG, Davignon D. Increased mortality associated with diabetic foot ulcer. Diabetic Med 1996; 13:967–72.
3. Krentz AJ, Acheson P, Basu A et al. Morbidity and mortality associated with diabetic foot disease: a 12-month prospective survey of hospital admissions in a single UK centre. Foot 1997; 7:144–7.
4. Tentolouris N, Al-Sabbagh S, Walker MG, Boulton AJM, Jude EB. Mortality in diabetic and non-diabetic patients after amputations performed from 1990 to 1995: a 5-year follow-up study. Diabetes Care 2004; 27:1598–1604.
5. Jude EB, Boulton AJM. End stage complications of diabetic neuropathy. Diabetes Rev 1999; 7:395–410.
6. Kumar S, Ashe HA, Parnell LN et al. The prevalence of foot ulceration and its correlates in type 2 diabetic patients: a population-based study. Diabetic Med 1994; 11:480–4.
7. Neil HA, Thompson AV, Thorogood M, Fowler GH, Mann JI. Diabetes in the elderly: the Oxford Community Diabetes Study. Diabetic Med 1989; 6:608–13.
8. Borssen B, Bergenheim T, Lithner F. The epidemiology of foot lesions in diabetic patients aged 15–50 years. Diabetic Med 1990; 7:438–44.
9. Abbott CA, Carrington AL, Ashe H et al. The North West Diabetic Foot Care Study: incidence of, and risk factors for, new diabetic foot ulceration in

a community-based patient cohort. Diabetic Med 2002; 19:377–84.

10. Moss SE, Klein R, Klein B. The prevalence and incidence of lower extremity amputation in a diabetic population. Arch Intern Med 1992; 152:610–13.
11. Ramsey SD, Newton K, Blough DK et al. Incidence, outcomes, and cost of foot ulcers in patients with diabetes. Diabetes Care 1999; 22:382–7.
12. Oyibo SO, Jude EB, Voyatzoglou D, Boulton AJM. Clinical characteristics of patients with diabetic foot problems: changing patterns of foot ulcer presentation. Pract Diabetes Int 2002; 19:10–12.
13. Most RS, Sinnock P. The epidemiology of lower extremity amputations in diabetic individuals. Diabetes Care 1983; 6:87–91.
14. Gujral JS, McNally PG, O'Malley BP, Burden AC. Ethnic differences in the incidence of lower extremity amputation secondary to diabetes mellitus. Diabetic Med 1993; 10:271–4.
15. Young MJ, Boulton AJ, MacLeod AF, Williams DR, Sonksen PH. A multicentre study of the prevalence of diabetic peripheral neuropathy in the United Kingdom hospital clinic population. Diabetologia 1993; 36:150–4.
16. Walters DP, Gatling W, Mullee MA, Hill RD. The prevalence of diabetic distal sensory neuropathy in an English community. Diabetic Med 1992; 9:349–53.
17. Backonja M, Beydoun A, Edwards KR et al. Gabapentin for the symptomatic treatment of painful neuropathy in patients with diabetes mellitus: a randomised controlled trial. JAMA 1998; 280:1831–6.
18. Rull JA, Quibrera R, Gonzalez-Millan H, Lozano Castaneda O. Sympathetic treatment of peripheral diabetic neuropathy with carbamazepine (Tegretol). Diabetologia 1969; 5:215–8.
19. Capsaicin Study Group. The effect of treatment with capsaicin on the daily activities of patients with painful diabetic neuropathy. Diabetes Care 1992; 15:159–65.
20. Boulton AJM, Scarpello JH, Ward JD. Venous oxygenation in the neuropathic diabetic foot: evidence of arteriovenous shunting. Diabetologia 1982; 22:6–8.
21. Young MJ, Breddy JL, Veves A, Boulton AJM. The prediction of diabetic neuropathic foot ulceration using vibration perception thresholds. A prospective study. Diabetes Care 1994; 17:557–60.
22. Rith-Najarian SJ, Stolusky T, Gohdes DM. Identifying diabetic patients at high risk for lower-extremity amputation in a primary health care setting. A prospective evaluation of simple screening criteria. Diabetes Care 1992; 15:1386–9.
23. Pecoraro RE, Reiber GE, Burgess EM. Pathways to diabetic limb amputation: basis for prevention. Diabetes Care 1990; 13:513–21.

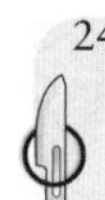

24. Reiber GE, Vileikyte L, Boyko EJ et al. Causal pathways for incident lower-extremity ulcers in patients with diabetes from two settings. Diabetes Care 1999; 22:157–62.
25. Boulton AJM, Malik RA, Arezzo JC, Sosenko JM. Diabetic somatic neuropathy: a technical review. Diabetes Care 2004; 27: in press.
26. National Diabetes Advisory Board. The prevention and treatment of five complications of diabetes: a guide for primary care practitioners. HHS publ. no. 83-8392. Atlanta, GA: Centers for Disease Control, 1983.
27. Strandness DE, Priest RE, Gibbons RE, Seattle MD. Combined clinical and pathological study of diabetic and non diabetic peripheral artery disease. Diabetes 1961; 13:366–72.
28. King TA, DePalma RG, Rhodes RS. Diabetes mellitus and atherosclerotic involvement of the profunda femoris artery. Surg Gynecol Obstet 1984; 159:553–6.
29. Jude EB, Oyibo SO, Chalmers N, Boulton AJM. Peripheral arterial disease in diabetic and non-diabetic patients: a comparison of severity and outcome. Diabetes Care 2001; 24:1433–7.
30. Karacagil S, Almgren B, Bowald S, Bergqvist D. Comparative analysis of patency, limb salvage and survival in diabetic and non-diabetic patients undergoing infrainguinal bypass surgery. Diabetic Med 1995; 12:537–41.
31. Weitz JL, Byrne J, Clagett GP et al. Diagnosis and treatment of chronic arterial insufficiency of the lower extremities: a critical review. Circulation 1996; 94:3026–49.
32. Pahlsson HI, Wahlberg E, Olotsson P, Swedenburg J. The toe pole-test for evaluation of arterial insufficiency in diabetic patients. Eur J Vasc Endovasc Surg 1999; 16:133–7.
33. Jacobs MJ, Ubbink DT, Kitslaar PJ et al. Assessment of the microcirculation provides additional information in critical limb ischaemia. Eur J Vasc Surg 1992; 6:135–41.

34. Ubels FL, Links TP, Sluiter WJ, Reitsma WD, Smit AJ. Walking training for intermittent claudication in diabetes. Diabetes Care 1999; 22:198–201.

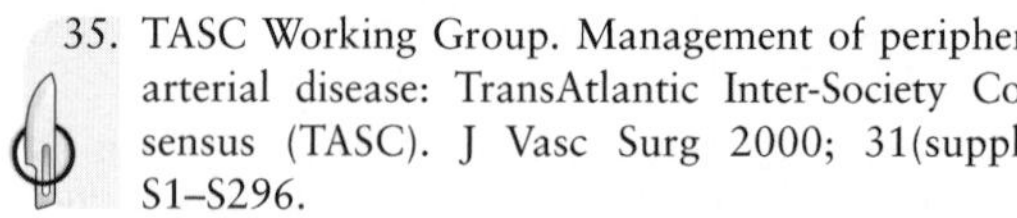

35. TASC Working Group. Management of peripheral arterial disease: TransAtlantic Inter-Society Consensus (TASC). J Vasc Surg 2000; 31(suppl.): S1–S296.
36. Robless P, Mikhailidis DP, Stansby G. Systematic review of antiplatelet therapy for the prevention of myocardial infarction, stroke or vascular death in patients with peripheral vascular disease. Br J Surg 2001; 88:787–800.
37. Chobanian AV, Bakris GL, Black HR et al. Seventh report of the Joint National Committee on Prevention, Detection, Evaluation and Treatment of high blood pressure. Hypertension 2003; 42:1206–52.

38. Heart Outcomes Prevention Evaluation Study Investigators. Effects of an angiotensin-converting enzyme inhibitor, ramipril, on cardiovascular events in high-risk patients. N Engl J Med 2000; 342:145–53.

    The HOPE study showed that the ACE inhibitor ramipril reduces cardiovascular morbidity and mortality in patients with peripheral arterial disease by around 25%.

39. Heart Protection Study Collaborative Group. MRC/BHF Heart Protection Study of cholesterol lowering with simvastatin in 20,536 high-risk individuals: a randomised placebo-controlled trial. Lancet 2002; 360:7–22.

    The Heart Protection Study showed that lowering total and LDL-cholesterol by 25% with a statin reduces cardiovascular mortality and morbidity in patients with peripheral arterial disease by around one-quarter.

40. British Medical Association and Royal Pharmaceutical Society of Great Britain. British National Formulary 43, March. London: BMA and RPSGB, 2002.
41. Chapman TM, Goa KL. Cilostazol. A review of its use in intermittent claudication. Am J Cardiovasc Drugs 2003; 3:117–38.
42. Hittel N, Donnelly R. Treating peripheral arterial disease in patients with diabetes. Diabetes Obes Metab 2002; 4(suppl. 2):S26–S31.
43. Rendell M, Cariski AT, Hittel N et al. Cilostazol treatment of claudication in diabetic patients. Curr Med Res Opin 2002; 18:479–87.
44. Van Schie CHM, Abbott CA, Vileikyte L et al. A comparative study of the Podotrack, a simple semi-quantitative device, and the optical pedobarograph in the assessment of pressures under the diabetic foot. Diabetic Med 1999; 16:154–9.
45. Veves A, Murray HJ, Young MJ, Boulton AJM. The risk of foot ulceration in diabetic patients with high foot pressures: a prospective study. Diabetologia 1992; 35:660–3.
46. Masson EA, Hay EM, Stockley I et al. Abnormal foot pressure alone does not cause ulceration. Diabetic Med 1989; 6:426–8.
47. Frykberg RG, Lavery LA, Pham H et al. Role of neuropathy and high foot pressures in diabetic foot ulceration. Diabetes Care 1998; 21:1714–19.
48. Stacpoole-Shea S, Shea G, Lavery L. An examination of plantar pressure measurements to identify the location of diabetic forefoot ulceration. J Foot Ankle Surg 1999; 38:109–15.
49. Boulton AJM. The pathogenesis of diabetic foot problems: an overview. Diabetic Med 1996; 13(suppl. 1):S12–S16.
50. Armstrong DG, Lavery LA. Plantar pressures are higher in diabetic patients following partial foot amputation. Ostomy Wound Manage 1998; 44:30–2.
51. Fernando DJ, Masson EA, Veves A, Boulton AJM. Relationship of limited joint mobility to abnormal foot pressures and diabetic foot ulceration. Diabetes Care 1991; 14:8–11.
52. Ctercteko GC, Dhanendran M, Hutton WC, Le Quesne LP. Vertical forces acting on the feet of diabetic patients with neuropathic ulceration. Br J Surg 1981; 68:608–14.
53. Boulton AJM, Hardisty CA, Betts RP et al. Dynamic foot pressure and other studies as diagnostic and management aids in diabetic neuropathy. Diabetes Care 1983; 6:26–33.
54. Murray HJ, Young MJ, Hollis S, Boulton AJM. The association between callus formation, high pressures and neuropathy in diabetic foot ulceration. Diabetic Med 1996; 13:979–82.
55. Young MJ, Cavanagh PR, Thomas G et al. The effect of callus removal on dynamic plantar foot pressures in diabetic patients. Diabetic Med 1992; 9:55–7.
56. Abouaesha F, van Schie CH, Griffiths GD, Young RJ, Boulton AJ. Plantar tissue thickness is related to peak plantar pressure in the high-risk diabetic foot. Diabetes Care 2001; 24:1270–4.
57. Young MJ, Coffey J, Taylor PM, Boulton AJM. Weight bearing ultrasound in diabetic and rheumatoid arthritis patients. Foot 1995; 5:76–9.
58. Flynn MD, Edmonds ME, Tooke JE, Watkins PJ. Direct measurement of capillary blood flow in the diabetic neuropathic foot. Diabetologia 1988; 31:652–6.
59. Rayman G, Hassan A, Tooke JE. Blood flow in the skin of the foot related to posture in diabetes mellitus. Br Med J 1986; 292:87–90.
60. Parkhouse N, Le Quesne PM. Impaired neurogenic vascular response in patients with diabetes and neuropathic foot lesions. N Engl J Med 1988; 318:1306–9.
61. Sapico FL, Bessman AN. Diabetic foot infections. In: Frykeberg RG (ed.) The high risk foot in diabetes mellitus. New York: Churchill Livingstone, 1991; p. 173.
62. Pecoraro RE, Chen MS. Ascorbic acid metabolism in diabetes mellitus. Ann NY Acad Sci 1987; 498:248–58.
63. Grossi EA, Esposito R, Harris LJ et al. Sternal wound infections and use of internal mammary artery grafts. J Thorac Cardiovasc Surg 1991; 102:342–6.
64. Edmonds ME, Blundell MP, Morris ME et al. Improved survival of the diabetic foot: the role of a specialized foot clinic. Q J Med 1986; 60:763–71.
65. Bailey TS, Yu HM, Rayfield EJ. Patterns of foot examination in a diabetes clinic. Am J Med 1985; 78:371–4.
66. Malone JM, Snyder M, Anderson G et al. Prevention of amputation by diabetic education. Am J Surg 1989; 158:520–3.

Educating diabetic patients can reduce foot ulceration and amputations.

67. Vileikyte L. Psychological aspects of diabetic neuropathic foot complications. An overview. Diabetes Metab Res Rev 2004; 20(suppl. 1):513–8.

68. Uccioli L, Faglia E, Monticone G et al. Manufactured shoes in the prevention of diabetic foot ulcers. Diabetes Care 1995; 18:1376–8.

69. van Schie CHM, Whalley A, Vileikyte L et al. Efficacy of injected liquid silicone in the diabetic foot to reduce risk factors for foot ulceration. Diabetes Care 2000; 23:634–8.

70. Veves A, Masson EA, Fernando DJ, Boulton AJM. Use of experimental padded hosiery to reduce abnormal foot pressures in diabetic neuropathy. Diabetes Care 1989; 12:653–5.

71. Schaff PS, Cavanagh PR. Shoes for the insensitive foot: the effect of a 'rocker bottom' shoe modification on plantar pressure distribution. Foot Ankle 1990; 11:129–40.

72. Patel VG, Wieman TJ. Effect of metatarsal head resection for diabetic foot ulcers on the dynamic plantar pressure distribution. Am J Surg 1994; 167:297–301.

73. Wagner FW Jr. The dysvascular foot: a system for diagnosis and treatment. Foot Ankle 1981; 2:64–122.

74. Lavery LA, Armstrong DG, Harkless LB. Classification of diabetic foot wounds. J Foot Ankle Surg 1996; 35:528–31.

75. Oyibo S, Jude EB, Tarawaneh I et al. Comparison of two diabetic foot ulcer classification systems: the Wagner and University of Texas systems. Diabetes Care 2001; 24:84–8.

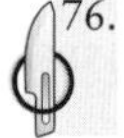

76. Armstrong DG, Nguyen HC, Lavery LA et al. Offloading the diabetic foot: a randomised clinical trial. Diabetes Care 2001; 24:1019–21.

Proper offloading of the diabetic foot ulcer was shown to enhance wound healing.

77. Shaw JE, Hsi WL, Ulbrecht JS et al. The mechanism of plantar unloading in total contact casts: implications for design and clinical use. Foot Ankle Int 1997; 18:809–17.

78. Knowlea EA, Armstrong DG, Hayat SA et al. Offloading diabetic foot wounds using the scotchcast boot: a retrospective study. Ostomy Wound Manage 2002; 48:50–3.

79. Lipsky BA, Pecoraro RE, Wheat LJ. The diabetic foot. Soft tissue and bone infection. Infect Dis Clin North Am 1990; 4:409–32.

80. Wheat LJ, Allen SD, Henry M et al. Diabetic foot infections. Bacteriologic analysis. Arch Intern Med 1986; 146:1935–40.

81. Tentolouris N, Jude EB, Smirnof I, Knowles EA, Boulton AJM. Methicillin-resistant *Staphylococcus aureus*: an increasing problem in a diabetic foot clinic. Diabetic Med 1999; 16:767–71.

82. Dang CN, Prasad YDM, Boulton AJM, Jude EB. Methicillin-resistant *Staphylococcus aureus* in the diabetic foot clinic: a worsening problem. Diabetic Med 2003; 20:159–61.

83. Park HM, Wheat LJ, Siddiqui AR et al. Scintigraphic evaluation of diabetic osteomyelitis: concise communication. J Nucl Med 1982; 23:569–73.

84. Keenan AM, Tindel NL, Alavi A. Diagnosis of pedal osteomyelitis in diabetic patients using current scintigraphic techniques. Arch Intern Med 1989; 149:2262–6.

85. Crerand S, Dolan M, Laing P et al. Diagnosis of osteomyelitis in neuropathic foot ulcers. J Bone Joint Surg Br 1996; 78:51–5.

86. Grayson ML, Gibbons GW, Balogh K, Levin E, Karchmer AW. Probing to bone in infected pedal ulcers. A clinical sign of underlying osteomyelitis in diabetic patients. JAMA 1995; 273:721–3.

87. Jude EB, Unsworth PF. Optimal treatment of infected diabetic foot ulcers. Drugs Aging 2004; 21:833–50.

88. Chantelau E, Tanudjaja T, Altenhofer F et al. Antibiotic treatment for uncomplicated neuropathic forefoot ulcers in diabetes: a controlled trial. Diabetic Med 1996; 13:156–9.

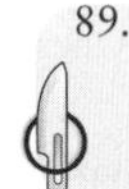

89. Lipsky BA, Baker PD, Landon GC, Fernau R. Antibiotic therapy for diabetic foot infections: comparison of two parenteral-to-oral regimens. Clin Infect Dis 1997; 24:643–8.

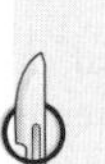

90. Grayson ML, Gibbons GW, Habershaw GM et al. Use of ampicillin/sulbactam versus imipenem/cilastatin in the treatment of limb-threatening foot infections in diabetic patients. Clin Infect Dis 1994; 18:683–93.

91. Lipsky BA, Itani K, Norden C. Linezolid Diabetic Foot Infections Study Group. Treating foot infections in diabetic patients: a randomized, multicentre, open-label trial of linezolid versus ampicillin–sulbactam/amoxicillin–clavulanate. Clin Infect Dis 2004; 38:17–24.

A large randomised trial showing the efficacy of the new antibiotic linezolid in the management of diabetic foot infections.

92. Perry CM, Jarvis B. Linezolid: a review of its use in the management of serious Gram-positive infections. Drugs 2001; 61:525–51.

93. Melzer M, Goldsmith D, Gransden W. Successful treatment of vertebral osteomyelitis with linezolid in a patient receiving hemodialysis and with persistent methicillin-resistant *Staphylococcus aureus* and vancomycin-resistant *Enterococcus* bacteremias. Clin Infect Dis 2000; 31:208–9.

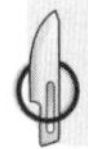

94. Wieman TJ, Smiell JM, Su Y. Efficacy and safety of a topical gel formulation of recombinant human platelet-derived growth factor-BB (becaplermin) in patients with chronic neuropathic diabetic ulcers. A phase III randomized placebo-controlled double-blind study. Diabetes Care 1998; 21:822–7.

Platelet-derived growth factor was shown to enhance healing of neuropathic foot ulcers compared with standard care alone.

95. Gentzkow GD, Iwasaki SD, Hershon KS et al. Use of dermagraft, a cultured human dermis, to treat diabetic foot ulcers. Diabetes Care 1996; 19:350–4.

96. Faglia E, Favales F, Aldeghi A et al. Adjunctive systemic hyperbaric oxygen therapy in treatment of severe prevalently ischemic diabetic foot ulcer. A randomized study. Diabetes Care 1996; 19:1338–43.

97. Veves A, Falanga V, Armstrong DG, Sabolinski ML. Graftskin, a human skin equivalent, is effective in the management of noninfected neuropathic diabetic foot ulcers: a prospective randomised multicentre clinical trial. Diabetes Care 2001; 24:290–5.

Graftskin was shown to enhance healing of neuropathic foot ulcers compared with standard care alone.

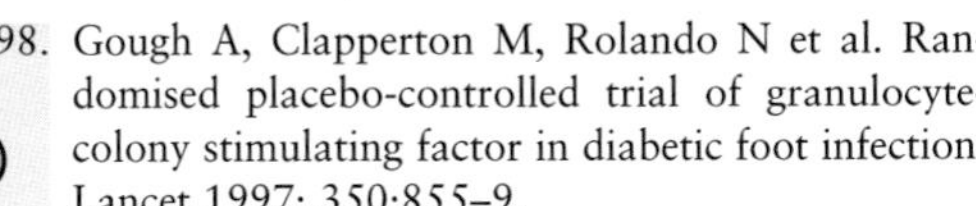

98. Gough A, Clapperton M, Rolando N et al. Randomised placebo-controlled trial of granulocyte-colony stimulating factor in diabetic foot infection. Lancet 1997; 350:855–9.

Granulocyte colony-stimulating factor was shown to enhance healing of infected neuropathic foot ulcers.

99. Thomas S, Jones M, Shutler S, Jones S. Using larvae in modern wound management. J Wound Care 1996; 5:60–9.

100. Thomas S. New drugs for diabetic foot ulcers: larval therapy. In: Boulton AJM, Connor H, Cavanagh PR (eds) The foot in diabetes, 3rd edn. Chichester: John Wiley & Sons, 2000; pp. 185–91.

101. Casu RE, Eisemann CH, Vuoclo T, Tellman RL. The major excretory/secretory protease from *Lucilia cuprina* larvae is also a gut digestive protease. Int J Parasitol 1996; 26:623–8.

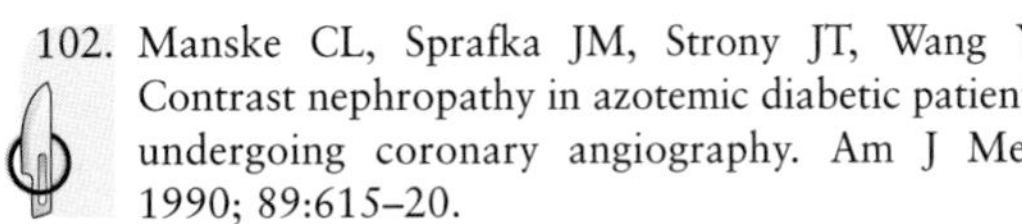

102. Manske CL, Sprafka JM, Strony JT, Wang Y. Contrast nephropathy in azotemic diabetic patients undergoing coronary angiography. Am J Med 1990; 89:615–20.

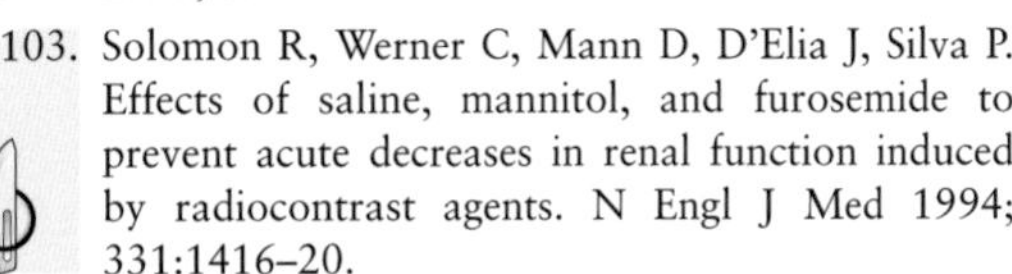

103. Solomon R, Werner C, Mann D, D'Elia J, Silva P. Effects of saline, mannitol, and furosemide to prevent acute decreases in renal function induced by radiocontrast agents. N Engl J Med 1994; 331:1416–20.

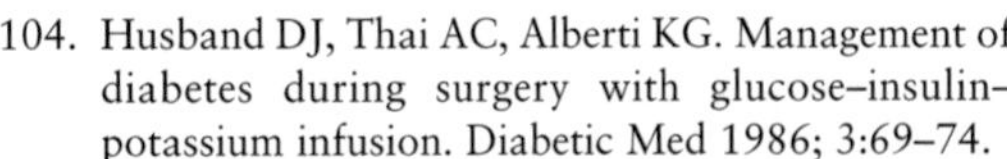

104. Husband DJ, Thai AC, Alberti KG. Management of diabetes during surgery with glucose–insulin–potassium infusion. Diabetic Med 1986; 3:69–74.

105. Cavanagh PR, Young MJ, Adams JE, Vickers KL, Boulton AJ. Radiographic abnormalities in the feet of patients with diabetic neuropathy. Diabetes Care 1994; 17:201–9.

106. Edmonds ME, Clarke MB, Newton S, Barrett J, Watkins PJ. Increased uptake of bone radiopharmaceutical in diabetic neuropathy. Q J Med 1985; 57:843–55.

107. Young MJ, Marshall A, Adams JE, Selby PL, Boulton AJ. Osteopenia, neurological dysfunction, and the development of Charcot neuroarthropathy. Diabetes Care 1995; 18:34–8.

108. Selby PL, Young MJ, Boulton AJ. Bisphosphonates: a new treatment for diabetic Charcot neuroarthropathy? Diabetic Med 1994; 11:28–31.

109. Jude EB, Selby PL, Mawer B et al. Pamidronate in diabetic Charcot neuroarthropathy: a randomised placebo controlled trial. Diabetologia 2001; 44:2032–7.

This trial showed the efficacy of bisphosphonates in treating acute Charcot neuroarthropathy.

CHAPTER

Eight

Revision vascular surgery

Christopher P. Gibbons

INTRODUCTION

Revision of vascular reconstructions is frequently required beyond the first 6 weeks because of progressive atherosclerosis, graft occlusion, aneurysm formation or infection. Up to 40% of infrainguinal bypass surgery grafts require reintervention within 5 years.[1] Revision surgery requires experience and judgement: it is technically more difficult because of fibrosis and the loss of easily definable tissue planes, necessitating careful sharp dissection to gain arterial control. Operating times, blood loss, infection rates and operative risk are increased.

GRAFT OCCLUSION

Graft thrombosis usually presents acutely but is occasionally heralded by increasing ischaemic symptoms. Its effect depends upon the bypass and the collateral circulation, ranging from mild claudication through critical ischaemia to an acutely threatened limb. Occasionally, simultaneous distal embolisation causes digital ischaemia (the blue toe syndrome) or gangrene. Whereas graft thrombosis in the first 6 weeks is generally due to technical error or poor run-off, most late occlusions result from intimal hyperplasia within the bypass or progressive inflow or run-off disease (see Chapter 4). Graft stenoses are usually asymptomatic and occur in 20–30% of infrainguinal vein grafts, mostly in the first year, but those greater than 70% (velocity >3 m/s or velocity ratio >3.0) compromise flow and often occlude if untreated.[2]

Factors influencing graft occlusion

LOCAL FACTORS

These are essentially the quality of the inflow, the run-off and the conduit itself (see Chapter 4).[3]

- Patency is better for suprainguinal than infrainguinal grafts and graft occlusion is more frequent in femerotibial than femeropopliteal bypasses.[3]

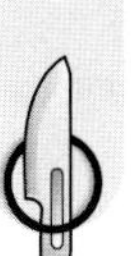

- Infrainguinal bypass patency of autologous vein is better than Dacron, polytetrafluoroethylene (PTFE) and human umbilical vein,[3–7] but heparin-bonded Dacron is better than PTFE.[8]
- Vein cuffs and patches[9] or an expanded hood[10] at the lower anastomosis improve PTFE graft patency.

- Xenograft or allograft conduits suffer from poor early patency and late aneurysm formation.[7,11–13]
- Larger vein (>4 mm diameter)[14,15] and prosthetic infrainguinal grafts (e.g. 8 mm rather than 6 mm) and those with higher perioperative flow have better patency.[16]

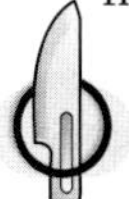

- Reversed and in situ vein grafts are equivalent.[14,17]

- Arm veins are similar to long saphenous vein provided angioscopically detected defects are corrected.[18–20]

- Splicing several veins does not compromise patency.[19]
- Stenoses are more significant in narrow vein grafts and relate to early postoperative flow defects[21,22] or a thickened wall[23] but not clamp injury.[15,24]
- The quality and number of run-off vessels strongly predicts outcome.[25,26]
- Bypasses for gangrene occlude more frequently than for ulceration or rest pain.[27]

GENERAL FACTORS

- Continued smoking increases graft thrombosis threefold to fivefold.[21,28,29]
- Diabetes[30] and renal failure[31] compromise patient survival but not graft patency.
- Raised fibrinogen, hyperlipidaemia,[28,32] thrombophilias (e.g. protein C, protein S or antithrombin III deficiency, antiphospholipid antibodies, factor V Leiden mutation) and increased platelet aggregation favour graft thrombosis[29,33–37]
- Graft occlusion and recurrent stenoses are commoner in women[38,39] and hormone replacement therapy potentiates this.[40]

Prevention of graft thrombosis

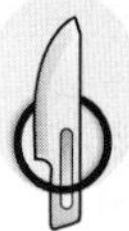

- Antiplatelet agents should promote graft patency but good evidence exists only for aspirin.[41,42] Aspirin is more effective for infrainguinal prosthetic grafts, whereas warfarin is better for vein grafts.[43]

- Radiotherapy may prevent intimal hyperplasia of prosthetic bypasses.[44]
- Duplex Doppler surveillance is generally recommended for infrainguinal vein but not prosthetic grafts[6,45] since most critical (>3 m/s) and many intermediate (2–3 m/s) stenoses occlude if untreated[2] and the outcome after revision is good,[46] although randomised trials are conflicting.[47]

Management of graft stenosis (the failing graft)

Stenoses of greater than 70% should be treated by either angioplasty or surgical revision. Short (<2 cm) midgraft or distal anastomotic stenoses may respond to angioplasty using high inflation pressures (up to 2020 kPa)[48] (**Fig. 8.1**) with good long-term patency[49] especially if cutting balloons are used.[50] However, proximal anastomotic, recurrent or multiple stenoses and those longer than 2–3 cm are probably better treated surgically (**Fig. 8.2**).[51,52] While stents are probably best avoided in vein grafts they may be useful for recurrent prosthetic anastomotic stenoses, and drug-eluting stents have shown promise for the prevention of recurrent intimal hyperplasia.[53] Angioplasty is probably less durable than surgical revision[54,55] but is less invasive and rarely compromises subsequent surgery.[56]

Longer vein graft stenoses may be bypassed using arm vein, contralateral long saphenous or femoral vein.[20] Tibial or distal popliteal anastomotic stenoses resistant to angioplasty are best treated by a jump graft to a fresh run-off vessel to avoid scar tissue and adherent tibial veins (**Fig. 8.2c**).

Management of the failed graft

If graft occlusion causes non-disabling claudication, a conservative approach is usually preferred. Mild ischaemia allows time for thrombolysis or elective surgery but an anaesthetic paralysed limb demands emergency revascularisation within 3–4 hours.

ROLE OF THROMBOLYSIS

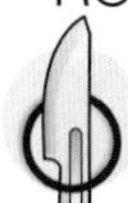

Thrombolysis is indicated for a viable limb within 14 days of graft occlusion provided the patient has not undergone surgery within 3 months.[57]

Caution is necessary in aortic grafts because of possible bleeding through the Dacron fabric.[59] For claudicants the risk of thrombolysis probably outweighs any benefit.[60] Otherwise, thrombolysis using recombinant tissue plasminogen activator via a pulse-spray catheter will achieve lysis in 70–80%, but recanalisation is more likely in recent occlusions (<4 days) and older grafts (>11 months).[61,62] Any underlying stenosis is corrected by angioplasty or early surgery.[63] However, the popularity of thrombolysis is reducing because of haemorrhagic complications, poor long-term patency and persistent ischaemia (see Chapter 9).[64–67]

AORTIC GRAFT THROMBOSIS

Chronic aortic graft occlusion presenting with recurrent claudication or rest pain allows elective or urgent investigation by intra-arterial digital subtraction angiography. Either computed tomography (CT) or ultrasound should be performed to eliminate infection as a cause for graft thrombosis. When acute aortic graft occlusion presents with threatened lower limbs, buttocks and pelvic organs, it is best to proceed directly to an axillo-bifemoral graft without angiography, provided the upper limb pulses are satisfactory.

A single occluded aorto-bifemoral graft limb can be thrombectomised through the femoral anastomotic hood with simultaneous pressure on the opposite groin to prevent contralateral embolisation. A No. 5 or 6 embolectomy catheter should clear a fresh occlusion but more organised thrombus

(a)
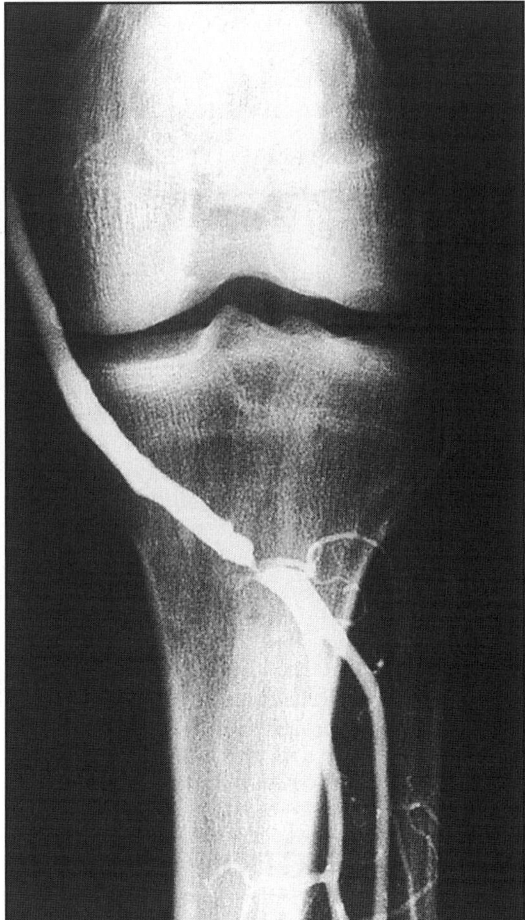
(b)
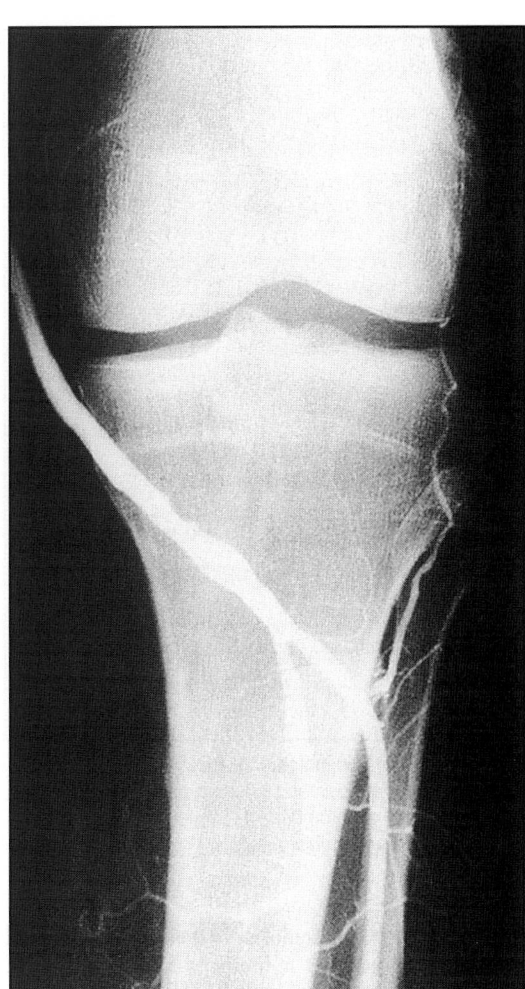

Figure 8.1 • Vein graft stenosis near the below-knee popliteal anastomosis **(a)** successfully treated by balloon angioplasty **(b)**.

requires a ring stripper or adherent clot catheter. Any run-off stenosis is corrected by extending the graft into the profunda femoris or superficial femoral artery (**Fig. 8.3**). If thrombectomy fails, a femoro-femoral crossover graft should be performed.

EXTRA-ANATOMICAL GRAFT THROMBOSIS

Thrombosis of a femoro-femoral graft or one limb of an axillo-bifemoral graft is usually due to outflow stenosis and can be managed by either thrombolysis and angioplasty or thrombectomy and graft revision/extension.

Complete axillo-bifemoral thrombosis results from an axillary anastomotic or subclavian stenosis, infection or pressure on the graft (e.g. during sleep). Preoperative duplex and angiography of the subclavian, axillary and run-off arteries are ideal, but if viability is compromised immediate surgery is required. Thrombolysis rarely succeeds because of the mass of thrombus. Thrombectomy is performed through incisions near the axillary and femoral anastomoses and any stenosis corrected. Scarring around the axillary vessels is best avoided by placing a fresh contralateral graft, as advocated by some authors.[68]

INFRAINGUINAL GRAFT THROMBOSIS

Ischaemia following infrainguinal graft thrombosis is usually worse for prosthetic than vein grafts because they often take out the run-off.[5] Duplex Doppler and intra-arterial digital subtraction angiography can be performed for viable limbs, and thrombolysis can be considered in patients aged under 80 years with a recent occlusion. Prosthetic grafts or vein grafts that have been occluded for less than a week can be thrombectomised, with revision

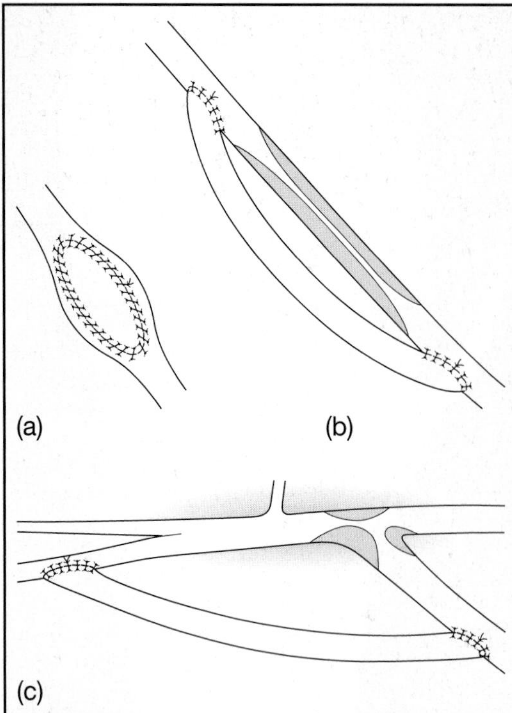

Figure 8.2 • **(a)** Vein patch angioplasty, **(b)** bypass of long vein graft stenosis and **(c)** jump graft around stenosed distal anastomosis of a femoro-popliteal bypass graft to the posterior tibial artery.

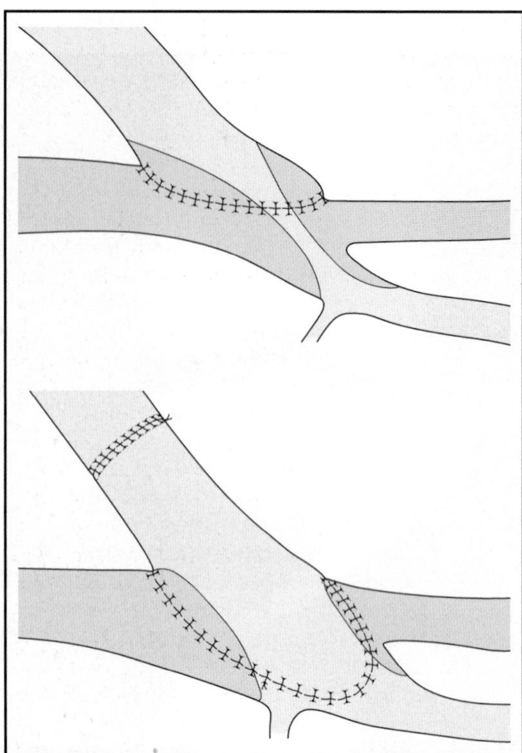

Figure 8.3 • Extension graft to one limb of an aorto-bifemoral graft to treat a stenosis at the profunda origin. In this case the superficial femoral artery is occluded.

of any underlying stenosis by vein patch, partial graft replacement or a jump graft (see **Fig. 8.2**). If recanalisation fails, a fresh bypass should be constructed, preferably with autologous vein.[69] Long-term anticoagulation is advisable.

A threatened limb demands revascularisation as soon as possible and within 6 hours. A tender 'woody' calf indicates muscle necrosis, and an ischaemic contracture or limb loss may occur even after successful revascularisation. Provided there is a good femoral pulse, on-table angiography can be performed after thrombectomy through incisions near the proximal and distal anastomoses with a No. 3 embolectomy catheter and repeated flushing with heparinised saline. Residual thrombus can be lysed by infusing 100 000 units of streptokinase or 10–15 mg of recombinant tissue plasminogen activator in 30 mL saline and clamping for 20 minutes.[70] Any defect must be revised otherwise rethrombosis is likely despite anticoagulation.

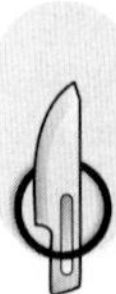

Following thrombectomy for acute ischaemia, four-compartment fasciotomy should be considered to relieve pressure and improve distal perfusion, especially if there is any calf swelling or tenderness (see Chapter 9).[71]

GRAFT INFECTION

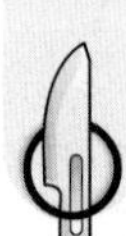

Graft infection is relatively uncommon (1–5%)[72] but has a high amputation risk (10–25%) and mortality (20%).[73] In a recent multicentre audit of 55 graft infections, 31% died, 33% underwent amputation and only 45% left hospital alive without amputation.[74]

Causes

Most graft infections originate at surgery[75] due to a breakdown of sterility or from pre-existing bacteria (e.g. mycotic aneurysms) but some occur by extension from superficial wound infections or from haematogenous spread.

Wound (and graft) infections are more likely in patients with tissue loss and in the elderly, obese and those undergoing reoperation during the same hospital admission. Preoperative shaving, open surgical drainage for more than 3 days, operations lasting over 2 hours,[76] emergency surgery, diabetes, steroids, renal failure, recent arteriography and wound haematoma are also risk factors.[77] Blood-borne bacteria from intravenous lines, or systemic infections may also cause graft sepsis.

Once infected a prosthesis acts as a foreign body, rendering bacteria inaccessible to antibiotics. Vein grafts are more resistant but direct bacterial erosion can occur, especially when exposed in an open wound.

Prevention

- Patients should be admitted as near to surgery as possible and isolated from patients with known infections, especially methicillin-resistant *Staphylococcus aureus* (MRSA).[78]
- Strict aseptic technique and laminar flow theatres minimise infection rates. Iodine-impregnated adhesive drapes help isolate the operative field.
- Prophylactic antibiotics reduce wound and graft infection.[79] Most use a cephalosporin or co-amoxiclav against staphylococci or coliforms but vancomycin or teicoplanin prophylaxis is probably wise[80–82] because of the high prevalence of MRSA[80] and considerable morbidity and mortality of MRSA graft infections.[83,84]

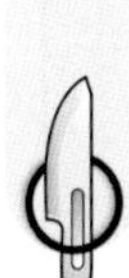

- Antibiotic-bonded grafts: rifampicin binds to gelatin-, collagen- or albumin-coated grafts and remains for at least 3 days.[85] Although rifampicin bonding is effective in experimental graft infection,[86] randomised clinical trials have failed to demonstrate any prophylactic effect.[87–89]

- Silver-coated grafts have in vitro antibacterial activity and reduced graft infection in an experimental model[90] but randomised clinical trials are required.

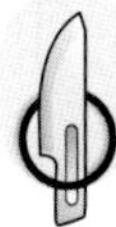

- Closed suction drainage removes potentially infected haematoma or seroma but two small randomised trials of inguinal wound drainage showed no advantage.[91,92]

- There is little consensus on the need for prophylactic antibiotics before other surgical or dental procedures in the presence of prosthetic grafts.[93]

Presentation

Szilagii et al.[94] classified postoperative vascular wound infections according to the depth of tissue involvement: type 1 involves the skin, type 2 the subcutaneous tissue and type 3 the graft itself. Prosthetic graft infection can present at any time from days to years after surgery with local abscesses and sinuses, graft exposure (**Fig. 8.4**, see also Plate 9, facing p. 116), thrombosis or anastomotic haemorrhage. Septic erosion of exposed vein grafts can occur at any point.

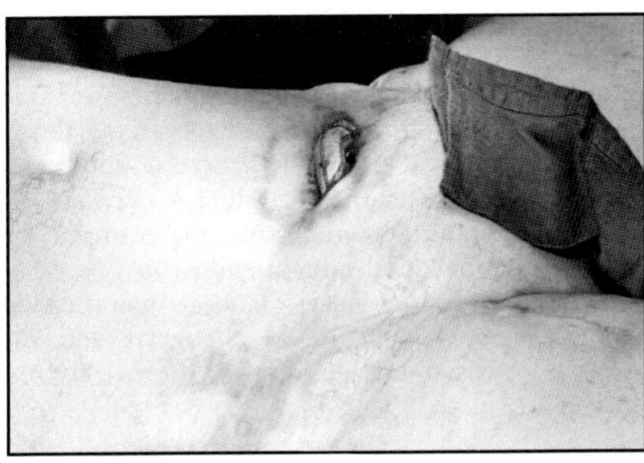

Figure 8.4 • A chronically exposed femoro-femoral bypass graft.

Infected aortic grafts can erode the fourth part of the duodenum or occasionally other parts of the bowel causing aorto-enteric fistulas, which may present with one or two sentinel gastrointestinal bleeds before the inevitable catastrophic haemorrhage. The mortality of aorto-enteric fistula is high (>50%), with recurrent infection or aortic stump disruption in over 25%.[95]

Bacteriology

Most graft infections are due to skin organisms. *Staphylococcus epidermidis* is the least virulent, producing a biofilm or an infected seroma after months or years. It is difficult to culture, requiring careful preparation of explanted graft material to dislodge adherent bacteria.[96] *Staphylococcus aureus* is more virulent and usually presents earlier. MRSA may have particularly high morbidity and mortality.[74,80] Streptococci, enterococci, coliforms, *Serratia marcescens*, *Pseudomonas* and *Bacteroides* are also causative organisms. Gram-negative species, especially *Pseudomonas*, are more likely to cause anastomotic haemorrhage.[77,97] Sometimes no organism is cultured from an obviously infected graft because of failure to isolate *Staph. epidermidis* or prior exposure to antibiotics.

Diagnosis

In most cases there is a perigraft abscess or sinus. Aspiration of frank pus or turbid fluid from around the graft and the subsequent culture of a causative organism are diagnostic. CT, magnetic resonance imaging (MRI) or ultrasound usually demonstrates perigraft fluid[98] and inflammation but can underestimate the extent of infection, especially if a sinus is present, when sinography may be useful.

For wholly intra-abdominal prostheses there may be few signs but the leucocyte count, erythrocyte sedimentation rate and C-reactive protein may be raised. Perigraft fluid after 3–6 months or gas beyond 7–10 days on ultrasound CT or MRI[98,99] suggests infection (**Fig. 8.5**). One in four anastomotic aneurysms[100] result from graft infection, but this is not always evident from CT. Where doubt exists, indium-labelled leucocyte scanning is occasionally helpful.[101] In aorto-enteric fistula, the graft may be seen eroding the duodenum at endoscopy.[102]

Definitive confirmation is made at operation by the presence of pus around the graft and the absence of tissue incorporation of knitted Dacron or PTFE grafts.

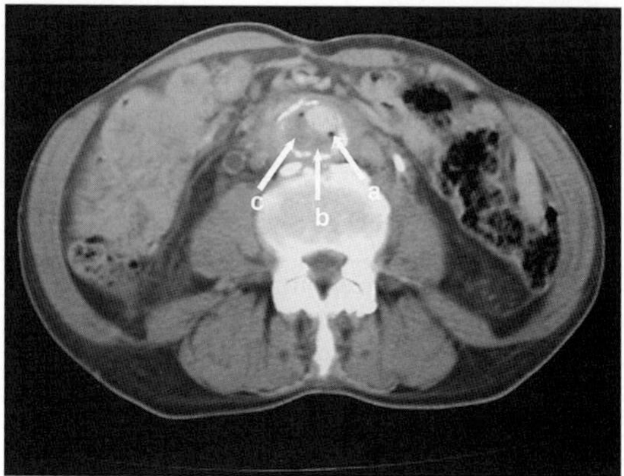

Figure 8.5 • CT scan with intravenous contrast of an aortoiliac graft showing perigraft gas **(a)** and fluid **(b)**. The left limb of the graft is occluded **(c)**.

Management

Once infection is confirmed, urgent treatment is required to pre-empt catastrophic haemorrhage or graft thrombosis. Conservative measures are rarely curative and after partial excision the remaining graft usually requires later replacement.[103] Radical graft excision with débridement and revascularisation, preferably with an autologous conduit, is the procedure of choice.

CONSERVATIVE MEASURES

- Prolonged antibiotic therapy may buy time during preparation for definitive surgery. Implantation of gentamicin-impregnated collagen foam or beads[104,105] is unlikely to succeed in established infection unless the prosthesis itself is removed.
- Antiseptic or antibiotic irrigation after drainage of a perigraft abscess has advocates but is rarely curative.[106,107]
- Muscle flaps: sartorius detached proximally and rotated medially will cover exposed femoral vessels (**Fig. 8.6**) but cannot reach above the inguinal ligament.[108,109] Rectus femoris, divided distally and reflected upwards under sartorius, will cover exposed femoro-femoral or axillo-femoral grafts (**Fig. 8.7**, see also Plate 10, facing p. 116).[110] Other techniques include rectus abdominis, gracilis, semimembranosus and gastrocnemius flaps.[111–114] However, if there is gross sepsis or haemorrhage, recurrent infection is frequent.[114]
- Greater omentum is useful for wrapping intra-abdominal grafts in order to prevent adherence to bowel but can also be brought through the abdominal wall or under the inguinal ligament to cover exposed femoral anastomoses.[115]
- Exposed infrainguinal grafts in the lower leg are particularly challenging. The risk of graft erosion is greatest with Gram-negative or MRSA infections.[116,117] Soleus or gastrocnemius flaps combined with split skin grafts or, alternatively, microvascular free flaps may provide successful cover[118] but it is usually easier to bypass the area with a fresh vein graft or re-route the graft in a deeper plane.
- Endovascular grafts will seal aorto-enteric fistulas in the short term but recurrent infection is likely.[119,120]

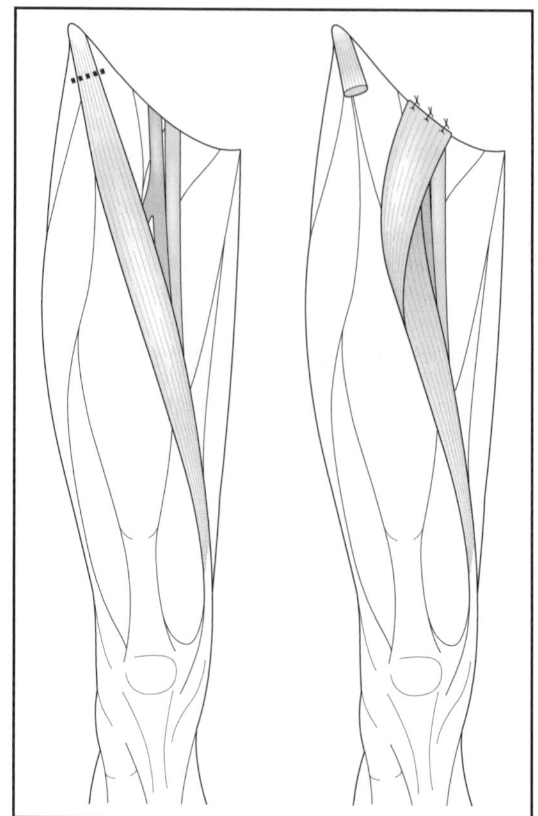

Figure 8.6 • The sartorius flap.

(a)

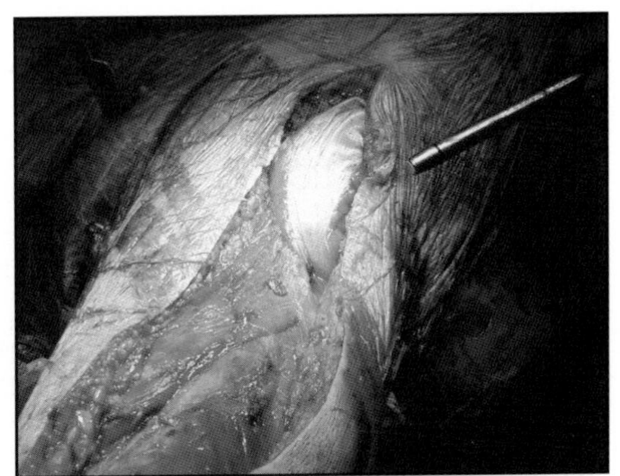

(b)

Figure 8.7 • Use of a rectus femoris flap to cover a femoral anastomosis: **(a)** after mobilisation of the flap; **(b)** with the flap in position over the anastomosis.

SIMPLE GRAFT EXCISION

The mainstay of treatment is excision of the infected graft but unless revascularisation is performed, limb loss is likely. After aortic graft excision, the proximal extent of the ischaemia may prevent even bilateral high above-knee amputations from healing so that revascularisation should almost always be attempted. For infrainguinal bypass, simple graft excision usually allows a satisfactory amputation and is sometimes the safest option in high-risk patients.

GRAFT EXCISION AND EXTRA-ANATOMICAL BYPASS

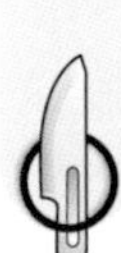

Revascularisation with a fresh prosthesis in a clean field and excision of the infected graft is the 'gold standard'. Unless there is acute haemorrhage, revascularisation should precede aortic graft excision as this reduces the risk of amputation from 45 to 11%.[73]

For aortic or aortoiliac graft infections, axillo-bifemoral or bilateral axillo-femoral grafts can be anastomosed to the common femoral artery but for aorto-bifemoral replacement the distal anastomosis must be to the superficial femoral or popliteal artery to ensure an uninfected field.

To avoid localised groin sepsis, iliofemoral grafts can be re-routed to the superficial femoral or popliteal artery via the obturator foramen[121,122] (**Fig. 8.8**), lateral to the femoral nerve under the inguinal ligament[123] or through a hole drilled in the ilium.[124] Subscrotal femoro-femoral grafts[125] and a lateral approach to the profunda femoris[126] may be occasionally useful. Replacement infrainguinal grafts can be tunnelled laterally.

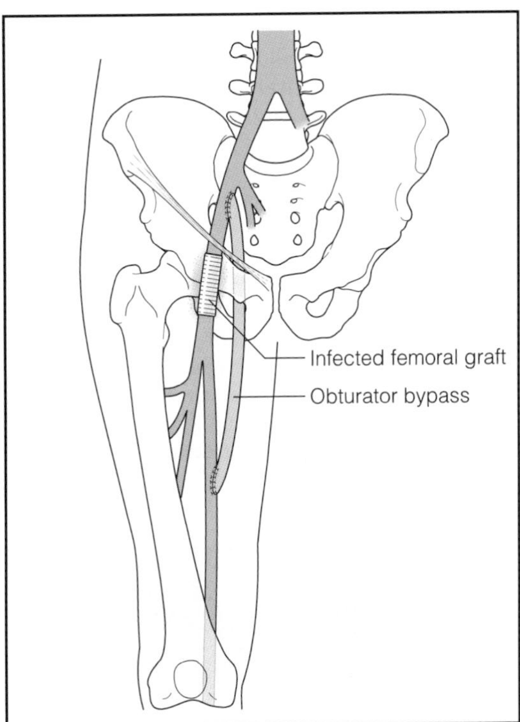

Figure 8.8 • Obturator bypass.

The infected field should be excluded by adhesive drapes during the extra-anatomical reconstruction and the wounds sealed before excising the infected prosthesis. All infected material should be removed and the arteriotomy closed, if necessary with a vein patch. The wounds should be thoroughly cleaned, irrigated with antiseptics and drained. Gentamicin-impregnated collagen foam may be helpful. Adequate antibiotic cover is essential during and for about 6 weeks after surgery.

The mortality is about 20%, with 10% limb loss. However, the extra-anatomical graft becomes reinfected in approximately 10%,[73,127–129] and the incidence of late thrombosis is higher than with in situ reconstructions.

IN SITU PROSTHETIC RECONSTRUCTION

An alternative is graft excision with débridement, with immediate prosthetic replacement. A rifampicin-bonded or silver-impregnated graft is used, although no good evidence of clinical effectiveness exists despite encouraging individual series.[130–133] Mortality, amputation and reinfection rates are similar to those of excision and extra-anatomical bypass[73] but most have reserved it for low-grade graft infections.

ALLOGRAFTS

There have been encouraging reports of in situ replacement of infected prosthetic grafts using cryopreserved arterial allografts, with 6% mortality, good long-term survival and few graft complications.[134] However, mortality is higher in other series, with up to 9% early graft ruptures and 10% late graft complications, including reinfection, rupture and aneurysms especially after graft–enteric fistulas.[135,136]

AUTOLOGOUS RECONSTRUCTION

In situ reconstruction using autologous vein offers the best prospect for eliminating infection.[110,137–141] Long saphenous vein, arm veins or even endarterectomised superficial femoral artery can be used to replace infected infrainguinal grafts but are too narrow for aortoiliac reconstruction.

The femoral vein has a thick wall and good calibre and can be harvested from below the profunda femoris to the knee with little morbidity.[142,143] (An 18% incidence of compartment syndrome requiring fasciotomy has recently been described in 264 limbs undergoing deep vein harvest.[144] However, I have yet to find this necessary after harvesting 54 deep veins.) One vein suffices for aortoiliac or femoro-femoral graft replacement but both are required for aorto-bifemoral or axillo-femoral grafts. Preoperative duplex is wise to confirm their patency and calibre (preferably >1 cm diameter).

Two or three teams operating together shorten operating time and are essential in patients with actively bleeding aorto-enteric fistulas in order to avoid excessive clamp times. Preoperative broad-spectrum antibiotic prophylaxis (e.g. co-amoxiclav, ciprofloxacin, teicoplanin and metronidazole or tazocillin, teicoplanin and metronidazole) is continued for 6 weeks and modified to cover any cultured organism.

In stable patients the femoral veins are first harvested (**Fig. 8.9**, see also Plate 11, facing p. 116) before exposing any femoral anastomosis to obtain distal control before aortic clamping. The graft is then excised, aspirating any pus and débriding the infected tissue. The native artery is trimmed back to uninfected tissue and the area washed repeatedly with povidone iodine and hydrogen peroxide. The new graft is fashioned using reversed (or antegrade valve-disrupted) femoral vein. Various configurations have been used, such as a trouser graft or an aorto-unifemoral graft with a femoro-femoral crossover, but the easiest is the inverted Y graft (**Fig. 8.10**, see also Plate 12, facing p. 116). Size discrepancy at the

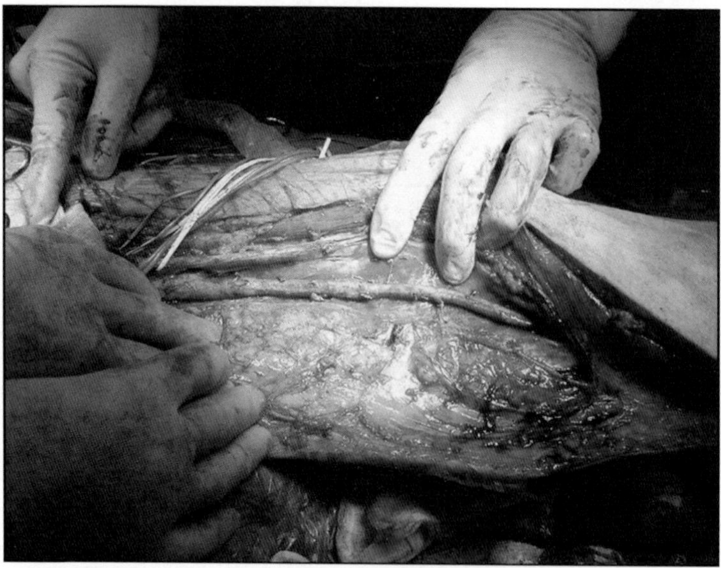

Figure 8.9 • Exposure of the femoral vein.

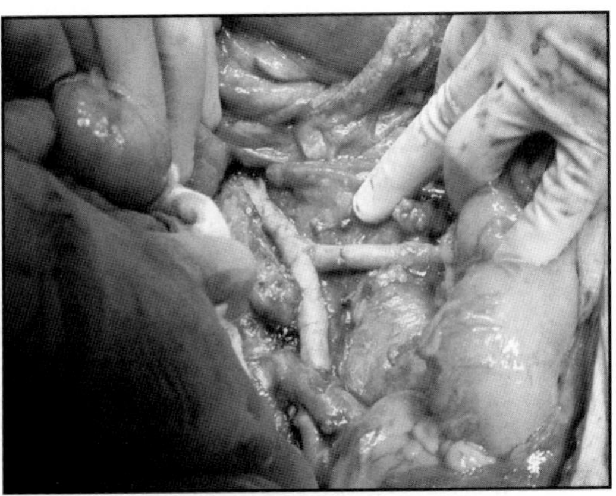

Figure 8.10 • Aortic reconstruction using femoral vein after excision of an infected aortic graft.

aortic anastomosis can be corrected by a variety of techniques (**Fig. 8.11**) but 'fish-mouthing' the vein is simple and avoids angulation. The vein is placed in a fresh tunnel and its upper part wrapped in omentum. Gentamicin-impregnated collagen foam is placed around it and the area drained. If skin cover is poor, a sartorius or rectus femoris flap will protect the femoral anastomosis.

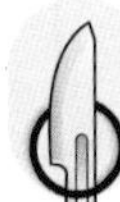

Mortality and limb loss are both about 10% following femoral vein replacement but infection is eliminated in the survivors,[110,137–141] making it the procedure of choice for most patients.

Postoperative duplex surveillance is recommended in order to detect anastomotic or graft stenoses, which can be treated by angioplasty or surgery.[110]

(a)

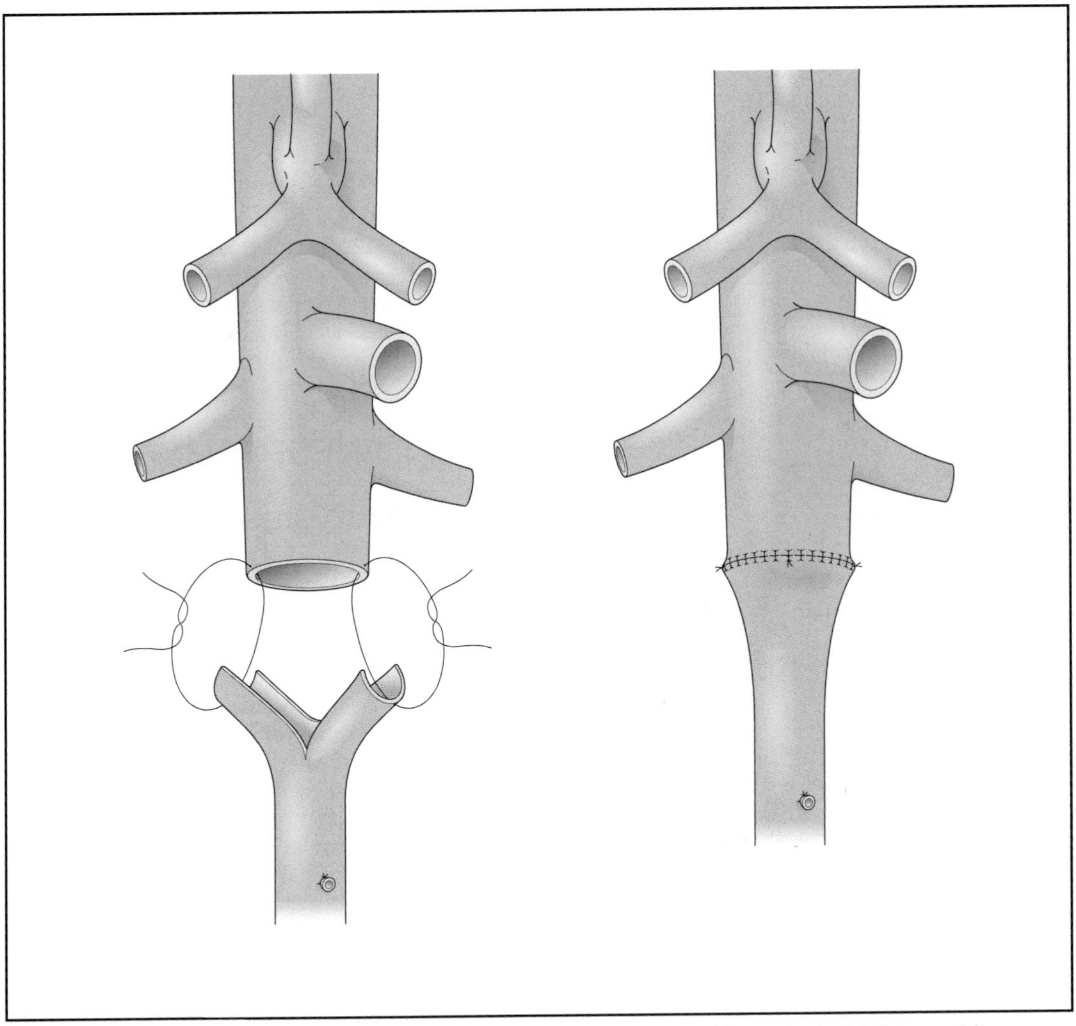

Figure 8.11 • Methods for correction of size discrepancy between the aorta and femoral vein: **(a)** 'fish-mouth' technique.

(b)

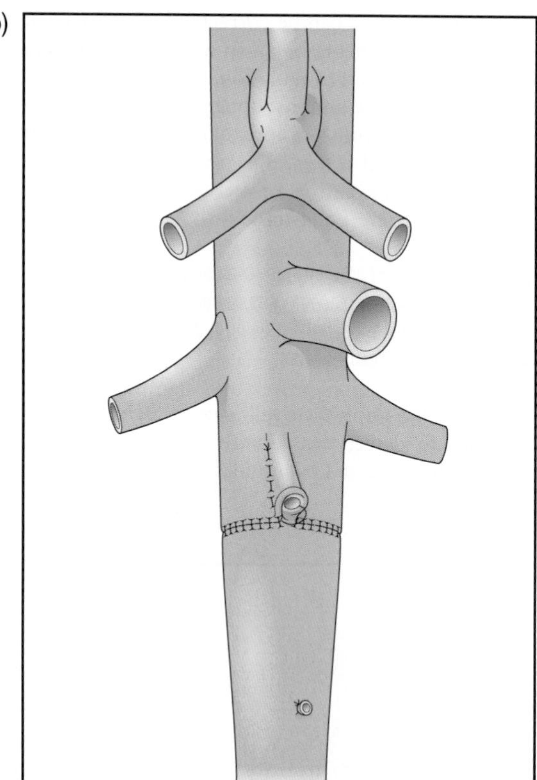

(c)

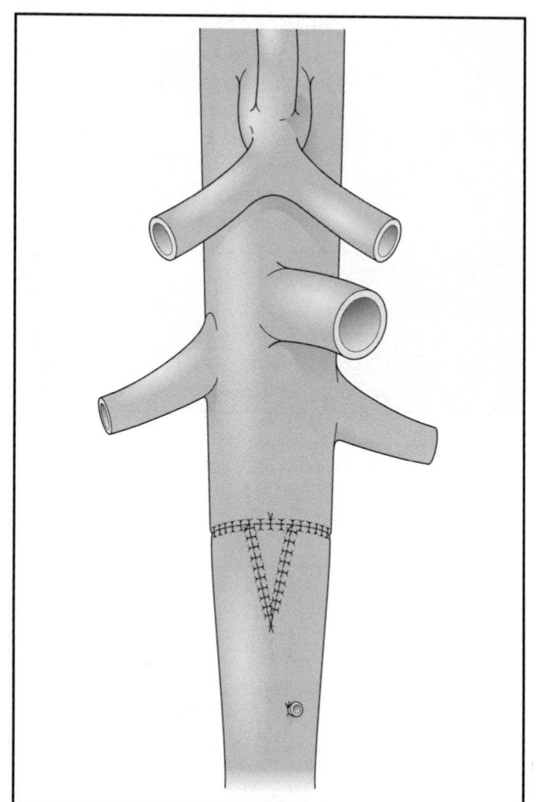

(d)

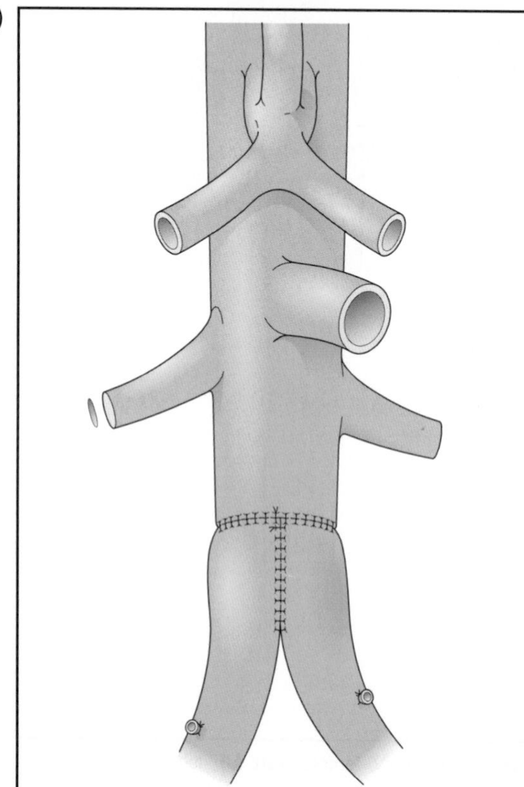

Figure 8.11 (*cont.*) • Methods for correction of size discrepancy between the aorta and femoral vein: **(b)** aortic plication; **(c)** venous gusset; **(d)** 'trouser' graft.

GRAFT ANEURYSMS

True aneurysms

Following repair of a true aneurysm, the adjacent artery may also become aneurysmal.[145] Aneurysms were frequent within some early PTFE grafts but manufacturing improvements have almost eliminated this.[146] Biological grafts such as the human umbilical vein graft frequently became aneurysmal before the addition of a Dacron wrap.[147] Xenografts such as bovine mesenteric vein and cryopreserved venous or arterial allografts are particularly subject to aneurysmal degeneration.[11–13]

Dacron undergoes late degradation and dilatation, which becomes clinically significant in 2–3%. After 5–10 years, disruption can occur at points of stress (e.g. under the inguinal ligament) causing false aneurysms,[148] which may present with haemorrhage or thrombosis. Distraction during shoulder abduction may cause spontaneous rupture[149,150] or axillary anastomotic disruption of PTFE axillofemoral grafts.[151,152] Vein graft aneurysms are rare but more frequent in bypasses for popliteal aneurysms than for occlusive disease.[153]

Information on the natural history of untreated graft aneurysms is lacking but repair is generally recommended and is essential for rupture, thrombosis or embolism. Treatment is either with a covered endovascular stent or by graft replacement.

False aneurysms

False aneurysms are essentially pulsating haematomas, which may occur at the arterial puncture site after angiography or at disrupted arterial anastomoses. Puncture-site aneurysms often thrombose spontaneously. Ultrasound-guided compression occludes over 80% and most others will thrombose following thrombin injection.[154] Direct surgical repair or a covered stent are rarely necessary.[155]

Anastomotic aneurysms result from mechanical distraction or graft infection.[100] They occur most commonly at femoral anastomoses, where the risks of rupture and thrombosis are size related,[156] and are one of the most frequent long-term complications of aortic grafts so that a routine 5-year CT scan is advisable.[157] Compression or thrombin injection is rarely applicable, and open repair with an interposition graft is wise, especially in the aorta,[158] although a covered stent may occasionally be used (**Fig. 8.12**).[159]

(a)

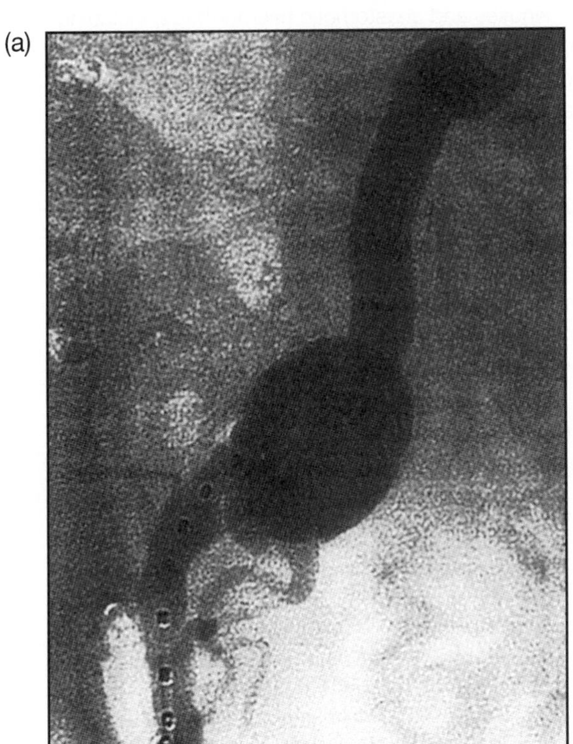

(b)

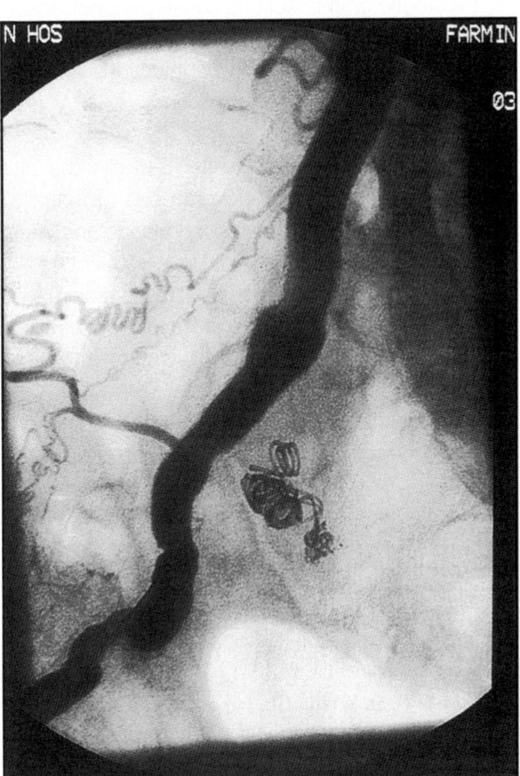

Figure 8.12 • Anastomotic aneurysm at the distal end of a previous aortoiliac bypass **(a)** treated by coil embolisation of the internal iliac artery and placement of a covered stent across the aneurysm **(b)**.

Key points

- Late graft occlusion is caused by intimal hyperplasia or progressive atherosclerotic stenosis of the inflow or run-off.
- Graft stenoses occur in 20–30% of infrainguinal vein grafts and those stenoses greater than 70% often progress to occlusion. Treatment is by angioplasty or surgery.
- The effects of graft occlusion depend on the collateral circulation and may result in an acutely threatened limb, the recurrence of claudication or critical ischaemia.
- Thrombolysis of occluded grafts may be attempted in patients aged under 80 years with critical ischaemia provided that limb viability is not threatened, that the patient has not undergone surgery within 3 months and that the occlusion is less than 14 days old.
- Graft infection results from a breakdown of sterility at surgery, by extension from a superficial wound infection or from blood-borne bacteria.
- Prosthetic graft infections cause perigraft abscesses, sinuses and anastomotic haemorrhage, including aorto-enteric fistula. Vein grafts may be eroded by infection, particularly in open wounds.
- *Staphylococcus epidermidis* infections are usually chronic. *Staphylococcus aureus* or Gram-negative infections tend to present early. MRSA and Gram-negative infections are more likely to cause anastomotic bleeding.
- Any fluid around a graft after 3–6 months or gas beyond 7–10 days on CT or ultrasound suggests infection. Aspiration of perigraft pus will usually secure the diagnosis.
- Prolonged antibiotic therapy, drainage and irrigation, or covering exposed grafts with muscle or omental flaps is rarely curative.
- Simple graft excision usually causes severe ischaemia leading to amputation or death.
- The 'gold standard' is extra-anatomical revascularisation followed by graft excision. However, graft excision and in situ revascularisation with autologous vein (e.g. femoral vein) has better patency and recurrent infection is rare.
- True aneurysms can occur within prosthetic or vein grafts or adjacent to previous aneurysms.
- False aneurysms may result from anastomotic distraction or infection. Treatment is usually surgical.

REFERENCES

1. Dawson I, van Bockel JH. Reintervention and mortality after infrainguinal reconstructive surgery for leg ischaemia. Br J Surg 1999; 86:38–44.
2. Mills JL Sr, Wixon CL, James DC et al. The natural history of intermediate and critical vein graft stenosis: recommendations for continued surveillance or repair. J Vasc Surg 2001; 33:273–8.
3. Gonzales-Farjardo JA, Vacquero C. Femorocrural bypass for limb salvage: real indications and results. In: Branchereau A, Jacobs M (eds) Critical limb ischaemia. Armonk, NY: Futura Publishing Company, 1999; pp. 165–81.

   A comprehensive review of the results and factors affecting patency of femoro-distal bypass.

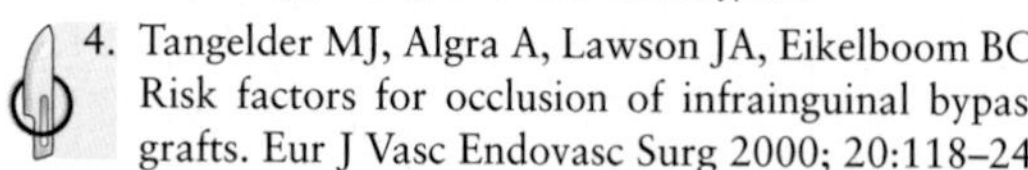
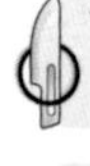

4. Tangelder MJ, Algra A, Lawson JA, Eikelboom BC. Risk factors for occlusion of infrainguinal bypass grafts. Eur J Vasc Endovasc Surg 2000; 20:118–24.

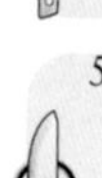

5. Jackson MR, Belott TP, Dickason T et al. The consequences of a failed femoropopliteal bypass grafting: comparison of saphenous vein and PTFE grafts. J Vasc Surg 2000; 32:498–504.

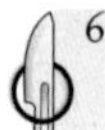

6. Trans-Atlantic Inter-Society Consensus (TASC). Management of peripheral arterial disease. Eur J Vasc Endovasc Surg 2000; 19(suppl. A).

   Authoritative consensus view and guidelines for the treatment of peripheral vascular disease.

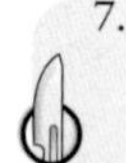

7. Paaske WP. Femoropopliteal reconstruction. In: Branchereau A, Jacobs M (eds) Critical limb ischaemia. Armonk, NY: Futura Publishing Company, 1999; pp. 147–64.

   A comprehensive review of femoro-popliteal bypass.

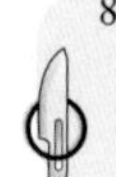

8. Devine C, Hons B, McCollum C. Heparin-bonded Dacron or polytetrafluoroethylene for femoro-popliteal bypass grafting: a multicenter trial. J Vasc Surg 2001; 33:533–9.

   A randomised controlled trial with 100 patients in each group showing a definite patency advantage of heparin-bonded Dacron over PTFE in femoro-popliteal bypass.

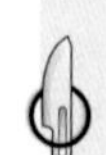

9. Stonebridge PA, Prescott RJ, Ruckley CV. Randomized trial comparing infrainguinal polytetrafluoroethylene bypass grafting with and without vein interposition cuff at the distal anastomosis. The Joint Vascular Research Group. J Vasc Surg 1997; 26:543–50.

A randomised controlled trial with 130 patients in each group showing a significant advantage for interposition vein cuffs in below-knee but not above-knee PTFE femoro-popliteal bypass.

10. Fisher RK, Kirkpatrick UJ, How TV et al. The distaflo graft: a valid alternative to interposition vein? Eur J Vasc Endovasc Surg 2003; 25:235–9.
11. Rossi G, Munteanu FD, Padula G et al. Non-anastomotic aneurysms in venous homologous grafts and bovine heterografts in femoropopliteal bypasses. Am J Surg 1976; 132:358–62.
12. Kovalic AJ, Beattie DK, Davies AH. Outcome of ProCol, a bovine mesenteric vein graft, in infra-inguinal reconstruction. Eur J Vasc Endovasc Surg 2002; 24:533–4.
13. Farber A, Major K, Wagner WH et al. Cryo-preserved saphenous vein allografts in infrainguinal revascularization: analysis of 240 grafts. J Vasc Surg 2003; 38:15–21.
14. Watelet J, Soury P, Menard JF et al. Femoro-popliteal bypass: in situ or reversed vein grafts? Ten-year results of a randomized prospective study. Ann Vasc Surg 1997; 11:510–19.

A small, 10-year, single-centre, randomised study with 50 patients in each group showing no difference between the patency of in situ and reversed vein grafts.

15. Idu MM, Buth J, Hop WC et al. Factors influencing the development of vein-graft stenosis and their significance for clinical management. Eur J Vasc Endovasc Surg 1999; 17:15–21.
16. Ihlberg LH, Alback NA, Lassila R, Lepantalo M. Intraoperative flow predicts the development of stenosis in infrainguinal vein grafts. J Vasc Surg 2001; 34:269–76.

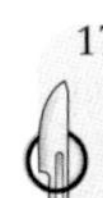

17. Wengerter KR, Veith FJ, Gupta SK et al. Prospective randomized multicenter comparison of in situ and reversed vein infrapopliteal bypasses. J Vasc Surg 1991; 13:189–97.

A relatively small multicentre study (60 patients in each group) that failed to show any advantage for in situ infrapopliteal bypass.

18. Faries PL, Arora S, Pomposelli FB et al. The use of arm vein in lower extremity revascularization: results of 520 procedures performed in eight years. J Vasc Surg 2000; 31:50–9.
19. Eugster T, Stierli P, Fischer G, Gurke L. Long-term results of infrainguinal reconstruction with spliced veins are equal to results with non-spliced veins. Eur J Vasc Endovasc Surg 2001; 22:152–6.
20. Gibbons CP, Osman HY, Shiralkar S. The use of alternative sources of autologous vein for infra-inguinal bypass. Eur J Vasc Endovasc Surg 2003; 25:93–4.
21. Gentile AT, Mills JL, Gooden MA et al. Identification of predictors for lower extremity vein graft stenosis. Am J Surg 1997; 174:218–21.
22. Ferris BL, Mills JL Sr, Hughes JD et al. Is early postoperative duplex scan surveillance of leg bypass grafts clinically important? J Vasc Surg 2003; 37:495–500.
23. Marin ML, Veith FJ, Panetta TF et al. Saphenous vein biopsy: a predictor of vein graft failure. J Vasc Surg 1993; 18:407–14.
24. Moody AP, Edwards PR, Harris PL. The aetiology of vein graft strictures: a prospective marker study. Eur J Vasc Surg 1992; 6:509–11.
25. Stewart AH, Lucas A, Smith FC et al. Pre-operative hand-held Doppler run-off score can be used to stratify risk prior to infra-inguinal bypass surgery. Eur J Vasc Endovasc Surg 2002; 23:500–4.
26. Ulus AT, Ljungman C, Almgren B et al. The influence of distal runoff on patency of infrainguinal vein bypass grafts. Vasc Surg 2001; 35:31–5.
27. Nasr MK, McCarthy RJ, Budd JS, Horrocks M. Infrainguinal bypass graft patency and limb salvage rates in critical limb ischemia: influence of the mode of presentation. Ann Vasc Surg 2003; 17:192–7.
28. Cheshire NJ, Wolfe JH, Barradas MA et al. Smoking and plasma fibrinogen, lipoprotein (a) and serotonin are markers for postoperative infra-inguinal graft stenosis. Eur J Vasc Endovasc Surg 1996; 11:479–86.
29. Giswold ME, Landry GJ, Sexton GJ et al. Modifiable patient factors are associated with reverse vein graft occlusion in the era of duplex scan surveillance. J Vasc Surg 2003; 37:47–53.
30. Wolfle KD, Bruijnen H, Loeprecht H et al. Graft patency and clinical outcome of femorodistal arterial reconstruction in diabetic and non-diabetic patients: results of a multicentre comparative analysis. Eur J Vasc Endovasc Surg 2003; 25:229–34.
31. Albers M, Romiti M, Pereira CAB et al. A meta-analysis of infrainguinal arterial reconstruction in patients with end-stage renal disease. Eur J Vasc Endovasc Surg 2001; 22:285–300.
32. Daida H, Yokoi H, Miyano H et al. Relation of saphenous vein graft obstruction to serum cholesterol levels. J Am Coll Cardiol 1995; 25:193–7.
33. Nielsen TG, Nordestgaard BG, von Jessen M et al. Antibodies to cardiolipin may increase the risk of failure of peripheral vein bypasses. Eur J Vasc Endovasc Surg 1997; 24:177–84.
34. Donaldson MC, Belkin M, Whittemore AD et al. Impact of activated protein C resistance on general vascular surgical patients. J Vasc Surg 1997; 25:1054–60.
35. Curi MA, Skelly CL, Baldwin ZK et al. Long-term outcome of infrainguinal bypass grafting in patients with serologically proven hypercoagulability. J Vasc Surg 2003; 37:301–6.
36. Fligelstone LJ, Cachia PG, Ralis H et al. Lupus anticoagulant in patients with peripheral vascular disease: a prospective study. Eur J Vasc Endovasc Surg 1995; 9:277–83.

37. Saad EM, Kaplan S, el-Massry S et al. Platelet aggregometry can accurately predict failure of externally supported knitted Dacron femoropopliteal bypass grafts. J Vasc Surg 1993; 18:587–94.

38. Henke PK, Proctor MC, Zajkowski PJ et al. Tissue loss, early primary graft occlusion, female gender, and a prohibitive failure rate of secondary infrainguinal arterial reconstruction. J Vasc Surg 2002; 35:902–9.

39. Watson HR, Schroeder TV, Simms MH, Horrocks M. Association of sex with patency of femorodistal bypass grafts. Eur J Vasc Endovasc Surg 2000; 20:61–6.

40. Timaran CH, Stevens SL, Grandas OH et al. Influence of hormone replacement therapy on graft patency after femoropopliteal bypass grafting. J Vasc Surg 2000; 32:506–16.

41. Dorffler-Melly J, Koopman MM, Adam DJ et al. Antiplatelet agents for preventing thrombosis after peripheral arterial bypass surgery. Cochrane Database Syst Rev 2003; CD000535.

An up-to-date systematic review concluding that aspirin has a slight beneficial effect on bypass patency.

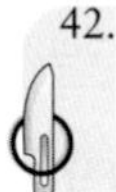

42. Towne JB. Anticoagulation to prolong lower limb bypass. In: Greenhalgh RM (ed.) The durability of vascular and endovascular surgery. London: WB Saunders, 1999; pp. 207–16.

A review of the evidence for anticoagulants and antiplatelet agents for prolonging graft patency.

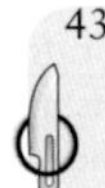

43. The Dutch Bypass Oral Anticoagulants or Aspirin Study. Efficacy of oral anticoagulants compared with aspirin after infrainguinal bypass surgery: a randomised trial. Lancet 2000; 355:346–51.

An important randomised controlled study of over 2500 patients showing that oral anticoagulation was better for the prevention of infrainguinal vein graft occlusion and for lowering the rate of ischaemic events, whereas aspirin was better for the prevention of non-venous graft occlusion and was associated with fewer bleeding episodes.

44. Hofmann WJ, Kopp M, Sedlmayer F et al. External beam radiation for prevention of intimal hyperplasia in peripheral arterial bypasses. Int J Radiat Oncol Biol Phys 2003; 56:1180–3.

45. Calligaro KD, Doerr K, McAffee-Bennett S et al. Should duplex ultrasonography be performed for surveillance of femoropopliteal and femorotibial arterial prosthetic bypasses? Ann Vasc Surg 2001; 15:520–4.

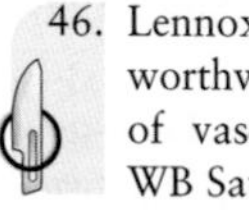

46. Lennox AF, Wolfe JHN. Vein graft surveillance is worthwhile. In: Greenhalgh RM (ed.) The durability of vascular and endovascular surgery. London: WB Saunders, 1999; pp. 317–31.

A useful source of evidence for graft surveillance.

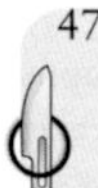

47. Beattie DK, Ellis M, Davies AH. Graft surveillance programmes. In: Beard JD, Murray S (eds) Pathways of care in vascular surgery. Shrewsbury: tfm Publishing, 2002; pp. 107–16.

A balanced review of the evidence for and against graft surveillance.

48. Schneider PA. Endovascular skills. Guidewires, catheters, arteriography, balloon angioplasty, stents. St Louis, Mo: Quality Medical Publishing, 1998; p. 196.

49. Avino AJ, Bandyk DF, Gonsalves AJ et al. Surgical and endovascular intervention for infrainguinal vein graft stenosis. J Vasc Surg 1999; 29:60–70.

50. Engelke C, Morgan RA, Belli AM. Cutting balloon percutaneous transluminal angioplasty for salvage of lower limb arterial bypass grafts: feasibility. Radiology 2002; 223:106–14.

51. Tong Y, Matthews PG, Royle JP. Outcome of endovascular intervention for infrainguinal vein graft stenosis. Cardiovasc Surg 2002; 10:545–50.

52. Houghton AD, Todd C, Pardy B et al. Percutaneous angioplasty for infrainguinal graft-related stenoses. Eur J Vasc Endovasc Surg 1997; 14:380–5.

53. Duda SH, Pusich B, Richter G et al. Sirolimus-eluting stents for the treatment of obstructive superficial femoral artery disease: six-month results. Circulation 2002; 106:1505–9.

54. Perler BA, Osterman FA, Mitchell SE et al. Balloon dilatation versus surgical revision of infra-inguinal autogenous vein graft stenoses: long-term follow-up. J Cardiovasc Surg (Torino) 1990; 31:656–66.

55. Alexander JQ, Katz SG. The efficacy of percutaneous transluminal angioplasty in the treatment of infrainguinal vein bypass graft stenosis. Arch Surg 2003; 138:510–13.

56. Lofberg AM, Karacagil S, Ljungman C et al. Distal percutaneous transluminal angioplasty through infrainguinal bypass grafts. Eur J Vasc Endovasc Surg 2002; 23:212–19.

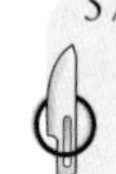

57. Comerota AJ, Weaver FA, Hosking JD et al. Results of a prospective, randomized trial of surgery versus thrombolysis for occluded lower extremity bypass grafts. Am J Surg 1996; 172:105–12.

Trial of 124 occluded grafts randomised to either surgery or thrombolysis showing an advantage for surgery in grafts occluded for more than 14 days but improved limb salvage and reduced magnitude of surgery in thrombolysed grafts occluded for less than 14 days.

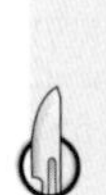

58. Braithwaite BD, Buckenham TM, Galland RB et al. Prospective randomized trial of high-dose bolus versus low-dose tissue plasminogen activator infusion in the management of acute limb ischaemia. Thrombolysis Study Group. Br J Surg 1997; 84:646–50.

A small trial (50 patients per group) showing that high-dose bolus therapy significantly accelerated thrombolysis with tissue plasminogen activator without compromising outcome, enabling thrombolysis to be used as primary therapy for many patients with acute critical ischaemia.

59. Pope M, Kalman PG. Aortic transgraft haemorrhage after systemic thrombolytic therapy. Ann Vasc Surg 1997; 11:292–94.

60. Braithwaite BD, Tomlinson MA, Walker SR et al. Peripheral thrombolysis for acute-onset claudication. Thrombolysis Study Group. Br J Surg 1999; 86:800–4.

61. Schwierz T, Gschwendtner M, Havlicek W et al. Indications for directed thrombolysis or new bypass in treatment of occlusion of lower extremity arterial bypass reconstruction. Ann Vasc Surg 2001; 15:644–52.

62. Berkowitz HD, Kee JC. Occluded infrainguinal grafts: when to choose lytic therapy versus a new bypass graft. Am J Surg 1995; 170:136–9.

63. Buckenham TM. Graft thrombolysis. In: Earnshaw JJ, Gregson RHS (eds) Practical peripheral arterial thrombolysis. Oxford: Butterworth-Heinemann, 1994; pp. 106–17.

A useful review of the radiological techniques for clearing thrombosed grafts.

64. Galland RB, Magee TR, Whitman B et al. Patency following successful thrombolysis of occluded vascular grafts. Eur J Vasc Endovasc Surg 2001; 22:157–60.

65. Nackman GB, Walsh DB, Fillinger MF et al. Thrombolysis of occluded infrainguinal vein grafts: predictors of outcome. J Vasc Surg 1997; 25:1023–31.

66. Aburahma AF, Hopkins ES, Wulu JT Jr, Cook CC. Lysis/balloon angioplasty versus thrombectomy/open patch angioplasty of failed femoropopliteal polytetrafluoroethylene bypass grafts. J Vasc Surg 2002; 35:307–15.

67. Richards T, Pittathankal AA, Magee TR, Galland RB. The current role of intra-arterial thrombolysis. Eur J Vasc Endovasc Surg 2003; 26:166–9.

68. Olson CJ, Edwards JM, Taylor LM et al. Repeat axillofemoral grafting as treatment for axillofemoral graft occlusion. Arch Surg 2002; 137:1364–7.

69. Landry GJ, Moneta GL, Taylor LM Jr et al. Choice of autogenous conduit for lower extremity vein graft revisions. J Vasc Surg 2002; 36:238–43.

70. Beard JD, Nyamekye I, Earnshaw JJ et al. Intra-operative streptokinase: a useful adjunct to balloon-catheter embolectomy. Br J Surg 1993; 80:21–4.

71. Jensen SL, Sandermann J. Compartment syndrome and fasciotomy in vascular surgery. A review of 57 cases. Eur J Vasc Endovasc Surg 1997; 13:48–53.

72. Seeger JM. Management of patients with prosthetic graft infection. Am Surg 2000; 66:166–7.

73. Yeager RA, Porter JM. Arterial and prosthetic graft infection. Ann Vasc Surg 1992; 5:485–91.

An excellent source of combined statistics on graft infection that is still relevant 13 years later.

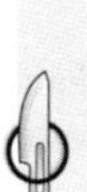

74. Naylor AR, Hayes PD, Darke S on behalf of the Joint Vascular Research Group. A prospective audit of complex wound and graft infections in Great Britain and Ireland: the emergence of MRSA. Eur J Vasc Endovasc Surg 2001; 21:289–94.

75. Jones L, Braithwaite BD, Davies B et al. Mechanism of late prosthetic vascular graft infection. Cardiovasc Surg 1997; 5:486–9.

76. Moro ML, Carrieri MP, Tozzi AE et al. Risk factors for surgical wound infections in clean surgery: a multicenter study. Italian PRINOS Study Group. Ann Ital Chir 1996; 67:13–19.

77. Hicks RJC, Greenhalgh RM. The pathogenesis of vascular graft infection. Eur J Vasc Endovasc Surg 1997; 14(suppl. A):5–9.

A short review of the causes and microbiology of graft infection.

78. Chalmers RT, Wolfe JH, Cheshire NJ et al. Improved management of infrainguinal bypass graft infection with methicillin-resistant *Staphylococcus aureus*. Br J Surg 1999; 86:1433–6.

79. Strachan CJ. Antibiotic prophylaxis in peripheral vascular and orthopaedic prosthetic surgery. J Antimicrob Chemother 1993; 31(suppl. B):65–78.

80. Earnshaw JJ. Methicillin-resistant *Staphylococcus aureus*: vascular surgeons should fight back. Eur J Vasc Endovasc Surg 2002; 24:283–6.

81. Santini C, Baiocchi P, Serra P. Perioperative antibiotic prophylaxis in vascular surgery. Eur J Vasc Endovasc Surg 1997; 14(suppl. A):13–14.

A short review of antibiotic prophylaxis in vascular surgery.

82. Mini E, Nobili S, Periti P. Does surgical prophylaxis with teicoplanin constitute a therapeutic advance? J Chemother 2000;12(suppl. 5):40–55.

83. Nasim A, Thompson MM, Naylor AR et al. The impact of MRSA on vascular surgery. Eur J Vasc Endovasc Surg 2001; 22:211–14.

84. Murphy GJ, Pararajasingam R, Nasim A et al. Methicillin-resistant *Staphylococcus aureus* infection in vascular surgical patients. Ann R Coll Surg Engl 2001; 83:158–63.

85. Lovering AM, White LO, MacGowan AP, Reeves DS. The elution and binding characteristics of rifampicin for three commercially available protein-sealed vascular grafts. J Antimicrob Chemother 1996; 38:599–604.

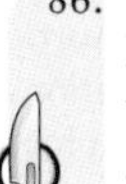

86. Sardelic F, Ao PY, Taylor DA, Fletcher JP. Prophylaxis against *Staphylococcus epidermidis* vascular graft infection with rifampicin-soaked, gelatin-sealed Dacron. Cardiovasc Surg 1996; 4:389–92.

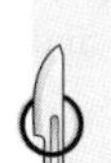

87. Earnshaw JJ, Whitman B, Heather BP on behalf of the Joint Vascular Research Group. Two-year results of a randomized controlled trial of rifampicin-bonded extra-anatomic dacron grafts. Br J Surg 2000; 87:758–9.

A small, multicentre, randomised, controlled trial that failed to show any prophylactic effect of rifampicin bonding on subsequent graft infection. However, the power of the study was low because of the infrequency of graft infection.

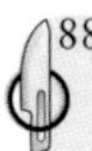

88. Pratesi C, Russo D, Dorigo W, Chiti E. Antibiotic prophylaxis in clean surgery: vascular surgery. J Chemother 2001; 13(special issue No. 1):123–8.

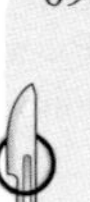

89. D'Addato M, Curti T, Freyrie A. Prophylaxis of graft infection with rifampicin-bonded Gelseal graft: 2-year follow-up of a prospective clinical trial. Italian Investigators Group. Cardiovasc Surg 1996; 4:200–4.

   A randomised controlled trial that failed to show any effect of rifampicin bonding in Dacron grafts but the power of the study was low, with only 5 of 296 infections in the rifampicin group compared with 7 of 304 in the control group.

90. Benvenisty AI, Tannenbaum G, Ahlborn TN et al. Control of prosthetic bacterial infection: evaluation of an easily incorporated, tightly bound, silver antibiotic PTFE graft. J Surg Res 1988; 44:1–7.

91. Dunlop MG, Fox JN, Stonebridge PA et al. Vacuum drainage of groin wounds after vascular surgery: a controlled trial. Br J Surg 1990; 77:562–3.

   A small randomised trial failing to show any value of drainage in groin incisions.

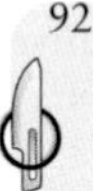

92. Healy DA, Keyser J III, Holcomb GW III et al. Prophylactic closed suction drainage of femoral wounds in patients undergoing vascular reconstruction. J Vasc Surg 1990; 10:18–19.

   Results similar to those of Dunlop et al. (91).

93. Baker KA. Antibiotic prophylaxis for selected implants and devices. J Calif Dent Assoc 2000; 28:620–6.

94. Szilagii DE, Smith RF, Elliott JP, Vrandecic MP. Infection in arterial reconstruction with synthetic grafts. Ann Surg 1972; 176:321–33.

95. Menawat SS, Gloviczki P, Serry RD et al. Management of aortic graft enteric fistulae. Eur J Vasc Endovasc Surg 1997; 14(suppl. A):74–81.

96. Selan L, Pasariello C. Microbiological diagnosis of aortofemoral graft infections. Eur J Vasc Endovasc Surg 1997; 14(suppl. A):10–12.

97. Calligaro KD, Veith FJ, Schwartz ML et al. Are gram-negative bacteria a contraindication to selective preservation of infected prosthetic arterial grafts? J Vasc Surg 1992; 136:337–45.

98. Orton DF, LeVeen RF, Saigh JA et al. Aortic prosthetic graft infections: radiologic manifestations and implications for management. Radiographics 2000; 20:977–93.

99. Spartera C, Morettini G, Petrassi C et al. Role of magnetic resonance imaging in the evaluation of aortic graft healing, perigraft fluid collection, and graft infection. Eur J Vasc Surg 1990; 4:69–73.

100. Clarke AM, Poskitt KR, Baird RN, Horrocks M. Anastomotic aneurysms of the femoral artery: aetiology and treatment. Br J Surg 1989; 76:1014–16.

101. Liberatore M, Iurilli AP, Ponzo F et al. Aortofemoral graft infection: the usefulness of ^{99m}Tc-HMPAO-labelled leucocyte scan. Eur J Vasc Endovasc Surg 1997; 14(suppl. A):27–9.

102. Baker MS, Fisher JH, van der Reis L, Baker BH. The endoscopic diagnosis of an aortoduodenal fistula. Arch Surg 1976; 111:304.

103. Becquemin JP, Qvarfordt P, Kron J et al. Aortic graft infection: is there a place for partial graft removal? Eur J Vasc Endovasc Surg 1997; 14(suppl. A):53–8.

104. Nielsen OM, Noer HH, Jorgensen LG, Lorentzen JE. Gentamicin beads in the treatment of localised vascular graft infection: long term results in 17 cases. Eur J Vasc Surg 1991; 5:283–5.

105. Holdsworth J. Treatment of infective and potentially infective complications of vascular bypass grafting using gentamicin with collagen sponge. Ann R Coll Surg Engl 1999; 81:166–70.

106. Almgren B, Eriksson I. Local antibiotic irrigation in the treatment of arterial graft infections. Acta Chir Scand 1981; 147:33–6.

107. Morris GE, Friend PJ, Vassallo DJ et al. Antibiotic irrigation and conservative surgery for major aortic graft infection. J Vasc Surg 1994; 20:88–95.

108. Sladen JG, Thompson RP, Brosseuk DT et al. Sartorius myoplasty in the treatment of exposed arterial grafts. Cardiovasc Surg 1993; 1:113–17.

109. Galland RB. Sartorius transposition in the management of synthetic graft infection. Eur J Vasc Endovasc Surg 2002; 23:175–7.

110. Gibbons CP, Ferguson CJ, Fligelstone LJ, Edwards K. Experience with femoro-popliteal veins as a conduit for vascular reconstruction in infected fields. Eur J Vasc Endovasc Surg 2003; 25:424–31.

111. Gomes MN, Spear SL. Pedicled muscle flaps in the management of infected aortofemoral grafts. Cardiovasc Surg 1994; 2:70–7.

112. Thomas WO, Parry SW, Powell RW et al. Management of exposed inguinofemoral arterial conduits by skeletal muscular rotational flaps. Am Surg 1994; 60:872–80.

113. Meland NB, Arnold PG, Pairolero PC, Lovich SF. Muscle-flap coverage for infected peripheral vascular prostheses. Plast Reconstr Surg 1994; 93:1005–11.

114. Calligaro KD, Veith FJ, Sales CM et al. Comparison of muscle flaps and delayed secondary intention wound healing for infected lower extremity arterial grafts. Ann Vasc Surg 1994; 8:31–7.

115. Kretschmer G, Niederle B, Huk I et al. Groin infections following vascular surgery: obturator bypass (BYP) versus 'biologic coverage' (TRP). A comparative analysis. Eur J Vasc Surg 1989; 3:25–9.

116. Ouriel K, Geary KJ, Green RM, DeWeese JA. Fate of the exposed saphenous vein graft. Am J Surg 1990; 160:148–50.

117. Kahn AM, Lad T, Tanuj L, Jacobs S. Methicillin resistant *Staphylococcus aureus* (MRSA) and autogenous saphenous vein grafts in femoro-popliteal bypass procedures. EJVES Extra 2002; 4:58–60.

118. Lepantalo M, Kallio M, Tukianen E. Wound and foot healing problems following distal bypass surgery. In: Branchereau A, Jacobs M (eds) Complications in vascular and endovascular surgery, part II. Armonk, NY: Futura Publishing Company, 2002; pp. 279–94.

119. Burks JA Jr, Faries PL, Gravereaux EC et al. Endovascular repair of bleeding aortoenteric fistulas: a 5-year experience. J Vasc Surg 2001; 34:1055–9.

120. Chuter TA, Lukaszewicz GC, Reilly LM et al. Endovascular repair of a presumed aortoenteric fistula: late failure due to recurrent infection. J Endovasc Ther 2000; 7:240–4.

121. Reddy DJ, Shin LH. Obturator bypass: technical considerations. Semin Vasc Surg 2000; 13:49–52.

122. Nevelsteen A, Mees U, Deleersnijder J, Suy R. Obturator bypass: a sixteen year experience with 55 cases. Ann Vasc Surg 1987; 1:558–63.

123. Sugawara Y, Sueda T, Orihashi K et al. Retrosartorius bypass in the treatment of graft infection after peripheral vascular surgery. J Vasc Surg 2003; 37:892–4.

124. Donayre CE, Ewbanks P, Ayers B et al. Iliac to popliteal artery bypass through the iliac wing: an alternative extracavitary route for management of complex groin injuries. Ann Vasc Surg 1999; 13:209–15.

125. Branchereau A, Ciosi G, Bordeaux J et al. Femorofemoral bypass through the perineum for infection complicating arterial revascularization of the lower limb. Ann Vasc Surg 1988; 2:43–9.

126. Naraynsingh V, Karmody AM, Leather RP, Corson JD. Lateral approach to the profunda femoris artery. Am J Surg 1984; 147:813–14.

127. Quinones-Baldrich WJ, Hernandez JJ, Moore WS. Long-term results following surgical management of aortic graft infection. Arch Surg 1991; 126:507–11.

128. Yeager RA, Taylor LM Jr, Moneta GL et al. Improved results with conventional management of infrarenal aortic infection. J Vasc Surg 1999; 30:76–83.

Sixty patients with aortic graft infection treated by axillo-bifemoral bypass and graft excision, with 13% mortality and 2-year limb salvage of 93%.

129. Seeger JM, Pretus HA, Welborn MB et al. Long-term outcome after treatment of aortic graft infection with staged extra-anatomic bypass grafting and aortic graft removal. Surgery 2000; 32:451–9.

130. Bandyk DF, Novotney ML, Johnson BL et al. Use of rifampicin-soaked gelatin-sealed polyester grafts for in situ treatment of primary aortic and vascular prosthetic infections. J Surg Res 2001; 95:44–9.

131. Naylor AR. Aortic prosthetic infection. Br J Surg 1999; 86:435–6.

132. Hayes PD, Nasim A, London NJM et al. In situ replacement of infected aortic grafts with rifampicin-bonded prostheses: the Leicester experience (1992–1998). J Vasc Surg 1999; 30:92–8.

133. Zegelman M, Gunther G. Infected grafts require excision and extra-anatomic reconstruction. Against the motion. In: Greenhalgh RM (ed.) The evidence for vascular and endovascular reconstruction. London: WB Saunders, 2002; pp. 252–8.

134. Vogt PR, Brunner-LaRocca HP, Lachat M et al. Technical details with the use of cryopreserved arterial allografts for aortic infection: influence on early and midterm mortality. J Vasc Surg 2002; 35:80–6.

135. Noel AA, Gloviczki P, Cherry KJ Jr et al. United States Cryopreserved Aortic Allograft Registry. Abdominal aortic reconstruction in infected fields: early results of the United States cryopreserved aortic allograft registry. J Vasc Surg 2002; 35:847–52.

136. Verhelst R, Lacroix V, Vraux H et al. Use of cryopreserved arterial homografts for management of infected prosthetic grafts: a multicentre study. Ann Vasc Surg 2000; 14:602–7.

137. Clagett GP, Valentine RJ, Hagino RT. Autogenous aortoiliac/femoral reconstruction from superficial femoral-popliteal veins: feasibility and durability. J Vasc Surg 1997; 25:255–70.

Excellent long-term results of femoral vein replacement for infected aortic grafts from one of the groups originating the technique.

138. Gordon LL, Hagino RT, Jackson MR et al. Complex aortofemoral prosthetic infections: the role of autogenous superficial femoropopliteal vein reconstruction. Arch Surg 1999; 134:615–21.

139. Nevelsteen A, Lacroix H, Suy R. Autogenous reconstruction with lower extremity deep veins: an alternative treatment of prosthetic infection after reconstructive surgery for aortoiliac disease. J Vasc Surg 1995; 22:129–34.

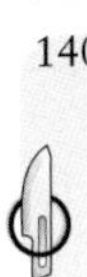

140. Daenens K, Fourneau I, Nevelsteen A. Ten-year experience in autogenous reconstruction with the femoral vein in the treatment of aortofemoral prosthetic infection. Eur J Vasc Endovasc Surg 2003; 25:240–5.

An up-to-date report of extensive experience from another pioneering centre.

141. Brown PM, Kim VB, Lalikos JF et al. Autologous superficial femoral vein for aortic reconstruction in infected fields. Ann Vasc Surg 1999; 13:32–6.

142. Coburn M, Ashworth C, Francis W et al. Venous stasis complications of the use of the superficial femoral and popliteal veins for lower extremity bypass. J Vasc Surg 1993; 17:1005–9.

143. Wells JK, Hagino RT, Bargmann KM et al. Venous morbidity after superficial femoral–popliteal vein harvest. J Vasc Surg 1999; 29:282–91.

144. Modrall JG, Sadjadi J, Ali AT et al. Deep vein harvest: predicting need for fasciotomy. J Vasc Surg 2004; 39:387–94.

145. Plate G, Hollier LA, O'Brien P et al. Recurrent aneurysms and late vascular complications following repair of abdominal aortic aneurysms. Arch Surg 1985; 120:590–4.

146. Biederer J, Muller-Hulsbeck S, Loose JR, Heller M. Late aneurysm formation in a femoro-popliteal polytetrafluoroethylene graft. Eur Radiol 1999; 9:1678–81.

147. Dardik H, Wengerter K, Qin F et al. Comparative decades of experience with glutaraldehyde-tanned human umbilical cord vein graft for lower limb revascularization: an analysis of 1275 cases. J Vasc Surg 2002; 35:64–71.

148. Reipe G, Chafke N, Morlock M, Imig H. Dilatation and durability of polyester grafts. In: Branchereau A, Jacobs M (eds) Complications in vascular and endovascular surgery, part 1. Armonk NY: Futura Publishing Company, 2000; pp. 35–43.

149. Taylor LM Jr, Park TC, Edwards JM et al. Acute disruption of polytetrafluoroethylene grafts adjacent to axillary anastomoses: a complication of axillofemoral grafting. J Vasc Surg 1994; 20:520–6.

150. Onoe M, Watarida S, Sugita T et al. Disruption of the expanded polytetrafluoroethylene (ePTFE) graft of axillofemoral by-pass. J Cardiovasc Surg (Torino) 1994; 35:165–8.

151. Brophy CM, Quist WC, Kwolek C, LoGerfo FW. Disruption of proximal axillobifemoral bypass graft anastomosis. J Vasc Surg 1992; 15:218–20.

152. White GH, Donayre CE, Williams RA et al. Exertional disruption of axillofemoral graft anastomosis. 'The axillary pullout syndrome'. Arch Surg 1990; 125:625–7.

153. Jones WT, Hagino RT, Chiou AC et al. Graft patency is not the only clinical predictor of success after exclusion and bypass of popliteal artery aneurysms. J Vasc Surg 2003; 37:392–8.

154. Morgan R, Belli AM. Current treatment methods for postcatheterization pseudoaneurysms. J Vasc Intervent Radiol 2003; 14:697–710.

155. Stella N, Pellicciotti A, Udini M. Endovascular exclusion of iatrogenic femoral artery pseudoaneurysm with the Wallgraft-Endoprosthesis. J Cardiovasc Surg (Torino) 2003; 44:259–62.

156. Levi N, Schroeder TV. True and anastomotic femoral artery aneurysms: is the risk of rupture and thrombosis related to the size of the aneurysms? Eur J Vasc Endovasc Surg 1999; 18:111–13.

157. Matsumura JS, Pearce WH, Cabellon A et al. Reoperative aortic surgery. Cardiovasc Surg 1999; 7:614–21.

158. Mulder EJ, van Bockel JH, Maas J et al. Morbidity and mortality of reconstructive surgery of noninfected false aneurysms detected long after aortic prosthetic reconstruction. Arch Surg 1998; 133:45–9.

159. Tiesenhausen K, Hausegger KA, Tauss J et al. Endovascular treatment of proximal anastomotic aneurysms after aortic prosthetic reconstruction. Cardiovasc Intervent Radiol 2001; 24:49–52.

CHAPTER

Nine

Management of acute lower limb ischaemia

Jonothan J. Earnshaw, Peter A. Gaines and Jonathan D. Beard

INTRODUCTION

There is no internationally accepted definition of acute leg ischaemia (ALI). The acutely bloodless limb with sensorimotor loss obviously falls within any definition but there is often a delay in the presentation and the ischaemia is not immediately limb-threatening. Chronic critical leg ischaemia is defined as rest pain of more than 2 weeks' duration (see Chapters 2 and 3).

It seems reasonable therefore to define ALI as deterioration in the blood supply of a previously stable leg that results in rest pain and/or other features of severe ischaemia of less than 2 weeks' duration. However, some overlap with chronic critical leg ischaemia is inevitable. The severity of ischaemia is often defined according to the SVS/ISCVS guidelines (**Table 9.1**),[1] although this classification seems difficult to use in clinical practice. It is simpler to group patients into the following categories:

- subcritical acute ischaemia (viable leg) where there is no neurological deficit and an audible arterial Doppler signal at the ankle;
- critical acute ischaemia (threatened leg) where there is no audible ankle Doppler signal and a partial neurological deficit;

Table 9.1 • Suggested classification of acute limb ischaemia

					Doppler signals	
Category	**Description**	**Capillary return**	**Muscle paralysis**	**Sensory loss**	**Arterial**	**Venous**
I Viable	Not immediately threatened	Intact	None	None	Audible	Audible
IIa Threatened	Salvageable if promptly treated	Intact/slow	None	Partial	Inaudible	Audible
IIb Threatened	Salvageable if immediately treated	Slow/absent	Partial	Partial/ complete	Inaudible	Audible
III Irreversible	Primary amputation	Absent Staining	Complete Tense compartment	Complete	Inaudible	Inaudible

Reprinted from J Vasc Surg. Rutherford RB, Flanigan DP, Gupta SK et al. Suggested standards for reports dealing with lower extremity ischemia: 1986; 4:80–94, with permission from Society for Vascular Surgery.

- irreversible acute ischaemia where the leg has a complete neurological deficit, tense muscles, with absent capillary return and no arterial or venous Doppler signal.[2]

In the Gloucestershire community survey done in 1994, the incidence of ALI was 1 per 6000 of the population per year, which means that an average district general hospital serving approximately 250 000 people should see 30–40 cases annually.[3] The condition is on the increase and there is evidence that the outcome is improved when patients are managed by a vascular service providing 24-hour cover.[4] ALI is associated with a high cost to the community because of the risk of amputation and prolonged hospitalisation. Costs are minimised and outcome optimised by accurate clinical assessment and an understanding of the available therapeutic options.

AETIOLOGY

ALI is the result of occlusion of a native artery or bypass graft. In situ thrombosis or embolism can cause native arterial occlusion (**Box 9.1**).

Box 9.1 • Aetiology of acute lower limb ischaemia

Thrombosis
Atherosclerosis
Popliteal aneurysm
Bypass graft occlusion
Thrombotic conditions
Embolism
Atrial fibrillation
Mural thrombosis
Vegetations
Proximal aneurysms
Atherosclerotic plaque
Rare causes
Dissection
Trauma (including iatrogenic)
External compression
Popliteal entrapment
Cystic adventitial disease
Compartment syndrome

Embolism

Until about 30 years ago, embolism caused most ALI. Emboli large enough to occlude major vessels usually arise in the heart. Rheumatic mitral valve disease was the most common cause, with large emboli forming in a dilated left atrium. In 80% of patients, atrial fibrillation due to ischaemic heart disease is now the origin of cardiac embolism; mural thrombus following acute myocardial infarction causes most of the remainder.[5] Less common sources of emboli include proximal aneurysms on atherosclerotic plaques, usually located in the thoracic or abdominal aorta. Whereas cardiac embolism usually consists entirely of platelet thrombus, embolism from proximal arteries can include atherosclerotic plaque or cholesterol-rich emboli. This has a much worse prognosis than cardiac embolism because embolectomy is less effective. Small particles of atheroembolism can pass to very distal vessels in the foot. This digital embolism can result in the 'acute blue toe syndrome'. In this condition, the embolic source should be identified and treated if possible (**Fig. 9.1**). Large emboli typically lodge at an arterial bifurcation, particularly in the common femoral or popliteal arteries (**Fig. 9.2**). Patients with cardiac embolism may also suffer from peripheral vascular disease as a result of the underlying process of atherosclerosis. This increases the difficulty in establishing the cause of the ischaemia and in revascularisation, which may be one reason why the prognosis for this condition remains poor.

Thrombosis

In situ thrombosis in a native artery is now the commonest cause of ALI. It is usually the result of critical flow arrest at the site of an atherosclerotic stenosis. The advancing age of the population and the commensurate increase in atherosclerosis explains the rising incidence of ALI. Acute native vessel arterial occlusion may be compounded by surgery (e.g. knee replacement destroying geniculate collateral vessels formed around a popliteal occlusion), heart failure or a thrombotic tendency (polycythaemia, dehydration, etc.). Acute thrombosis of a popliteal aneurysm poses the highest risk to the leg. Typically, this occurs in elderly men in association with aneurysms elsewhere (50% have an aortic aneurysm) or generalised arterial ectasia. Popliteal aneurysms usually commence in the above-knee popliteal artery and extend distally to the tibial trifurcation. As they enlarge they can fill with lamellar thrombus, which may cause either acute thrombosis or distal embolisation that occludes the tibial vessels. The latter will place the

(a)

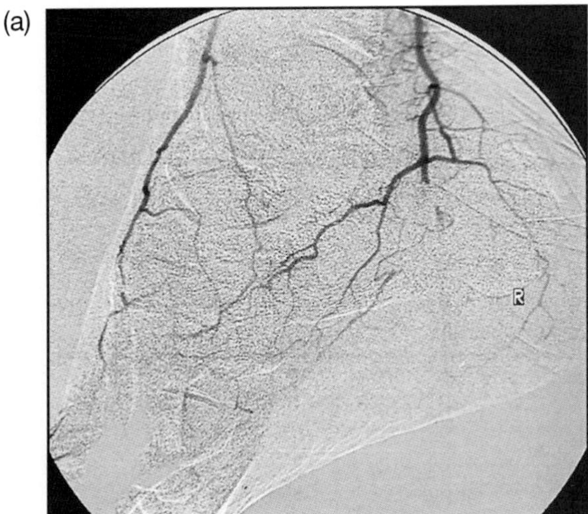

(b)

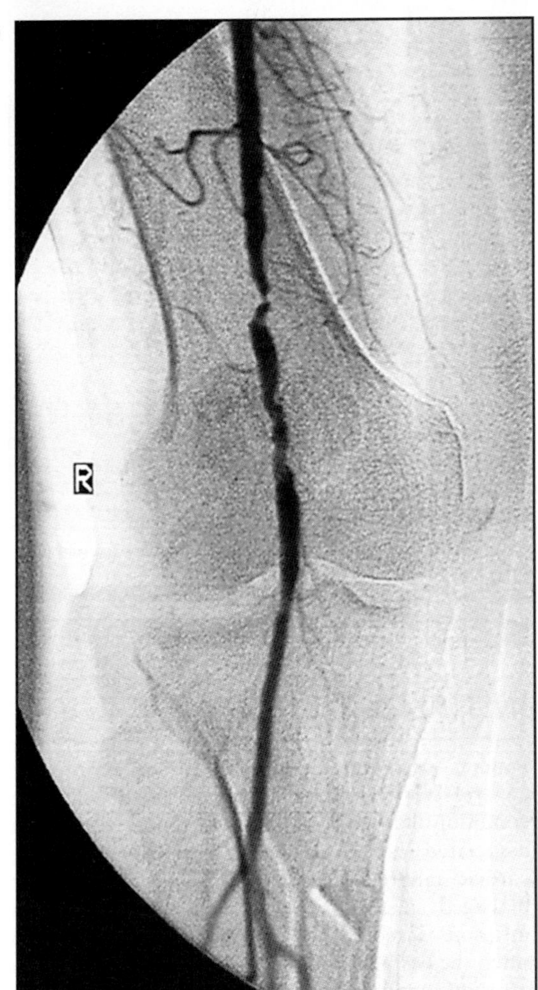

Figure 9.1 • 'Blue toe syndrome' due to digital and pedal arterial atheroembolism **(a)** from a proximal atherosclerotic stenosis **(b)**. Note the acute cut-off of the posterior tibial artery. Ultrasonography excluded a popliteal aneurysm and the lesion was treated by balloon angioplasty.

leg in extreme jeopardy. In 20% of patients with ALI, a source for the embolus cannot be found.

The increasing use of bypass grafts for arterial insufficiency means that surgeons often have to deal with acute graft thrombosis. Grafts occlude for a variety of reasons. Graft occlusion within 1 month of insertion is usually the result of technical problems at the time of surgery or poor distal run-off. Graft occlusion within 1 year of placement is often caused by myointimal hyperplasia at an anastomosis or the development of stenoses within a vein graft. Occlusion after 1 year is usually due to progression of distal atherosclerosis. Prosthetic grafts have a higher occlusion rate than autogenous vein grafts (see Chapters 3 and 8).

Spontaneous native arterial thrombosis occasionally occurs without an underlying flow-limiting stenosis and these patients should be investigated for an intrinsic clotting abnormality, e.g. anti-phospholipid syndrome, activated protein C deficiency (see Chapter 17), or malignancy.

Other causes

Occasionally, acute arterial occlusion may be due to arterial dissection, trauma, extrinsic compression or compartment syndrome. In a young patient with acute popliteal artery occlusion, either popliteal entrapment or cystic adventitial disease should be considered.

CLINICAL FEATURES

The severity of ischaemia at presentation is the most important factor affecting outcome of the leg.[2,6] Complete occlusion of a proximal artery in the absence of preformed collateral vessels (as in cardiac embolism) results in the classical clinical presentation of pain, paralysis, paraesthesia, pallor, pulselessness and a perishingly cold leg. The pain is severe and frequently resistant to analgesia. Calf pain and tenderness with a tense muscle compartment indicates muscle necrosis and critical (often irreversible) ischaemia. Sensorimotor deficit including muscle paralysis and paraesthesia are indicative of muscle and nerve ischaemia with the potential for salvage with prompt treatment. Initially the leg is white with empty veins but after 6–12 hours vasodilatation occurs, probably caused by hypoxia of the smooth muscle. The capillaries then fill with stagnant deoxygenated blood, resulting in a mottled appearance that blanches on digital pressure (**Fig. 9.3**). If flow is not restored rapidly, the arteries distal to the occlusion fill with propagated thrombus and the capillaries rupture, resulting in a fixed blue staining of the skin that is a sign of irreversible ischaemia. These features are typical

(a)

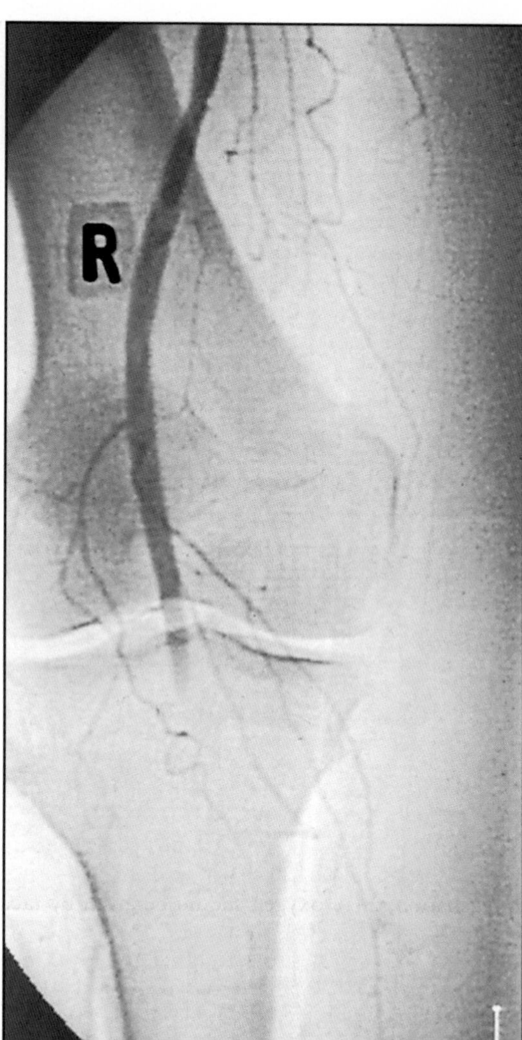

(b)

Figure 9.2 • Arteriogram demonstrating an embolus lodged in the bifurcation of the common femoral artery **(a)** with further emboli occluding the distal profunda and popliteal artery **(b)**.

of an acute arterial occlusion in the absence of existing collaterals and suggest an embolic cause. When arterial occlusion occurs as part of a chronic process where collaterals have developed, typically the leg is less severely ischaemic. Patients with peripheral atherosclerosis deteriorate in a stepwise fashion as thrombosis supervenes on an existing arterial plaque. Patients often report a sudden change in symptoms, which progress over a few days: the foot often has a dusky hue with slow capillary return. Previous claudication or absent pulses in the contralateral foot help make a clinical diagnosis of in situ thrombosis. Palpation of a mass in either popliteal fossa suggests thrombosis of a popliteal aneurysm.

INITIAL MANAGEMENT

Patients presenting with ALI are often in poor general health, which is one reason why the condition has such a high mortality rate from associated cardiovascular disease. Dehydration, cardiac failure, hypoxia and pain should all be managed in the standard way. An intravenous infusion is required for rehydration and is also often the best means of providing analgesia with an infusion pump. If thrombolysis is an option, intramuscular analgesia should be avoided because of the risk of bleeding. Intravenous heparin (5000 units) should be given immediately followed by systemic heparinisation, principally to restrict propagation

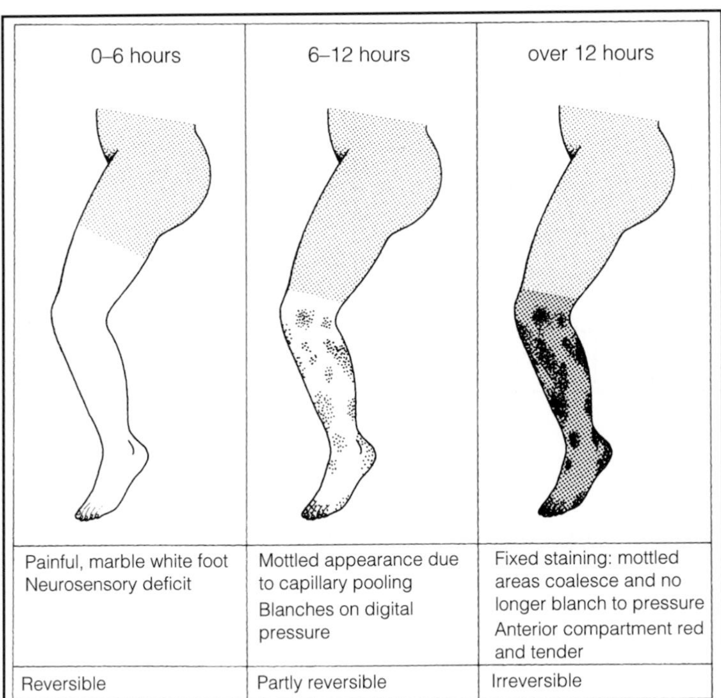

Figure 9.3 • Clinical outcome after acute leg ischaemia.

of thrombus, although there is also evidence that it improves the prognosis.[7] In order to improve oxygenation, 24% oxygen should be given by face mask.

Venous blood should be taken for full blood count, urea, electrolytes and glucose. An ECG and chest radiograph may be of value in diagnosing and managing cardiac arrhythmias and heart failure. If a primary thrombotic tendency is suspected, investigation of this should be delayed as the diagnostic tests are inaccurate in the face of fresh thrombus.

When clinical examination suggests that an aortic aneurysm or popliteal aneurysm may be the cause of ALI, then duplex ultrasound imaging is indicated.

REVASCULARISATION

The clinical assessment of the severity of limb ischaemia will largely dictate the most appropriate form of therapy (**Fig. 9.4**).

Irreversible leg ischaemia

A small number of patients will present in a moribund state or with irreversible leg ischaemia (muscle paralysis, tense swollen fascial compartments, fixed skin staining). Terminal care may be the kindest option. For the irreversibly ischaemic leg revascularisation is, by definition, inappropriate and may be dangerous. This includes the patient who develops ALI while being treated for another condition, usually as an inpatient on an elderly care ward. Prognosis is particularly dismal in this group.[3] Surviving patients should be resuscitated and stabilised before considering amputation.

Acute critical ischaemia

The acute white leg with sensorimotor deficit requires urgent intervention to prevent limb loss. Although the differentiation between thrombosis and embolus is often difficult, it is in this group of patients that embolism is more likely. An acute white leg with no prior history of claudication, normal contralateral pulses and a probable embolic source, such as atrial fibrillation, would indicate that embolisation is the likely cause. Urgent surgery is indicated in these patients, after resuscitation, without the need for preoperative arteriography, which simply wastes time. Groin exploration with balloon catheter embolectomy and on-table arteriography is indicated (see below). There is some debate about whether preoperative angiography provides beneficial information when the femoral pulse is absent, as it may help to exclude alternative

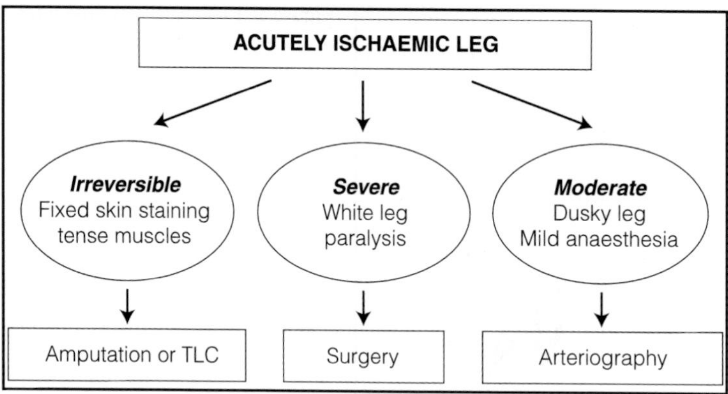

Figure 9.4 • Clinical approach to the management of the acutely ischaemic leg.

diagnoses, such as dissection, and to plan appropriate surgery. An alternative is to proceed directly to operation but to prepare both groins so that a femoral crossover graft can be inserted if adequate inflow cannot be achieved using an embolectomy catheter.

Acute subcritical ischaemia

The majority of patients presenting with ALI have acute onset of rest pain but no paralysis and no, or only mild, sensory loss. The cause is often acute thrombosis of either an atherosclerotic artery or graft. Because the leg is not immediately threatened, time is available to plan appropriate intervention using arteriography (**Fig. 9.5**). The alternative in these patients is intervention with surgery or percutaneous thrombolysis. Thromboembolectomy is unlikely to reopen an artery occluded by thrombus and atherosclerotic plaque; formal arterial bypass is more likely to be needed.

Thrombolysis is arguably less invasive than revascularisation surgery. It has the capacity to open small as well as large arteries. It may also uncover the cause of the in situ thrombosis, such as an arterial stenosis, which can be treated by angioplasty to produce a lasting outcome.

Some patients are admitted to hospital with acute thrombosis of a peripheral artery (usually the superficial femoral) but have only claudication and no ischaemic pain at rest. Thrombolysis might appear an attractive option to treat the claudication, but the risks are as high as in patients with limb-threatening ischaemia.[8] Reverting to the principles described by Blaisdell, i.e. initial anticoagulation followed by management depending on the progression of ischaemia, reduces the risk to both life and limb.[7]

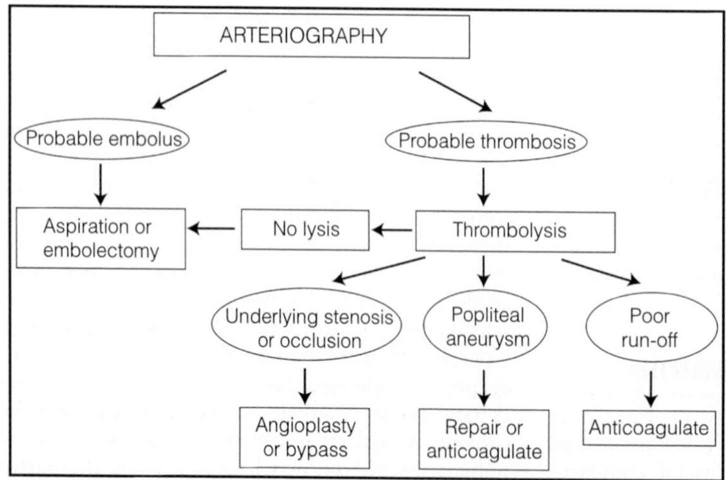

Figure 9.5 • Treatment pathways following arteriography.

Choice between surgery and thrombolysis: the evidence

There remains considerable controversy about the individual roles of surgery and thrombolysis for ALI. A review of 42 studies (most non-randomised) by Diffin and Kandarpa[9] suggested that thrombolysis was associated with substantially better limb salvage and mortality rates than surgery. There are three major randomised studies from which to draw harder evidence.[10–15] The New York study was the first to show that thrombolysis improves survival in patients with limb-threatening ischaemia of less than 14 days.[10] This study was small and the advantage was due to the high incidence of cardiorespiratory deaths following emergency surgery. The STILE study was much larger and included patients with ischaemia for longer than 14 days.[11] This study has been much criticised because of the failure of one-third of the radiologists to insert a catheter successfully for peripheral thrombolysis. The study introduced the concept of amputation-free survival but failed to show any significant improvement in this primary endpoint between the treatment groups. In the subgroup of patients with ischaemia for fewer than 14 days, thrombolysis reduced the rate of amputation. Subsequent analysis of patients from this study up to 1 year revealed that thrombolysis was better initial treatment for graft occlusions, whereas surgery was more effective and durable for native vessel occlusions.[12,13] However, few of the patients in the STILE study had critical ischaemia. The TOPAS trial was designed, using lessons learned from the above studies, to try to settle this debate. In the first phase, an optimal dose of thrombolytic therapy was selected (urokinase 4000 IU/hour)[14] and in phase II this was compared with urgent surgery in 544 patients.[15] Amputation-free survival was similar in both groups at 6 months and 1 year (72% and 65% for urokinase vs. 75% and 70% for surgery, respectively), though thrombolysis reduced the need for open surgical procedures.

In conclusion, both surgery and thrombolysis seem effective and the choice should be made on an individual basis for each patient, taking into account the skills and experience available in the vascular unit.

Peripheral arterial thrombolysis

Thrombus dissolution is achieved by stimulating the conversion of fibrin-bound plasminogen into the active enzyme plasmin. Plasmin is a non-specific protease capable of degrading fibrin and producing thrombus dissolution.

In contrast to the thrombolytic treatment of acute myocardial infarction, systemic infusion of thrombolytic agents for ALI results in a poor success rate and unacceptable complications. By selectively placing a catheter within the thrombus via the percutaneous route and delivering the thrombolytic agent locally, the concentration of agent is maximised and plasmin is less likely to be neutralised by circulating antiplasmins. The dose of thrombolytic agent can be optimised to the minimum level that results in a local effect without producing systemic thrombolysis and the attendant complications.

CONTRAINDICATIONS (Box 9.2)

Perhaps the only absolute contraindication to lysis is active internal bleeding. Most other contraindications are relative, where the risk of complications from thrombolysis must be weighed against the potential benefits of limb salvage. It is unwise to consider thrombolysis within 2 weeks of surgery or within 2 months of a stroke. Dacron grafts may take 3 months to seal, and if they do not become fully incorporated they may become porous if thrombolytic therapy is employed. Care should be exercised when using thrombolysis to open Dacron grafts within the abdomen where manual compression is not possible should bleeding occur. The presence of cardiac thrombus theoretically increases the likelihood of systemic embolisation during thrombolysis, but there is no evidence that patient selection based on echocardiography affects management or outcome.

Box 9.2 • Contraindications to thrombolysis

Active internal bleeding
Known pregnancy
Stroke within 2 months
Transient ischaemic attack within 2 months
Known intracerebral tumour, aneurysm or arteriovenous malformation
Severe bleeding tendency
Craniotomy within 2 months
Vascular surgery within 2 weeks
Abdominal surgery within 2 weeks
Puncture of a non-compressible vessel or biopsy within 10 days
Previous gastrointestinal haemorrhage
Trauma within 10 days

TECHNIQUE

All patients should have adequate analgesia and a cannula inserted for venous access, analgesia and hydration. The extent of occlusive disease needs to be defined by arteriography or duplex imaging before intervention. The number of arterial punctures should be kept to a minimum to reduce the risk of puncture-site bleeding during treatment. The initial diagnostic approach is tailored to the distribution of disease. If there is an absent femoral pulse in the affected leg but a palpable femoral pulse on the contralateral side, then it is reasonable to anticipate an iliac artery occlusion. In this situation, a contralateral femoral puncture will provide access for the diagnostic arteriogram and subsequently the iliac thrombosis can be approached from the same puncture site using a crossover technique (**Fig. 9.6**). If there is a normal femoral pulse on the side of acute ischaemia, then initial diagnostic information may be provided by intravenous digital subtraction angiography or duplex imaging. As long as adequate inflow can be ensured using one of these methods, an antegrade puncture should be attempted to treat occlusions below the femoral bifurcation so that adjuvant procedures such as angioplasty or thrombus aspiration can be performed from the same side (**Fig. 9.6**). An occluded arterial bypass graft is optimally accessed from the native artery proximal to the graft so that any stenoses can be treated via the same puncture site. However, this is not always possible for technical reasons, although direct puncture of the most proximal accessible part of the graft results in a high success rate from thrombolysis. Once access has been achieved, a guidewire should be passed through the occlusion; indeed, the ability to do this implies the presence of soft thrombus and is a good predictor of success (guidewire traversal test). The catheter used to deliver the lytic agent is then placed within the thrombus.

Several techniques are described for delivering thrombolysis. The low-dose infusion method involves running the thrombolytic drug through the catheter over several hours. This may be combined

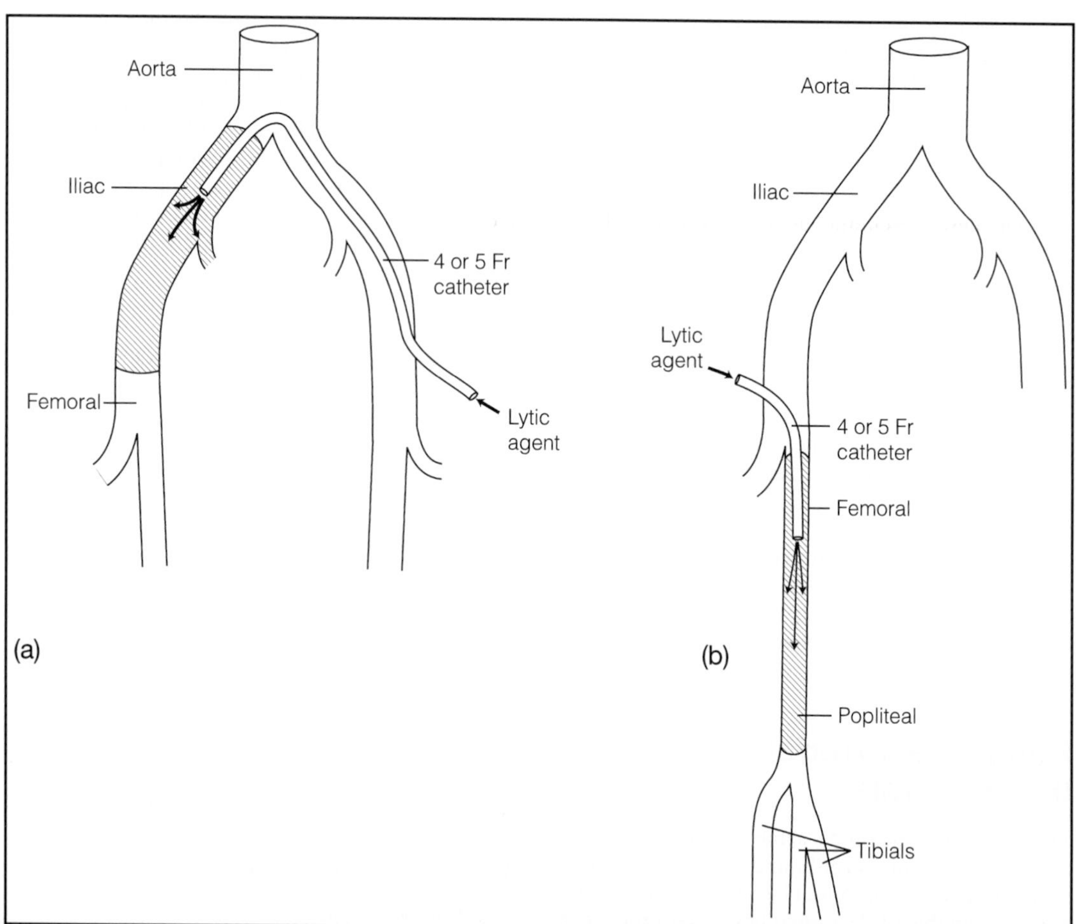

Figure 9.6 • Technique of percutaneous thrombolysis: **(a)** contralateral and **(b)** ipsilateral transfemoral approaches.

with an initial high-dose bolus. More recently, high-dose techniques have been described that accelerate the rate of thrombus dissolution.[16] This may be achieved by administering a number of high-dose boluses sequentially or by using the 'pulse spray' technique.[17] The latter involves high-pressure injection of tiny pulses of lytic agent through a catheter with multiple side holes, and thus it combines enzymatic thrombolysis with mechanical disruption. The high-dose techniques accelerate thrombolysis and allow patients to be treated within the normal working hours of a radiology department. Several randomised trials comparing low-dose and accelerated methods of thrombolysis have found that limb salvage rate and complication rates appear similar, though accelerated methods are quicker.[16–18] Experienced radiologists use both high- and low-dose techniques to treat the majority of patients with ALI; the high-dose technique allows treatment of more severe ischaemia in patients where surgery is not possible and rapid revascularisation is required.

Additional endovascular techniques are being developed that can be used as adjuncts to peripheral thrombolysis. Aspiration embolectomy is a technique for percutaneous aspiration of thrombus by hand using a large end-hole catheter. This can debulk an occlusive thrombus and assists thrombolysis by reducing the time taken to restore distal perfusion.[19] In expert hands, aspiration embolectomy may obviate the need for additional thrombolysis (**Fig. 9.7**).

Other new percutaneous devices can achieve mechanical thrombectomy.[20] A variety of devices have been described that are intended to remove, fragment or disperse thrombus in arteries, veins and bypass grafts. Some devices simply macerate thrombus into particles so small that they are removed by natural fibrinolysis (e.g. Amplatz Thrombectomy Device). Others include a clot aspiration system to remove fragments of thrombus and prevent distal embolisation (e.g. Angiojet). Thrombolysis is often required as a supplement after mechanical thrombectomy. The most recent devices combine the benefits of both methods. In the Trellis Thrombectomy System, the occluded segment of artery is isolated by proximal and distal balloons. An oscillating wire fragments the thrombus while a thrombolytic infusion helps to dissolve it before the liquefied material is aspirated from the islolated segment. These devices are all expensive and have not yet reached general use.

Three drugs are currently available for peripheral thrombolysis: streptokinase, urokinase and tissue plasminogen activator (t-PA). Appropriate dose regimens are shown in **Box 9.3**. There are very few high-quality trials to determine which drug is most effective. One small series suggested that t-PA was more effective than streptokinase.[21] In addition,

Box 9.3 • Suggested drug regimens for thrombolysis

Slow infusion
Streptokinase 5000 units/hour
Tissue plasminogen activator (t-PA) 0.5 mg/hour
Urokinase* 4000 IU/min for 2 hours, then 2000 IU/min for 2 hours, then 1000 IU/min
Pulsed spray
t-PA 0.3 mg per pulse every 30 seconds
Urokinase 5000 IU per pulse every 30 seconds
High-dose bolus
t-PA 5-mg bolus every 10 min three times, then 3.5 mg/hour for up to 4 hours, then (if required) as for slow infusion

*Urokinase is not currently available.

streptokinase has the potential to cause anaphylaxis and is ineffective in patients previously exposed to streptococcal infections or who have been treated with streptokinase before, because of the production of inactivating antibodies. Many radiologists have abandoned streptokinase on clinical grounds, and t-PA is the agent of choice in the UK. In North America, many radiologists preferred urokinase, but it has not been widely available due to manufacturing difficulties in the past few years. The STILE trial suggested that urokinase and t-PA had equivalent activity[11] and this was confirmed in unpublished manufacturers' data. Further randomised data would be helpful but cost considerations and availability largely determine the choice between urokinase and t-PA.

Heparin is often administered systemically before and after thrombolysis to counteract the associated prothrombotic tendency, although no good evidence is available to support its routine use. Some data from trials of the thrombolytic treatment of acute stroke suggest that heparin may increase haemorrhagic complications. An alternative is concurrent administration of low-dose heparin (200 units/hour) via the proximal arterial sheath while delivering the thrombolytic agent via an end-hole catheter to an occlusion below the inguinal ligament. Heparin should be given routinely for 48 hours after completion of thrombolysis. Consideration will then be needed to determine whether individual patients need lifelong anticoagulation with warfarin. No data exist to guide appropriate therapy. Thrombolysis should be considered a diagnostic process aimed at exposing the underlying flow-limiting lesion (**Fig 9.7**). This should be found in the majority of patients using biplanar arteriography. If no

(a)

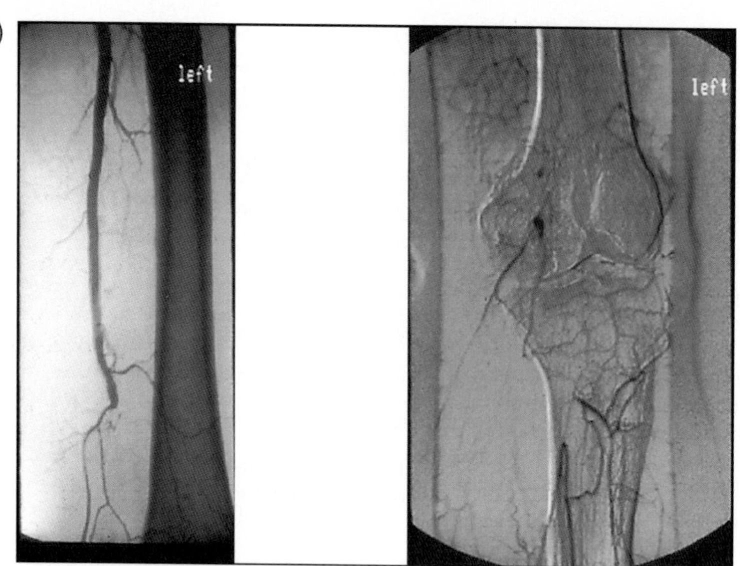

(b)

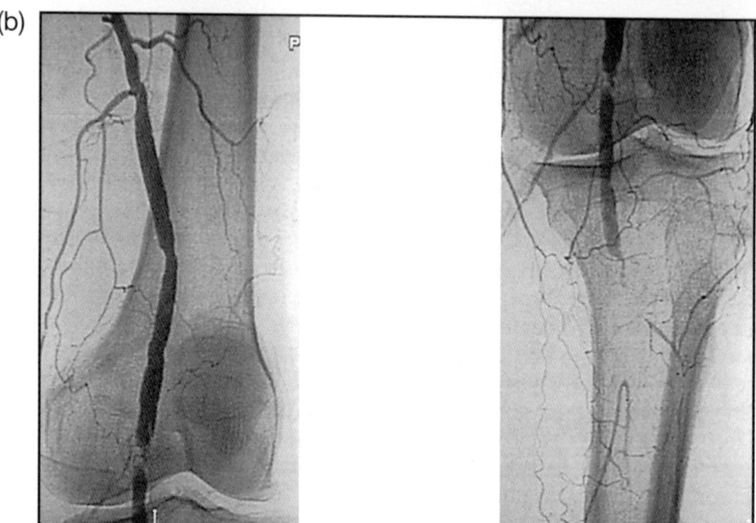

(c)

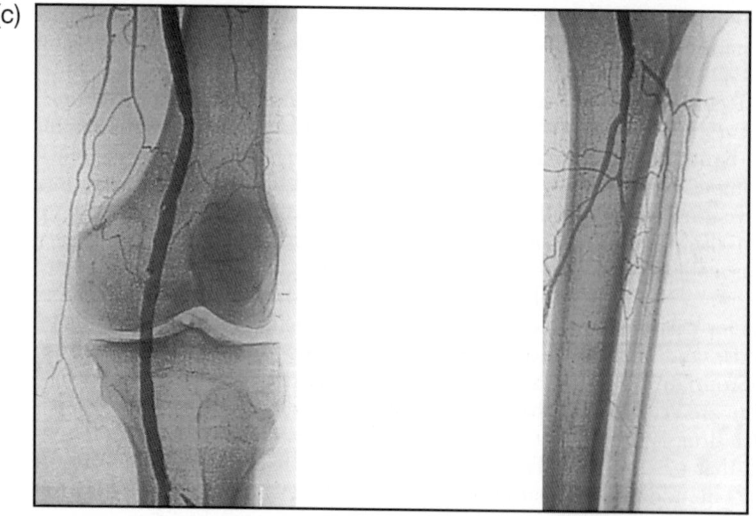

Figure 9.7 • **(a)** Arteriography demonstrates an occlusion of the popliteal artery extending into the tibial vessels. **(b)** Thrombolysis reveals a popliteal stenosis but persistent occlusion of the tibial trifurcation. **(c)** The stenosis was treated by balloon angioplasty and the thrombus aspirated from the tibial vessels using an aspiration catheter.

abnormality is detected, duplex ultrasonography of the suspect arterial segment often proves diagnostic. The majority of lesions can be managed by angioplasty or stent placement. Where the disease appears too extensive, surgical reconstruction may be required, particularly when an anastomotic stenosis results in graft occlusion.

ALI due to a popliteal aneurysm remains a difficult clinical problem. The bulk of thrombus within the aneurysm restricts the use of thrombolysis because of the high risk of massive distal embolisation, the slow clearance and large amount of residual thrombus after recanalisation. If thrombolysis does have a role to play, then it is to open run-off vessels for distal bypass grafting. This is achieved by placing a catheter through the popliteal artery into a tibial vessel and then lysing it until a distal vessel becomes patent for bypass. Alternatively, urgent surgery may be performed with on-table angiography and thrombolysis to clear the run-off (see later).

COMPLICATIONS

There are significant risks associated with percutaneous thrombolytic therapy, most of which can be attributed to the fragile health of the patients and their advanced systemic atherosclerosis. Myocardial infarction and stroke are the commonest causes of death. The rate of reported adverse outcomes is variable, depending on the condition of the patients treated. In the review by Diffin and Kandarpa, principally of North American articles, the mortality rate after thrombolysis was 4% at 30 days.[9] The British Thrombolysis Study Group (TSG) database, which includes over 1100 episodes of thrombolysis (mostly for limb-threatening ischaemia), records a 12.4% mortality rate at 30 days.[22] Other large series report intermediate results.[23–26] Major haemorrhage occurs in approximately 9% of patients, usually at a groin puncture site but occasionally retroperitoneal or intra-abdominal. If major haemorrhage occurs during thrombolysis, aprotinin is an effective plasmin inhibitor and the administration of whole blood, fresh frozen plasma and, in particular, fibrinogen concentrate will replenish the clotting factors. Stroke is seen in approximately 3% of patients (2.3% in the TSG database). Most occur after thrombolysis, during therapeutic anticoagulation. About half are thrombotic rather than haemorrhagic. If a stroke occurs, cerebral haemorrhage should be excluded by urgent computed tomography. If haemorrhage is not the cause, then a clinical decision needs to be made whether to persist with thrombolysis to salvage the affected limb, with possible additional benefits to the intracerebral circulation.

Minor haemorrhage is common (approximately 40% of infusions) and usually occurs at the groin puncture site. It can be managed by direct compression or by exchanging the catheter system for a larger catheter or sheath. Distal embolisation during thrombolysis is a nuisance, occurring in 4% of patients, and is usually managed by either aspiration thromboembolectomy or continued lysis. Reperfusion damage has been reported in 2% and pericatheter thrombosis in 1%.

OUTCOME

Diffin and Kandarpa[9] report successful thrombolysis in 70% of treatments, with limb salvage in 93%, although many patients in the collected review did not have limb-threatening ischaemia. The TSG database records complete lysis in 45.5% and clinically useful lysis in a further 27.9% of infusions, leading to a limb salvage rate of 75.2%; 12.4% of patients required an amputation and 12.4% died.[22] Thrombolysis was similarly effective in bypass grafts and native vessels. The outcome seems dependent on the nature of the lesion treated and the clinical state of the patient. Patients with subcritical ischaemia appear less likely to need amputation than patients with critical ischaemia including a neurosensory deficit. In addition, the following are more likely to predict failure of thrombolysis: inability to traverse the occlusion with a guidewire or place a catheter within the thrombus, diabetes, multilevel disease, vein graft occlusion, advancing age and female sex.[27] In the long term, approximately 75% of successfully opened native vessels remain patent at 1 year and 55% at 2 years.[28,29] When an identifiable lesion is found after graft thrombolysis, the 2-year patency is approximately 85%. Long-term patency is less good where no underlying lesion is found in native vessels or grafts. In addition, successfully treated iliac occlusions and emboli have a better long-term outlook.

There is currently great interest in trying to improve the results of peripheral thrombolysis. It is unlikely that advances in techniques will make a significant difference as no one method can be shown to be superior. A consensus group has met and produced a document containing all the available evidence and made recommendations for thrombolytic treatment.[30] Other scoring systems may be used to try to identify patients unlikely to survive after thrombolysis.[31]

Detailed analysis of available data and large databases may help identify patients at greater risk of a poor outcome from thrombolysis. A detailed statistical analysis of the TSG database has shown that the following factors were associated with reduced amputation-free survival: increasing patient age, increasing severity of ischaemia (Fontaine grade and presence of a sensorimotor deficit), shorter duration of ischaemia, and diabetes.[22] Being on warfarin at the time of the occlusion improved the chance of amputation-free survival. The risk of death after thrombolysis was highest in patients with an embolic occlusion, women, older patients and those with ischaemic heart disease. Amputation risk was highest in younger men, legs with a sensorimotor deficit, and graft and thrombotic occlusions.

Surgical management

With the increasing age of the population, underlying atherosclerosis often complicates ischaemia even if the cause is primarily embolic. Consequently, complex secondary procedures may well be necessary if initial balloon catheter embolectomy fails (**Fig. 9.8**). It is therefore advisable that an experienced vascular surgeon performs or supervises the operation. Local anaesthesia may be preferred in a slim patient with a clear-cut embolus and high cardiac risk. However, an anaesthetist should always be present to monitor the ECG and oxygen saturation, administer sedation or analgesia and convert to general anaesthesia if required. Obesity, patient confusion and the likelihood of additional procedures seem good reasons for general anaesthesia.

BALLOON CATHETER EMBOLECTOMY

Both groins and the entire leg should be prepared to permit surgical access and arteriography. The foot should be placed in a sterile transparent bag for easy inspection. The common femoral artery bifurcation is exposed via an oblique groin incision, which reduces wound-healing problems, and the vessels controlled with Silastic slings. Clamps

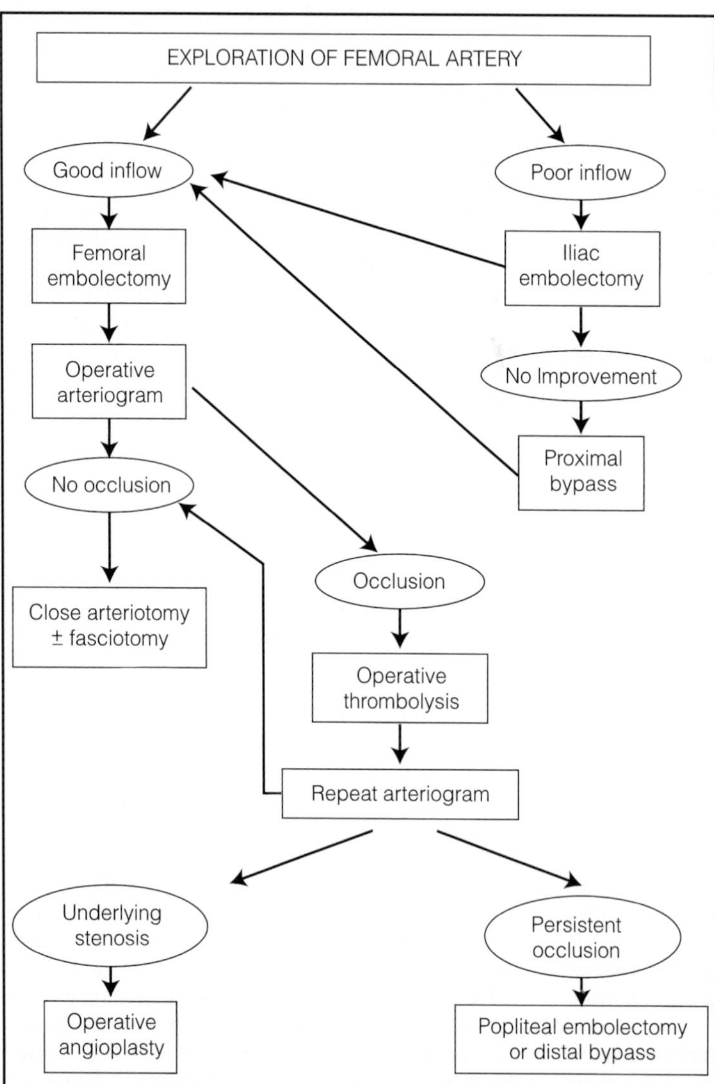

Figure 9.8 • Possible treatment pathway required when exploring the femoral artery.

should be avoided initially because they fragment thrombus that may otherwise be removed intact. A transverse arteriotomy is made in the common femoral artery proximal to the bifurcation, avoiding any obvious plaque (**Fig. 9.9**). A transverse arteriotomy is easier to close without narrowing and it can be converted to a diamond shape for proximal anastomosis if a bypass is required. Any thrombus at the bifurcation can be removed by gentle suction or forceps and momentary release of the sling or clamp.

If pulsatile inflow is not present, then a 4 Fr or 5 Fr balloon catheter is passed proximally up into the aorta, inflated and withdrawn. Pressure should be applied to the contralateral femoral artery during this procedure to prevent contralateral embolisation. If good inflow cannot be achieved, then a femorofemoral or axillo-femoral bypass will be required. A saddle embolus can usually be retrieved by bilateral femoral embolectomy. Next, a 3 Fr or 4 Fr balloon catheter is passed as far distally as possible down both the profunda and superficial femoral arteries. Force should not be used if resistance is met as dissection or perforation may result. The balloon is inflated only as the catheter is withdrawn and the amount of inflation adjusted to avoid excessive intimal friction. The procedure is repeated until no more thromboembolic material can be retrieved. Conventional embolectomy is performed blind and the surgeon has no control over the direction of the catheter past the popliteal trifurcation. Use of an end-hole balloon catheter permits selective catheterisation of the tibial arteries, over a guidewire, under fluoroscopic control (**Fig. 9.10**).

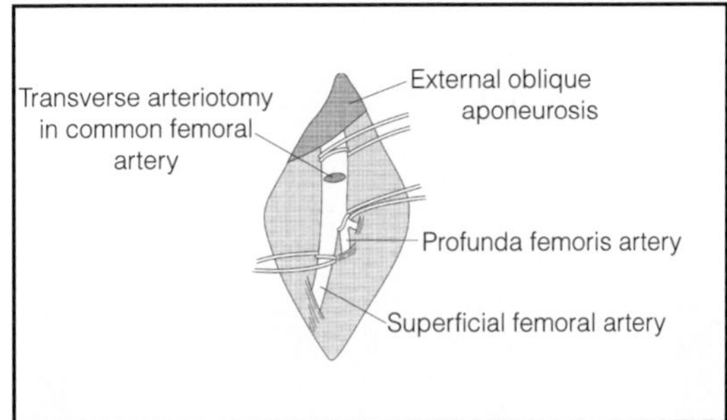

Figure 9.9 • Exploration of the femoral artery using Silastic slings to control the vessels and a transverse arteriotomy proximal to the common femoral bifurcation.

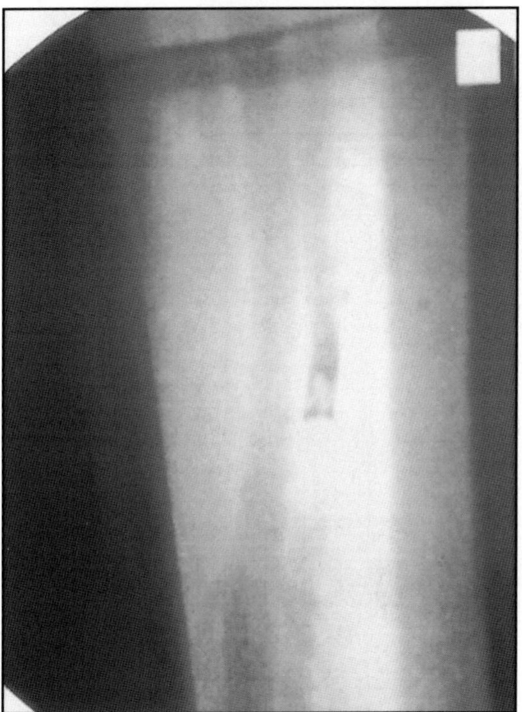

Figure 9.10 • Angiographically controlled balloon catheter embolectomy. The balloon occluding the lumen and the thrombus above it can be seen as negative images against the contrast-filled artery.

COMPLETION ARTERIOGRAPHY

A completion arteriogram should always be performed because persistent thrombus may be present even if the catheter passes to the foot;[32] backbleeding is of no prognostic value as it may arise from established proximal collaterals. Many theatres now have excellent fluoroscopic facilities capable of high-quality arteriography. If this is not available, place a radiography film cassette wrapped in a sterile towel under the leg and infuse 20 mL of contrast medium down the superficial femoral artery via an umbilical catheter with the inflow clamped before exposing the film. The distal arteries are irrigated with 100 mL of heparin saline and if no thrombus is present on the arteriogram, the arteriotomy is repaired with 5/0 prolene. On removing the clamps the foot should become pink with palpable pulses.

FAILED EMBOLECTOMY

If the arteriogram shows persistent occlusion, then streptokinase 100 000 units or t-PA 15 mg in 100 mL heparin saline can be infused via an umbilical catheter over 30 minutes and the arteriogram repeated (**Fig. 9.11**). This often results in complete lysis and reduces the need for popliteal exploration.[33] The technique may also be used to lyse residual thrombus in the tibial arteries during bypass of a popliteal aneurysm.[34] If an underlying stenosis of the superficial femoral artery is revealed, then on-table angioplasty may be attempted. Persistent distal occlusion requires exploration of the below-knee popliteal artery and either popliteal embolectomy or distal bypass. The origins of the anterior tibial artery and tibioperoneal trunk should

(a)

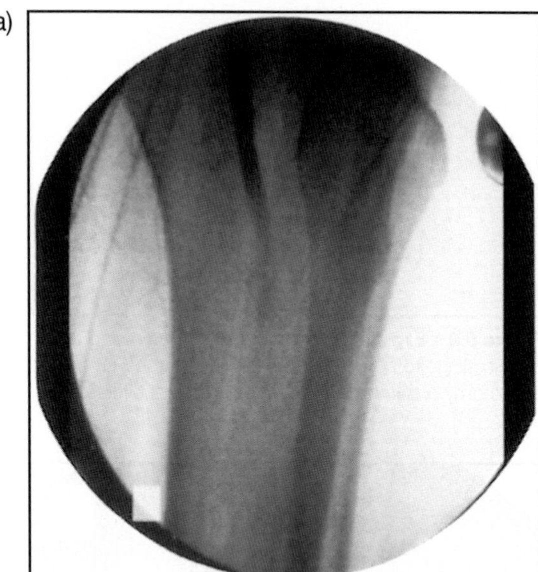

(b)

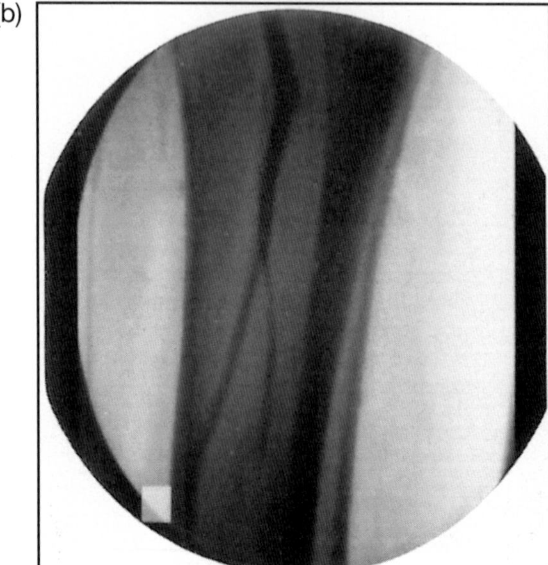

Figure 9.11 • Completion angiogram after embolectomy showing persistent occlusion of the popliteal trifurcation **(a)** and complete lysis after intraoperative thrombolysis **(b)**.

be controlled with slings and selective embolectomy performed via a longitudinal arteriotomy. The popliteal arteriotomy requires repair with a vein patch.

Further management

Revascularisation of an ischaemic leg results in a sudden venous return of blood with low pH and a high potassium concentration. The anaesthetist must be prepared to correct these, as hypotension and arrhythmias may occur. Reperfusion of a large mass of ischaemic tissue results in a systemic inflammatory reaction caused by neutrophil activation. This may cause multiple organ dysfunction including renal and pulmonary failure. Renal function may be further impaired by myoglobinuria, which is helped by maintaining a good diuresis.

Revascularisation of ischaemic muscle can result in considerable swelling within the fascial compartments of the leg. This compartment syndrome will lead to further muscle and nerve damage if not relieved. All muscle compartments should be decompressed via full-length skin and fascial incisions from knee to ankle if any muscle tenseness is present at the time of embolectomy or subsequently.[35] The anterior fasciotomy should be made about two finger-breadths lateral to the anterior border of the tibia, which avoids the peroneal nerve. The posterior fasciotomy incision is done in a line about two finger-breadths posterior to the medial condyle of the femur and the medial malleolus, which avoids the long saphenous vein. A split-skin graft can be applied to the defects later.

After embolectomy, anticoagulation with heparin and then warfarin is continued as this reduces the risk of recurrent embolism, especially if atrial fibrillation is present.[36–38] There is little guidance about the role of anticoagulation in patients who are not fibrillating and have no other obvious cause. Results of a search for proximal sources of emboli using echocardiography and aortic ultrasound may indicate the need for lifelong anticoagulation, but in many patients an individual decision will need to be made based on the risks of warfarinisation and the state of the distal circulation.

OVERALL PROGNOSIS

There has been little change in overall outcome from ALI because the improvements in radiological and surgical techniques have been balanced by increasing atherosclerotic arterial disease in ever older patients. A Swedish population study demonstrated that between 1965 and 1983 there was an increasing incidence of ALI, without any improvement in amputation rates or survival,[39] although outcome after treatment in a university hospital was better than in a district hospital.[40] A recent prospective survey by the Vascular Surgical Society of Great Britain and Ireland that included 539 episodes in 474 patients recorded a limb salvage rate of 70% and an overall mortality rate of 22%.[41] An analysis of patients taken from the National Inpatient Sample in the USA recorded an amputation rate of 12.7% and a mortality rate of 9%.[26] Patients with embolism have a higher mortality rate due to their underlying cardiac disease. In contrast, those with thrombosis are at increased risk of amputation. Patients with a high mortality rate after embolectomy are characterised by:[37]

- poor cardiac function;
- associated peripheral vascular disease;
- short duration of symptoms;
- the need for amputation.

The amputation risk appears higher in patients with a longer duration of ischaemia and poor pre-operative and postoperative cardiac function.[42] Patients with ALI are often elderly and within this group there is a cohort of individuals whose leg problem heralds the end of life. It is important to recognise this group and to offer appropriate palliative care rather than aggressive intervention.[43]

CONCLUSIONS

Although there have been huge changes in the therapeutic options for patients with ALI, there remains debate over the optimal management. Clinical trials in this area are difficult to organise and are often flawed by the great variation in the condition of the patients and their legs. However, further stratification of existing data could help define which occlusions are most suitable for thrombolysis or surgery. A clear comparison between the different drugs available and delivery techniques would help. New drugs will undoubtedly become available with improved safety profiles. In future, thrombolysis combined with other endovascular techniques may enhance its effectiveness.

Key points

- Patients with ALI have high morbidity and mortality rates.
- Optimal management is based on the severity of the ischaemia at presentation.
- Randomised trials have failed to show superiority of thrombolysis or surgery as primary management for all cases.
- Current research is starting to show which patients benefit most from intra-arterial thrombolysis.
- The best results are achieved when management is agreed jointly by a team consisting of vascular surgeon and interventional radiologist using available expertise and local guidelines.

REFERENCES

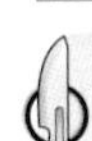

1. Rutherford RB, Flanigan DP, Gupta SK et al. Suggested standards for reports dealing with lower extremity ischemia. J Vasc Surg 1986; 4:80–94.

   Definitive standards for all scientific research.

2. Earnshaw JJ, Hopkinson BR, Makin GS. Acute critical ischaemia of the limb: a prospective evaluation. Eur J Vasc Surg 1990; 4:365–8.
3. Davies B, Braithwaite BD, Birch PA et al. Acute leg ischaemia in Gloucestershire. Br J Surg 1997; 84:504–8.
4. Clason AE, Stonebridge PA, Duncan AJ et al. Acute ischaemia of the lower limb: the effect of centralising vascular surgical services on morbidity and mortality. Br J Surg 1989; 76:592–3.
5. Earnshaw JJ. Demography and aetiology of acute leg ischaemia. Semin Vasc Surg 2001; 14:86–92.
6. Jivegard L, Holm J, Schersten T. Acute limb ischaemia due to arterial embolism or thrombosis: influence of limb ischaemia versus pre-existing cardiac disease on postoperative mortality rate. J Cardiovasc Surg (Torino) 1988; 29:32–6.
7. Blaisdell FW, Steele M, Allen RE. Management of lower extremity arterial ischaemia due to embolism and thrombosis. Surgery 1978; 84:822–34.
8. Braithwaite BD, Tomlinson MA, Walker SR et al. Peripheral thrombolysis for acute-onset claudication. Br J Surg 1999; 86:800–4.

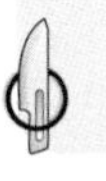

9. Diffin DC, Kandarpa K. Assessment of peripheral intraarterial thrombolysis versus surgical revascularization in acute lower limb ischemia: a review of limb salvage and mortality statistics. J Vasc Intervent Radiol 1996; 7:57–63.

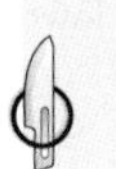

10. Ouriel K, Shortell CK, DeWeese JA et al. A comparison of thrombolytic therapy with operative revascularisation in the initial treatment of acute peripheral arterial ischaemia. J Vasc Surg 1994; 19:1021–30.

    Intra-arterial thrombolysis was associated with a reduction in cardiorespiratory complications and a corresponding increase in survival.

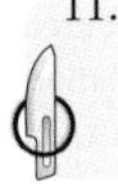

11. The STILE Investigators. Results of a prospective randomized trial evaluating surgery versus thrombolysis for ischaemia of the lower extremity. Ann Surg 1994; 220:251–68.

    There were similar outcomes at 30 days, but patients with ischaemia for less than 14 days had improved amputation-free survival after thrombolysis.

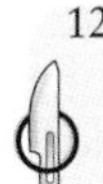

12. Comerota AJ, Weaver FA, Hosking JD et al. Results of a prospective randomized trial of surgery versus thrombolysis for occluded lower extremity bypass grafts. Am J Surg 1996; 172:105–12.

    Patients with ischaemia for less than 14 days did better after surgery, those with shorter-duration ischaemia did better after thrombolysis.

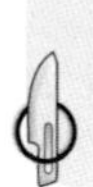

13. Weaver FA, Comerota AJ, Youngblood M et al. Surgical revascularisation versus thrombolysis for nonembolic lower extremity native artery occlusions: results of a prospective randomized trial. J Vasc Surg 1996; 24:513–23.

Surgical revascularisation was more effective and durable than lysis for native vessel occlusions.

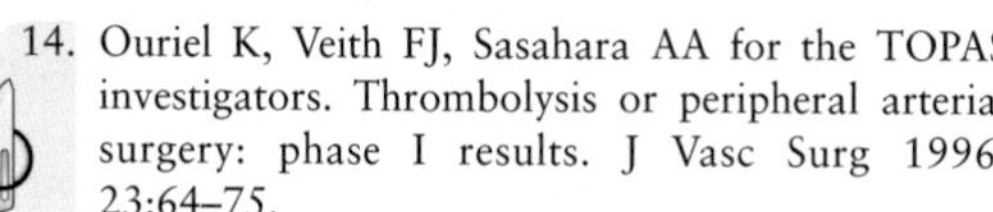

14. Ouriel K, Veith FJ, Sasahara AA for the TOPAS investigators. Thrombolysis or peripheral arterial surgery: phase I results. J Vasc Surg 1996; 23:64–75.

This study was designed to find the optimum dose of urokinase for the second phase of the trial.

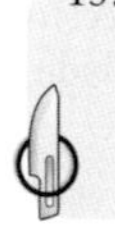

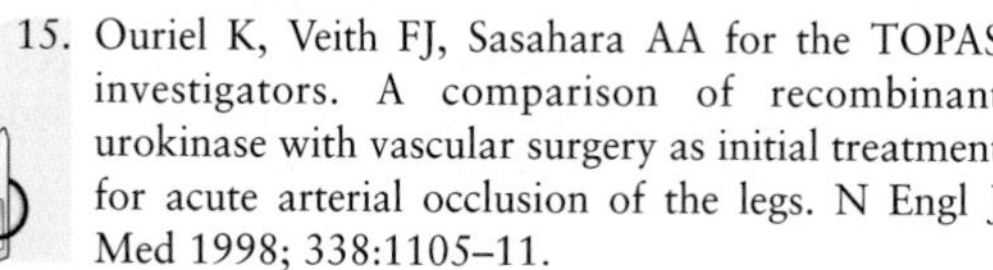

15. Ouriel K, Veith FJ, Sasahara AA for the TOPAS investigators. A comparison of recombinant urokinase with vascular surgery as initial treatment for acute arterial occlusion of the legs. N Engl J Med 1998; 338:1105–11.

This was the largest of the thrombolysis studies and included 544 patients; the results were similar up to 1 year in both groups.

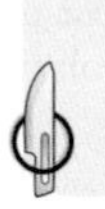

16. Braithwaite BD, Buckenham TM, Galland RB, Heather BP, Earnshaw JJ on behalf of the Thrombolysis Study Group. Prospective randomized trial of high-dose bolus versus low-dose tissue plasminogen activator infusion in the management of acute limb ischaemia. Br J Surg 1997; 84:646–50.

High-dose bolus therapy significantly accelerated thrombolysis without compromising outcome.

17. Yusuf SW, Whitaker SC, Gregson RHS et al. Prospective randomised comparative study of pulse spray and conventional local thrombolysis. Eur J Vasc Endovasc Surg 1995; 10:136–41.

Pulse spray lysis was quicker.

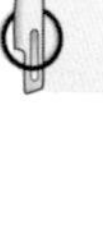

18. Kandarpa K, Chopra PS, Arung JE, Meyerovitz MF, Goldhaber SZ. Intra-arterial thrombolysis of lower extremity occlusion: prospective randomized comparison of forced periodic infusion and conventional slow continuous infusion. Radiology 1993; 188:861–7.

There was no difference in success or complication rates but forced periodic infusion was quicker.

19. Cleveland TJ, Cumberland DC, Gaines P. Percutaneous aspiration thromboembolectomy to manage the embolic complications of angioplasty and as an adjunct to thrombolysis. Clin Radiol 1994; 49:549–52.

20. Haskal ZJ. Mechanical thrombectomy devices for the treatment of acute peripheral arterial occlusions. Rev Cardiovasc Med 2002; 3(suppl. 2):S45–S52.

21. Berridge DC, Gregson RHS, Hopkinson BR, Makin GS. Randomized trial of intra-arterial recombinant tissue plasminogen activator, intravenous recombinant tissue plasminogen activator and intra-arterial streptokinase in peripheral thrombolysis. Br J Surg 1991; 78:988–95.

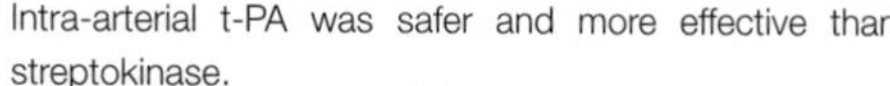

Intra-arterial t-PA was safer and more effective than streptokinase.

22. Earnshaw JJ, Whitman B, Foy C on behalf of the Thrombolysis Study Group. National Audit of Thrombolysis for Acute Leg Ischaemia (NATALI): clinical factors associated with early outcome. J Vasc Surg 2004; 39:1018–25.

23. Mori KW, Bookstein JJ, Heeney DJ et al. Selective streptokinase infusion: clinical and laboratory correlates. Radiology 1983; 148:677–82.

24. Graor RA, Risius B, Denny KM et al. Local thrombolysis in the treatment of thrombosed arteries, bypass grafts, and arteriovenous fistulas. J Vasc Surg 1985; 2:404–14.

25. Hess H, Mietaschk A, Bruckl R. Peripheral arterial occlusions: a 6-year experience with local low-dose thrombolytic therapy. Radiology 1987; 163:753–8.

26. Eliason JL, Wainess RM, Proctor MC et al. A national and institutional experience in the contemporary treatment of acute lower extremity ischaemia. Ann Surg 2003; 238:382–9.

27. Ouriel K, Shortell CK, Azodo MVU, Guiterrez OH, Marder VJ. Acute peripheral arterial occlusions: predictors of success in catheter-directed thrombolytic therapy. Radiology 1994; 193:561–6.

28. McNamara TO, Bomberger RA. Factors affecting initial and six month patency rates after intra-arterial thrombolysis with high dose urokinase. Am J Surg 1986; 152:709–12.

29. Durham JD, Rutherford RB. Assessment of long-term efficacy of fibrinolytic therapy in the ischaemic extremity. Semin Intervent Radiol 1992; 9:166–73.

30. Working Party on Thrombolysis in the Management of Limb Ischemia. Thrombolysis in the management of lower limb peripheral arterial occlusion: a consensus document. J Am Coll Cardiol 1998; 81:207–18.

Recommendations from expert surgeons and radiologists.

31. Neary B, Whitman B, Foy C, Heather BP, Earnshaw JJ. Value of POSSUM physiology scoring to assess the outcome after thrombolysis for acute leg ischaemia. Br J Surg 2001; 88:1344–5.

32. Bosma HW, Jorning PJG. Intraoperative arteriography in arterial embolectomy. Eur J Vasc Surg 1990; 4:469–72.

33. Beard JD, Nyamekye I, Earnshaw JJ, Scott DJA, Thompson JF. Intraoperative streptokinase: a useful adjunct to balloon catheter embolectomy. Br J Surg 1993; 80:21–4.

34. Thompson JF, Beard J, Scott DJA, Earnshaw JJ. Intraoperative thrombolysis in the management of thrombosed popliteal aneurysm. Br J Surg 1993; 80:858–9.

35. Ernst CB. Fasciotomy in perspective. J Vasc Surg 1989; 9:829–30.

36. Hammarsten J, Holm J, Shersten T. Positive and negative effects of anticoagulant treatment during and after arterial embolectomy. J Cardiovasc Surg 1978; 19:373–9.

37. Ljungman C, Adami H-O, Bergqvist D, Sparen P, Bergstrom R. Risk factors for early lower limb loss after embolectomy for acute arterial occlusion: a population-based case–control study. Br J Surg 1991; 78:1482–5.

38. Campbell, Ridler BM, Szymanska TH. Two year follow-up after acute thromboembolic leg ischaemia: the importance of anticoagulation. Eur J Vasc Endovasc Surg 2000; 19:169–73.

39. Ljungman C, Adami H-O, Bergqvist D, Berglund A, Persson I. Time trends in incidence rates of acute, non-traumatic extremity ischaemia: a population based study during a 19-year period. Br J Surg 1991; 78:857–60.

40. Ljungman C, Holmberg L, Bergqvist D, Bergstrom R, Adami H-O. Amputation risk and survival after embolectomy for acute arterial ischaemia. Time trends in a defined Swedish population. Eur J Vasc Endovasc Surg 1996; 11:176–82.

41. Campbell WB, Ridler BMF, Symanska TH on behalf of the Vascular Surgical Society of Great Britain and Ireland. Current management of acute leg ischaemia: results of an audit by the Vascular Surgical Society of Great Britain and Ireland. Br J Surg 1998; 85:1498–503.

42. Dreglid EB, Stangeland LB, Eide GE, Trippestaed A. Patient survival and limb prognosis after arterial embolectomy. Eur J Vasc Surg 1987; 1:263–71.

43. Braithwaite BD, Davies B, Birch PA, Heather BP, Earnshaw JJ. Management of acute leg ischaemia in the elderly. Br J Surg 1998; 85:217–20.

CHAPTER

Ten

Vascular trauma

Jacobus van Marle and
Dirk A. le Roux

INTRODUCTION

Trauma is a major health and social problem and is the main cause of death in people up to the age of 38 years.[1] Fewer than 10% of patients with polytrauma have associated vascular injuries, but these injuries can cause significant morbidity and mortality.[2] Surgery for vascular trauma has evolved from military conflicts, with valuable lessons learned particularly from the Korean and Vietnam wars.[3,4] With a decline in military conflicts, civilian trauma now constitutes the majority of vascular injuries. The incidence and type of vascular trauma differs between various societies. In most European countries today the major emphasis in the management of vascular trauma has shifted towards blunt (traffic accidents) and iatrogenic injuries.[5] In contrast, South Africa has seen an unprecedented increase in violence over the last 20 years, and injuries presenting at trauma centres have also changed from predominantly stab and blunt trauma to injuries caused by firearms.[6]

Complex vascular injuries have a high morbidity and mortality and may present some of the most challenging problems for the surgeon. A clear understanding of the pathophysiology of vascular trauma and a logical approach to the management of trauma in general, and vascular injuries in particular, are essential for a favourable outcome.

MECHANISM OF INJURY

Vascular injuries are classified according to the mechanism of the injury (**Box 10.1**). Direct trauma to the artery accounts for the majority of blunt vascular injuries. Indirect trauma is usually the result of shearing and distraction forces following dislocation of major joints, displaced long-bone fractures, and acceleration/deceleration injuries as seen with high-speed motor vehicle accidents and falls from a height. The usual result of blunt trauma to the arterial wall is disruption of the intima followed by thrombosis. The arterial intima is the least elastic layer of the arterial wall and gives way first. This intimal tear may cause immediate obstruction due to an intimal flap or may predispose to thrombosis and delayed obstruction. As the vessel is stretched further, progressive layers of the media are disrupted until the continuity of the vessel is maintained only by the elastic adventitia or there is complete disruption.

Box 10.1 • Mechanisms of injury

Blunt injury
Direct
Indirect
Penetrating injury
Stab
Missile
Low velocity
High velocity
Shotgun
Bomb blasts
Iatrogenic injury

Penetrating trauma results in either partial or complete transection of a vessel or penetrating or perforating wounds. Bleeding is often brisk and peripheral flow is interrupted. In penetrating trauma the damage can be either localised and confined to the tract of the injury, as seen with stab and low-velocity missile injuries, or extensive as seen with high-velocity missiles. The injury transfer involved with high-velocity missiles causes a cavitation effect, with total tissue destruction around the missile tract and, surrounding this, an area of doubtful tissue viability, all of which results in extensive associated soft tissue trauma.[7] Shotgun injuries also cause extensive local tissue destruction with often multiple sites of perforation. Bomb blasts cause complex injuries due to the combination of extensive local tissue trauma, high-velocity fragments and thermal injury.

Iatrogenic injuries are becoming increasingly important and account for more than 40% of vascular trauma in many European countries.[5] This has been attributed to the increase in percutaneous transluminal vascular procedures and, to a lesser extent, laparoscopic procedures.[8,9]

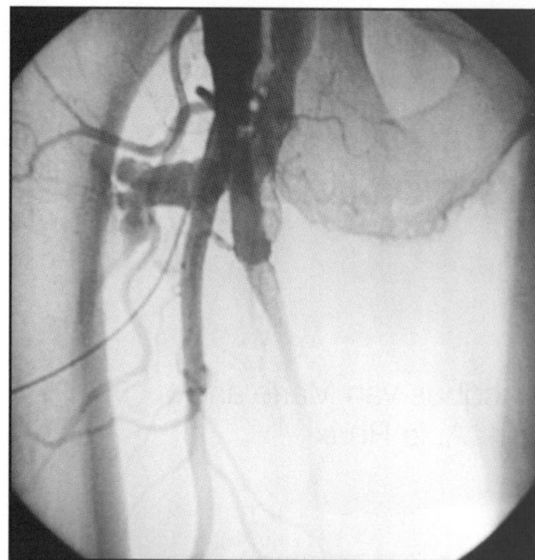

Figure 10.1 • Arteriovenous fistula of the right femoral vessels following iatrogenic injury after diagnostic cardiac catheterisation.

SEQUELAE OF VASCULAR INJURIES

Vascular injuries have significant sequelae (**Box 10.2; Figs 10.1** and **10.2**). A contused artery may be patent initially but thrombose later. Propagation of clot may cause progressive ischaemia by obstructing essential collaterals. Acute ischaemia leads to nerve myelin degeneration and axial retraction within 4–6 hours, with discoid degeneration of muscle cells at 6 hours and marked impairment of contractility at 12 hours.[10] Most of the muscle impairment is irreversible after 12 hours.

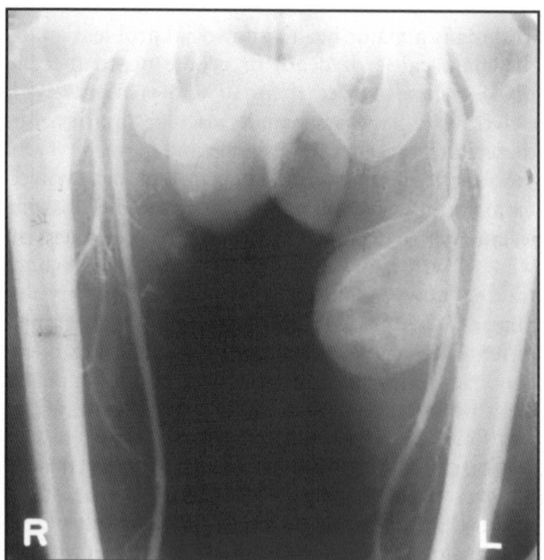

Figure 10.2 • False aneurysm of the left thigh after gunshot wound.

Box 10.2 • Sequelae of vascular injuries

- Acute haemorrhage
  - Overt external bleeding
  - Contained (e.g. in muscle compartment)
  - Concealed (e.g. pleural cavity)
- Hypovolaemia, shock
- Haematoma with or without secondary infection
- Delayed bleeding and rebleeding
- Thrombosis: acute or delayed
- Ischaemia: acute or delayed
- Arteriovenous fistula (see **Fig. 10.1**)
- Pseudoaneurysm formation (see **Fig. 10.2**)

Concomitant fractures, dislocations, injuries to accompanying veins and nerves, soft tissue trauma and contamination of the wound with foreign material serve to compound vascular injury. Other determinants of the final outcome are the level of vascular injury, the quality of the collateral circulation and pre-existing occlusive arterial disease.

CLINICAL ASSESSMENT

History

Information regarding the mechanism of the trauma, blood loss prior to hospital admission and underlying vascular disease should be obtained.

Examination

Initial assessment should be carried out according to advanced trauma life support (ATLS) principles and life-threatening conditions managed. Vascular injury may present with any of the sequelae listed in **Box 10.2**. Clinical signs of vascular injuries can be divided into hard and soft signs.

Hard signs of vascular injury

- Active pulsatile bleeding.
- Shock with ongoing bleeding.
- Absent distal pulses.
- Symptoms and signs of acute ischaemia.
- Expanding or pulsating haematoma.
- Bruits or thrill over the area of injury.

Soft signs of vascular injury

- History of severe bleeding.
- Diminished distal pulse.
- Injury of anatomically related structures.
- Small non-expanding haematoma.
- Multiple fractures and extensive soft tissue injury.
- Injury in anatomical area of major blood vessel.

Distal pulses may be difficult to evaluate in patients with extensive soft tissue trauma, swelling and multiple wounds.

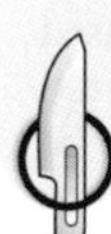

A diminished or absent pulse is due to arterial occlusion until proven otherwise and should not be attributed to vascular spasm, external compression or any other ill-defined factor. Arterial Doppler pressure measurement is a useful supplement to the clinical examination. The arterial pressure index (API) (systolic arterial pressure in the injured limb divided by systolic pressure in an uninvolved arm) of more than 0.9 reliably excludes significant occult arterial injury.[11]

Signs of acute arterial insufficiency (ischaemia) include pulse deficit (absent/diminished pulse), pain, pallor, paraesthesia and paralysis. Neurological deficit must be evaluated carefully in order to distinguish between ischaemic neuropathy and direct injury to the nerve. Tender swollen muscle compartments are signs of prolonged ischaemia, whereas demarcation and skin blisters are indicative of a non-salvageable limb.

Diagnosis

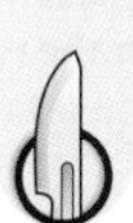

The value and accuracy of a thorough clinical examination in predicting significant vascular injury has been reported in various series.[12,13] Special investigations should only be performed in patients who have been adequately resuscitated and who are haemodynamically stable. Haemodynamic instability, active bleeding and an expanding haematoma are indications for immediate surgery.

RESUSCITATION AND INITIAL MANAGEMENT

A detailed description of resuscitation falls outside the scope of this chapter. ATLS guidelines are followed, with priorities being a patent airway, effective ventilation, arrest of bleeding and restoration of blood volume. The resuscitation of the unstable patient in urgent need of surgery may be best conducted in the operating room.

The amount and timing of fluid resuscitation is important. Moderate fluid replacement is superior to unlimited/uncontrolled fluid resuscitation, which may lead to increased intravascular pressure, decreased blood viscosity and loss of the haemostatic plug, with resultant increased bleeding and mortality.[14,15]

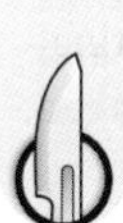

Permitting moderate hypotension (systolic blood pressure between 70 and 90 mmHg) and limiting fluid administration until operative control of bleeding are well-established principles for ruptured abdominal aortic aneurysms and may equally apply in major vascular trauma.

Active bleeding is an indication for urgent exploration, but can usually be temporarily controlled by direct pressure. Blind clamping of vessels in the depth of a wound is contraindicated. Tourniquets should only be used under exceptional circumstances and then only for short periods.

Fractures must be stabilised during the period of resuscitation and diagnostic investigation in order to protect blood vessels and other soft tissue from further trauma. Preliminary reduction of a displaced fracture or dislocation may improve distal circulation.

SPECIAL INVESTIGATIONS

Plain radiography

Plain radiographs are usually taken for associated skeletal injuries. A high index of suspicion for vascular trauma should exist with dislocations and displaced fractures. Chest radiography is valuable in patients with chest trauma.

Arteriography

Arteriography replaced mandatory surgical exploration for exclusion of vascular trauma in the 1980s.

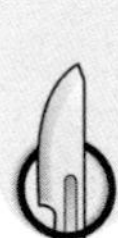

The routine use of arteriography for excluding vascular injury in the absence of hard clinical signs is no longer warranted, especially in extremity trauma.[16,17] However, arteriography is still indicated for the following conditions in the haemodynamically stable patient: multiple fractures, extensive soft tissue injury, shotgun injuries, zone 1 and 3 neck injuries, and thoracic and abdominal injuries.

Surgical intervention should not be delayed by arteriography where vascular injury is evident and the patient unstable or the limb is at ischaemic risk.

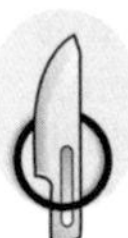

On-table arteriography in the operating room should be performed in vascular injuries to the extremity where surgery cannot be delayed and the additional information is considered valuable.[18]

Ultrasound

Duplex Doppler examination has been described in the evaluation of extremity vascular trauma and neck and abdominal injuries. It is mostly used as a screening test in the absence of hard signs and for follow-up evaluation in patients managed expectantly.

Helical computed tomography

Helical computed tomography (CT) is valuable in blunt cervical, abdominal and thoracic injuries.

Magnetic resonance angiography

The use of magnetic resonance angiography (MRA) in trauma is limited due to time constraints and inaccessibility to the patient during the examination.

GENERAL PRINCIPLES OF MANAGEMENT OF VASCULAR INJURY

Procedures are performed under general anaesthesia in a well-equipped theatre and with proper illumination. Blood products should be available and arrangements for intraoperative autotransfusion should be made where further bleeding is expected. The value of prophylactic antibiotics in vascular surgery is established.

Adequate exposure is vital for obtaining proximal and distal control of injured vessels. This often requires inclusion of adjacent anatomical areas in the operative field, e.g. preparing the neck in thoracic injuries (and vice versa) and the abdomen in groin injuries. An uninjured leg is prepared for possible vein harvesting should bypass be required. Vascular control must be achieved proximally and distally before directly approaching the area of injury. Bleeding may be temporarily arrested by digital compression until clamps have been applied.

The artery should be carefully inspected. In blunt and high-velocity trauma there is often extensive intimal damage, and careful débridement of the vessel is necessary until normal-appearing intima is found. Antegrade and retrograde flow should be evaluated. Arteries are cleared of clot by careful passage of embolectomy catheters followed by irrigation with heparin/saline solution.

After débridement of the artery, repair/reconstruction is completed by a technique suitable to the specific lesion. Simple laceration of the vessel wall is repaired by lateral suture, provided it does not lead to stenosis, when patch graft angioplasty is indicated. Where more than 50% of the circumference of a vessel wall is damaged, this area should be excised followed by end-to-end anastomosis. This requires mobilisation of the proximal and distal arterial stumps to achieve approximation without tension. Failing this, an interposition graft is indicated. Although autogenous vein is the preferred conduit for reconstruction, prosthetic material may be used in exceptional circumstances.[19,20] Intraluminal shunts can be used to maintain antegrade flow during repair.[21]

Completion angiography should be performed where possible to document a technically perfect repair and to assess the distal arterial tree. Vascular injuries are often associated with other injuries, which are addressed once vascular repair has been completed. Proper débridement of the wound area should be performed, with removal of all devitalised and contaminated tissue. Where contaminated wounds are left open, the vascular repair must be covered by soft tissue. Repeated wound inspections are performed, with delayed primary suture when the wound is clean.

ENDOVASCULAR MANAGEMENT OF VASCULAR TRAUMA

Advances in peripheral angiography and newer imaging modalities such as helical CT have led to more accurate diagnosis, obviating the need for mandatory surgical exploration in vascular trauma. Minimally invasive techniques are used more frequently in all aspects of surgery and endovascular procedures have become an integral part of the elective treatment of peripheral vascular disease. The application of these techniques in the injured patient has many potential advantages. Endovascular treatment obviates the need for general anaesthesia. Surgical trauma, with further blood loss, hypothermia, etc., is avoided. It is not necessary to cross-clamp major vessels, preventing distal ischaemia and subsequent reperfusion injury. The main advantage of interventional treatment is the option of approaching complex arterial lesions in anatomically challenging locations from a remote site. A difficult exploration in an injured area is avoided, with less potential damage to surrounding structures including collaterals. Opening a contained haematoma, releasing the tamponade effect and inducing fresh bleeding is also avoided. All the above may lead to decreased morbidity and mortality and shorter hospital stay.

Endovascular techniques are increasingly applied in vascular trauma, but there are still certain limitations. These techniques are usually not applicable, mainly due to time constraints, in patients with active bleeding, in those who are haemodynamically unstable or where there is end-organ ischaemia. Endovascular techniques should also not be used where there are existing compression symptoms, in the presence of infected wounds or where concomitant injuries exist that would require open exploration, e.g. penetrating abdominal injuries. There are also some technical restrictions: (i) inability to traverse the lesion by guidewire, (ii) where intraluminal clot prevents the safe passage of a guidewire due to the danger of distal embolisation or (iii) where luminal discrepancy exists between the proximal and distal involved segments.

Endovascular/interventional techniques are used to manage vascular trauma in three ways.

1. *To obtain definite haemostasis*. Damaged vessels are embolised using a variety of substances including haemostatic agents (gel foam), coils and balloons. This technique was originally described in 1972 for managing significant bleeding following pelvic fractures, and has since become the standard method of treatment.[22,23] Angiographic embolisation is now a recognised option in the management of traumatic lesions of non-essential inaccessible vessels in the cervical, pelvic and limb regions.[24] This technique is also used to control bleeding due to penetrating and blunt trauma of the liver, kidneys and spleen.[25–27]
2. *To obtain vascular control*. A balloon placed in the damaged vessel at the time of diagnostic angiography can be used to temporarily occlude vessels. This technique is especially valuable in relatively inaccessible regions where temporary balloon occlusion limits the extent of the exposure to obtain surgical control.[28] Inflow control of the subclavian artery obviates the need for sternotomy, whereas balloon occlusion of the external iliac artery avoids laparotomy or retroperitoneal exposure for proximal control of femoral artery injuries. This technique is also valuable in managing vascular injuries in zones 1 and 3 of the neck.[28] Occlusion balloons have been placed in the abdominal aorta in the management of ruptured aortic aneurysms and this same technique may be applied in vascular trauma to prevent exsanguinating bleeding until permanent treatment can be effected.
3. *For vascular repair*. The experience gained with stentgrafts in elective management of peripheral vascular disease is increasingly applied in trauma. The most important indication for stentgrafts is inaccessible vessels in anatomically challenging locations where stentgraft repair would obviate the need for major surgical procedures. The use of endovascular repair in vascular trauma is justified in injuries of the thoracic aorta, thoracic outlet vessels, internal carotid and vertebral arteries (**Fig. 10.3**).[29–33] Abdominal vascular injuries rarely present with haemodynamic stability and are usually associated with concomitant bowel injuries requiring laparotomy. Endovascular management is usually not indicated for trauma to the extremity vessels, which are best addressed by conventional open surgical techniques.

Long-term durability remains one of the major concerns in the endovascular treatment of peripheral vascular disease. In-stent stenosis, graft migration, stent breakage and endoleaks are well-known complications of stentgraft repair. This is of concern in the younger population who are the main victims of trauma. Although early results are promising, long-term follow-up and randomised prospective trials comparing standard surgery with endovascular grafting will be necessary before the generalised use of these devices can be recommended.

CERVICAL VASCULAR INJURIES

The cervical vessels are involved in 25% of patients with head or neck trauma and carotid artery injury constitutes 5–10% of all arterial injuries.[34] The mortality and morbidity of these injuries remain high despite advances in diagnosis and treatment.

(a)

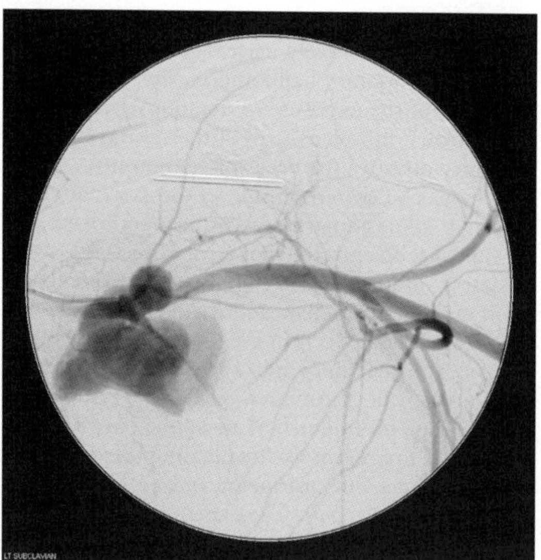

(b)

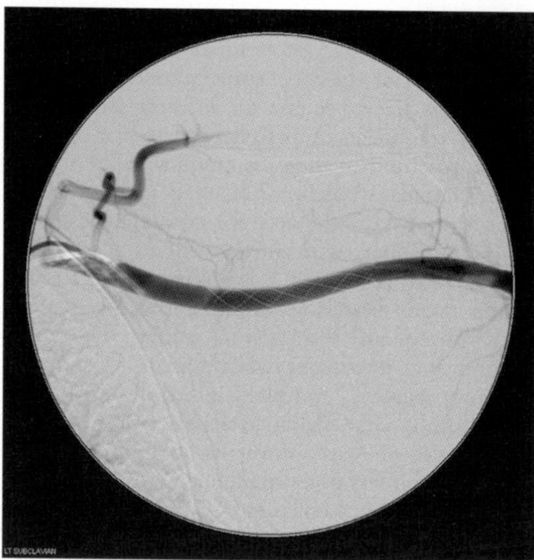

Figure 10.3 • False aneurysm of left subclavian artery after infraclavicular stab wound **(a)** repaired by means of a covered stentgraft **(b)**.

Mortality for carotid injuries ranges from 10 to 31%, with permanent neurological deficit ranging from 16 to 60%.[35,36]

Mechanism

More than 90% of carotid injuries are caused by penetrating trauma. Blunt trauma is caused by a direct blow to the artery, hyperextension, hyperrotation, or contusion by bone fragments associated with fractures of the mandible, temporal bone or cervical spine.

Penetrating injury may cause partial or complete transection with thrombosis of the vessel or pseudoaneurysm. Pseudoaneurysm may have an acute or delayed onset, with progressive enlargement causing compression of the aerodigestive tract or brachial plexus. An arteriovenous fistula develops where there is adjacent arterial and venous perforation and is often accompanied by pseudoaneurysm. Intimal injury can be caused by the shock wave of a high-velocity missile. The vessel is microscopically intact with minimal bruising but on opening the vessel there is an intimal tear with superimposed thrombosis.[37]

Blunt trauma of the carotid and vertebral arteries may cause a variety of lesions: intimal flaps, intramural haematoma, dissection, complete disruption of arterial wall with pseudoaneurysms, arteriovenous fistulas and total occlusion.

Neurological sequelae are caused by hypoperfusion (transected or thrombosed vessels) or embolisation from thrombus, pseudoaneurysm or arteriovenous fistula.

Clinical signs

The neck has been divided into three anatomical zones in order to standardise diagnosis and management of cervical vascular injuries (**Fig.10.4**).[38]

Rapidly expanding cervical haematoma, absent carotid pulse and a bruit or thrill are hard signs indicative of vascular injury. Soft signs that may indicate an associated vascular injury and which warrant further investigation include active bleeding from wounds of the neck or the pharynx, a deficit of the superficial temporal artery pulse, ipsilateral Horner's sign, dysfunction of cranial nerves IX–XII, a widened mediastinum, fractures of the skull base and temporal bone, and fractures and dislocation of the cervical spine. Neurological deficit may be present but obscured due to concomitant

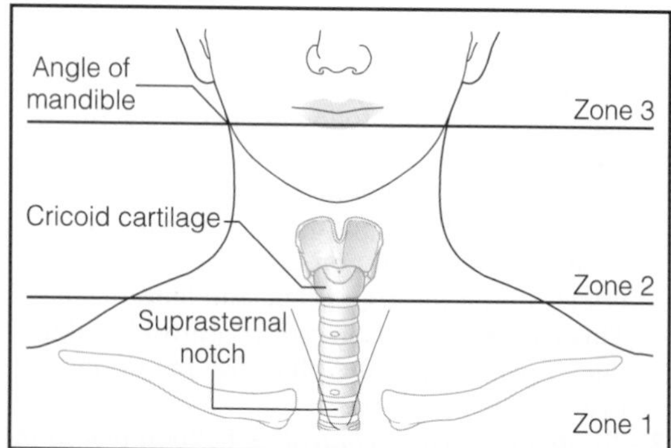

Figure 10.4 • Zones of the neck.

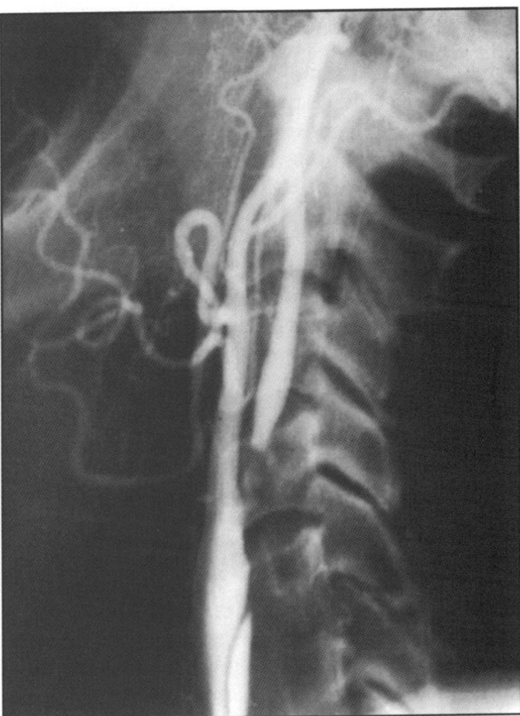

Figure 10.5 • Dissection of the common carotid artery with blunt trauma to the neck following a motor vehicle accident.

head injury, shock or the use of alcohol or drugs. About 50% of patients with established blunt injury to the carotid and vertebral arteries could initially be asymptomatic, but 43–58% of these will eventually develop neurological signs after hospital admission (**Fig. 10.5**).[39,40]

Diagnosis

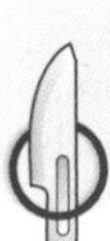

Patients with active bleeding and a compromised airway require immediate exploration, while those who are haemodynamically stable and have a patent airway should undergo further appropriate investigations.

Anteroposterior chest radiography can provide valuable information regarding associated haemothorax or pneumothorax, widening of the mediastinum, surgical emphysema of the neck with concomitant aerodigestive tract injuries, etc.

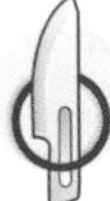

Duplex Doppler examination is extremely useful for investigating zone 2 vascular injuries and is now the preferred diagnostic modality.[41,42]

However, duplex scanning has limitations in zones 1 and 3 due to anatomical constraints. Arch angiography remains the gold standard for the diagnosis of cervico-mediastinal and zone 3 vascular injuries. It provides information regarding suspected injuries to other vessels and is important for proper planning of the surgical procedure and evaluation for possible endovascular treatment.

CT of the brain should be used to investigate patients with associated head trauma, bone injuries of the spine and skull, and neurological deficit. CT of the brain is a good predictor of outcome: patients who have an infarct on initial CT on admission have a high mortality with poor chance of neurological recovery compared with those who have a normal CT on admission.[39] MRA may be valuable in carotid artery and vertebral artery dissection.[43]

Management

Mandatory exploration of all penetrating neck injuries has been replaced by a selective approach.[44]

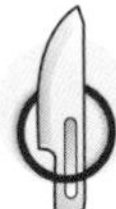

Active pulsatile haemorrhage, expanding cervical haematoma and airway compromise are indications for urgent surgical exploration.

Some low-velocity penetrating injuries may be managed expectantly with careful observation, provided there is no active bleeding and the distal circulation is normal. These injuries include intimal defects, small pseudoaneurysms (<5 mm) and non-obstructive intimal flaps. This selective non-operative management is advocated by Stain et al.[44] and Frykberg et al.,[45] whereas Robbs[46] believes that all perforations, as well as small pseudoaneurysms, should be dealt with as the consequences of late haemorrhage are highly significant in terms of morbidity.

Most patients with carotid artery injuries are best managed by primary arterial repair, regardless of contralateral neurological status.[36,47,48] Neurological deficit is only a contraindication to surgical repair in a deeply comatose patient with a dense neurological deficit, arterial occlusion and a huge infarct on cerebral CT; these patients have poor outcome regardless of treatment.[48] All other patients with associated neurological deficit would benefit from arterial repair, with improved mortality and final neurological status.[36,47,48]

Most blunt injuries of the carotid and vertebral arteries result in intimal disruption, with dissection and/or thrombosis, and the immediate goal of management is to restore cerebral perfusion and to prevent embolisation. Systemic anticoagulation is therefore the treatment of choice, because it limits the formation, propagation and/or embolisation of the thrombus. Intravenous heparin is administered in the acute phase, followed by oral anticoagulation for at least 3 months.[49,50]

Operative technique

Detailed description of operative technique falls outside the scope of this chapter and the reader is referred to the standard textbooks of operative surgery.[51] The general principles of management include the following.

1. The patient should be in a supine position with a bolster between the scapulae and with the neck extended and the head rotated to the contralateral side. The patient must be draped to allow access from the base of the skull to the xiphisternum.
2. Zone 2 injuries are explored by the standard carotid incision overlying the anterior border of the sternocleidomastoid muscle.
3. Zone 1 injuries may require a median sternotomy.
4. Various techniques have been described to improve exposure of the distal internal carotid artery in zone 3 injuries.
5. Some authors recommend routine shunting to maintain antegrade flow. We only make use of intraluminal shunts during complicated repairs of the internal carotid artery.
6. The external carotid artery can be safely ligated if the internal carotid artery is patent. Internal carotid artery ligation is only allowed when the distal vessel is thrombosed with no back-bleeding following extraction of thrombus.
7. Minor venous injuries can be managed by lateral suture repair, but complex venous repair is not indicated as there is a high occlusion rate and it increases the magnitude of the operative procedure. Ligation of the jugular vein can be performed without significant sequelae.[52]
8. In the presence of associated injuries to the trachea and oesophagus, the vascular repair should be protected by soft tissue interposition (sternocleidomastoid muscle).

Vertebral artery injuries

The occurrence of vertebral artery injury is low, with the reported incidence in penetrating neck trauma ranging from 1 to 7.4%. Gunshot wounds are the most common mechanism of injury.[53,54] Blunt injury of the vertebral artery is even less common and is caused by fractures of the lateral mass of the cervical vertebrae involving the foramen transversarium, vertebral fractures, ligamentous cervical spine injury, or severe and sudden rotation and/or hyperextension of the head. These injuries are seen with motor vehicle accidents and near-hanging injuries and have also been described during extreme chiropractic manipulation.[55]

The majority of patients with vertebral artery injuries have associated injuries of the cervical spine, spinal cord and other vascular structures in the neck or aerodigestive tract.[56] Helical CT angiography has a high sensitivity and specificity for detecting injury of the vertebral artery and is being used increasingly in penetrating neck trauma.[57]

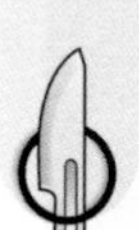

Angiographic embolisation is the treatment of choice in the majority of patients with vertebral artery injuries.[32] Operative management is only indicated for severe active bleeding or when embolisation has failed. Haemodynamically stable patients with a thrombosed vertebral artery do not need any intervention.

A detailed description of surgical approaches to, and management of, vertebral artery injuries is given by Demetriades et al.[32] and Hatzitheofilou et al.[58]

THORACIC VASCULAR INJURIES

Penetrating trauma is responsible for more than 90% of thoracic vascular injuries.[59] Blunt aortic injuries account for 10–15% of motor vehicle accident fatalities;[60] 70–90% of patients sustaining these injuries will die before reaching a hospital.[61] The proximal descending aorta is most commonly involved in these injuries. The site of insertion of the ligamentum arteriosum, just distal to the origin of the left subclavian artery, is the typical point of injury. Frontal deceleration is the most common mechanism causing blunt thoracic injury, but recent studies have also implicated side-impact collisions.[62] Deceleration or compression injury may also involve the brachiocephalic trunk, the pulmonary veins and the vena cava.

Clinical presentation and initial management

Patients with penetrating thoracic vascular trauma are usually haemodynamically unstable, often with continuing haemorrhage into the pleural cavity or the mediastinum. These patients should be taken rapidly for urgent thoracotomy and a precise diagnosis of vascular injury is only made intra-operatively. Patients with blunt thoracic trauma may initially be haemodynamically stable and the injury may not be immediately apparent due to the high incidence of concomitant trauma. The following clinical findings may be associated with underlying thoracic great vessel injury:[63]

- shock/hypotension;
- difference in blood pressure or pulses between the two upper extremities (brachiocephalic trunk or subclavian artery injury);

- difference in blood pressure between upper and lower extremities (pseudocoarctation syndrome);
- expanding haematoma at the thoracic outlet;
- left flail chest;
- intrascapular murmur;
- palpable fracture of the sternum;
- palpable fracture of the thoracic spine;
- external evidence of major chest trauma;
- history indicating deceleration or compression injury to the chest.

Diagnostic studies

The number and type of diagnostic studies performed will be determined by the patient's haemodynamic stability and general status as well as the type of aortic lesion and concomitant injuries.

CHEST RADIOGRAPHY

A frontal chest radiograph is an important screening tool and should be obtained in all patients with penetrating and suspected blunt thoracic trauma. In patients with penetrating injuries, radio-opaque markers are useful for identifying entrance and exit sites.

A widened mediastinum on chest radiography is associated with more than 90% of thoracic aortic injuries, with a 90% sensitivity and 95% negative predictive value.[64,65] Other radiographic findings associated with blunt injuries of the descending aorta include the following.[63]

1. Mediastinal findings:
   - **(a)** Widening of the mediastinum greater than 8 cm
   - **(b)** Obliteration of the aortic knob contour
   - **(c)** Depression of the left main stem bronchus greater than 140°
   - **(d)** Loss of the paravertebral pleural line
   - **(e)** Lateral displacement of the trachea
   - **(f)** Deviation of a nasal gastric tube
   - **(g)** Calcium laying of the aortic knob.
2. Fractures of sternum and scapula, clavicle fracture in a polytrauma patient and multiple rib fractures.
3. Other findings on anteroposterior chest radiograph: apical pleural haematoma (apical cap), massive left haemothorax, ruptured diaphragm.
4. Findings on a lateral chest radiograph: anterior displacement of trachea, loss of the aorto-pulmonary window.

Positive findings on chest radiography are indications for further advanced diagnostic studies, mainly angiography and helical CT.

ANGIOGRAPHY

Aortography is required to detect, localise and determine the extent of aortic injury and provides important information that may influence operative strategy as different thoracic incisions may be required for different injuries. It is indicated in penetrating thoracic trauma for suspected injury to the innominate, carotid or subclavian arteries, but only if the patient is haemodynamically stable. The proximity of a missile trajectory to the brachiocephalic vessels may in itself be an indication for arteriography even without any physical findings of vascular injury.[63]

HELICAL CT

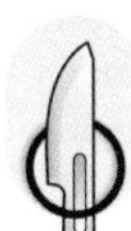

Helical CT is no longer used just as a screening procedure to select patients for angiography but is considered a definitive diagnostic procedure that recognises aortic injury and rupture.[66,67]

It is less invasive, faster to obtain and more readily available compared with angiography and has a further advantage that it can provide important information regarding associated lesions. However, the relative inaccessibility to the patient during examination limits its use in unstable patients.

OTHER IMAGING MODALITIES

Transoesophageal echocardiography and intravascular ultrasound may be used as complementary modalities in selected patients, but routine use of these techniques is limited.

Treatment

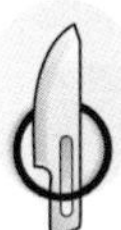

Indications for urgent surgery are haemodynamic instability, increasing haemorrhage from chest tubes and radiographic evidence of an expanding haematoma.

An initial large volume of blood drained from a chest tube (>1500 mL) or ongoing haemorrhage of more than 200–300 mL/hour may also indicate great vessel injury and may be an indication for thoracotomy. Certain selected patients who are haemodynamically stable may benefit from a delayed repair.

The current indications for delayed aortic repair in the haemodynamically stable patient include trauma to the central nervous system with coma, respiratory failure from lung contusion, body surface burns, blunt cardiac injury, visceral injury that will undergo non-operative management, retroperitoneal haematoma, contaminated wounds, hypothermia, coagulopathy and other conditions that can be corrected to improve the outcome of operative repair, age 50 years or older and medical comorbidities.[68–70]

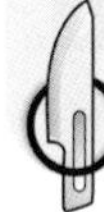

Certain minimal aortic lesions, for example intimal defects, small intimal flaps and pseudoaneurysms, may be managed non-operatively with close observation.[71] Patients selected for initial non-operative management should be closely monitored, with systolic blood pressure kept below 120 mmHg or mean arterial pressure below 80 mmHg. Aronstam et al.[72] reported on the beneficial effect of beta-blockade in patients with a blunt aortic injury, and intravenous beta-blockade titrated to heart rate is currently included in many protocols.

Surgical repair

Adequate exposure for proximal and distal control of the great vessels is mandatory. Skin preparation should include the anterior neck, thorax, abdomen and a lower extremity. There are four basic surgical approaches.

1. Left anterolateral thoracotomy is indicated for the hypotensive unstable patient with an undiagnosed injury. The patient is placed in the supine position and a left anterior thoracotomy performed through the fourth intercostal space. If wider exposure is needed, the incision may be extended medially across the sternum or posteriorly.
2. Posterolateral thoracotomy through the fourth intercostal space or bed of the fifth rib gives excellent exposure to most of the left hemithorax. The incision may be extended across the sternum or into the abdomen for further exposure to manage accompanying injuries.
3. A median sternotomy is indicated for injuries to the ascending aorta, transverse aortic arch, innominate and proximal carotid and right subclavian arteries. The incision may be extended into the neck to improve exposure of the arch and the brachiocephalic branches.
4. The proximal left subclavian artery is approached via a median sternotomy or through an anterolateral thoracotomy in the third intercostal space with a separate supraclavicular incision to provide distal control if required.

The main controversial issue in the repair of thoracic aortic injuries is whether distal circulatory support should be used. Many authors still advocate a simple clamp-and-repair technique without the use of systemic anticoagulation or shunts.[73,74] However, others advocate the use of distal circulatory support, of which left heart bypass between the left atrium and distal aorta or femoral artery seems to be the most promising.[75] Regardless of the technique used, paraplegia occurs in approximately 8% of patients and no prospective randomised trial has as yet identified the superiority of any single method.[63]

Endovascular repair

Endovascular stentgrafts have been used with success in the treatment of descending thoracic aortic aneurysms and acute type B dissections (**Fig. 10.6**).[76,77] These techniques have been successfully applied in traumatic aortic injuries,

(a)

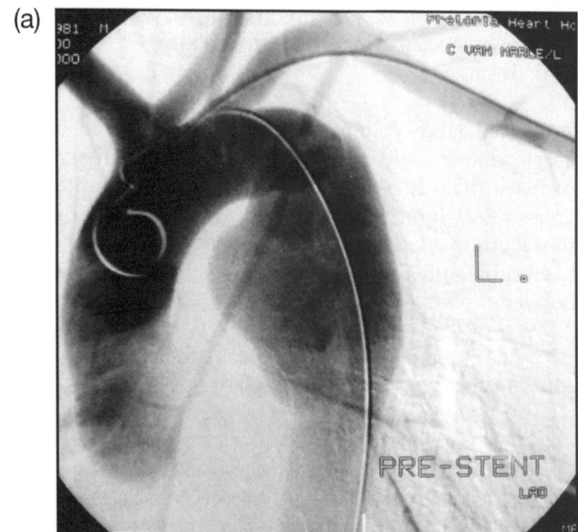

(b)

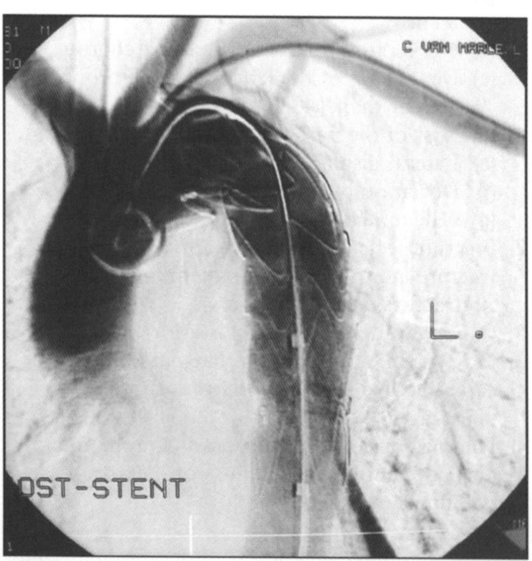

Figure 10.6 • Thoracic aneurysm after blunt injury to the chest **(a)** treated with a covered aortic stentgraft **(b)**.

with a high technical success rate and significantly lower morbidity and mortality.[29,78]

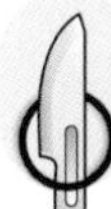

Endovascular repair of traumatic aortic rupture is the preferred treatment in patients who are haemodynamically stable and have appropriate anatomy.

ABDOMINAL VASCULAR INJURIES

Penetrating trauma accounts for 90–95% of abdominal vascular injuries (**Fig. 10.7**), with a high mortality due to the nature of these injuries as well as associated injuries to other intra-abdominal organs.[79] It is important to consider intra-abdominal injury with all penetrating injuries from the nipples to the upper thighs.

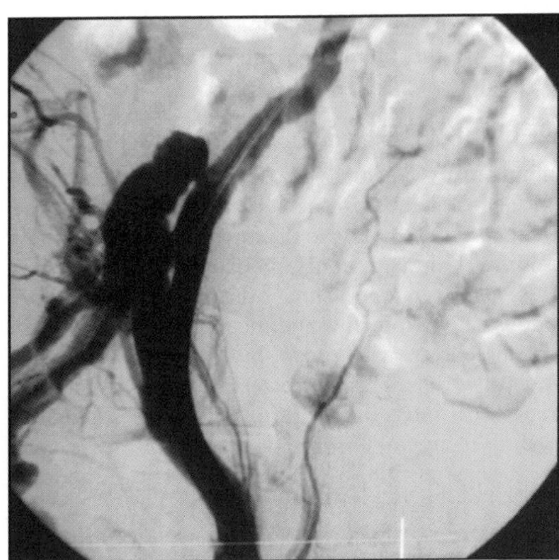

Figure 10.7 • Fistula of left common iliac artery after a penetrating injury (gunshot wound to the abdomen).

Diagnosis

The unstable patient with a possible abdominal vascular injury requires immediate surgery. The stable patient should be investigated according to the injuries. Plain abdominal radiography using radio-opaque markers is of value in establishing the trajectory of missiles in penetrating injuries. Arteriography and CT have little if any role in the diagnosis of penetrating abdominal vascular injury.[80]

Management

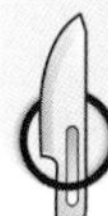

The surgeon should be ready to enter the abdominal cavity rapidly at induction of anaesthesia. A generous laparotomy incision is required from xiphisternum to suprapubis. Four-quadrant packing of the abdomen is performed as soon as it is entered and the proximal aorta is controlled at the diaphragmatic crus. Once control of the vascular injury is obtained, resuscitation with blood products can be instituted. Bowel injuries are temporarily controlled until vascular repair is effected.

Different surgical exposures are used for specific injuries. The Mattox manoeuvre (left paracolic incision, mobilising the splenic flexure descending and sigmoid colon to the right) allows access to the supracoeliac aorta, coeliac axis with its branches to the left, superior mesenteric artery (SMA), inferior mesenteric artery, left renal artery and left iliac vessels. The Cattell–Braasch or extended Kocher manoeuvre allows access to infrahepatic inferior vena cava, right renal vein, portal system and right iliac vessels. The infrarenal aorta may also be approached via the root of the descending mesocolon. The iliac arteries are exposed via separate incisions lateral to the caecum and sigmoid respectively, avoiding injury to the ureters as they cross the common iliac arteries. The iliac veins may only be accessible after dividing the arteries that lie anterior to them.

AORTIC INJURIES

Simple lacerations can simply be oversewed. An interposition polyester or polytetrafluoroethylene (PTFE) graft may be employed if necessary in the uncontaminated field. In the 'damage control' scenario, a temporary shunt using a sterile thoracostomy tube can be placed. Definitive repair is performed once the patient is stable and all physiological parameters are normal.[81] In severe contamination, a graft made of panelled saphenous vein may be used, or the aorta is ligated and an extra-anatomical bypass (e.g. axillo-femoral) performed.[82]

ILIAC INJURIES

These injuries can be repaired using primary suturing or interposition grafting. In the case of severe contamination, ligation and femoro-femoral bypass is an accepted technique.[82]

COELIAC TRUNK AND BRANCHES

Injuries to these structures are usually dealt with by primary ligation.[82]

SUPERIOR MESENTERIC ARTERY

Fullen et al.[83] divided the SMA into four zones; injuries to the first two zones (i.e. SMA trunk to the origin of the middle colic artery) should be treated with primary repair whenever possible.

INFERIOR MESENTERIC ARTERY

Injuries to the inferior mesenteric artery can usually be ligated.[83]

RENAL ARTERY INJURY

Blunt injury is usually caused by the acceleration/deceleration mechanism, which causes thrombosis of the vessels. One should attempt to repair these injuries within 12 hours, since renal viability after this period is very slim.[82] Proximal injuries are approached from the midline through the base of the mesentery, while distal injuries are approached laterally. Repair is performed by either primary repair or interposition grafting using saphenous vein.

INFERIOR VENA CAVA

The inferior vena cava (IVC) consists of four parts: infrarenal, suprarenal, retrohepatic and intrapericardial. The retrohepatic and intrapericardial portions are usually affected by blunt trauma. Approximately 50% of patients die before reaching hospital and the in-hospital mortality ranges between 20 and 57%.[84,85]

Wounds in the infrahepatic IVC can be temporarily controlled by means of digital pressure or intraluminal balloon catheters. When clamps are applied, one should be aware of the abundant lumbar collateral circulation.

Repair is effected by means of lateral suture or, when there are large defects, even prosthetic material. The anterior laceration in a through-and-through lesion may need to be extended so that the posterior defect can be repaired first. In dire attempts to save an exsanguinating patient this part of the IVC may be ligated.

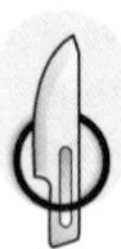

The retrohepatic IVC should be approached with extreme caution and if haemorrhage can be controlled with packing this should be the method of treatment.

Various strategies to repair these injuries have been described but the prognosis is still dismal, with a reported mortality of 70–90%.[85,86] The Shrock shunt, which is inserted through the right atrium, can be used to control these injuries temporarily. We use a modified technique by inserting an endotracheal tube through the infrahepatic IVC and inflating the balloon in the right atrium.

Total hepatic isolation (Heany manoeuvre) is associated with a high mortality, especially in an exsanguinated patient. Venous repair is by means of ligation of hepatic veins or direct repair.

PELVIC VASCULAR INJURIES

Haemorrhage is the primary cause of death in patients with pelvic fractures.[87] The common iliac, external iliac and common femoral arteries and corresponding veins are the source of catastrophic blood loss in only about 1% of pelvic fractures and require open surgery.

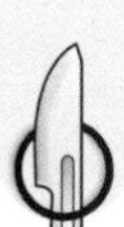

The major sources of bleeding are branches of the internal iliac artery, venous radicles, bone and soft tissues. These injuries associated with pelvic fractures are treated with transcatheter embolisation.[22,23]

Angiography is of little value in penetrating injuries and appropriate surgical intervention should be carried out without delay.

EXTREMITY VASCULAR TRAUMA

The incidence of peripheral vascular injury depends on the extent and type of trauma, ranging from 0.6–3.6% for isolated extremity fractures, 7.3% for polytrauma patients to 25–30% for all penetrating injuries of the extremities;[2,88,89] 23–50% of patients with dislocations or fractures of the knee have popliteal artery injuries. The risk of limb loss is greatest following blunt trauma and injuries from high-velocity missiles or close-range shotgun wounds.[90]

Diagnosis

Any extremity injury warrants a complete physical examination of the injured extremity and distal vessels.

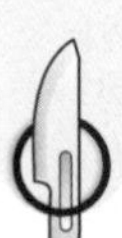

The absence of hard signs of vascular injury reliably excludes surgically significant arterial injury and does not require arteriography.[12,91,92] Arteriography for proximity injury is indicated only in patients with shotgun injuries and multiple fractures (**Fig. 10.8**).[93]

Although ischaemia may not be present initially, it may develop rapidly if thrombosis supervenes. The occurrence of delayed thrombosis stresses the importance of regular reassessment of the peripheral circulation for at least 24 hours after orthopaedic injury.[94] There may be a role for duplex Doppler studies in patients with soft signs of vascular injury or with proximity injuries.[95]

General principles of management

1. Restoration of perfusion to an extremity with an arterial injury should generally be performed in less than 6 hours in order to maximise limb salvage.[96]

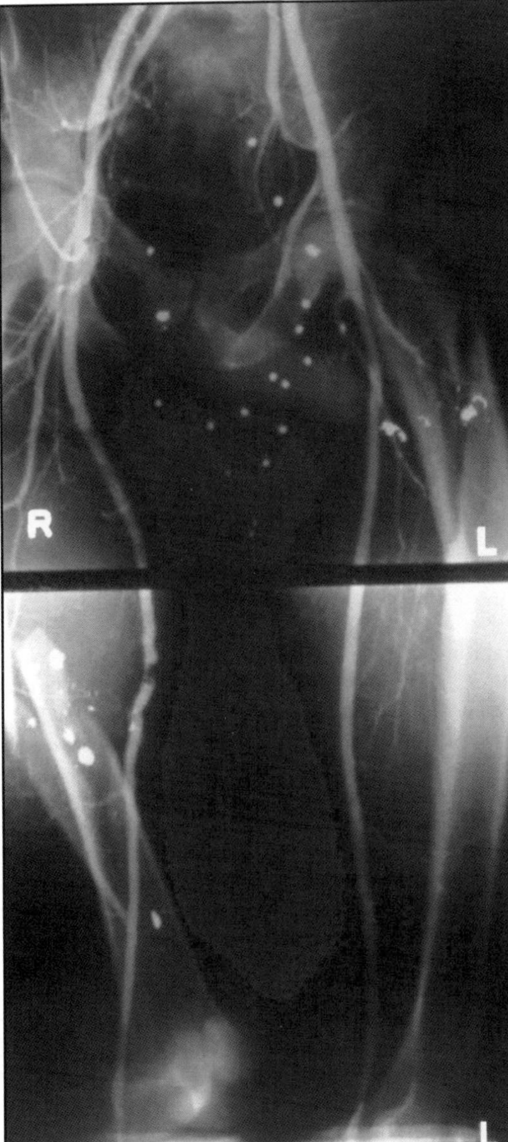

Figure 10.8 • Arteriogram of the pelvis and thighs to assess level of arterial injury after shotgun wound.

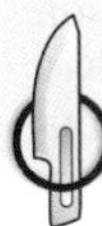

2. Non-operative observation of asymptomatic non-occlusive arterial injuries is acceptable.[12] These injuries can be defined as small pseudoaneurysms, intimal flaps or irregularities, small arteriovenous fistulas, and haemodynamic insignificant narrowings of the vessels. Should subsequent repair of these injuries be required, it can be done without significant increase in morbidity.[12]

3. Simple arterial repairs do better than grafts. If complex repair is required, vein grafts appear to be the best choice.[97,98] PTFE is an acceptable conduit when no vein is available and may even be used in a contaminated field.[19,20] Effort should be made to cover the graft with soft tissue.

4. Temporary shunting is valuable for maintaining antegrade flow in order to allow stabilisation of unstable fractures and/or dislocations prior to definitive arterial repair (**Fig. 10.9**).[21]
5. Early four-compartment lower leg fasciotomy should be applied liberally. Although this procedure is not indicated for all patients, careful and repeated examination of the limb with a high index of suspicion is mandatory. Indications for fasciotomy include (i) ischaemic time greater than 4–6 hours, (ii) signs of acute ischaemia, (iii) extensive soft tissue injuries, (iv) combined arterial and venous injuries, (v) intracompartmental bleeding and (vi) increased compartmental pressure. Measurement of compartment pressures is an important adjunct, but must be done in all compartments, and should be interpreted in the context of each individual patient because tissue perfusion is a balance between compartment pressure and blood pressure. Acceptable compartment pressures have been defined as absolute compartment pressures of less than 20 mmHg and at least 30 mmHg less than mean arterial pressure.[99]

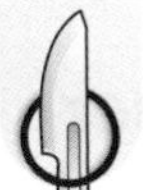

6. Completion arteriogram should be performed after arterial repair to assess patency and technical perfection of the repair.

7. Although amputation rates increase with longer ischaemia times, quantifying the relationship is difficult because amputation rates also depend on other factors such as extent of soft tissue damage, the capacity of collaterals, pre-existing arterial disease and the vessels injured.[100]
8. In certain cases primary amputation may be considered. Scoring systems such as the mangled extremity severity score (MESS) have been developed to help predict outcome of limb salvage procedures.[101] A MESS score of 7 or more has a predicted amputation rate of 100%. Given the significance of amputation, delaying the procedure even by a day or two is preferred as it allows careful examination of the limb and discussion with the patient and family.
9. Reperfusion injury and renal protection: measures should be taken to protect against the systemic effects of reperfusion injury and subsequent renal damage by creating a diuresis of at least 1.5–2 mL/kg per hour with the administration of adequate volumes of normal saline. Mannitol, which has a diuretic as well as a radical scavenger effect, is added. Urine is alkalinised by administering 8.5% sodium

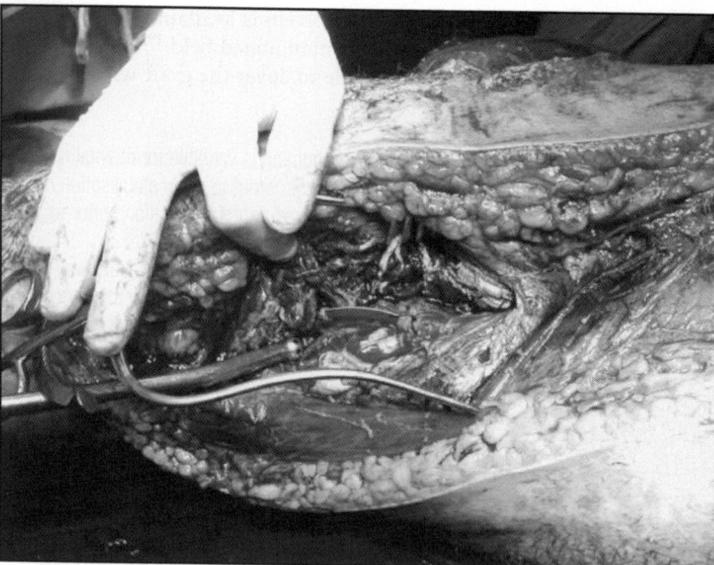

Figure 10.9 • Temporary shunt in right superficial femoral artery, allowing distal perfusion while external fixator is applied to the femur, following a motorcycle accident.

bicarbonate to prevent precipitation of myoglobin crystals in the renal tubuli. Measures to treat hyperkalaemia may be required. Serum myoglobin levels should be monitored regularly.

Vascular injuries to the upper extremity (Fig. 10.10)

The majority of injuries are to the brachial artery, and 90% of injuries are due to penetrating trauma.[102] Upper extremity vascular injuries are usually not life-threatening but significant morbidity may occur. Return of function is often related to associated nerve injury. Timely restoration of blood flow is essential to optimise outcome. Venous injuries to the arm rarely require repair and even injuries to the brachial and axillary veins may be ligated because the collateral venous network is extensive.

SUBCLAVIAN AND AXILLARY INJURIES (Fig. 10.11)

All patients with periclavicular trauma should be evaluated for possible vascular injury. Most of these injuries are caused by penetrating trauma. The presence of a peripheral pulse does not reliably exclude significant proximal arterial injury.[103] A difference in blood pressure of more than 20 mmHg between the upper limbs or an API of less than 0.9 warrants further investigation. The brachial plexus is injured in about one-third of patients with subclavian or axillary artery injuries due to the anatomical proximity of the neurovascular structures. A thorough neurological assessment should be performed.

Duplex Doppler reliably assesses arterial and venous injuries.[103] However, there are certain limitations, for example visualising the origin of the subclavian artery. Arteriography has a diagnostic role in evaluating superior mediastinal injuries or where duplex Doppler is inconclusive, and also has a therapeutic role in embolisation or stentgraft repair.

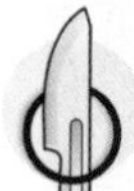

Promising results have been obtained with endovascular repair of pseudoaneurysms and arteriovenous fistulas in selected patients.[30]

Where surgical repair is required, the neck and chest should be included in the operative field. The patient is placed supine and the arm is draped free and abducted to 30°. The head is turned to the other side. The standard incision starts at the sternoclavicular joint and extends over the medial half of the clavicle, curving over the deltopectoral groove. For proximal subclavian injuries this incision can be combined with a median sternotomy. The proximal left subclavian artery can also be approached via a left anterior thoracotomy through the third intercostal space. The so-called 'trapdoor' incision (supraclavicular incision, upper third median sternotomy and left anterior thoracotomy) is not recommended due to significant postoperative morbidity.

The axillary artery is exposed through an infraclavicular incision between the clavicular and sternal parts of the pectoralis major muscle. Dividing the

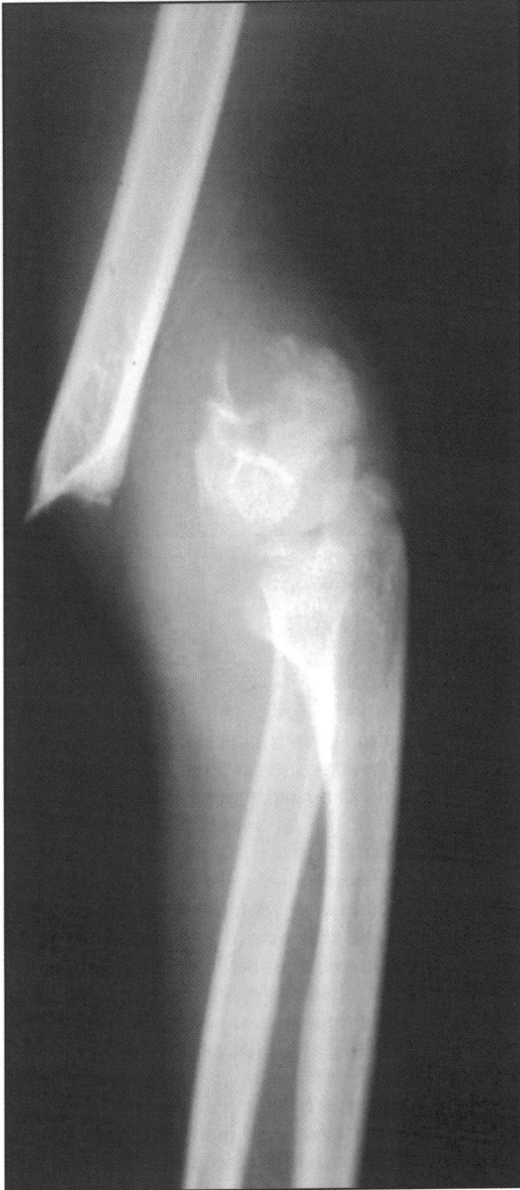

Figure 10.10 • Fractures of the supracondylar humerus are often associated with vascular injuries and should alert the physician to the possibility of a vascular injury.

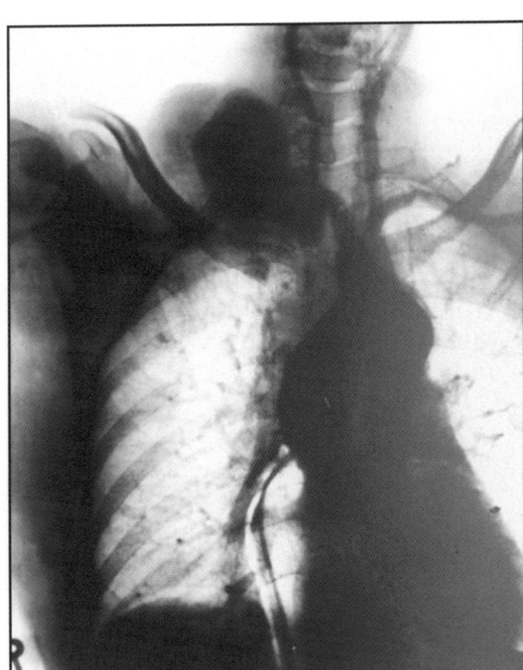

Figure 10.11 • False aneurysm of the right subclavian artery after penetrating trauma to the base of the neck. Patient presented with a pulsatile mass 6 months after the initial injury.

clavicle should be avoided whenever possible due to postoperative morbidity.

Vascular injuries to the lower limb

These injuries are often associated with skeletal injuries, of which posterior dislocation of the knee, proximal tibial fractures and supracondylar femur fractures are the most common. Immediate arterial repair should be performed when the skeletal injury is stable and not significantly displaced. When there is instability or severe displacement or where extreme orthopaedic manipulation is anticipated, a temporary shunt should be placed to restore blood flow while the orthopaedic repair is completed, after which definite arterial repair is performed.

FEMORAL VESSEL INJURIES (Fig. 10.12)

Injuries to the femoral artery are usually clinically apparent and tend to result from penetrating trauma. Patients may have significant exsanguination from arterial injuries, which should be controlled with direct pressure. Bleeding from the femoral triangle can be difficult to control, particularly if both the artery and vein are injured. Blind clamping in this area is strongly discouraged because of the danger of injuring adjacent nerves and vessels. The supra-inguinal region can be entered through a separate incision above the inguinal ligament to obtain proximal control of vessels.

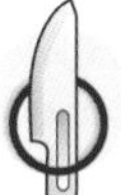

Common femoral artery injuries should always be repaired as ligation has a 50% amputation rate.[100]

Effort should be made to repair the common femoral vein.

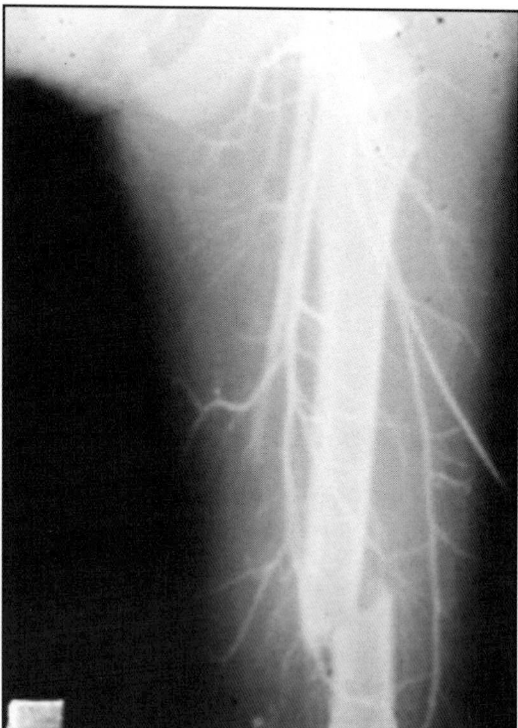

Figure 10.12 • Fracture of left femur with an on-table arteriogram showing disruption of the left superficial femoral artery.

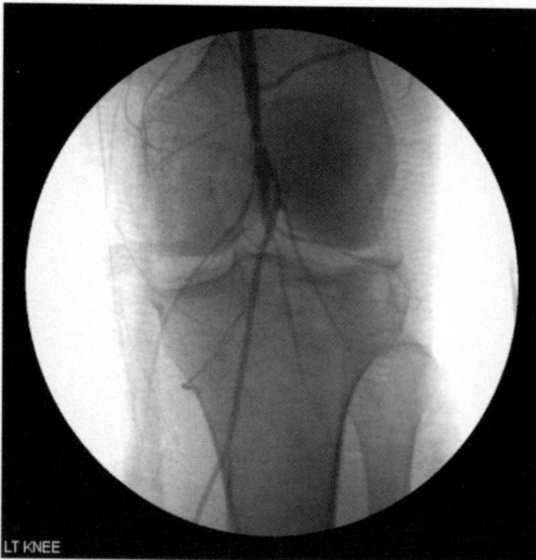

Figure 10.13 • Popliteal artery injury after posterior dislocation of the left knee.

POPLITEAL ARTERY (Fig. 10.13)

The lower leg is almost totally dependent on the popliteal artery. An amputation rate of up to 16% after popliteal artery injury has been reported in a recent series.[100] In regions with a low incidence of penetrating trauma, most popliteal injuries result from blunt mechanisms.

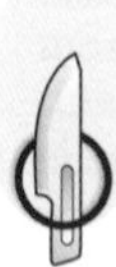

The association between posterior knee dislocation and popliteal artery disruption is well known. All patients with posterior knee dislocations should have a complete neurovascular examination of the affected limb.

Most popliteal artery injuries present with hard signs of arterial injury. The absence of hard signs is usually sufficient to rule out injuries to the popliteal artery and arteriography is not mandatory.[104] Patients who are managed expectantly should be closely observed, with regular reassessment of the peripheral circulation. This approach substantially reduces cost and resource use without adverse impact on the patient. However, there is a major school of thought that still advocates routine arteriography in all patients with documented knee dislocations.[105]

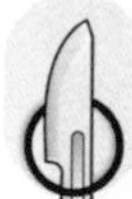

Injury to popliteal veins should be repaired in order to minimise postoperative swelling and compartment syndrome and to improve the patency of arterial repairs.

Compartment syndrome is a major risk factor for amputation following popliteal artery injury.[101] There is evidence that fasciotomy performed at the time of arterial repair, but before the development of compartment syndrome (prophylactic fasciotomy), may lower amputation rates, particularly in patients with long preoperative delays, extensive injuries, injuries of the artery and vein, and venous injuries treated with ligation.[106]

Single tibial vessels may be ligated if there is documented collateral flow distally.[107]

Venous injuries

Venous injuries found during exploration for associated arterial injury should be repaired, but only if the repair itself can be done simply (e.g. lateral suture repair) and only if it will not significantly delay treatment of associated injuries or destabilise the patient's condition. Complex venous repair, such as panelled or spiral vein grafts, may only be attempted if the patient is haemodynamically stable. All veins, including the IVC, can be tied off in cases of haemodynamic instability, but with the subsequent complications of venous hypertension and leg oedema.

Key points

- A high index of suspicion should be maintained regarding possible vascular injuries in the trauma patient.
- A thorough clinical examination is accurate in predicting significant vascular injury.
- Special investigations should only be performed in adequately resuscitated and haemodynamically stable patients.
- Haemodynamic instability, active bleeding and an expanding haematoma are indications for immediate surgery.
- The absence of hard signs of arterial injury justifies an expectant non-operative approach with careful observation.
- Restoration of arterial blood supply should be achieved as soon as possible; temporary intra-arterial shunts are valuable in this regard.
- Adequate surgical exposure is vital for proper management of vascular injuries.
- Fasciotomy should be applied liberally in lower-extremity vascular trauma.
- Endovascular treatment is useful in managing arterial lesions in anatomically challenging locations and is currently indicated for injuries of the descending thoracic aorta, proximal aortic arch branches and distal internal carotid and vertebral arteries.

REFERENCES

1. Trunkey DD. Overview of trauma. Surg Clin North Am 1982; 62:3–7
2. Herberer G, Becker HM, Ditmer H et al. Vascular injuries in polytrauma. World J Surg 1983; 7:68–79.
3. Hughes CW. Arterial repair during the Korean war. Ann Surg 1958; 147:555–61.
4. Rich NM, Baugh JH, Hughes CW. Acute arterial injuries in Vietnam: 1000 cases. J Trauma 1970; 10:359–69.
5. Fingerhut A, Leppäniemi AK, Androulakis GA et al. The European experience with vascular injuries. Surg Clin North Am 2002; 82:175–88.
6. Bowley DMG, Degiannis E, Goosen J, Boffard D. Penetrating vascular trauma in Johannesburg South Africa. Surg Clin North Am 2002; 82:221–36.
7. Levien LJ. Ballistics of bullet injury. In: Champion HR, Robbs JV, Trunkey D (eds) Robb and Smith's operative surgery, 4th edn. London: Butterworths, 1989; pp. 106–10.
8. Bergqvist D, Johnson K, Weibull H. An analysis of complications of percutaneous transluminal angioplasty of extremity and renal arteries. Acta Radiol 1987; 28:3–12.
9. Bergqvist D, Bergqvist A. Vascular injuries during gynecologic surgery. Acta Obstet Gynecol Scand 1987; 66:19–23.
10. Malan E, Taltoni G. Physio- and anatomo-pathology of acute ischaemia of the extremity. J Cardiovasc Surg (Torino) 1963; 4:212–25.

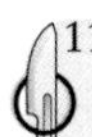

11. Johansen K, Lynch K. Non-invasive vascular tests reliably exclude occult arterial trauma in injured extremities. J Trauma 1991; 31:515–22.

    In this prospective study it was shown that an API of more than 0.9 has a negative predictive value of 99% for excluding significant arterial trauma. Reserving arteriography for limbs with an API of less than 0.9 is safe, accurate and cost-effective.

12. Dennis JW, Frykberg ER, Veldenz HC et al. Validation of non-operative management of occult vascular injuries and accuracy of physical examination alone in penetrating extremity trauma: 5–10 year follow up. J Trauma 1998; 44:243–53.

    Prospective study with 10-year follow-up proving the accuracy of clinical assessment and conservative management of occult vascular trauma.

13. Gonzalis RP, Falimirski ME. The utility of physical examination in proximity penetrating extremity trauma. Ann Surg 1999; 65:784–9.
14. Bickell WH, Wall MJ, Pepe PE et al. Immediate vs delayed fluid resuscitation for hypotensive patients with penetrating torso injuries. N Engl J Med 1994; 331:1105–9.
15. Stern SA, Dronen SC, Birrer P et al. Effect of blood pressure on haemorrhage, volume and survival in a near fatal model incorporating a vascular injury. Am J Emerg Med 1995; 13:269–75.
16. Rose SC, Moore EE. Trauma angiography: the use of clinical findings to improve patient selection and case preparation. J Trauma 1988; 28:240–5.
17. Weaver FA, Yellin AE. Is arterial proximity a valid indication for arteriography in penetrating extremity trauma? A prospective study. Arch Surg 1990; 125:1256–60.

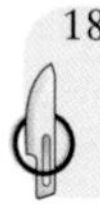

18. O'Gorman RB, Feliciano DV. Emergency centre arteriography in the evaluation of suspected peripheral vascular injuries. Arch Surg 1984; 119:568–73.

19. Lau JM, Mattox KL, Beale AL, de Bakey MC. Use of substitute conduits in traumatic vascular surgery. J Trauma 1977; 17:541–6.

20. Shah DM, Leather RP, Carson JD, Karmody AM. Polytetra fluoro-ethylene grafts in the rapid reconstruction of acute contaminated peripheral vascular injuries. Am J Surg 1984; 148:229–33.

21. Barros D'Sa AAB. Complex vascular and orthopedic injuries. J Bone Joint Surg 1992; 74:176–8.

This paper discusses the problems encountered with, and management of, complex vascular and orthopaedic injuries, advocating the use of temporary arterial and venous shunts for improving outcome.

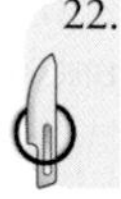

22. Margolis MN, Rien EG, Waltman AC et al. Arteriography in the management of haemorrhage from pelvic fractures. N Engl J Med 1972; 287:317–21.

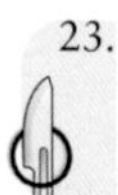

23. Panetta T, Sclafani SJA, Goldstein AS et al. Percutaneous transcatheter embolization for massive bleeding from pelvic fractures. J Trauma 1985; 25:1021–9.

24. Coldwell DM, Stokes KR, Jakes WF. Embolotherapy: agents, clinical applications and techniques. Radiographics 1994; 14:623–43.

25. Mervis SE, Pais SO. Trauma radiology: part 3. Diagnostic and therapeutic angiography in trauma. Intensive Care Med 1994; 9:244–56.

26. Carrillo EH, Spain DA, Wohltmann D et al. Interventional techniques are useful adjuncts in non-operative management of hepatic injuries. J Trauma 1999; 46:619–22.

27. Sclafani SJ, Shafton GW, Scalea TM et al. Non-operative salvage of CT diagnosed splenic injury: utilization of angiography for triage and embolization for hemostases. J Trauma 1995; 39:818–25.

28. Scalea TM, Sclafani SJ. Angiographically placed balloons for arterial control: a description of a technique. J Trauma 1991; 31:1671–7.

29. Lachat M, Phammatter T, Witzke H et al. Acute traumatic aortic rupture: early stentgraft repair. Eur J Cardiothorac Surg 2002; 21:956–63.

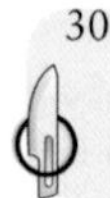

30. Du Toit DF, Strauss DC, Blaszczyk M et al. Endovascular treatment of penetrating thoracic outlet arterial injuries. Eur J Vasc Endovasc Surg 2000; 19:489–95.

The authors give an overview of the clinical problem and discuss the technique used.

31. Gomez CR, May AK, Terry JB et al. Endovascular therapy of traumatic injuries of the extracranial cerebral arteries. Crit Care Clin 1999; 15:789–809.

32. Demetriades D, Theodorou D, Asensio J. Management options in vertebral arteries injuries. Br J Surg 1996; 83:83–6.

33. Parodi JC, Schonholz C, Ferreira LM, Berghen J. Endovascular stent-graft treatment of traumatic arterial lesions. Ann Vasc Surg 1999; 13:121–9.

34. Kumar SR, Weaver FA, Yellin AE. Cervical vascular injuries: carotid and jugular venous injuries. Surg Clin North Am 2001; 81:1331–44.

35. McKevitt EC, Kirkpatrick AW, Vertisi L et al. Blunt vascular neck injuries: diagnosis and outcomes of extra-cranial vessel injury. J Trauma 2002; 53:472–6.

36. Weaver FA, Yellin AE, Wagner WH et al. The role of arterial reconstruction in penetrating carotid injuries. Arch Surg 1988; 123:1106–11.

37. Robbs JV. Basic principles in the surgical management of vascular trauma. In: Greenhalgh RM (ed.) Vascular and endovascular techniques, 4th edn. London: WB Saunders, 2001; pp. 455–65.

38. Robbs JV, Keanin J. Exploration of the neck. In: Champion HR, Robbs JV, Trunky D (eds) Robb and Smith's operative surgery, 4th edn. London: Butterworths, 1989; pp. 166–72.

39. Coggbill TH, Moore EE, Meissner M et al. The spectrum of blunt injury to the carotid artery: a multi-centre perspective. J Trauma 1994; 37:473–9.

40. Biffl WL, Moore EE, Offner PJ, Birch JM. Blunt carotid and vertebral arterial injuries. World J Surg 2001; 25:1036–43.

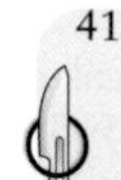

41. Fry WR, Dot JA, Smith RS et al. Duplex scanning replaces arteriography and operative exploration in the diagnosis of potential cervical vascular injury. Am J Surg 1994; 168:693–5.

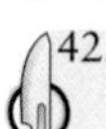

42. Corr P, Abdool-Carim AT, Robbs J. Colour-flow ultrasound in the detection of penetrating vascular injuries of the neck. S Afr Med J 1999; 80:644–6.

This prospective study demonstrates the sensitivity of colour-flow ultrasound as a screening investigation to detect vascular injuries following penetrating neck trauma.

43. Levy C, Laissy JP, Raveau V et al. Carotid and vertebral artery dissections: three-dimensional time-of-flight MR angiography and MR imaging vs conventional angiography. Radiology 1994; 190:97–103.

44. Stain SC, Yellin AE, Weaver FA et al. Selective management of non-occlusive arterial injuries. Arch Surg 1989; 124:1136–40.

45. Frykberg ER, Crump JM, Dennis JW et al. Non-operative observation of clinically occult arterial injuries: a prospective evaluation. Surgery 1991; 109:85–96.

46. Robbs J. Penetrating injury to the blood vessels of the neck and mediastinum. In: Branchereai A, Jacobs M (eds) Vascular emergencies. New York: Futura, 2003; pp. 39–48.

47. Kuehne JP, Weaver FA, Papanicolao U et al. Penetrating trauma of the internal carotid artery. Arch Surg 1996; 131:942–7.

48. Robbs JV, Human RR, Rajaruthnam P et al. Neurologic deficit and injuries involving the neck arteries. Br J Surg 1983; 70:220–2.

49. Fabian TC, Pattern JH Jr, Croce MA et al. Blunt carotid injury. Importance of early diagnosis and anticoagulation therapy. Ann Surg 1996; 223:513–25.

50. Biffl WL, Moore EE, Ryu RK et al. The unrecognized epidemic of blunt carotid arterial injuries: early diagnosis improves neurologic outcome. Ann Surg 1998; 228:462–70.

51. Robbs JV. Injuries to the vessels of the neck and superior mediastinum. In: Champion HR, Robbs JV, Trunky D (eds) Robb and Smith's operative surgery, 4th edn. London: Butterworths, 1989; pp. 529–38.

Description of operative technique with good illustrations.

52. Nair R, Robbs JV, Muckart D. Management of penetrating cervico-mediastinal venous trauma. Eur J Vasc Endovasc Surg 2000; 19:65–9.

53. Stein A, Seward P. Penetrating wounds of the neck. J Trauma 1976; 7:238–47.

54. Demetriades D, Theodorou D, Cornwill E et al. Evaluation of penetrating injuries of the neck: prospective study of 223 patients. World J Surg 1997; 21:41–8.

55. Nadgir RN, Loevner LA, Ahmed T et al. Simultaneous internal carotid and vertebral artery dissection following chiropractic manipulation: case report and review of the literature. Neuroradiology 2003; 45:311–14.

56. Biffl WL, Moore E, Elliot J et al. The devastating potential of blunt vertebral artery injuries. Ann Surg 2000; 231:672–81.

57. Munera F, Solo J, Palacio D et al. Diagnosis of arterial injuries caused by penetrating trauma to the neck: comparison of helical CT angiography and conventional angiography. Radiology 2000; 216:556–62.

58. Hatzitheofilou C, Demetriades D, Melissas J et al. Surgical approaches to vertebral artery injuries. Br J Surg 1988; 75:234–7.

59. Mattox KL, Feliciano DV, Burch J et al. Five thousand seven hundred and sixty cardiovascular injuries in 4459 patients. Epidemiologic evolution 1958–1978. Ann Surg 1989; 209:698–707.

60. Williams JS, Graff JA, Uku JM et al. Aortic injury in the vehicular trauma. Ann Thorac Surg 1994; 57:726–30.

61. Hunt PJ, Baker CC, Lentz CW et al. Thoracic aortic injuries: management and outcome of 144 patients. J Trauma 1996; 40:547–56.

62. Katyal D, McLellan B A, Brenneman FD et al. Lateral impact motor vehicle collisions: significant cause for blunt traumatic rupture of the thoracic aorta. J Trauma 1997; 42:769–72.

63. Wall MJ, Hirshberg AH, Le Maire SA et al. Thoracic aortic and thoracic vascular injuries. Surg Clin North Am 2001; 81:1375–93.

Comprehensive review article with extensive reference list.

64. Hilgenberg AD, Logan DL, Akins CW et al. Blunt injuries of the thoracic aorta. Ann Thorac Surg 1992; 53:233–9.

65. Patel NH, Stephens KE, Mirvis SE et al. Imaging of acute thoracic aortic injury due to blunt trauma: a review. Radiology 1998; 209:335–48.

66. Chiesa R, Castellano R, Lucci C et al. Traumatic rupture of the thoracic aorta. In: Branchereau A, Jacobz M (eds) Vascular emergencies. Centura Publishing Company, 2003; pp. 107–23.

67. Noveline R, Rhea GT, Rao PM et al. Helical CT in emergency radiology. Radiology 1999; 213:321–9.

68. Magissano R, Nathens A, Alexandrova NA et al. Traumatic rupture of the thoracic aorta: should one always operate immediately? Ann Vasc Surg 1995; 9:44–52.

69. Walker WA, Pate JW. Medical management of acute traumatic rupture of the aorta. Ann Thorac Surg 1990; 50:965–7.

70. Esterra A, Mattox KL, War MJ. Thoracic aortic injury. Semin Vasc Surg 2000; 4:345–52.

71. Fischer RG, Oria RA, Mattox KL et al. Conservative management of aortic lacerations due to blunt trauma. J Trauma 1990; 30:1562–6.

72. Aronstam EN, Domez AC, O'Connell J et al. Recent surgical and pharmacological experience with acute dissecting and traumatic aneurysms. J Thorac Cardiovasc Surg 1970; 59:231–8.

73. Mattox KL, Holtzman M, Pickard R et al. Clamp/repair: a safe technique for treatment of blunt injury to the descending thoracic aorta. Ann Thorac Surg 1985; 40:456–63.

74. Sweeney MS, Young DH, Frasier OH et al. Traumatic aortic transsections: eight year experience with a 'clamp-sew' technique. Ann Thorac Surg 1997; 64:384–9.

75. Read RA, Moore EE, Moore FA et al. Partial left heart bypass for thoracic aortic repair. Arch Surg 1993; 128:746–52.

76. Dake MD, Muller DC, Semba CP et al. Transluminal placement of endovascular stentgrafts for the treatment of descending thoracic aortic aneurysms. N Engl J Med 1994; 331:1729–34.

77. Nienaber CA, Fattori R, Lund G et al. Non-surgical reconstruction of thoracic aortic dissection by stentgraft placement. N Engl J Med 1999; 340:1539–45.

78. Thompson CS, Rodriguez JA, Ramaiah VG et al. Acute traumatic rupture of the thoracic aorta

treated with endo-luminal stentgrafts. J Trauma 2002; 52:1173–7.

79. Demetriades D, Theodoru D, Murray J et al. Mortality and prognostic factors in penetrating injuries of the aorta. J Trauma 1996; 40:761–3.

80. Asensio JA, Lejarraga M. Abdominal vascular injuries. In: Demetriades D, Asensio JA (eds) Trauma handbook. Austin, TX: Landes Biosciences, 2000; pp. 356–62.

81. Aucar JA, Hirshberg A. Damage control for vascular injuries. Surg Clin North Am 1997; 77:853–62.

A good review of the different techniques in vascular damage control.

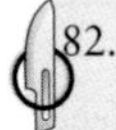
82. Asensio JA. Abdominal vascular injuries. Surg Clin North Am 2001; 81:1395–416.

83. Fullen WD, Hunt J, Altemeier WA. The clinical spectrum of penetrating injury to the superior mesenteric arterial circulation. J Trauma 1972; 12:656–64.

84. Asensio JA. Operative management and outcome of 302 vascular injuries. Am J Surg 2001; 180:528–34.

85. Burch JM, Feliciano DV, Mattox KL. Injuries to the inferior vena cava. Am J Surg 1998; 156:548–52.

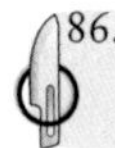
86. Buckman RF, Bradley M. Injuries to the inferior vena cava. Surg Clin North Am 2001; 81:1431–48.

An excellent review of the management options of this difficult clinical problem.

87. Rohtenberger DA, Fischer RP, Perry JF Jr. Major vascular injuries secondary to pelvic fractures. Am J Surg 1978; 136:660–2.

88. Connoly J. Management of fractures associated with arterial injuries. Am J Surg 1971; 120:331–4.

89. Lim RC, Miller SC. Management of acute civilian vascular injuries. Surg Clin North Am 1982; 62:113–19.

90. Seller JG, Richardson JD. Amputation after extremity injury. Am J Surg 1986; 152:260–4.

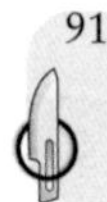
91. Frykberg ER, Dennis JW, Bishop K et al. The reliability of physical examination in the evaluation of penetrating extremity trauma for vascular injury: results at one year. J Trauma 1991; 31:502–11.

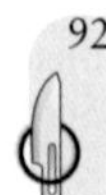
92. Frykberg ER, Crump JM, Vines FS et al. A reassessment of the role of arteriography in penetrating proximity trauma: a prospective study. J Trauma 1989; 29:1041–52.

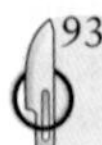
93. Meyer JP, Lim LT, Schuler JJ et al. Peripheral vascular trauma from close range shotgun injuries. Arch Surg 1985; 120:1126–31.

94. Meak AC, Robbs JV. Vascular injury with associated bone and joint trauma. Br J Surg 1984; 71:341–4.

95. Schwartz M, Weaver F, Yellin A et al. The utility of color flow Doppler examination in penetrating extremity arterial trauma. Am Surg 1993; 59:375–8.

96. The EAST Practice Management Guidelines Work Group. Practice management guidelines for penetrating trauma to the lower extremity. http://www.east.org

This website supplies practice guidelines according to literature searches and level of evidence.

97. Keen RR, Meyer JP, Durham JR et al. Autogenous vein graft repair of injured extremity arteries: early and late results with 134 consecutive patients. J Vasc Surg 1991; 13:664–8.

98. Martin LC, McKenney MG, Sosa JL et al. Management of lower extremity arterial trauma. J Trauma 1994; 37:591–8.

99. Mabee JR, Bostwick TL. Pathophysiology and mechanisms of compartment syndrome. Orthop Rev 1993; 22:175–81.

100. Hafez HM, Woolgar J, Robbs JV. Lower extremity arterial injury: results of 550 cases and review of risk factors associated with limb loss. J Vasc Surg 2001; 33:1212–19.

The authors review the factors associated with limb loss in their extensive experience of more than 500 cases.

101. Johansen K, Daines M, Howey T, Helfet D, Hansen ST Jr. Objective criteria accurately predict amputation following lower extremity trauma. J Trauma 1990; 30:568–72.

102. Hunt CA, Kingsley JR. Upper extremity trauma. South Med J 2000; 93:466–8.

103. Demetriades D, Ascensio JA. Subclavian and axillary vascular injuries. Surg Clin North Am 2001; 81:1357–73.

104. Miranda FE, Dennis JW, Frykberg ER et al. Confirmation of the safety and accuracy of physical examination in the evaluation of knee dislocation for injury of the popliteal artery: a prospective study. J Trauma 2000; 49:247–52.

105. Thal ER, Snyder WH, Perry MO. Vascular injuries of the extremities. In: Rutherford (ed.) Vascular surgery, 4th edn. Philadelphia: WB Saunders, 1994; pp. 713–35.

106. Fainzilber G, Roy-Shapira A, Wall MJ Jr, Mattox KL. Predictors of amputation for popliteal artery injuries. Am J Surg 1995; 170:568–70.

107. Padberg FT, Rubelowsky JJ, Hernandez-Maldonado JJ et al. Infrapopliteal arterial injury: prompt revascularization affords optimal limb salvage. J Vasc Surg 1992; 16:877–85.

CHAPTER

Eleven

Vascular disorders of the upper limb

Jean-Baptiste Ricco and
Jean-Michel Cormier

INTRODUCTION

Arterial diseases of the upper limb are relatively rare in comparison with those involving the lower extremity, with the exception of embolism. The good collateral supply around the shoulder and elbow explains why chronic occlusive disease is commonly asymptomatic, but acute occlusion due to embolism can result in limb-threatening ischaemia. In addition, thoracic outlet syndrome, axillo-subclavian vein thrombosis and occupational vascular problems should be considered as part of vascular diseases of the upper extremity. In this chapter we do not review vasospastic disorders, connective tissue disease, vasculitis and Raynaud's disease, as these are covered in Chapter 12, nor vascular trauma (covered in Chapter 10). The main causes of upper limb vascular disease are summarized in **Box 11.1**.

CLINICAL EXAMINATION

Vascular assessment of the upper limb should include the thoracic outlet. Palpation and auscultation of the supraclavicular region may help to detect a cervical rib, a subclavian stenosis or aneurysm. The arm pulses should be examined with the arm placed in the neutral position and then in abduction and external rotation (surrender position) in order to detect arterial thoracic outlet compression. Pulse palpation is important and must include the axillary, brachial, radial and ulnar pulses. The blood pressure should be measured in both arms, preferably using a hand-held Doppler. A difference of more than 15% is abnormal.

Examination of hand ischaemia is not complete unless an Allen test is performed. The examiner compresses the radial and ulnar arteries at the wrist. The examiner then asks the subject to clench the fist in order to empty the hand of blood. The radial artery is then released and the hand is observed for return of colour. The test is then repeated for the ulnar artery. The test is normal if refilling of the hand is complete within less than 10 seconds. Any portion of the hand that does not blush is an indication of incomplete continuity of the palmar arch. The nail folds should be examined for infarcts and splinter haemorrhages.

OCCLUSIVE DISEASE

Occlusive lesions of the brachiocephalic and subclavian arteries occur in relatively young patients with mean ages ranging from 50 to 60 years. These lesions are much less frequent than those involving the carotid bifurcation.[1] Atherosclerosis is the predominant cause in Europe, with Buerger's disease and Takayasu's arteritis far behind. The symptoms of occlusive disease of the upper extremities include muscle fatigue and ischaemic rest pain. Digital necrosis or atheroembolisation is less common than in the lower extremities, accounting for no more than 5% of patients with limb ischaemia.[2]

Brachiocephalic artery

Stenotic lesions of the brachiocephalic artery are uncommon and may be asymptomatic in 13–22% of patients.[3,4] Symptomatic patients may present

Box 11.1 • Causes of upper-limb vascular diseases

ARTERIAL OBSTRUCTION
Large artery
Atherosclerosis
Radiotherapy
Thoracic outlet syndrome
Arteritis (giant cell, Takayasu's)
Small artery
Atherosclerosis
Connective tissue disease
Myeloproliferative disease
Buerger's disease
Vibrating tools
ARTERIAL VASOSPASM
Large artery
Ergot-containing medications and other pharmacological causes
Small artery
Raynaud's disease
Vibrating tools
Embolism: proximal sources
Heart
Ulcerated arterial plaques (aortic arch, brachiocephalic and subclavian arteries)
Aneurysm (brachiocephalic, subclavian, axillary, brachial, ulnar arteries)
Thoracic outlet syndrome
Subclavian–axillary vein thrombosis
Primary: Paget–Schroetter syndrome (thoracic outlet syndrome)
Secondary: catheter, hypercoagulable states
Hypercoagulable states
Heparin antibodies
Deficiencies of antithrombin III, proteins C and S
Antiphospholipid syndrome
Malignancy
Cryoglobulinaemia
Aneurysms

with ischaemia of the right upper extremity, carotid territory symptoms or vertebrobasilar symptoms. The percentage of patients presenting with upper extremity or neurological symptoms is variable (53.8% and 76.9% respectively in the Mayo Clinic experience[5]). The diagnosis is suspected by physical examination (i.e. right supraclavicular/cervical bruit, absent right subclavian or axillary pulse) and confirmed by duplex scanning, conventional angiography or computed tomography (CT) or magnetic resonance angiography (MRA). Most patients (61–84%) with brachiocephalic artery occlusion have multiple lesions of the aortic arch vessels.[6] This should be kept in mind when planning treatment.

Stenotic lesions of the brachiocephalic artery may be approached by median sternotomy with direct bypass grafting from the aortic arch, or indirectly by extra-anatomical bypass such as subclavian–subclavian, contralateral carotid–carotid or subclavian–carotid bypass.

Extra-anatomical bypasses have a lower morbidity and mortality but direct bypass from the aortic arch offers an excellent source of inflow and is more durable.

AORTO-BRACHIOCEPHALIC BYPASS

A median sternotomy is used with extension into the neck to allow exposure of the subclavian and common carotid arteries. The left brachiocephalic vein is identified with division of the inferior thyroid and internal mammary vein (**Fig. 11.1a**). A partial occluding clamp or two curved clamps are applied to the ascending aorta proximal to the brachiocephalic artery in order to avoid the risk of fracturing atheromatous plaque (**Fig. 11.1b**). An 8–10 mm prosthetic graft is anastomosed at this site with deep suture placement in the aortic wall (**Fig. 11.1c**). Once the anastomosis is completed, a clamp is applied across the graft and systemic heparin is given. The brachiocephalic artery is clamped, sectioned and the proximal stump oversewn. The patent distal artery is spatulated and the graft attached in an end-to-end fashion (**Fig. 11.1d**). Air is evacuated from the graft by back-bleeding the subclavian artery, then flow is released into the arm and then into the carotid artery. The mortality of direct bypass ranges from 5.8 to 8% in Kieffer's and Berguer's series with a primary patency rate at 5 years of 94% in both series.

BRACHIOCEPHALIC ENDARTERECTOMY

This operation also has good results, although the proximal location of the disease with extension into the aortic arch makes this technique hazardous in some patients. Attempts to remove an orifice

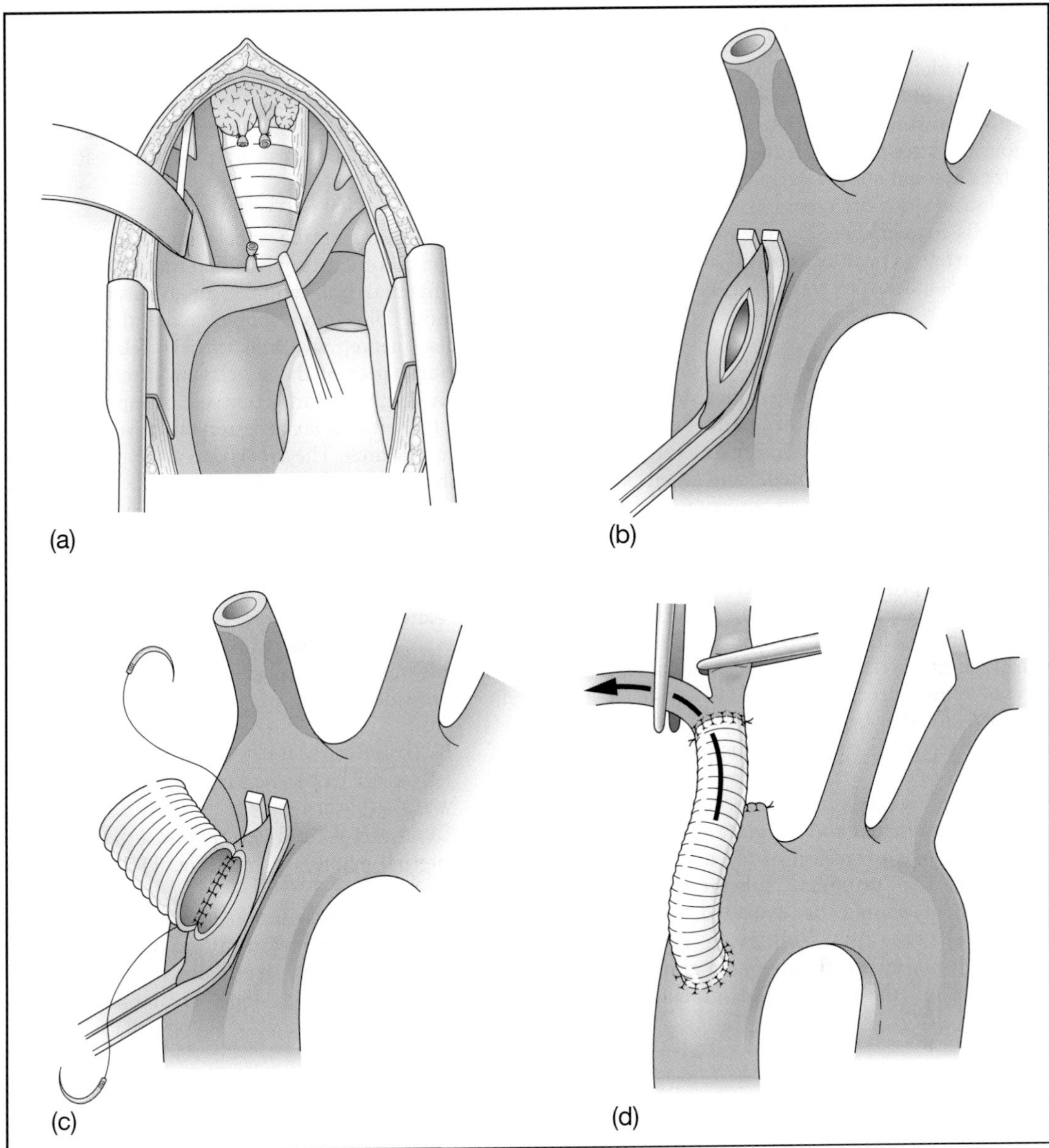

Figure 11.1 • **(a)** The left brachiocephalic vein is retracted to expose the brachiocephalic artery. **(b)** A clamp is applied laterally to the ascending aorta. **(c)** A polyester graft is implanted on the ascending thoracic aorta proximal to the brachiocephalic artery. **(d)** Completed bypass. Flow is released into the arm and then into the common carotid artery.

lesion may initiate an aortic dissection or distal embolisation. For this reason bypass is preferred for all brachiocephalic lesions except for those located in the distal segment.

ENDOVASCULAR TREATMENT

Percutaneous transluminal angioplasty (PTA)/stenting of the brachiocephalic artery is being performed with increased frequency. The approach may be percutaneous from either the groin or arm, or through an anterolateral cervical approach with clamping of the right common carotid artery to avoid atheroembolisation during the subsequent procedure.

On the basis of recent data, and in selected patients, intraoperative balloon angioplasty of stenosis of the innominate artery with stent placement is a safe and effective alternative to conventional operations.[7]

Subclavian artery

Symptomatic lesions of the subclavian artery are associated in 72% of cases with concomitant lesions of carotid and vertebral vessels.[1] The indications for intervention are those of vertebrobasilar insufficiency and upper extremity ischaemia. Atheroembolisation is quite common in this location.[8] If surgery is contemplated and the ipsilateral common carotid artery is healthy, carotid–subclavian bypass or carotid–subclavian transposition is the method of choice.

CAROTID–SUBCLAVIAN BYPASS

Access is achieved by a horizontal supraclavicular incision with division of both heads of the sternomastoid muscle. Scalenus anterior and phrenic nerve are exposed, and then scalenus anterior is sectioned near its insertion into the first rib (**Fig. 11.2a**). The internal jugular vein is freed to allow retraction in either direction. On the left side, take care to protect the thoracic duct or ligate it. The carotid sheath is opened, safeguarding the vagus nerve. After heparinisation, the common carotid artery is clamped as low as possible. A vein or polytetrafluoroethylene (PTFE) graft is then attached to the lateral aspect of the common carotid artery in an end-to-side fashion (**Fig. 11.2b**). The graft under arterial tension is then passed behind the jugular vein. Graft length should be cautiously estimated and the graft attached end-to-side to the superior aspect of the distal subclavian artery. If the proximal subclavian lesion is ulcerated, it should be excluded by proximal ligation. If the distal subclavian artery is too diseased for distal implantation, the graft should be passed behind the clavicle and implanted on the axillary artery exposed via a short infraclavicular incision.

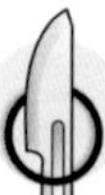

Prosthetic carotid–subclavian bypass has an excellent patency in this location. Postoperative mortality is less than 1%, with a primary patency of 95% at 10 years.[9]

CAROTID TRANSPOSITION

Reimplantation of the subclavian artery into the common carotid artery is an alternative that avoids graft material but requires an extensive cervical dissection. Dissection should avoid the recurrent laryngeal nerve, which is closely related to the posterior aspect of the subclavian artery. Systemic heparin is given and a curved clamp is applied across the left subclavian artery as close as possible to the aortic arch. The subclavian artery is transected and the proximal stump oversewn. The site of anastomosis to the common carotid artery should be chosen to avoid kinking and angulation of the vertebral artery. The clamps on the common carotid artery should be rotated anteriorly to present the posterolateral surface for anastomosis with the subclavian artery (**Fig. 11.3**). An ellipse is excised from this wall and the subclavian artery anastomosed in end-to-side fashion.

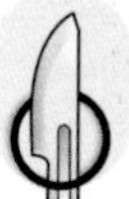

Subclavian–carotid reimplantation is an excellent technique. Postoperative mortality is less than 1%, with a long-term patency of 100% in the series of Sandman et al.[10] and Kretschmer et al.[11]

CROSSOVER GRAFTS

Subclavian revascularisation may also be achieved by crossover subclavian–subclavian or axillo-axillary bypass. These grafts are relatively simple to construct, although their greater length and

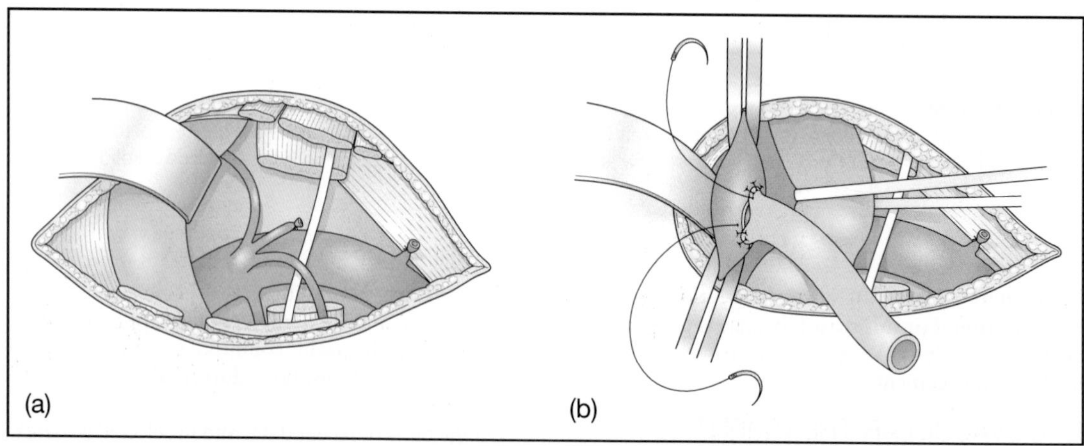

Figure 11.2 • **(a)** Cervical approach for carotid–subclavian bypass. The sternomastoid muscle is divided and the subclavian artery is exposed by sectioning the scalenus anterior. **(b)** A PTFE graft is anastomosed to the lateral aspect of the left common carotid artery.

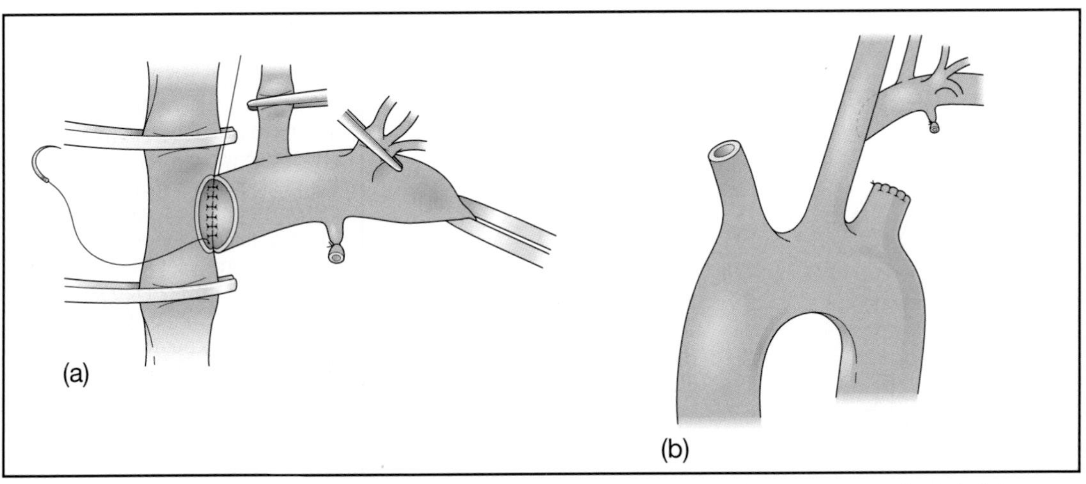

Figure 11.3 • Carotid–subclavian transposition: **(a)** clamps on the common carotid artery are rotated anteriorly to present the posterolateral surface for anastomosis with the subclavian artery; **(b)** end-to-side anastomosis completed.

reversed angle of take-off may reduce durability. Furthermore, problems may arise if subsequent median sternotomy is needed for coronary bypass. The donor and recipient arteries are exposed by a short supraclavicular incision on either side (**Fig. 11.4**). A tunnel is created from one side of the neck to the other passing behind the sternomastoid muscles and anterior to the carotid vessels. Cross-over axillo-axillary bypass is easier to perform but the graft has to pass subcutaneously over the sternum, which risks compression or erosion.

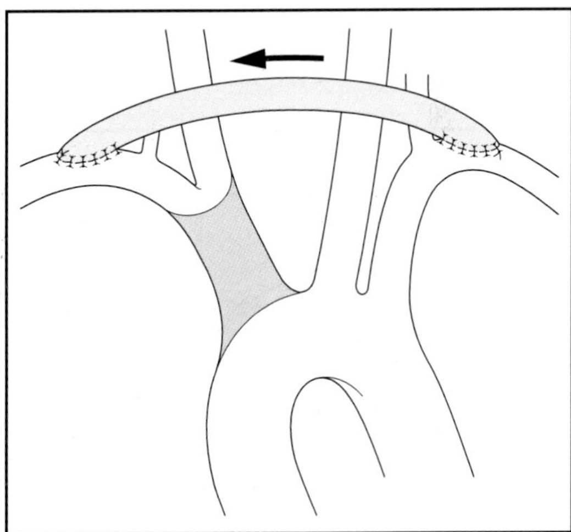

Figure 11.4 • Brachiocephalic artery occlusion. Revascularisation by a cross-subclavian PTFE graft. Tunnelisation is done behind the sternomastoid muscles and anterior to the carotid vessels.

ENDOVASCULAR TREATMENT

PTA of subclavian artery stenosis is a safe and relatively simple procedure to perform. Access is usually obtained from the femoral artery and the lesion dilated to 5–8 mm (**Fig. 11.5**). Because there is usually retrograde flow in the vertebral artery, stroke is rare. When there is not retrograde flow, an occlusion balloon may be placed in the vertebral artery from the arm while the stenosis is dilated from the groin. Simple stenoses are adequately dilated by balloon. Occlusions are more difficult to cross from the groin and usually require an approach from the arm. In addition, because of the bulk of disease, balloon-expandable stents are usually placed (**Fig. 11.6**).

Martinez et al.[12] studied 17 patients and reported a 94% procedural success rate with 81% primary patency at 6 months. Westerband et al.[13] reviewed their experience on subclavian stenting in 14 patients with stenoses leading to flow reversal through a patent in situ internal mammary artery graft. Mean follow-up was 29 months, with two restenoses and an assisted primary patency rate of 100%. Motarjeme[7] studied 112 patients who underwent percutaneous treatment of 151 lesions in the brachiocephalic, subclavian, carotid and vertebral arteries and reported excellent mid-term results for stenotic lesions but only moderate success for subclavian occlusion, with only 46% recanalisation.

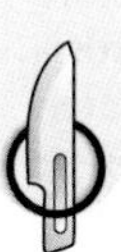

PTA with or without stenting is an appropriate treatment for symptomatic patients with localised subclavian artery stenosis. However, long-term patency of subclavian artery PTA series is inferior to that obtained with carotid–subclavian bypass or transposition.

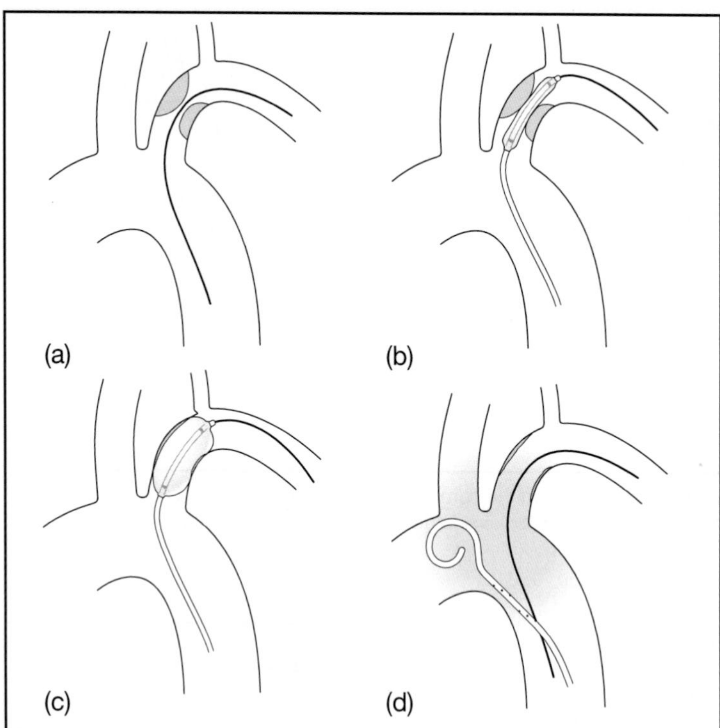

Figure 11.5 • Antegrade approach from the femoral artery: **(a)** the guidewire is placed through the subclavian stenosis; **(b)** balloon is advanced over the guidewire; **(c)** balloon angioplasty; **(d)** arteriography through another catheter introduced from a remote site (e.g. the other femoral artery) or from the guiding catheter if this has been used. Copyright (2003) from Endovascular Skills by Schneider PA. Reproduced by permission of Routledge/Taylor & Francis Group, LLC.

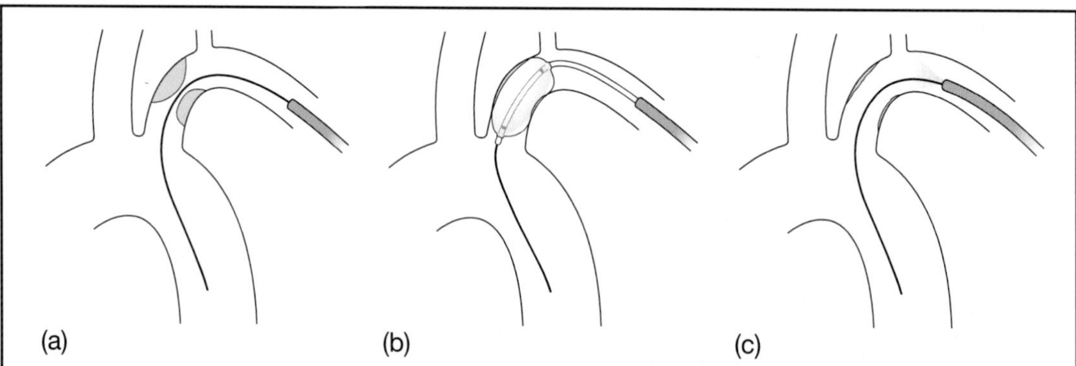

Figure 11.6 • Retrograde approach from the brachial artery by percutaneous puncture or cut-down if stenting is necessary: **(a)** the guidewire is placed through the subclavian stenosis; **(b)** balloon is advanced over the guidewire and balloon angioplasty performed; **(c)** arteriography completed by withdrawing the balloon with the same catheter. Copyright (2003) from Endovascular Skills by Schneider PA. Reproduced by permission of Routledge/Taylor & Francis Group, LLC.

Upper arm arteries

Patients with chronic atherosclerotic occlusion of the axillary or brachial arteries usually present with fatigue on using the arm. Many of these patients have radiation-induced occlusive disease. More severe ischaemia with rest pain or digital necrosis is uncommon unless there have been repeated episodes of embolism due to proximal ulceration or aneurysmal lesion. Direct reconstructive surgery is feasible since the occlusive lesions tend to be segmental with preserved distal patency. Axillo-brachial occlusions are managed by a bypass procedure if symptoms justify it. These sites can usually be approached by limited incisions (**Fig. 11.7a**) and the bypass tunnelled subcutaneously between the two (**Fig. 11.7b**). Autogenous saphenous vein is the preferred graft material. When unavailable, the basilic or cephalic vein may be considered. Upper limb bypass using saphenous vein has a 5-year

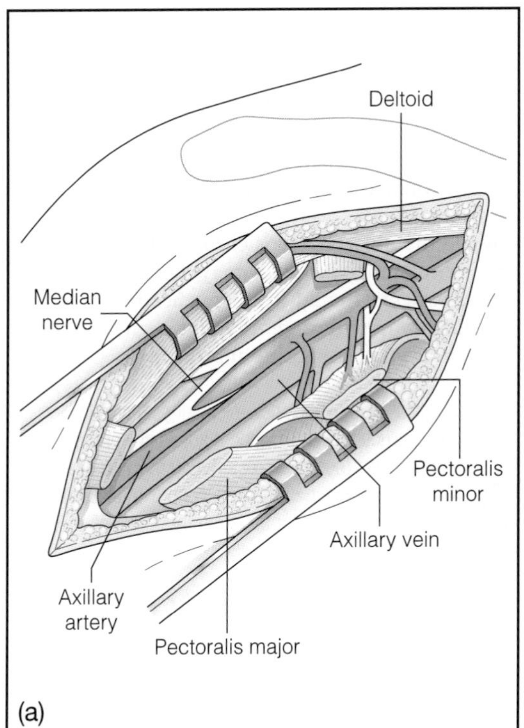

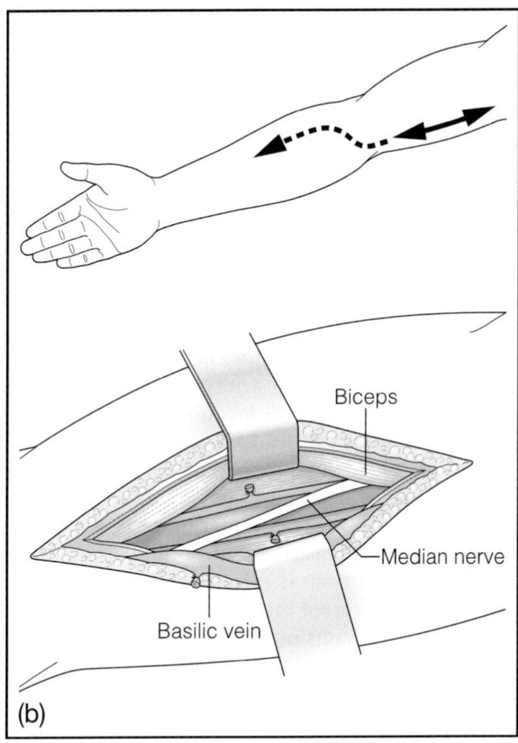

Figure 11.7 • **(a)** Axillary artery approach. The pectoralis minor muscle is divided and the neurovascular bundle is exposed. If access to the axillobrachial junction is needed, pectoralis major tendon should also be resected. **(b)** Brachial artery approach. Incision along the medial border of the biceps. If necessary, the bicipital aponeurosis is divided to expose the brachial artery division.

patency rate of 60–90%.[14] PTFE has a lower patency rate at this level.

Lower arm and hand arteries

The causes of chronic occlusion in the forearm or hand vessels include atherosclerosis, Buerger's disease, immunological and connective tissue disorders (see Chapter 12) and occupational trauma. Arch angiography, to exclude proximal embolising disease, and selective arteriography are essential in evaluating these patients with distal disease. Most patients with distal disease and severe digital ischaemia can be managed conservatively. Avoidance of cold and abstinence of tobacco are essential. Vasodilator or sympatholytic agents may also be employed. Patients with digital necrosis may require local débridement or amputation if gangrene is extensive. Some patients with radial, ulnar or palmar arch occlusion and critical ischaemia may be managed, if run-off is present, by vein graft bypass using microsurgical techniques. Cervicodorsal sympathectomy by thoracoscopy may also be considered in patients with severe distal forearm ischaemia. However, results of sympathectomy have often been disappointing, particularly in patients with diffuse arteritis.

ANEURYSMAL DISEASE

True aneurysms of the upper limb arteries are uncommon. The subclavian artery is the most frequent site, usually caused by thoracic outlet compression, These patients may present with distal ischaemia, embolisation or acute thrombosis. False aneurysms from trauma or infection often produce motor or sensory impairment as a result of brachial plexus compression. Subclavian artery aneurysms are best managed by a combined supraclavicular and infraclavicular approach (see later).

An aberrant right subclavian artery arising from the descending thoracic aorta is a common anomaly. Rarely, the artery compresses the oesophagus against the trachea, producing a condition described as dysphagia lusoria, and aneurysmal degeneration, known as Kommerrell's diverticulum, may also occur. The largest experience has been reported by Kieffer et al.;[15] their 33 patients with aberrant right subclavian arteries included 13 cases of Kommerell's diverticulum. Because of the possibility of rupture, resection of the aneurysmal artery with prosthetic reconstruction via a thoracic approach is recommended. As this technique carries a high postoperative mortality, aortic stentgrafts have been tried in this location with limited success.

Upper arm artery aneurysms

Axillary artery aneurysms are usually caused by blunt or penetrating trauma. Degenerative or congenital aneurysms are rare in this location. False aneurysms of the axillary artery occur with humeral fractures and anterior dislocation of the shoulder. These aneurysms can lead to neurological complications because of compression of the brachial plexus. Duplex scan and arteriography allow an accurate diagnosis. The axillary artery is exposed by a deltopectoral incision with section of pectoralis minor. The aneurysm is resected followed by interposition of a reversed saphenous vein.

Mycotic aneurysms of the brachial artery require interruption of the artery above and below the infected area with complete débridement. Immediate revascularisation may not be necessary in this location because of the good collateral supply of the arm. If needed an extra-anatomical bypass should be performed through a separate clean field. Endovascular stentgrafts have also been used to treat these aneurysms in an emergency.[16]

Lower arm and hand artery aneurysms

Radial artery aneurysms are usually due to inadequate compression or infection following removal of intra-arterial blood pressure cannulas. If the Allen test shows good filling of the hand from the ulnar artery, then the radial artery can simply be ligated above and below the aneurysm. If not, reconstruction using a vein graft will be required.

ULNAR ARTERY ANEURYSM OR HYPOTHENAR HAMMER SYNDROME

It is important to recognise an ulnar artery aneurysm because it may lead to digital necrosis. The condition known as hypothenar hammer syndrome develops in workers who suffer repetitive trauma to their hands, i.e. carpenters and pipe fitters. Those who play sports such as volleyball or karate are also at risk. The pathophysiology is related to the vascular anatomy of the hand. The distal ulnar artery is vulnerable to external trauma between the distal margin of Guyon's canal and the palmar aponeurosis. Over this short distance, the artery lies anterior to the hook of the hamate bone and is covered only by the palmaris brevis muscle and the skin (**Fig. 11.8**). Trauma of the ulnar artery at this level causes thrombosis or aneurysm formation and distal embolisation in the fourth and fifth fingers, with pain, coldness and cyanosis. The thumb is always spared because of its radial blood supply. Angiography with magnification is essential in these patients.

When the ulnar artery is chronically thrombosed, calcium channel blockers may be helpful. In all cases, patients should avoid further hand trauma. Satisfactory long-term results have been reported by Vayssairat et al. using this approach.[17]

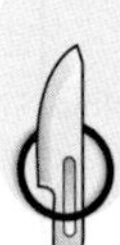

Surgical therapy includes microsurgical arterial reconstruction with or without adjunctive preoperative thrombolytic therapy to restore patency to digital arteries. Resection of the aneurysm with placement of an interposition vein graft is the treatment of choice.

UPPER LIMB EMBOLISM

Embolic arterial occlusion is the major cause of acute upper limb ischaemia; upper limb emboli represent 20–32% of major peripheral emboli.[18] A cardiac origin is found in 90% of the cases and is related to arrhythmia, myocardial infarction, valvular disorder or ventricular aneurysm. Noncardiac sources include ulcerative atherosclerotic plaques or aneurysms in the arch or subclavian–axillary arteries and thoracic outlet compression. The brachial bifurcation is the most frequently involved site for an embolus to lodge. Clinical examination and duplex scan can locate the level of the arterial occlusion. Preoperative conventional angiography or CT angiography is indicated in order to exclude a proximal arterial embolic lesion if a cardiac source is not evident. Immediate systemic heparinisation is essential to limit the propagation of thrombus and to prevent recurrent embolism.

Most emboli can be retrieved through a distal brachial transverse arteriotomy. This site has the advantage that both forearm arteries can be directly cannulated. An S-shaped incision is made in the antecubital fossa and the brachial artery division exposed by dividing the bicipital aponeurosis. A transverse arteriotomy is made proximal to the bifurcation. It is important to clear both forearm vessels with a 2 Fr Fogarty catheter (**Fig. 11.9**). Heparin saline is then instilled distally, and after confirming proximal patency the arteriotomy is closed with 6/0 prolene interrupted sutures. At this time, on-table angiography should be performed. If there is retained distal thrombus, the ulnar and radial artery can be opened at the wrist and a 2 Fr Fogarty catheter passed distally. Alternatively,

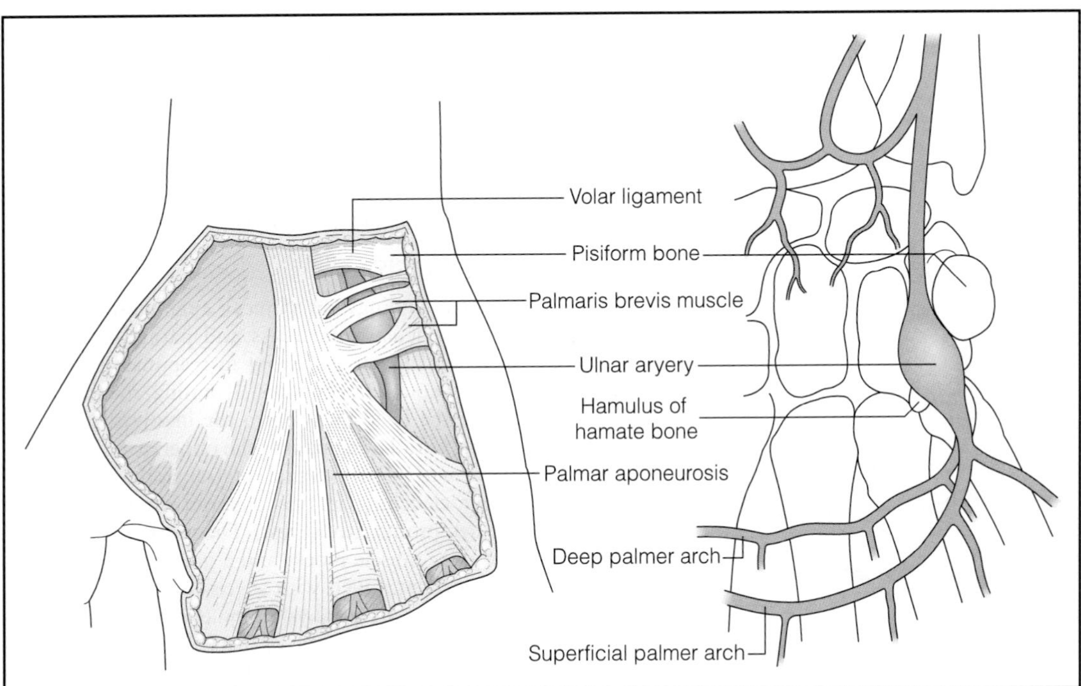

Figure 11.8 • Anatomy of the hypothenar hammer syndrome. The distal ulnar artery is exposed to external trauma in this short distance. The ulnar artery courses on top of the hook of the hamate bone and is only covered by the palmaris brevis muscle. From Clagett GP. Upper extremity aneurysms. In: Rutherford RB (ed.) Vascular surgery, 5th edn. Philadelphia: WB Saunders, 2000; p. 1364, with permission.

intraoperative thrombolysis can be used (see Chapter 9). Emboli in the axillary or subclavian arteries may also be removed by the same approach using transbrachial retrograde catheterisation. However, sometimes a large proximal embolus cannot be removed via the brachial arteriotomy, in which case an axillary or subclavian embolectomy will be required. Percutaneous thrombectomy has also been used in this situation with success.

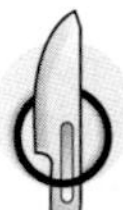

Brachial embolectomy should be performed under local anaesthesia with monitoring by an anaesthetist present in the operating room.

Other causes of acute ischaemia

The pharmacological causes of upper extremity ischaemia are summarized in **Box 11.2**. Inadvertent arterial injection by drug abusers often results in intense vasospasm due to particulate micro-embolism. Intra-arterial infusion of prostacyclin analogues such as iloprost or other vasodilators may help. Forearm compartment syndrome is rare except in this situation and requires fasciotomy. Limb loss is common.

Box 11.2 • Upper extremity ischaemia due to pharmacological history

- Ergot poisoning
- Beta-blockers
- Drug abuse, cocaine use
- Dopamine overdose
- Cytotoxic drugs

THORACIC OUTLET SYNDROME

Thoracic outlet syndrome describes a variety of symptoms caused by compression of the brachial plexus or subclavian vessels at the thoracic outlet. In the majority of cases, symptoms are neurological with pain and weakness resulting from C8 or T1 root compression. Arterial or venous symptoms resulting from compression are uncommon, accounting for 5% of cases in large published series.[19]

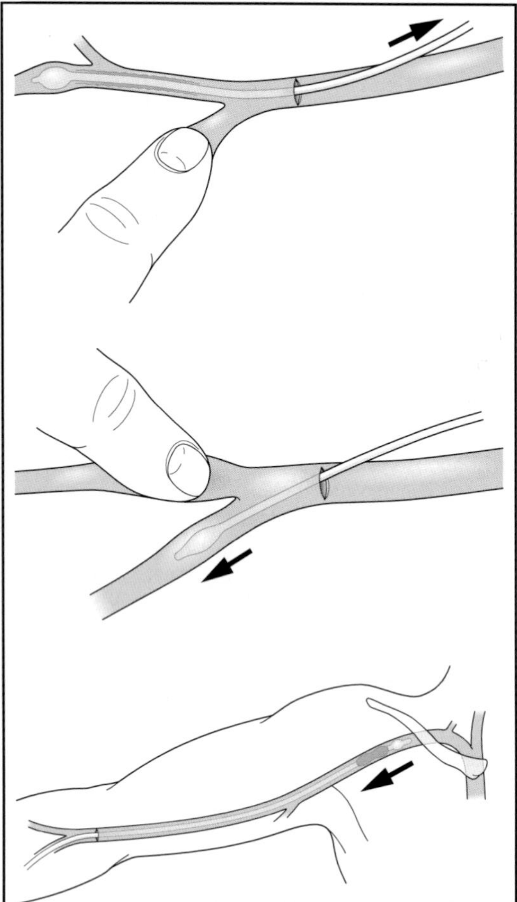

Figure 11.9 • Brachial artery embolectomy. A transverse arteriotomy is performed. A Fogarty catheter is directed into the radial and ulnar arteries in turn using alternate digital compression. A subclavian–axillary embolectomy is carried out by retrograde catheterisation from the antecubital fossa.

Neurogenic thoracic outlet compression syndrome

The neurovascular bundle may be compressed between the first rib and the clavicle as a result of a low-lying shoulder girdle or loss of muscle tone. Other anatomical factors include congenital fibromuscular bands crossing the thoracic outlet that tent up the brachial plexus, and abnormalities/hypertrophy of the scalene muscles. Bony lesions may also be the cause. These include cervical ribs, a broad first rib, and fracture or exostoses of the first rib or clavicle. The scalene triangle is the commonest site of nerve compression. It contains the brachial plexus and the subclavian artery. Neurogenic thoracic outlet compression syndrome (N-TOCS) probably represents a repetitive stress injury as there are well-defined at-risk occupations (e.g. typists) and sports (e.g. swimming). Most patients with N-TOCS are in the 25–45-year age group and 70% of them are women. The symptoms are arm pain, paraesthesia and weakness, with involvement of all the nerves of the brachial plexus or with specific patterns related to the upper plexus (median nerve) or lower plexus (ulnar nerve).

DIAGNOSIS

Positive findings on clinical examination include supraclavicular tenderness and paraesthesia in the ipsilateral upper extremity in response to pressure over the scalene muscles. Rotating the head and tilting the head away from the involved side often produces radiating pain in the upper arm. Abducting the arm to 90° in external rotation and repeated slow finger clenching in this position often reproduces the symptoms (Roos' test). Diagnostic tests include a scalene muscle block, and a good response to this test correlates well with successful surgical decompression.[20] Neurophysiology testing is helpful in excluding other sites of nerve compression, e.g. carpal tunnel syndrome. There is a reduction in the sensory action potential of the medial cutaneous nerve of the forearm, prolonged F-wave conduction and the EMG shows motor unit drop-out in the thenar muscles. Duplex scanning is a useful surrogate marker if it shows arterial compression in the stress position. Cervical spine films may detect cervical or abnormal first ribs but will not detect non-bony causes of compression. Magnetic resonance imaging is more useful for excluding cervical disc lesions than confirming N-TOCS.

TREATMENT

Therapy for N-TOCS should always begin with non-operative treatment, including postural exercises and physiotherapy. Patients should avoid heavy lifting and working with the arm above shoulder level. Conservative treatment should be continued for several months. The majority of patients will improve significantly and will not require surgery. Indications for surgery include failure of conservative therapy after several months and persisting disabling symptoms that interfere with work and activities of daily living. The goal of surgery is to decompress the brachial plexus. Transaxillary first rib resection is the most common operation performed for N-TOCS.

Transaxillary resection of first rib

The technique described by Roos[21] is indicated for neurogenic complications of TOCS and can be summarized as follows. The patient is placed in the lateral position leaving the arm free. The assistant elevates the shoulder by applying upward traction on the upper arm. This manoeuvre opens up the

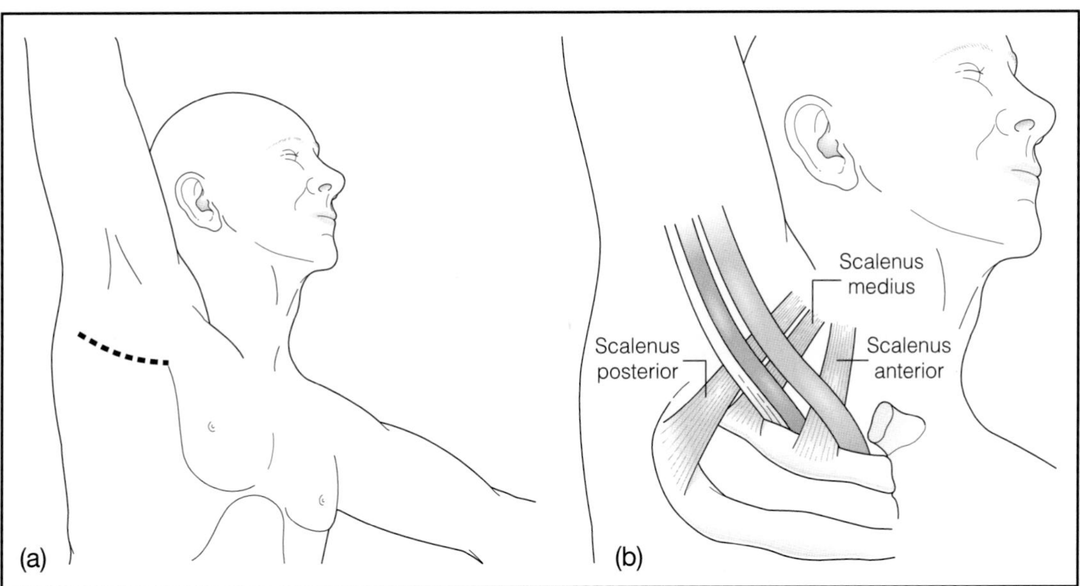

Figure 11.10 • Transaxillary resection of the first rib: **(a)** operative position and skin incision; **(b)** the neurovascular bundle is pulled away from the first rib by traction on the arm.

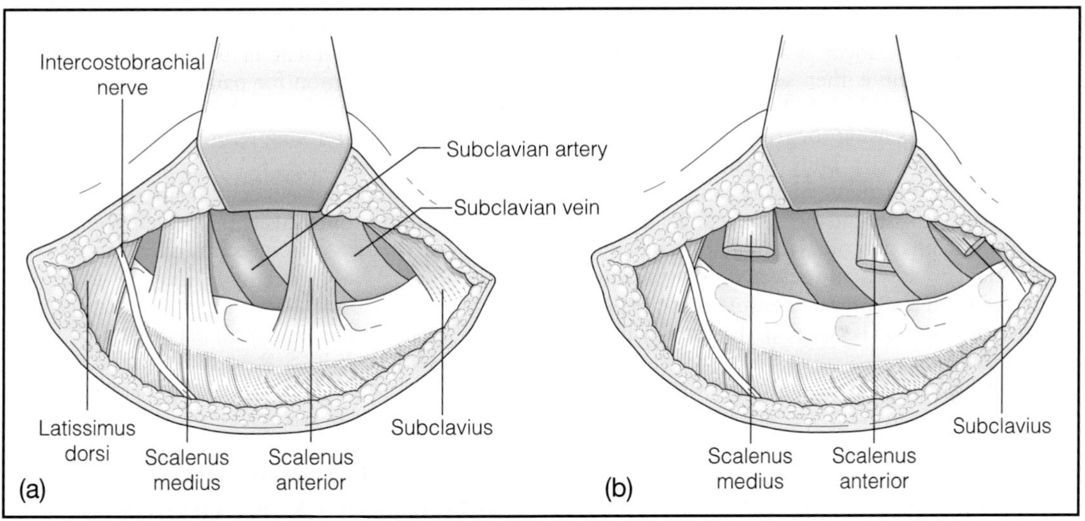

Figure 11.11 • Transaxillary resection of the first rib: **(a)** exposure of the first rib, scalene muscles and subclavian–axillary vessels; **(b)** detachment of the scalenus anterior, medius and subclavius muscles from the first rib.

costoclavicular space and pulls the neurovascular bundle away from the first rib. A horizontal skin incision is made at the lower border of the axillary line over the third rib (**Fig. 11.10**). From here the dissection extends proximally toward the apex of the axilla. The intercostal nerve emerging from the second intercostal space should be preserved. The fascial roof of the axilla is opened to expose the anterior portion of the first rib. Scalenus anterior is separated from the artery with a right-angled forceps and sectioned at its attachment to the first rib (**Fig. 11.11**). The tendon of the subclavius muscle is divided with care because of its close relation with the subclavian vein. The scalenus medius is then pushed off the rib using a blunt elevator. The intercostal muscles are similarly detached from the lower part of the rib and the pleura is dropped back from the operative zone. The rib is then sectioned at the chondrocostal junction and maintained by bone-holding forceps to distance it from the neurovascular bundle (**Fig. 11.12**). With the arm elevated, the T1 root is identified at the neck of the

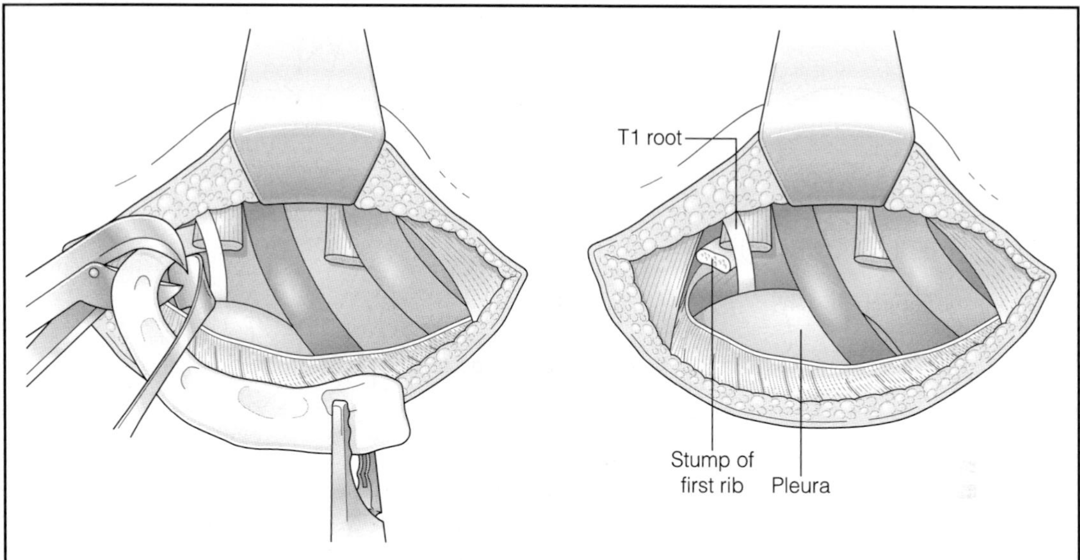

Figure 11.12 • Transaxillary resection of the first rib. **(a)** Exposure of the first rib. The rib has been disarticulated at the chondrocostal junction. T1 root is protected by a retractor. **(b)** Extraperiosteal resection of the first rib is complete.

first rib. The T1 root is displaced medially with care and an angled rib shear is set as far posteriorly as possible. The rib is then sectioned. This section is completed to within 1–2 cm of the vertebral transverse process using rongeurs. The stump must be smooth since sharp bony spicules may lacerate the plexus. Any remaining fibrous bands around the plexus or vessels should be resected. In the same way, the scalenus anterior is pulled down between the subclavian vessels and resected. Serum saline is then injected in the wound to ensure that the pleura is intact. The wound is closed in the usual way with suction drainage.

Complications of transaxillary rib resection include subclavian vein or artery injury, extrapleural haematoma or brachial plexus injury. The most serious complication is brachial plexus injury. Traction of the arm or damage to the T1 root by the rib shear or by retraction can be responsible for this complication. To avoid this, the T1 root should always be in view during posterior rib manipulation.

Other operative techniques for N-TOCS include a supraclavicular approach (see later). Axelrod et al.[22] reported the results of surgery in 170 patients operated for N-TOCS. No major operative complication occurred in these patients who underwent decompression via a supraclavicular approach. Only 11% of patients experienced minor complications, most commonly the need for chest tube placement as a result of pneumothorax. At short-term follow-up (10 months), most patients had improved pain levels (80%) and range of motion (82%). However, at long-term follow-up (47 months), residual symptoms were present in 65% of patients, and 35% took medication for pain. Nonetheless, 64% said they were satisfied with the result. Lepantalo et al.[23] performed a long-term follow-up after first rib resection (average 6.1 years) in which the examiners were independent from the surgeons. One month postoperatively, 77% were found to be improved whereas at long-term follow-up this was only 37%.

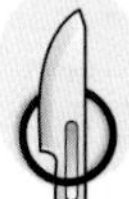

Controversy still exists concerning the surgical treatment of N-TOCS, and a randomized study of thoracic outlet surgery versus conservative treatment is lacking in this indication.

Arterial thoracic outlet compression syndrome

Arterial complications are often associated with bony abnormalities, including a complete cervical rib or fracture callus of the first rib or clavicle. The initial arterial lesion is fibrotic thickening with intimal damage and poststenotic dilation, leading to aneurysmal degeneration with mural thrombus and the risk of embolisation (**Fig. 11.13**). Most emboli are small and localised in the hand vessels, with pallor, paraesthesia and coldness suggestive of Raynaud's syndrome. If unrecognised, severe digital ischaemia with gangrene may occur. Early recognition of this condition is essential and a duplex scan should be performed in all patients with unilateral Raynaud's syndrome and asymptomatic patients

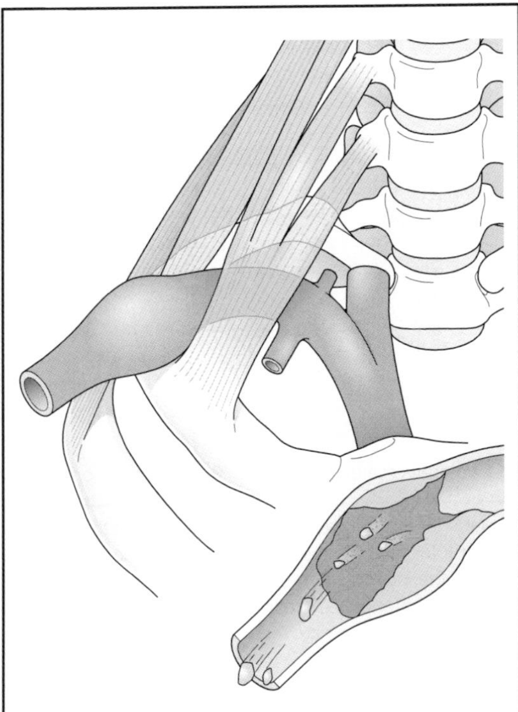

Figure 11.13 • Anatomy of a cervical rib with compression of the subclavian–axillary artery and poststenotic aneurysm with mural thrombus and distal embolisation. From Clagett GP. Upper extremity aneurysms. In: Rutherford RB (ed.) Vascular surgery, 5th edn. Philadelphia: WB Saunders, 2000; p. 1359, with permission.

with a cervical bruit. Loss of the radial pulse during Adson's manoeuvre (abduction and external rotation of the shoulder) is not very reliable as it is found in as many as 50% of normal subjects. The arteriographic changes may be obvious but may sometimes be minimal, with moderate dilation beyond a bony abnormality at the thoracic outlet and radiological evidence of distal embolisation. Subclavian stenosis is not always evident on anteroposterior view and oblique stress views are often necessary.

SURGICAL MANAGEMENT

The transaxillary approach previously described, largely used for isolated rib resection in the presence of neurological syndromes, does not offer satisfactory exposure of the subclavian–axillary artery and is contraindicated in the management of arterial complications. The transclavicular approach allows wide exposure of the supraclavicular and axillary region a significant cosmetic and functional impairment. Hopefully, the same surgical procedure can be done without dividing the clavicle using a combined supraclavicular and infraclavicular approach, the only indications for clavicular resection are arterial complications due to malunion or hypertrophic callus of the clavicle.

Combined supraclavicular and infraclavicular approach

The combined supraclavicular and infraclavicular approach offers a complete exposure. The infraclavicular dissection is commenced first with an S-shaped incision. Pectoralis major is detached from the upper sternum and clavicle (**Fig. 11.14**). Pectoralis

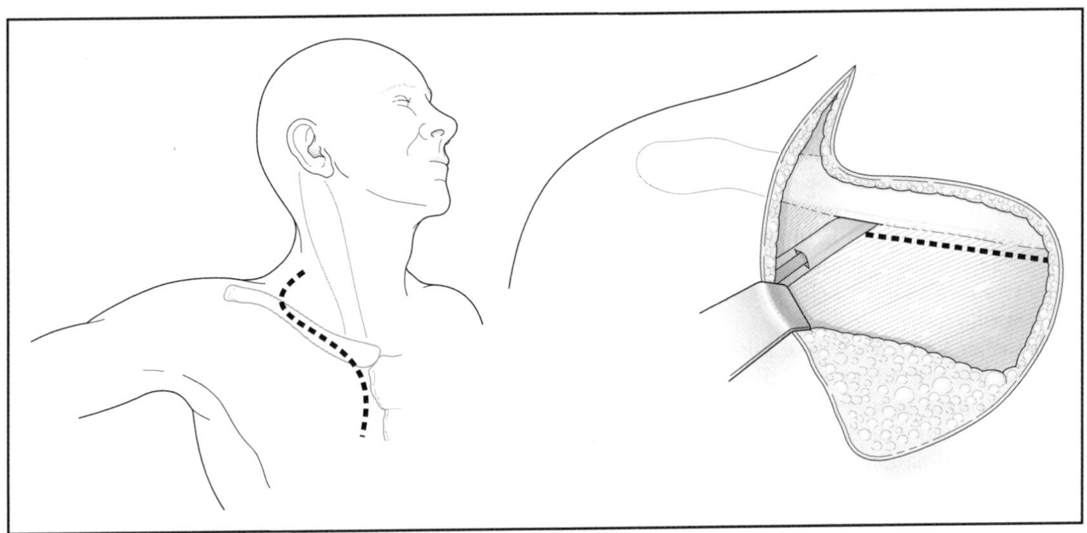

Figure 11.14 • Combined supraclavicular and infraclavicular approach for first rib resection. Skin incision and section of the pectoralis major from the clavicle.

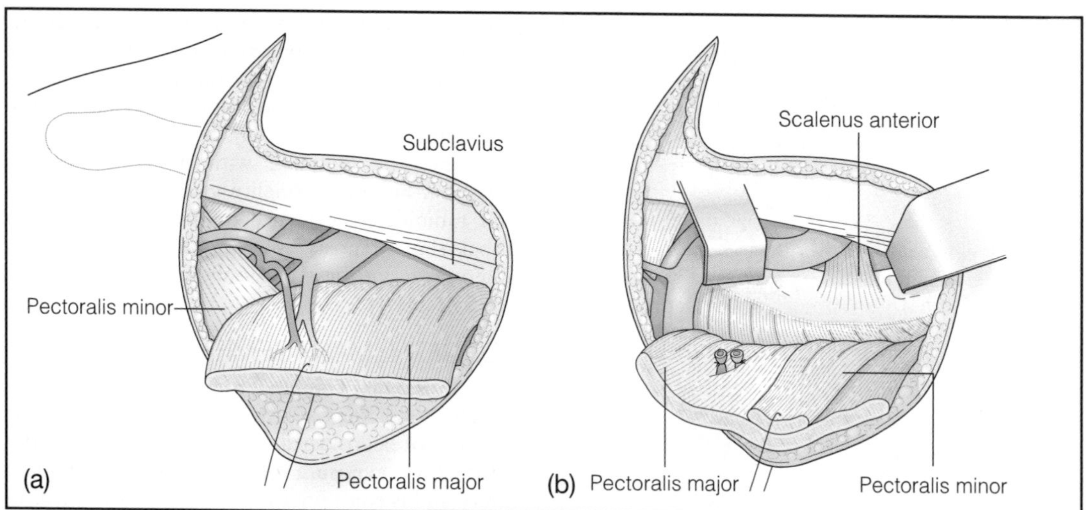

Figure 11.15 • Combined supraclavicular and infraclavicular approach for first rib resection. **(a)** Exposure of the proximal axillary vessels. The axillary vessels are held aside with a retractor to show the first rib and insertion of the scalenus anterior. **(b)** The infraclavicular dissection with detachment of the intercostal muscles from the first rib. The anterior portion of the rib will be removed and the first rib stump will be shortened via the supraclavicular exposure not shown here.

minor is then sectioned and the clavipectoral fascia opened to expose the subclavius and the anterior segment of the two first ribs. The subclavius is resected and the artery and the axillary vein are then freed behind the clavicle. Via a supraclavicular incision, the clavicular head of the sternomastoid and the external jugular vein are divided to expose the scalenus anterior and the phrenic nerve. The scalenus anterior is then sectioned near the first rib. The subclavian artery and vein are freed (**Fig. 11.15**). The intercostal muscles are detached from the lower border of the first rib and the rib is disarticulated at the costochondral junction. The rib is then sectioned without attempting to reach the posterior segment. Access to the rib stump is achieved via the supraclavicular exposure by reflecting the brachial plexus laterally and the artery medially. The scalenus medius is then detached from the first rib and, after protecting the T1 root, the rib is sectioned near the transverse process. If a complete cervical rib is present, the tip is disarticulated via the infraclavicular exposure, the remaining part being removed above the clavicle with the stump of the first rib.

In patients with aneurysm or poststenotic dilation secondary to first rib or cervical rib, there is often sufficient length of artery to permit resection of the arterial lesion and direct anastomosis (**Fig. 11.16**). When arterial lesions are more extensive, graft replacement is required using reversed great saphenous vein or PTFE if no vein is available. Intraoperative angiography is recommended in all cases. In patients with a recent distal embolic event, catheter embolectomy should be attempted through a transverse brachial arteriotomy or, if this is ineffective, through a radial or ulnar arteriotomy at the wrist using a No. 2 Fogarty catheter. If embolectomy is impossible, a distal bypass using the great saphenous vein may be needed in an attempt to revascularise one of the forearm arteries including the interosseous artery. Additional sympathectomy may also be considered where there is extensive long-standing distal embolic occlusion. Difficulty in clearing the distal arterial bed accounts for the incomplete revascularisation observed in advanced cases with disabling ischaemic sequelae.

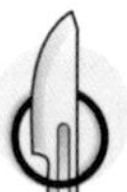

Arterial reconstruction and first rib or cervical rib resection is indicated in all patients with arterial complications of thoracic outlet syndrome.

SUBCLAVIAN–AXILLARY VEIN THROMBOSIS

Spontaneous or effort-related thrombosis in a fit young patient is known as Paget–Schroetter syndrome, the first cases being published separately by these two authors over a century ago. Hughes, who in 1949 collected 320 cases and recognised the distinct entity, coined the eponym. As the indications for central venous access have increased, so has the incidence of catheter-related subclavian–axillary vein thrombosis (SVT).[24]

Acute deep venous thrombosis (DVT) of the upper limb has many causes, with treatment and prog-

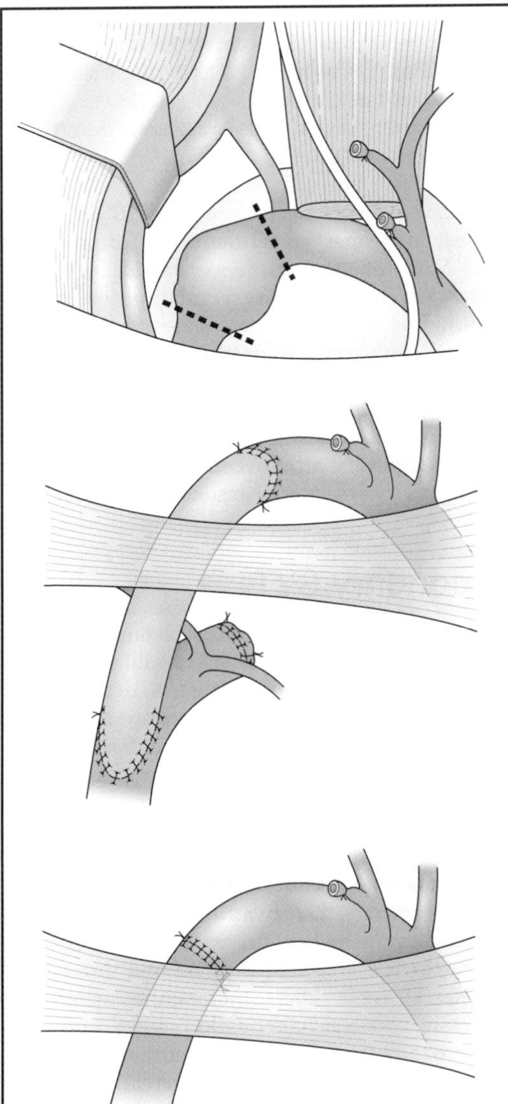

Figure 11.16 • Combined supraclavicular and infraclavicular approach for first rib resection with poststenotic aneurysm. Exposure of the subclavian and axillary vessels. Depending on the extent of arterial resection, end-to-end anastomosis or graft replacement is done.

nosis depending on the specific cause. SVT can be divided into two groups, primary and secondary. Primary SVT (Paget–Schroetter syndrome) is due to anatomical venous compression in the thoracic outlet during exercise (V-TOCS) and comprises about 25% of all cases. Secondary SVT is the result of multiple aetiological factors, although in most series trauma due to central venous catheters dominates this category (40% of all cases of SVT). SVT is responsible for 1–4% of all cases of DVT. Monreal et al.[25] reported a 15% incidence of pulmonary emboli in 30 consecutive patients with SVT who were investigated with ventilation–perfusion scanning.

Primary SVT

In a review of the literature, Hurlbert and Rutherford[26] reported a male to female ratio of 2:1, with an average age of 30 years for patients with primary SVT. Primary SVT represents only 3.5% of all cases of TOCS. Venous thrombosis is seen three times more frequently in the right than the left venous system, but bilateral venous compression also occurs frequently. Thrombosis is believed to be caused by repetitive trauma from compression. Virtually every patient has some degree of upper extremity swelling associated with pain that worsens with exertion. Some patients may have cyanosis of the arm. Unlike lower-extremity DVT, symptoms in the upper extremity are more related to venous obstruction than reflux. Venous outflow through the collateral vessels is limited, resulting in venous hypertension, swelling and even venous claudication. Venous gangrene is an extremely rare complication of SVT.

DIAGNOSIS

Clinically, the arm may be swollen and cyanosed with dilated shoulder girdle collateral veins. Duplex is the first-line investigation of choice and has a sensitivity of 94% and a specificity of 96% compared with venography.[27] MRA has poor sensitivity for non-occlusive thrombi and short-segment occlusion. CT has been used to diagnose upper-extremity DVT but its specificity and sensitivity are undetermined. Venography is still considered as the reference in evaluating SVT. The basilic vein is the preferred site for injection, with the arm abducted at 30°. The cephalic vein is not used because it joins directly with the subclavian vein and may miss an axillary vein thrombosis.

TREATMENT

For many years, treatment of SVT relied on rest and elevation of the upper limb with anticoagulant therapy. However, the morbidity associated with this conservative treatment is high. More recently, investigators have realised that many patients with SVT have compression at the thoracic outlet.

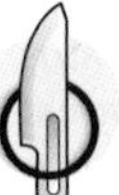

It has become accepted that treatment of primary upper-extremity DVT requires restoration of patency and removal of extrinsic compression.

Initially, in patients with primary SVT, subclavian vein patency was restored by open thrombectomy associated with first rib resection.[28] Although now supplanted by thrombolysis, open thrombectomy has proved effective and should be considered in patients with contraindications or failure of thrombolysis therapy.

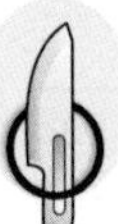

Thrombolytic therapy produces less morbidity than open thrombectomy in primary SVT, but carries poor long-term outcome if not combined with thoracic outlet decompression.

Catheter-directed techniques of thrombolysis allow for immediate venous evaluation and assess extrinsic compression with positional venography after thrombolysis.[29] However, Sheeran et al.[30] have shown that recanalisation of the vein by thrombolysis without decompression of the thoracic outlet is not adequate, with 55% of patients remaining symptomatic. Conversely, Machleder[31] reported the success of this combined treatment, with 86% of 36 patients becoming asymptomatic. The appropriate time interval between thrombolysis and thoracic outlet decompression is still under discussion. Machleder waited 3 months, whereas Lee et al.[32] recommended immediate first rib resection within 4 days after thrombolysis. Waiting too long risks rethrombosis, whereas operating immediately risks bleeding due to the thrombolytic agent.

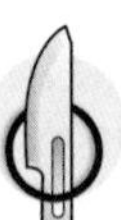

In thoracic outlet syndrome with SVT, it seems logical to recommend early complete treatment with thrombolysis and first rib resection.[33]

Specific problems may arise in some patients after thrombolysis. In a small group, no residual lesion or compression is seen on positional venography after thrombolysis. In these cases, anticoagulation therapy is recommended without thoracic outlet decompression. In other patients, intrinsic stenosis is seen on venography after thrombolysis. In these cases operative vein bypass or patch angioplasty with first rib resection is needed and should be performed in the days after thrombolysis because the risk of rethrombosis appears to be quite high.

Recently, percutaneous balloon angioplasty with or without stenting has been suggested. The results of this technique without thoracic outlet decompression are poor, with a 1-year primary patency of 35%.[34] Obviously, this technique does not obviate the need for surgery because thoracic outlet decompression is still needed. Even after thoracic outlet decompression, some venous stenoses are resistant to dilation or present intrinsic elastic recoil. Various types of stents have been used to treat residual stenoses, but acceptable results have been seen only in patients who had thoracic outlet decompression. In addition, venous stents underneath the clavicle are known to fracture.

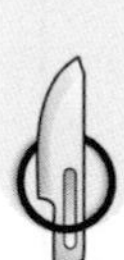

The long-term patency rate of stenting in primary SVT plus thoracic outlet compression is unknown. As surgery is always needed for thoracic outlet decompression, it seems logical to repair the subclavian vein with patch angioplasty or a short autogenous bypass.

In many patients seen more than 10 days after the onset of primary upper-limb DVT, thrombolysis fails. Most of these patients should be treated conservatively with anticoagulation unless the occlusion is short. In these cases, open thrombectomy with vein reconstruction and first rib resection can be recommended with acceptable results.[35] The technique used involves internal jugular vein transposition or cephalic vein bypass with a temporary arteriovenous fistula. Prosthetic bypass has shown inferior results in this location.

Secondary SVT

The common denominator for secondary SVT is central venous catheterisation. Overall, one-third of patients with central-line catheters develop SVT, although only 15% of them are symptomatic. The aetiology of catheter-associated thrombosis is multifactorial, but may be related to the fibrin sheath that forms around the catheter. The method of insertion, size, composition and duration of use of the catheter are also important. A reduced rate of thrombosis has been found with soft and more flexible catheters. Large catheters used for haemodialysis have a higher incidence of SVT. Another risk factor is the type of fluid infused through the catheter. Cancer chemotherapeutic agents are aggressive to vascular endothelium and may increase the risk of thrombosis. Furthermore, many patients with central-line catheters also have systemic risk factors for thrombosis, i.e. malignancy, sepsis, congestive heart failure and prolonged bed rest.

Symptomatic patients have oedema and distended veins around the shoulder. Pulmonary embolism is not uncommon, with 16% of patients positive on ventilation–perfusion scan.[36] Therapy guidelines are based on observational reports as no controlled studies are available. In all cases, anticoagulation using intravenous heparin via the affected arm is indicated to prevent clot extension until the catheter is removed. Thrombolytic therapy has a role in reopening thrombosed catheters. Prevention of thrombus formation has been emphasized, and for high-risk patients it may be advantageous to administer low-dose coumadin[37] or low-molecular-weight heparin to reduce the risk of catheter-associated thrombosis.

Key points

- Vascular diseases of the upper limb are rare in comparison to those involving the lower limbs, with the exception of arterial embolism.
- Clinical examination, including the Allen test, is important.
- There are good mid-term results of endovascular treatment of supra-aortic trunk stenoses.
- The long-term results of carotid bypass or carotid transposition are excellent.
- It is important to consider arterial disease in the work environment, e.g. hypothenar hammer syndrome.
- There is controversy concerning the diagnosis and treatment of N-TOCS.
- The combined supraclavicular and infraclavicular approach for first rib resection and arterial bypass is of value in the treatment of patients with arterial thoracic outlet compression syndrome.
- Early thrombolytic therapy combined with surgical thoracic outlet decompression is indicated in patients with primary SVT.

REFERENCES

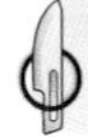

1. Fields WS, Lemak NA. Joint study of extracranial artery occlusion. Subclavian steal. A review of 168 cases. JAMA 1972; 222:1139–43.
2. McCarthy WJ, Flinn WR, Yao JST et al. Results of bypass grafting for upper limb ischemia. J Vasc Surg 1986; 3:741–6.

   Between 1978 and 1984, the authors performed 33 bypass grafts to relieve hand and forearm ischaemia in 27 patients. A reversed saphenous vein graft was used in 22 cases and PTFE in the remaining 11 procedures. Follow-up of 31 grafts from 6 to 72 months (mean 35.5 months) revealed an overall patency rate of 73% at 2 years and 67% at 3 years. More proximal grafts fared better: the 2-year patency rate was 83% for grafts at or above the brachial artery but only 53% for bypass distal to the brachial bifurcation.

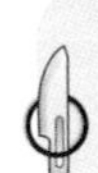

3. Kieffer E, Sabatier J, Koskas F et al. Atherosclerotic innominate artery occlusive disease: early and long term results of surgical reconstruction. J Vasc Surg 1995; 20:326–37.

   During a 20-year period (1974–93), the authors operated on 148 patients with brachiocephalic (innominate) artery atherosclerotic occlusive disease. Approach was through a median sternotomy in 135 (91%) patients. Endarterectomy was performed in 32 (22%) patients, whereas 116 (78%) patients underwent bypass. Eight (5.4%) patients died in the perioperative period. There were five (3.4%) perioperative strokes. Mean follow-up was 77 months. Survival was 51.9% at 10 years. The probability of freedom from ipsilateral stroke was 98.6% at 10 years. The primary patency rate was 98.4% at 10 years. In conclusion, surgical reconstruction of brachiocephalic artery atherosclerotic occlusive disease yields acceptable rates of perioperative complications with excellent long-term patency and freedom from neurological events and reoperation.

4. Berguer R, Morasch M, Kline R. Transthoracic repair of innominate and common carotid artery disease. Immediate and long-term outcome of 100 consecutive surgical reconstructions. J Vasc Surg 1998; 27:34–8.
5. Cherry KJ, McCullough JL, Hallett JW, Pairolero P. Technical principles of direct innominate artery revascularization. A comparison of endarterectomy and bypass grafts. J Vasc Surg 1989; 9:718–24.
6. Reul GL, Jacobs MJHM, Gregoric ID et al. Innominate artery occlusive disease. Surgical approach and long-term results. J Vasc Surg 1991; 14:405–12.
7. Motarjeme A. Percutaneous transluminal angioplasty of supra-aortic vessels. J Endovasc Surg 1996; 3:171–81.
8. Rapp JH, Reilly LM, Goldstone J et al. Ischemia of the upper extremity. Significance of proximal arterial disease. Am J Surg 1986; 152:122–6.

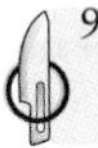

9. Vitti MJ, Thompson BW, Read RC et al. Carotid–subclavian bypass. A twenty-two years experience. J Vasc Surg 1994; 20:411–18.

   A retrospective review of 124 patients who underwent carotid–subclavian bypass from 1968 to 1990 was done to assess primary patency and symptom resolution. Graft conduits were PTFE in 44 (35%) and Dacron in 80 (65%) cases; 30-day mortality was 0.8%, 30-day primary patency was 100%. Primary patency rate was 95% at 10 years. Survival rate was 59% at 10 years. Symptom-free survival rate was 87% at 10 years. Carotid–subclavian bypass appears to be a safe and durable procedure for relief of symptomatic occlusive disease of the subclavian artery.

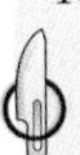

10. Sandmann W, Kniemeyer HW, Jaeschock R et al. The role of subclavian–carotid transposition in surgery for supra-aortic occlusive disease. J Vasc Surg 1987; 5:53–8.

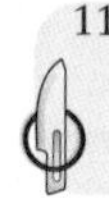

11. Kretschmer G, Teleky B, Marosi L et al. Obliterations of the proximal subclavian artery. To bypass or to anastomose? J Cardiovasc Surg (Torino) 1991; 32:334–9.
12. Martinez R, Rodrigo-Lopez J, Torruella R et al. Stenting for occlusion of the subclavian arteries. Tex Heart Inst J 1997; 24:23–7.
13. Westerband A, Rodriguez JA, Ramaiah VG et al. Endovascular therapy in prevention and management of coronary–subclavian steal. J Vasc Surg 2003; 38:699–704.
14. Brunkwall J, Berqvist D, Bergentz SE. Long term results of arterial reconstruction of the upper extremity. Eur J Vasc Surg 1994; 8:47–53.

15. Kieffer E, Bahnini A, Koskas F. Aberrant subclavian artery: surgical treatment in thirty-three adult patients. J Vasc Surg 1994; 19:100–10.

    The authors reviewed their experience with surgery for aberrant subclavian arteries (ASA). During a 16-year period they surgically treated 33 adult patients with ASA. Twenty-eight patients had a left-sided aortic arch with a right ASA, whereas five had a right-sided aortic arch with a left ASA. Eleven patients had dysphagia caused by oesophageal compression, five patients had ischaemic symptoms, ten patients had aneurysms of the ASA, and seven patients had an ASA arising from an aneurysmal thoracic aorta. In all cases the distal subclavian artery was revascularised, most often by direct transposition into the ipsilateral common carotid artery. The cervical approach was combined with a median sternotomy or a left thoracotomy in 17 patients. Aortic cross-clamping was required in 12 patients to perform the transaortic closure of the origin of the ASA with patch angioplasty or prosthetic replacement of the descending thoracic aorta. Cardiopulmonary bypass was used in six patients. Four patients died after operation. Satisfactory clinical and anatomical results were obtained in the remaining 29 patients. Provision should be made for cardiopulmonary bypass in patients with aneurysm of ASA or associated aortic aneurysm.

16. Sullivan TM, Bacharach JM, Perl J et al. Endovascular management of unusual aneurysms of the axillary and subclavian arteries. J Endovasc Surg 1996; 3:389–95.

    Aneurysms of the upper extremity arteries are uncommon and may be difficult to manage in emergency with standard surgical techniques. The authors report the exclusion of three axillary–subclavian aneurysms with covered stents. Palmaz stents were covered with either PTFE (two cases) or brachial vein and deployed to exclude pseudoaneurysms in one axillary and two left subclavian arteries. Endovascular exclusion of axillary and subclavian aneurysms with covered stents may offer a useful alternative to operative repair in patients with ruptured aneurysm or significant comorbidities.

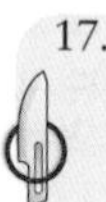

17. Vayssairat M, Debure C, Cormier J-M et al. Hypothenar hammer syndrome. Seventeen cases with long-term follow-up. J Vasc Surg 1987; 5:838–42.

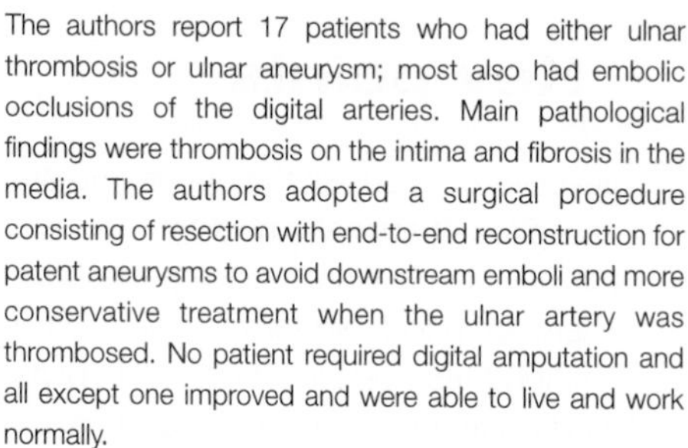

    The authors report 17 patients who had either ulnar thrombosis or ulnar aneurysm; most also had embolic occlusions of the digital arteries. Main pathological findings were thrombosis on the intima and fibrosis in the media. The authors adopted a surgical procedure consisting of resection with end-to-end reconstruction for patent aneurysms to avoid downstream emboli and more conservative treatment when the ulnar artery was thrombosed. No patient required digital amputation and all except one improved and were able to live and work normally.

18. Haimovici H. Cardiogenic embolism of the upper extremity. J Cardiovasc Surg (Torino) 1982; 23:209–15.
19. Sanders RJ, Cooper MA, Hammond SL et al. Neurogenic thoracic outlet syndrome. In: Rutherford RB (ed.) Vascular surgery, 5th edn. Philadelphia: WB Saunders, 2000; pp. 1184–99.
20. Sanders RJ, Haug CE. Thoracic outlet syndrome: a common sequela of neck injuries. Philadelphia: JB Lippincott, 1991; p. 93.
21. Roos DB. Thoracic outlet and carpal tunnel syndrome. In: Rutherford RB (ed.) Vascular surgery, 2nd edn. Philadelphia: WB Saunders, 1984; pp. 708–24.

22. Axelrod DA, Proctor MC, Geisser ME et al. Outcomes after surgery for thoracic outlet syndrome. J Vasc Surg 2001; 33:1220–5.

    This study determined whether there is an association between psychological and socioeconomic characteristics and long-term outcome of operative treatment for patients with sensory N-TOCS. Multivariate logistic regression models were developed as a means of identifying independent risk factors for postoperative disability. Operative decompression of the brachial plexus via a supraclavicular approach was performed for upper extremity pain and paraesthesia, with no mortality and minimal morbidity in 170 patients. After an average follow-up period of 47 months, 65% of patients reported improved symptoms, and 64% of patients were satisfied with their operative outcome. However, 35% of patients remained on medication and 18% of patients were disabled. Preoperative factors associated with persistent disability include major depression, being unmarried and having less than a high-school education. Operative decompression was beneficial for most patients. The impact of the preoperative treatment of depression on the outcome of TOCS decompression should be studied prospectively.

23. Lepantalo M, Lindgren KA, Leino E et al. Long-term outcome after resection of the first rib for thoracic outlet syndrome. Br J Surg 1989; 76:1255–6.

24. Rutherford RB, Hurlbert SN. Primary subclavian–axillary vein thrombosis. Consensus and commentary. Cardiovasc Surg 1996; 4:420–3.

    Fifteen multiple-choice questions concerning options in the management of primary subclavian–axillary vein thrombosis were discussed by a panel of experts and then voted upon by 25 attending vascular surgeons with experience in subclavian–axillary vein thrombosis. The large majority favoured or agreed upon (i) early clot removal for active healthy patients with a need/desire to use the involved limb in work or sport; (ii) catheter-directed thrombolysis as initial therapy; (iii) further therapy based on follow-up positional venography; (iv) surgical relief of demonstrated thoracic outlet compression after a brief period of anticoagulant therapy; (v) conservative therapy if post-lysis venogram showed either no extrinsic compression or a short residual occlusion; and (vi) intervention for residual intrinsic lesions with over 50% narrowing.

25. Monreal M, Lafoz E, Ruiz J et al. Upper extremity deep venous thrombosis and pulmonary embolism. Chest 1991; 99:280–3.

The authors prospectively evaluated the prevalence of pulmonary embolism in 30 consecutive patients with proved DVT of the upper extremity. Ten patients had primary DVT and 20 patients had catheter-related DVT. Ventilation–perfusion lung scans were routinely performed at the time of hospital admission in all but one patient. Lung scan findings were normal in nine of ten patients with primary DVT. In contrast, perfusion defects were considered highly suggestive of pulmonary embolism in four patients with catheter-related DVT. The authors conclude that pulmonary embolism is not a rare complication in upper-extremity DVT and that patients with catheter-related DVT seem to be at higher risk.

26. Hurlbert SN, Rutherford RB. Subclavian–axillary vein thrombosis. In: Rutherford RB (ed.) Vascular surgery, 5th edn. Philadelphia: WB Saunders, 2000; pp. 1208–21.

27. Koksoy C, Kuzu A, Kutlay J et al. The diagnostic value of colour doppler ultrasound in central venous catheter related thrombosis. Clin Radiol 1995; 50:687–9.

28. DeWeese JA, Adams JT, Gaiser DL. Subclavian venous thrombectomy. Circulation 1970; 42:158–63.

29. Lokanathan R, Salvian AJ, Chen JC et al. Outcome after thrombolysis and selective thoracic outlet decompression for primary axillary vein thrombosis. J Vasc Surg 2001; 33:783–8.

30. Sheeran SR, Hallisey MJ, Murphy TP et al. Local thrombolytic therapy as part of a multidisciplinary approach to acute axillo-subclavian vein thrombosis (Paget–Schroetter syndrome). J Vasc Intervent Radiol 1997; 8:253–60.

31. Machleder HI. Evaluation of a new treatment strategy for Paget–Schroetter syndrome: spontaneous thrombosis of the axillary–subclavian vein. J Vasc Surg 1993; 17:305–17.

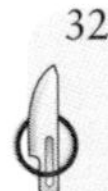

32. Lee MC, Grassi CJ, Belkin M et al. Early operative intervention following thrombolytic therapy for primary subclavian vein thrombosis. An effective treatment approach. J Vasc Surg 1998; 27:1101–8.

The authors conducted a study to determine an acceptable treatment approach to primary subclavian vein thrombosis. A retrospective review evaluated 11 patients in an 8-year period. All patients with occlusion received urokinase therapy and underwent surgical decompression within 5 days of thrombolytic therapy. Five percutaneous transluminal angioplasties were attempted before operative intervention. Eleven decompressions were performed. All patients received coumadin for 3–6 months after the operation. Urokinase therapy established wide venous patency in 9 of 11 extremities treated, with the remaining two requiring thrombectomy. One patient who underwent transluminal angioplasty before the operation had rethrombosis, and the remaining four showed no improvement in venous stenosis after the intervention. Eight of nine extremities treated by first rib resection and one of two treated by scalenectomy were free of residual symptoms at follow-up. The authors conclude that preoperative use of percutaneous balloon angioplasty is ineffective and should be avoided in this setting. Surgical intervention within days of thrombolysis enables patients to return to normal activity sooner.

33. Urschel HC, Razzuk MA. Paget–Schroetter syndrome: what is the best management? Ann Thorac Surg 2000; 69:1663–9.

The authors evaluated the results of 312 extremities in 294 patients with Paget–Schroetter syndrome to provide the basis for optimal management. Group I (35 extremities) was initially treated with anticoagulants only. Twenty-one developed recurrent symptoms after returning to work, requiring transaxillary resection of the first rib. Thrombectomy was necessary in eight. Group II (36 extremities) was treated with thrombolytic agents initially, with 20 requiring subsequent rib resection after returning to work. Thrombectomy was necessary in only four. Of the most recent 241 extremities (group III), excellent results accrued using thrombolysis plus prompt first rib resection for those evaluated during the first month after occlusion (199). The results were only fair for those seen later than 1 month (42). The authors conclude that early diagnosis (less than 1 month), expeditious thrombolytic therapy and prompt first rib resection are critical for the best results.

34. Glanz S, Gordon DH, Lipkowitz GS et al. Axillary and subclavian vein stenosis. Percutaneous angioplasty. Radiology 1988; 168:371–3.

35. Sanders RJ, Cooper MA. Surgical management of subclavian vein obstruction, including six cases of subclavian vein bypass. Surgery 1995; 118:856–63.

36. Monreal M, Raventos A, Lerma R et al. Pulmonary embolism in patients with upper extremity DVT associated with venous central lines. A prospective study. Thromb Haemost 1994; 72:548–50.

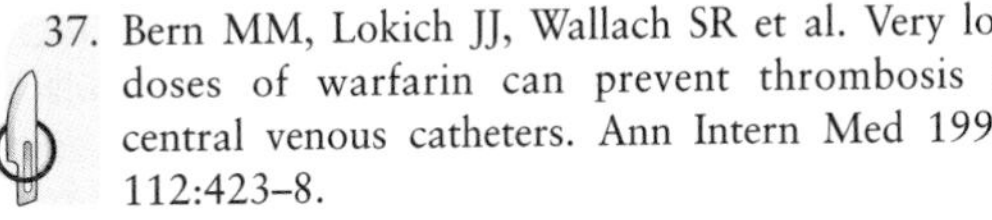

37. Bern MM, Lokich JJ, Wallach SR et al. Very low doses of warfarin can prevent thrombosis in central venous catheters. Ann Intern Med 1990; 112:423–8.

The goal of this study was to determine whether very low doses of warfarin are useful in thrombosis prophylaxis in patients with central venous catheters. Patients at risk for thrombosis associated with chronic indwelling central venous catheters were prospectively and randomly assigned to receive, or not to receive, 1 mg of warfarin beginning 3 days before catheter insertion and continuing for 90 days. Subclavian, innominate and superior vena cava venograms were done at onset of thrombosis symptoms or after 90 days in the study. A total of 121 patients entered the study, and 82 patients completed the study. Of 42 patients completing the study while receiving warfarin, four had venogram-proven thrombosis. All four had symptoms from thrombosis. Of 40 patients completing the study while not receiving warfarin, 15 had venogram-proven thrombosis and 10 had symptoms from thrombosis ($P < 0.001$). In conclusion, very low doses of warfarin can protect against thrombosis without inducing a haemorrhagic state. This approach may be applicable to other groups of patients.

CHAPTER

Twelve

Primary and secondary vasospastic disorders and vasculitis

Jill J.F. Belch and
Dean Patterson

INTRODUCTION

There are many inflammatory and vasospastic disorders that can present with ischaemia and thus come to the attention of the vascular clinician. These include Raynaud's phenomenon (RP) plus any associated connective tissue disorder, and the vasculitides. Because of the systemic nature of these diseases, medical practitioners of all disciplines will be involved in the management of these conditions at some stage in their career. Unfortunately, there is considerable overlap in the presenting features of these conditions and this can make diagnosis difficult. However, recent advances in immunopathological testing now allow the majority of disorders to be classified. On the other hand, the discovery of new autoantibodies makes the study of these disorders more difficult for the non-specialist. The aim of this chapter is to provide the vascular clinician with a grounding of knowledge in these disorders so that the initial diagnosis can be made. It describes the most common manifestations of these diseases, outlines their investigation (with particular emphasis on diagnostic autoantibody tests) and briefly delineates their treatment.

VASOSPASM

Vasospasm is the key feature of RP. Maurice Raynaud's original description was of episodic digital ischaemia induced by cold and emotion.[1] The classical manifestation of pallor preceding cyanosis and rubor reflects the initial vasospasm (**Fig. 12.1**), followed by deoxygenation of the static

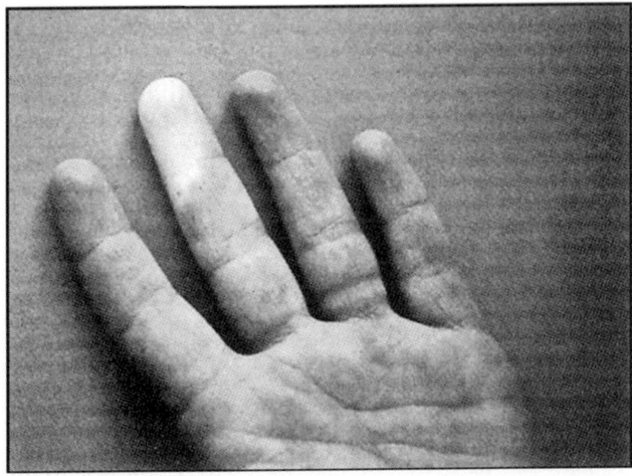

Figure 12.1 • Digital pallor due to vasospasm.

venous blood (cyanosis) and then reactive hyperaemia (rubor) with the return of blood flow. It is now known that the full triphasic colour change is not essential for the diagnosis of RP, and a history of cold-induced blanching with subsequent reactive hyperaemia can still reflect significant vasospasm. In addition, other stimuli can provoke an attack, for example chemicals (including drugs and those in tobacco smoke[2]), trauma and hormones. In addition to the digits, the vasospasm may involve the nose, tongue and ear lobes. Other organs may also be involved. A decrease in lung,[3] oesophageal[4] and myocardial[5] perfusion has been shown after cold challenge, which suggests systemic vasospasm, and these patients have a higher incidence of migraine and angina.[6]

RP is nine times more common in women, with an overall population prevalence of about 10%. In the recently published Framingham Offspring Study, the prevalence of RP was 9.6% in women and 5.8% in men. However, it may affect 20–30% of young women.[7] There also appears to be a familial predisposition, which is more marked if the age of onset of RP is under 30 years.[8] Despite this clear familial link, no candidate genes for this condition have yet been found,[9] although there is hope that proteomics will help unravel the mystery.[10]

Nomenclature: phenomenon, syndrome or disease

Inconsistent terminology is a major problem for clinicians managing RP. Europeans use RP as a blanket term for all cold-related vasospasm, with secondary Raynaud's syndrome (RS) being associated with another disease, and primary Raynaud's disease (RD) where it occurs in isolation. However, American and Australasian researchers use the syndrome and phenomenon interchangeably,[11] and differentiate the types of RP by indicating whether primary RP or secondary RP. The former classification has been used in this chapter.

It is probable that many patients with mild disease never present to their general practitioners but of those who do, most will have primary RD. Patients with more severe disease are likely to be referred to a hospital specialist, and an early marker for secondary RS is the severity of vasospastic attacks,[12] although the RP may precede associated systemic disease by more than 20 years.[13] Hospital practitioners are therefore more likely to see a higher proportion of RS, and the important challenge is to differentiate between the primary and secondary conditions in order to facilitate early management of the underlying associated disorder.

The secondary associations of RS are shown in **Box 12.1**. Of the connective tissue diseases (CTDs), systemic sclerosis is the most frequent association, but RS also occurs in the other diseases in this group and these are discussed in more detail later. In the hyperviscosity syndromes, such as myeloma, the prevalence is similar to the normal population but the symptomatology tends to be more severe.

Occupational RS is also well recognised and a relatively common form is hand–arm vibration syndrome (HAVS) (previously known as vibration white finger). As the name suggests, it occurs in workers exposed to vibrating instruments such as chain saws, pneumatic road drills and buffing machines. An estimated 1.5 million workers in the USA use vibratory tools.[14] Before these tools were regulated, 90% of exposed workers developed symptoms of HAVS. Among American shipyard workers, 71% of full-time pneumatic grinders complained of white fingers[15] and in Japan 9.6% of forest workers had symptoms of this syndrome.[16] However, by using lighter chain saws and reduced vibration, the frequency of clinical problems in Finnish forest workers was reduced from 40 to 5%.[17] The duration of exposure is important, with a latent period of often less than 5 years of full-time work. The severity of symptoms correlates with the length of exposure.[17] Vasospasm is not limited to the hands and has also been described in the toes.[18] It is likely that vibration-induced damage of the endothelium underlies this condition.[19] In approximately one-quarter of cases, the symptoms may

Box 12.1 • Conditions associated with Raynaud's phenomenon

Connective tissue diseases
Systemic sclerosis
Systemic lupus erythematosus
Rheumatoid arthritis
Mixed connective tissue diseases
Sjögren's syndrome
Dermatomyositis/polymyositis
Obstructive
Atherosclerosis (especially thromboangiitis obliterans)
Microemboli
Thoracic outlet syndrome (especially cervical ribs)
Drug therapy
Beta-blockers
Cytotoxics, e.g. bleomycin
Ciclosporin
Ergotamine and other antimigraine therapies
Sulfasalazine
Occupational
Vibration white finger disease
Vinyl chloride disease
Ammunition workers (outside work)
Frozen food packers
Miscellaneous
Hypothyroidism
Cryoglobulinaemia
Reflex sympathetic dystrophy
Malignancy

resolve if a job change is effected early in the course of the disease.[20]

In the UK, HAVS has been a prescribed industrial disease since 1985. Patients may be eligible for industrial injuries disablement benefits administered by the Department of Social Security if they fulfil certain criteria.[21] There is currently no specific legislation to control vibration at work but a European Directive on physical agents at work has been proposed and is still being evaluated.

Other occupation-related causes of RP include vinyl chloride disease, which is estimated to occur in 3% of workers exposed to this chemical. Ammunition workers also develop RP outside their work environment when the vasodilatory effects of nitrates are removed.

Atherosclerotic obstructive arterial disease is a common cause of RP in those over 60 years of age, particularly in men, and screening and treatment of known risk factors like hyperlipidaemia are recommended. Various drugs may precipitate or exacerbate RP (e.g. beta-blockers for angina) and alternative drug therapies may be more appropriate (e.g. calcium channel blockers such as nifedipine). Vasospasm is also a feature of reflex sympathetic dystrophy and thoracic outlet syndrome, particularly occurring in the presence of a cervical rib (see Chapter 11).

Pathophysiology

The precise mechanism that causes Raynaud's is unknown but three aetiological factors are considered to be important: (i) neurogenic; (ii) interactions between blood cells and the blood vessel wall; and (iii) inflammatory and immunological responses. It is likely that these mechanisms are interdependent and interact closely to produce the symptoms.

NEUROGENIC

Most studies have focused on the peripheral nervous system. In patients with RP, α-adrenergic receptor sensitivity and density are increased[22] and the responsiveness of β-adrenergic presynaptic receptors in the peripheral vessels is also increased.[2] The role of the central sympathetic nervous system is not clear. Support for its involvement comes from work showing that local vibration in one hand induces vasoconstriction in the other, which is abolished by proximal nerve blockade.[23] Furthermore, central sympathetic vasoconstriction produced by body cooling is required to produce vasoconstriction, and body cooling alone may produce vasospasm in the absence of local digital cooling.[24] In contrast, Freedman et al.[22] were unable to demonstrate changes in the response to reflex cooling or indirect heating following α- and β-adrenergic receptor blockade.

INTERACTIONS BETWEEN BLOOD AND BLOOD VESSEL WALLS

Microcirculatory flow depends on an intact and functioning endothelium, plasma factors and the cellular elements of blood. Activated platelets aggregate and form clumps that can obstruct flow. They may also release vasoconstrictive substances like thromboxane A_2 and serotonin, causing further platelet aggregation. Red blood cells (RBCs) appear less deformable in RP and cold temperatures further increase RBC stiffness.[25] Rigid RBCs and white blood cells (WBCs) may impede the microcirculation, and activated WBCs aggregate and adhere within the microcirculation and can narrow the vascular lumen. Additionally, WBC activation increases the formation of free radicals, which may be prothrombotic.[26] Elevated fibrinogen and globulin levels increase plasma viscosity and reduce blood flow. Increased platelet aggregation, rigid RBCs and activated WBCs have all been reported in patients with RS, together with raised plasma viscosity and reduced fibrinolysis.[27]

The intact endothelium is a functioning organ that produces many substances important in maintaining blood flow. Damage to it may impair blood flow in RP. Factor VIII von Willebrand factor (VWF) antigen is released following vascular damage and is increased in patients with RP.[28] VWF is active in the clotting cascade and platelet activation and may contribute to reduced blood flow. Tissue plasminogen activator is active in fibrinolysis and levels are reduced in RP, with a subsequent reduction in fibrinolysis.[27]

Endothelial vasoconstrictor/vasodilator production may also be impaired in RP. Prostacyclin (PGI_2) levels are increased in RP in the secondary form,[29] although RS appears to be resistant to the effects of PGI_2.[30] Endothelin is a potent vasoconstrictor and elevated levels have been demonstrated in RP,[31] whereas nitric oxide levels appear to be reduced.[32] Endothelium-dependent responses are abnormal in RP (e.g. to acetylcholine) but the blood vessel responds normally to endothelium-independent vasodilatation.[33] This suggests that endothelial dysfunction plays a major part in RP.

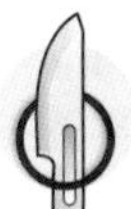

This is supported by the finding that endothelin-1 is related to sympathetic hyperactivity, which is more involved in primary Raynaud's than in HAVS.[34]

Inhibition of endothelial growth by tumour necrosis factor and lymphotoxin may also be important.

Most of these abnormalities are seen in patients with RS except for the increase in VWF, which occurs in the primary disease also. It is possible therefore that these are a consequence rather than the cause of the disorder. Nevertheless, they may still augment the impairment of blood flow and their correction by drug therapy may produce clinical benefit.

INFLAMMATORY AND IMMUNOLOGICAL MECHANISMS

Most cases of severe RS occur when associated with CTD, and disordered immunology and inflammation are found in these patients. Interestingly, however, abnormal WBC behaviour also occurs in HAVS,[27] which has no clear immunological/inflammatory basis.

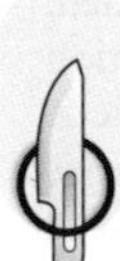

The serum level of soluble vascular cell adhesion molecules is significantly increased in patients with HAVS while the levels of intercellular adhesion molecule and E-selectin are not altered, an indication of endothelial damage.[35]

Tumour necrosis factor and lymphotoxin inhibit endothelial growth, stimulate fibroblast growth and collagen synthesis, and promote the release of vWF from endothelial cells. They have therefore been linked theoretically to the high levels of vWF in RS. Oxidative stress, important in both vascular disease and the inflammatory process, is augmented in RS.[26,36] However, more work is required in this area and current drug treatment is directed mainly at the haemorheological abnormalities.

Clinical features

The initial feature is episodic and demarcated blanching of extremities produced in response to cold or temperature change, and also to emotion. Digital artery spasm is the cause of this pallor. Although many people may complain of cold hands with some mild poorly delineated colour changes, they do not necessarily have RP but probably cold-induced closure of the arteriovenous shunts in the skin only, which decreases cutaneous blood flow and limits body heat loss. Patients with RP subsequently experience the cyanotic phase and/or the redness of the reactive hyperaemia phase. This last phase may be associated with rewarming paraesthesia and pain. RP is therefore characterised by being biphasic or triphasic, and usually affects the fingers and toes though finger symptoms tend to be more prominent. This may be asymmetrical in that, for example, only one or two digits may be affected on each hand, although all digits may be equally affected. As documented earlier, other extremities such as the ears, tongue and nose may also be affected, but a bluish discoloration in isolation is due to acrocyanosis and not RP. The occurrence of other skin-related problems, e.g. digital ulcers and recurrent chilblains, suggests secondary RP perhaps associated with CTD. Likewise, an onset in children under 10 years of age, an older adult onset (>30 years) and perennial attacks also suggest secondary RP.

Investigations

These should be directed at confirming the diagnosis of RP, if appropriate, and differentiating between the primary and secondary disease with elucidation of the underlying cause. In the majority of patients, the diagnosis of RP is made clinically from the history and examination if they present during a Raynaud's attack. Objective measures of blood flow are not usually required unless the clinical findings are vague. There are a variety of techniques available, many involving cold challenge but there is no gold standard because of practical difficulties and interindividual differences.

The test we use most involves the measurement of digital systolic blood pressure changes before and after local cooling at 15°C. A pressure drop of greater than 30 mmHg is considered to be significant,[36] but precautions are required to avoid false-negative results. Ideally, patients should not be tested if they have had a Raynaud's attack earlier in the day as they may still be in the reactive hyperaemia stage and relatively protected from further vasospasm. In practice, the test may be carried out 2–3 hours after an attack if there is good clinical recovery. All vasoactive medication should be stopped for 24 hours before testing and testing should be avoided during mid-cycle in premenopausal women as poor flow can occur during ovulation.[37] Patients should be warm and not vasoconstricted prior to baseline measurements and this is best done by resting in a temperature-controlled laboratory for 30 minutes prior to testing. In warmer weather, additional total body cooling may be required as a warm body may protect a patient from the vasospastic effects of localised digital cooling.

Strain gauge plethysmography is the usual method of measuring digital systolic blood pressure. Considerable operator skill is required and flow cannot be measured. Photoplethysmography with more sophisticated Doppler ultrasound equipment allows the measurement of the pressure at which blood flow returns.

Computerised thermography uses skin temperature as an indicator of finger blood flow. This technique allows dynamic measurement of all phases of the attack but results must be interpreted with care as skin temperature is also dependent on venous and arterial blood temperature.

Associated diseases should be sought by carrying out screening blood tests. A full blood count, urea and electrolytes and urinalysis should detect anaemia of chronic disease and renal disease, and thyroid function tests detect hypothyroidism.

Erythrocyte sedimentation rate (ESR) or plasma viscosity and rheumatoid antibody and antinuclear antibody tests help to detect associated CTD. Other tests, for example for cryoglobulins, may be carried out if appropriate. A chest radiograph will show basal fibrosis associated with CTD and a bony cervical rib.

Nail-fold capillaroscopy can be performed using an ophthalmoscope at high power. Normal vessels are not visualised (**Fig. 12.2**) but abnormally enlarged vessels, for example as seen in systemic sclerosis, will be seen quite easily (**Fig. 12.3**). These may also be examined by formal high-power microscopy but it should be noted that nail-fold changes also occur with trauma and in diabetes mellitus. The combination of abnormal nail-fold vessels and an abnormal immunological test has a 90% prediction value for later CTD.[9] Using structured classification systems, nail-fold patterns may be useful in assessing progression of the CTD.[38]

Management

A proportion of patients with mild disease will not require drug treatment. Associated disorders such as hypothyroidism should be treated and causative drug therapy (e.g. beta-blockers for hypertension) changed. Good symptomatic relief can be achieved in many patients despite the current lack of cure. A suggested management plan is shown in **Fig. 12.4**.

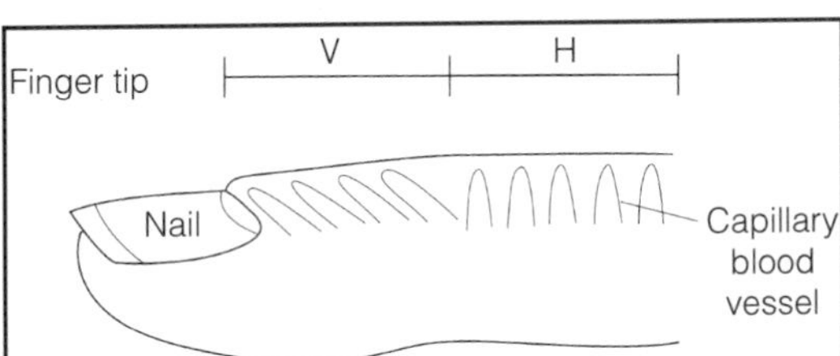

Figure 12.2 • Diagram of nail-fold vessels. V, vessels becoming parallel, visible if enlarged; H, vessels perpendicular, not visible.

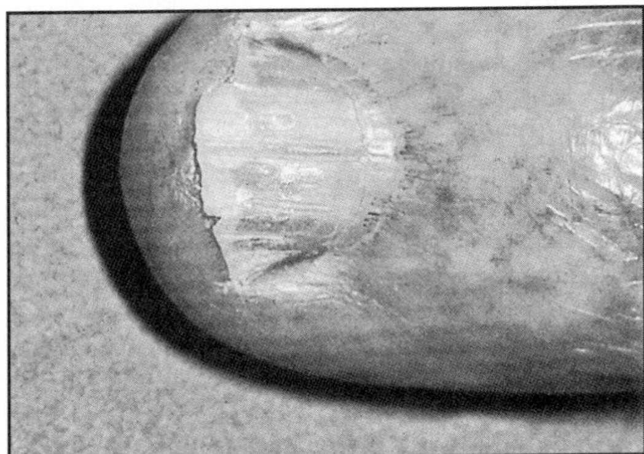

Figure 12.3 • Enlarged nail-fold capillaries in a patient with systemic sclerosis.

GENERAL MEASURES

Explanation of the disorder and reassurance is important in these patients who are often apprehensive about their condition. The Raynaud's and Scleroderma Association in the UK issues free information booklets, and local self-help groups can be invaluable for support.

Smokers should stop cigarette smoking. Pocket-sized thermochemical warming agents are available and convenient to use. Electrically heated gloves and socks are ideal for some and provide warmth for up to 3 hours. However, they require heavy batteries to be worn around the waist and are cumbersome, which means elderly patients may not be able to carry the battery. Newer designs are becoming available with the batteries inserted in a pocket on the gloves or socks themselves and should be more acceptable for many patients. Nevertheless, patients should be warned that the heat may irritate existing skin ulcers. 'Abel' shoes, available from surgical appliance suppliers, are padded and broad fitting and therefore warm while relieving pressure around the toes. Good ulcer care with early and adequate treatment of infection is important. It should be noted that the usual signs of infection, i.e. warmth, erythema and pus formation, may be absent because of poor blood flow. A high index of suspicion is required.

DRUG THERAPY

This should be offered when symptoms are severe enough to interfere with work or lifestyle. Most patients with RS and some with RD will fall into this category. A selection of the drugs used in the treatment of RP is shown in **Box 12.2**.

Calcium channel blockers

These drugs are vasodilatory. Nifedipine is the gold standard and the most frequently prescribed drug, and has additional antiplatelet[39] and anti-WBC activity. However, its use is limited by the vasodilatory effects of flushing, headache and ankle swelling. These will be attenuated by using the slow-release, or 'retard', preparations and starting with 10 mg once daily gradually increasing to a maximum of 20 mg t.d.s. if required.[40] Apart from ankle swelling, the vasodilatory adverse effects often abate with continued use. Nifedipine has no licence for use in pregnancy and patients should be advised accordingly. Other potentially useful calcium blockers include amlodipine,[41] diltiazem[42] and

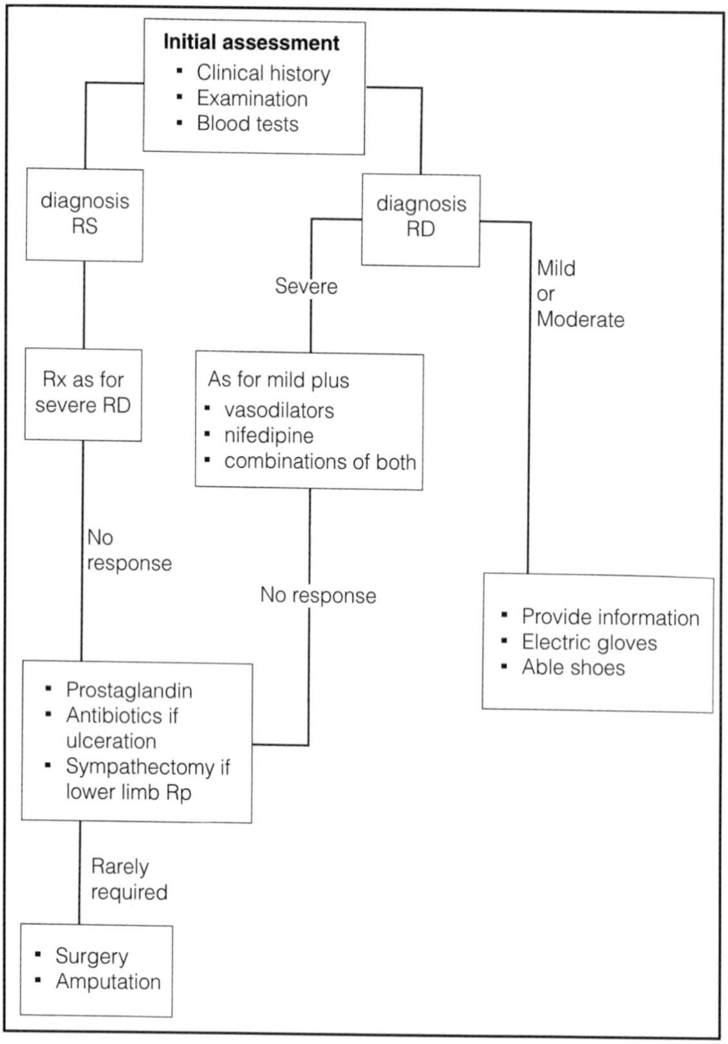

Initial assessment
- Clinical history
- Examination
- Blood tests

diagnosis RS

diagnosis RD

Severe

Mild or Moderate

Rx as for severe RD

As for mild plus
- vasodilators
- nifedipine
- combinations of both

No response

No response

- Provide information
- Electric gloves
- Able shoes

- Prostaglandin
- Antibiotics if ulceration
- Sympathectomy if lower limb Rp

Rarely required

- Surgery
- Amputation

Figure 12.4 • Flow chart for the management of Raynaud's phenomenon.

isradipine.[43] These tend to have less vasodilatory effects but at the expense of efficacy. Verapamil appears to be ineffective.

Other vasodilators

Naftidrofuryl oxalate (Praxilene) is a mild peripheral vasodilator with a serotonin receptor antagonist effect. An oral dose of 200 mg t.d.s. has been evaluated in many studies and mild improvement can be expected in terms of severity of pain and duration of attacks.

It is our experience that patients with primary RD respond better to vasodilators than those with RS, the limiting factor often being adverse effects at higher doses. Occasionally, we also find that a combination of a low-dose calcium blocker with a vasodilator such as naftidrofuryl can produce benefit while minimising the adverse effects seen with higher doses of either drug given in isolation.

Prostaglandins

Prostaglandins like PGI_2 and PGE_1 have potent vasodilatory and antiplatelet effects but are both very unstable and require intravenous administration. Iloprost is a stable prostacyclin analogue that is effective in RP.[44] It is given intravenously for 6 hours daily for 3–5 days per treatment. The dose is gradually increased during each 6-hour period to a maximum tolerated dose, which should never be greater than 2 ng/kg per min. It is often less than this, particularly in women, because of flushing, headache or rarely hypotension. The same maximum dose is used each day. It is probably equipotent with nifedipine but remains a second choice in Europe because of its parenteral mode of administration and lack of licence in some countries. Newer studies of oral iloprost,[45] oral limaprost[46] and oral beraprost[47] have been encouraging and these may become available in the relatively near future.

Box 12.2 • Commonly used drugs in the treatment of Raynaud's phenomenon

Nifedipine
Slow-release or retard preparation preferred, 10 mg b.d. then t.d.s.
Change to 20 mg b.d. then t.d.s. if required
Capsule as 'rescue medication' crushed under tongue if chronic dosing not tolerated
Can be combined at low dose (e.g. 10 mg once daily) with vasodilator if higher dose not tolerated
Naftidrofuryl
Initially 100 mg t.d.s. then 200 mg t.d.s. if required
Inositol nicotinate
Start at 500 mg t.d.s. increasing to forte 750 mg b.d. if required
Maximum dose is 1 g q.i.d.
Administer for a 3-month trial
Pentoxifylline
400 mg b.d. increasing to t.d.s. if required
Moxisylyte (thymoxamine)
40 mg q.d.s. increasing to 80 mg q.d.s.
Discontinue if no response in 2 weeks

Other drugs

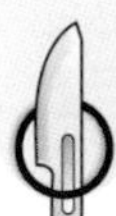

Case reports and pilot studies suggest interesting areas for future work. Sildenafil improved pulmonary hypertension and peripheral blood flow in a patient with scleroderma-associated lung fibrosis and RP,[48] while *Ginkgo biloba* extracts[49] and selective serotonin reuptake inhibitors[50] have been demonstrated in pilot studies to be of benefit.

SYMPATHECTOMY

This involves the injection of phenol into the sympathetic chain. Lumbar sympathectomy has an important role in intractable RP of the feet and is often worth considering. Cervical sympathectomy has a poor response and a high relapse rate and is no longer indicated for upper limb RP. The more selective digital sympathectomy is popular in some specialised centres but long-term follow-up results have yet to be published.

Conclusion

RP is a common condition affecting 10% of the female population. Differentiation between primary and secondary RP is important for the correct management strategy. Satisfactory symptomatic relief is possible with a combination of drug therapy and non-pharmacological aids despite the lack of a cure. Surgery may be appropriate in some cases with an obstructive, bony or fibrous cervical rib. Treatment of associated CTD is also important. Occupational RP can sometimes be improved by change of job or a change in work techniques and this should always be considered.

CONNECTIVE TISSUE DISEASE

The commonest disease associations with RS are the CTDs. **Box 12.3** lists these disorders and indicates the relevant incidence of RP. It is found in the majority of patients with systemic sclerosis and mixed CTD. At present, the frequency with which these secondary conditions are recognised varies widely in reported studies and may depend in part on the doctor's referral pattern and the thoroughness with which the screen for a CTD is undertaken.[11] Their early detection can be difficult but recently more clearly defined abnormalities have been documented in RP that have a strong link with disease progression to CTD. These include certain clinical features, the presence of abnormal nail-fold vessels as previously described, and abnormal tests of immunology.

The American Rheumatism Association (ARA) criteria for CTDs have high specificity but low sensitivity for the diseases. Thus patients who do not fulfil the ARA criteria for a particular CTD but who have a single feature of the disease, for example sclerodactyly, digital pitting or photosensitivity, are likely with time to develop fully established CTD.[51] Thus isolated features of CTD occurring in association with RP should arouse clinical suspicion. The age of onset of RP may also be important. As stated, RP is common among young women and most of these probably have primary RD. When RP develops in older subjects, the likelihood of an underlying

Box 12.3 • Incidence of Raynaud's phenomenon in connective tissue disorders

Systemic sclerosis	95%
Systemic lupus erythematosus	29–40%
Polymyositis/dermatomyositis	40%
Sjögren's syndrome	33%
Mixed connective tissue disease	85%
Rheumatoid arthritis	10%

CTD is increased. Kallenberg[52] reports a study in which the median age of onset of vasospastic symptoms in RD was 14 years, and 36 years in patients with definite CTD. About 80% of patients presenting with onset of RP at the age of 60 years or above also have an associated condition,[53] but the incidence of CTD is the same as in the general population. The larger numbers of secondary cases reflect a higher proportion of patients with atherosclerosis (29% vs. 5% in the total Raynaud's population), and to a lesser extent hyperviscosity syndromes secondary to malignancy. Conversely, RP occurring in very young children, though rare, is usually due to an underlying CTD.[54] Other suspicious symptoms that should alert the clinician to the likelihood of secondary RS include the presence of digital ulceration. Digital ulceration does not occur in RD. The recurrence of chilblains in adults may also raise suspicions, as should the occurrence of severe attacks persisting throughout the summer.[55] Furthermore, asymmetrical colour change with fewer digits affected suggests RS rather than RD.[56]

The above clinical symptoms can act as a guide to the future development of CTD and suggest that close monitoring of the patient with repeated observations of nail-fold vessels and immunopathological testing may be of value.

RP is a frequent accompanying symptom of CTDs. In some of these the RP is reported as merely consisting of a biphasic or triphasic colour change with minimal discomfort. In other conditions RP is the most significant symptom, with the patients complaining of pain, ulcers and even gangrene. The likeliest group of patients to be seen by the vascular clinician are those suffering from limited systemic sclerosis. This is because Raynaud's is severe in systemic sclerosis, thus meriting hospital referral. Furthermore, it often predates the other symptoms of connective tissue disease by many years. Thus a high index of suspicion for this particular disorder must be held by those seeing patients as a result of their vasospastic symptomatology. For an in-depth review of the CTDs, readers should consult other specialist texts.

VASCULITIS

Vasculitis is the term used to describe the group of conditions characterised by inflammation within the blood vessel wall and possibly damage to vessel integrity. The vasculitic process may involve only one or many blood vessels and therefore organ systems. In general, the clinical features result in ischaemia of the tissues supplied by the damaged vessel. These symptoms are often accompanied by the constitutional symptoms of fever, weight loss and anorexia that result from widespread inflammation. The vasculitic conditions may have a range of vessel involvement, from a mild obliterative disorder to necrotising vasculitis. **Table 12.1** shows some of the common vasculitides, stratified by the size of the vessel most commonly involved. The classification of vasculitis is confusing as there is considerable clinical overlap between the different vasculitic syndromes and often the cause of the vasculitis is unknown. Because the diagnosis of vasculitis still requires histological confirmation in most cases, the classification based on the size of the

Table 12.1 • Relationship between vasculitis classification and vessel size

Type of vasculitis	Aorta and branches	Large and medium-sized arteries	Medium-sized muscular arteries	Small muscular arteries	Arterioles, capillaries and venules
Takayasu's arteritis	✓				
Buerger's disease (thromboangiitis obliterans)	✓	✓			
Giant cell arteritis (temporal arteritis)	✓	✓			
Polyarteritis nodosa		✓	✓		
Wegener's granulomatosis			✓	✓	
Connective tissue disorders				✓	✓
Rheumatoid vasculitis				✓	✓
Cutaneous vasculitis (leucocytoclastic/allergic)					✓

predominant vessel involved and the type of inflammatory change is most frequently used.

Takayasu's arteritis

This is an inflammatory and obliterative arteritis that primarily affects the large elastic arteries. It affects all levels of the aorta, its branches and the pulmonary arteries. The disorder has a striking female predominance, affecting women five to nine times more frequently than men.[57] It usually presents between 10 and 30 years of age, although case reports of older patients have been published. The disease symptomatology can be divided into two phases: the acute systemic phase (pre-pulseless) and the chronic obliterative (pulseless) phase. The acute symptoms are often non-specific and are those one would expect to see with a generalised inflammatory process and include fatigue and malaise, weight loss and fever. Arthralgia and myalgia are common. The symptoms of the chronic phase are the result of the obliterative arterial lesion and depend on which vessels are affected. Possible findings include diminished or absent arterial pulses, vascular bruits, hypertension, inequality of blood pressure between arms and legs, and abnormalities on auscultation of the heart. Upper limb claudication can occur in association with the reduced or absent upper limb pulses (see Chapter 9).

Laboratory studies in Takayasu's arteritis reflect the inflammatory nature of the disorder. The ESR is elevated in the majority of patients during active disease. Conventional arteriography and magnetic resonance angiography[58] play an important role in the diagnosis of this disease, and the findings can include vessel occlusion and stenosis, aneurysm formation and the development of collaterals around occlusions. All levels of the aorta as well as its major branches may be involved and should be visualised. Pulmonary artery involvement has been seen in up to half of patients with this disorder. Biopsy during the early phase shows granulomatous inflammation with patchy involvement of the vessel wall. Later, the changes are characterised by intimal proliferation and band fibrosis of the adventitia and media.

During the acute inflammatory phase immunosuppression with corticosteroids and/or cyclophosphamide has been found to be effective in halting the angiographic progression.[59] Symptomatic management of the patient is also important and symptoms such as hypertension should be treated aggressively. Therapeutic response is best assessed by improvement in symptoms, a fall in ESR and improvement in serial angiographic studies. Surgery may be required to bypass stenosed or occluded segments of vessels that are producing significant ischaemia.[60]

Buerger's disease (thromboangiitis obliterans)

Buerger's disease is the clinical syndrome characterised by segmental thrombotic occlusions of the small and medium-sized arteries usually of the distal lower limb but occasionally also involving the upper extremities. Buerger's disease usually occurs in young smokers and is frequently associated with both RP and superficial migratory thrombophlebitis. Although previously mainly described in young men, the increased incidence of smoking in women has caused an increase in Buerger's disease in this sex.[61] In a recent review the changing pattern of this disease was recorded, confirming the increased prevalence of Buerger's disease in women.[62] It also documented that older patients (>40 years of age) are being more frequently diagnosed.

In the acute lesion, the internal elastic lamina of the arteries is almost always intact. Thrombus fills the vessel lumen and is hypercellular with an infiltration of lymphocytes, fibroblasts and later giant cells. There is no vessel wall necrosis or vascular wall calcification and atheromatous plaques and aneurysms are both absent. The consistent presence of an acute hypercellular occlusive thrombus is the hallmark of this disease.

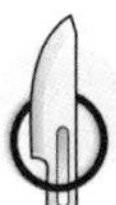

Altered haemorheological parameters have been detected in thromboangiitis obliterans, opening up some new therapeutic avenues.[63]

The symptoms of Buerger's disease are usually related to lower extremity ischaemia and include rest pain and tissue loss. Claudication is a rare symptom, but when present is usually confined to the foot. Femoral or popliteal pulses are usually present but the pedal pulses are absent.[64] The diagnosis of Buerger's disease depends to a great extent on the exclusion of other conditions, particularly early-onset atherosclerosis and immune disorders.

Investigation of the lower limb ischaemia reveals angiographically normal vessels proximal to the popliteal. The tibial and peroneal vessels are frequently normal to a point of sudden occlusion. Tortuous corkscrew collaterals may reconstitute patent segments of the distal tibial or pedal vessels (**Fig. 12.5**).

Tobacco abstinence is the cornerstone of management for Buerger's disease. In patients who do manage to stop smoking the appearance of new lesions and gangrene requiring amputation is unusual.[64] However, persistent smoking leads to continued progression of the disease. Upper limb RP, finger ulceration and gangrene is treated as described earlier (see **Fig. 12.4**). There have been a large number of medical treatments proposed for the treatment of Buerger's disease affecting the lower

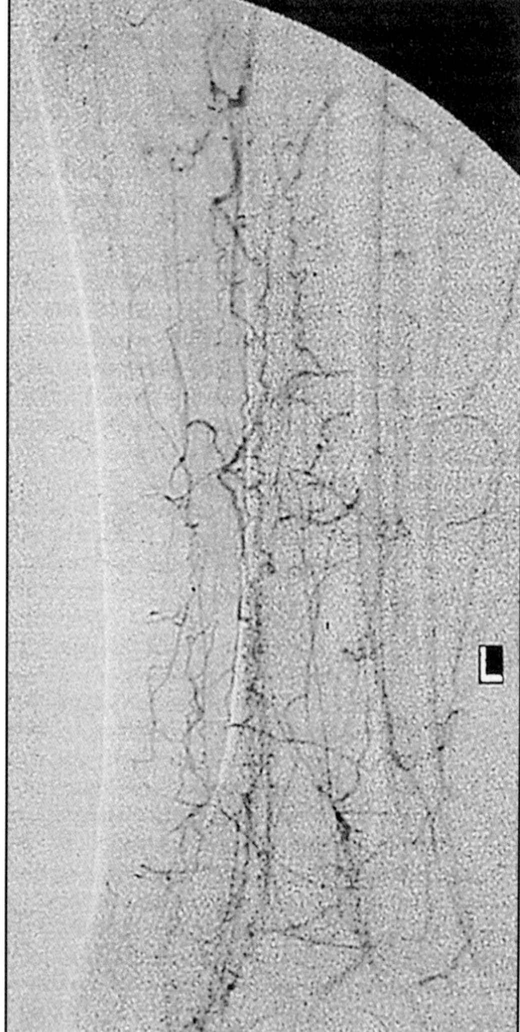

Figure 12.5 • Corkscrew collaterals in Buerger's disease.

limb and the variety of the treatments proposed testifies to the fact that none are completely satisfactory and nearly all lack documentary efficacy. Corticosteroids,[65] antiplatelet therapy and iloprost infusions[66] are just a few of the treatments that have been used. The evidence for corticosteroid therapy is tenuous, while that for the use of iloprost and aspirin-like compounds is more convincing. Further research is required into the benefits of the various medical treatment regimens currently available.

Giant cell arteritis

Giant cell arteritis, or temporal arteritis, is a systemic granulomatous vasculitis that predominantly affects large and medium-sized blood vessels. It usually involves the cranial branches of the aorta. It is most often seen in patients over 50 years of age and is an important preventable cause of blindness. However, it is recognised that temporal arteritis is a disease with many different manifestations and extracranial presentations are not uncommon. Among the vasculitic disorders, temporal arteritis is one of the more commonly occurring disorders though it is still relatively rare. The estimated overall incidence rate in persons older than 50 years of age is approximately 17 per 100 000 annually.[67] There is a three to five times higher incidence in women than in men. The risk of this disease occurring is increased in smokers and patients with already established atherosclerotic disease.[68]

Temporal arteritis may present acutely or insidiously. Although headaches and sudden blindness are the classical symptoms, constitutional symptoms such as fever, weight loss and fatigue may be the earliest manifestations.[69] Headaches are the usual complaint and these may be localised to the area overlying the superficial temporal arteries or may be generalised, resembling tension headaches. Scalp tenderness can also be a prominent feature and this can produce difficulty for the patients when combing their hair or sleeping at night on a pillow. This symptom is secondary to the involvement of the superficial temporal and occipital arteries. Jaw claudication occurs in approximately half of patients with this disease. This results from facial and maxillary artery involvement. Tongue claudication and dysphagia have also been reported and rarely glossitis and tongue necrosis is seen.[70] Sudden visual loss is a consequence of disease in the ophthalmic or posterior ciliary artery. Once blindness is established it is irreversible, but amaurosis fugax, a warning sign of impending blindness, is responsive to steroids. Pulmonary, renal and neurological symptomatology have also been reported as has synovitis, but cutaneous or limb vessel manifestations are rare. This disease is therefore unlikely to present to the vascular clinician.

The diagnosis of temporal arteritis is made by finding an elevated acute-phase response such as the ESR. However, it should be noted that the ESR is not necessarily always elevated in patients with this disorder. The diagnostic hallmark of temporal arteritis is a biopsy that shows granulomatous inflammation (**Fig. 12.6**). Because of the intermittent or skip pattern of the lesions, biopsy can be negative in 50% of cases. Thus a negative biopsy in the setting of a high suspicion for the disease does not rule out the disease and should not preclude steroid therapy. On occasions a trial of steroid therapy can in itself be used to make the diagnosis. Corticosteroids are the mainstay of treatment. This therapy is efficacious in preventing but not reversing blindness.[71]

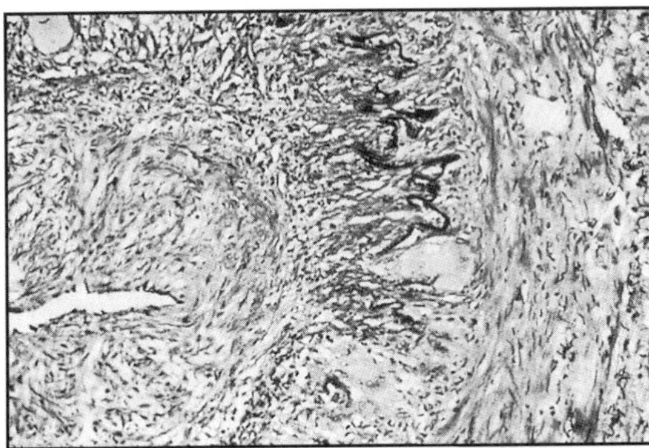

Figure 12.6 • Temporal artery biopsy demonstrating granulomatous inflammation and disruption of the internal elastic lamina.

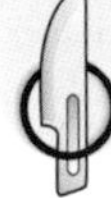

In studies of cytotoxic agents, methotrexate has been used as a corticosteroid-sparing drug in patients with polymyalgia rheumatica and giant cell arteritis, with conflicting results.[72,73] However, this drug may be tried in patients who are taking high doses of corticosteroids to control active disease and who have serious adverse effects from the steroids. Subjects with a raised platelet count are at higher risk of visual loss and should be treated effectively.[74] ESR/plasma viscosity and C-reactive protein (CRP) are generally used to monitor disease activity but anticardiolipin antibodies if present may also be of benefit if there is confounding pathology that will increase ESR/CRP (e.g. infection).[75] Levels of interleukin (IL)-6 may be a sensitive indicator of active disease in polymyalgia rheumatica;[76] however, a recent paper suggests that in GCA, subjects with a raised titre of IL-6 may in fact be at lower risk of ischaemic events.[77] Calcium and vitamin D supplementation should be given with corticosteroid therapy in all patients. In patients with reduced bone mineral density, bisphosphonates are recommended.[78]

Polyarteritis nodosa

Polyarteritis nodosa (PAN) is a unique process characterised by a systemic necrotising vasculitis involving the small and medium-sized muscular arteries. The prevalence of PAN ranges between 5 and 77 per million population, with the higher incidence being reported in hepatitis B hyperendemic populations.[79] PAN is twice as common in men than women and the average age of diagnosis is between 40 and 60 years, although PAN has been seen in both children and the elderly.

The symptoms reported depend on the vessels affected. The presenting symptoms are often constitutional, such as malaise, abdominal pain, weight loss, fever and myalgia. Organ involvement can occur at the same time or may develop later in the disease process. Renal disease with proteinuria and progressive renal failure occurs in about 70% of patients.[80] Hypertension is a frequent finding. Gastrointestinal involvement is common and manifests as abdominal pain, nausea and vomiting. Acute events such as infarction of the bowel, perforation and haemorrhage are rare but produce the high mortality associated with this condition. Skin manifestations include nail-fold infarcts (**Fig. 12.7**), palpable purpura and livedo reticularis (**Fig. 12.8**). Damage to the blood vessel wall can result in aneurysm formation. Mononeuritis multiplex is common and other important sites of involvement include the retina and testes. Laboratory findings can be non-specific, making the diagnosis difficult, but include anaemia, elevated ESR and a positive test for antineutrophil cytoplasmic antibody (ANCA). Hepatitis B surface antigen and antibodies should be measured in all patients with PAN. Angiography may be diagnostic, showing the characteristic findings of saccular or fusiform aneurysms and arterial

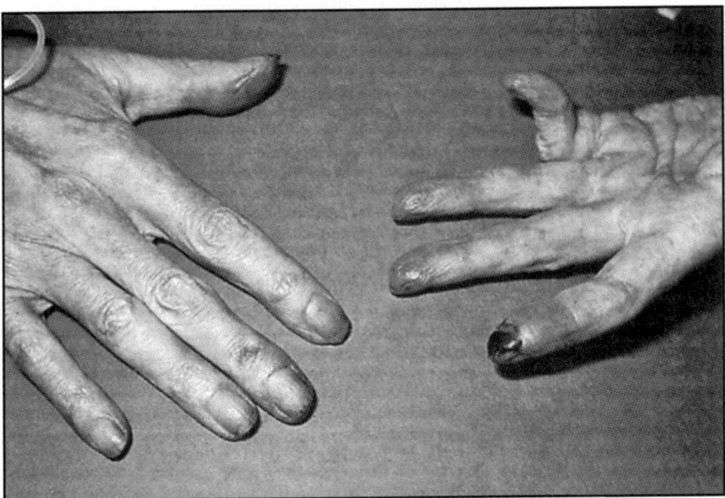

Figure 12.7 • Digital infarct in polyarteritis nodosa.

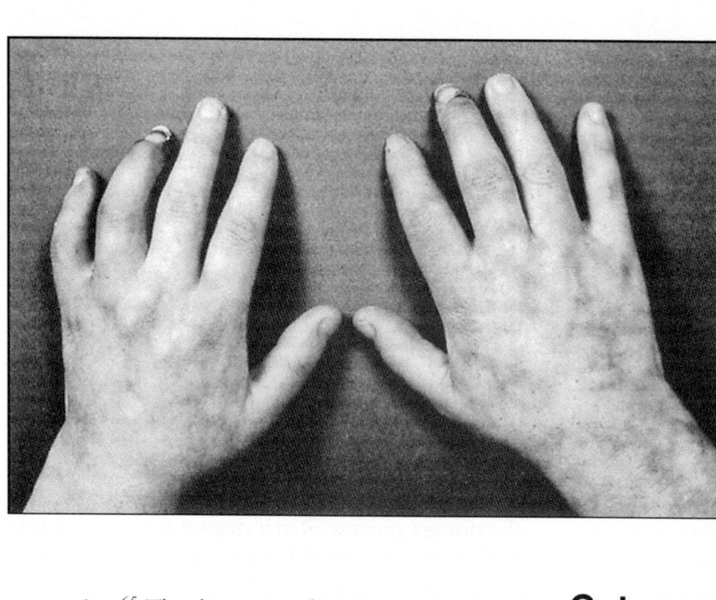

Figure 12.8 • Livedo reticularis in polyarteritis nodosa.

narrowing.[65] The diagnosis of PAN must be based on the demonstration of vasculitis by angiography or biopsy.

Corticosteroids are the cornerstone of treatment and cyclophosphamide can be added if the disease proves difficult to control.

Wegener's granulomatosis

Wegener's granulomatosis is a form of vasculitis that involves mainly the medium and small arteries and veins of the upper and lower respiratory tract and kidneys. Although it is a systemic necrotising granulomatous vasculitis, it is classically associated with the triad of upper respiratory tract, lung and kidney involvement. The manifestations and severity of the disease at presentation are variable but cutaneous vascular symptoms tend to be less frequently seen.[81] These consist of cutaneous ulceration, subcutaneous nodules and palpable purpura.

Laboratory findings show an inflammatory response. Sinus radiographs or computed tomography may show evidence of mucosal thickening, sinus opacification or air–fluid levels. Chest radiography may also be abnormal. Diagnosis is made through biopsy. The finding of elevated blood c-ANCA levels is strongly associated with Wegener's granulomatosis and these should be measured in cases of clinical suspicion.

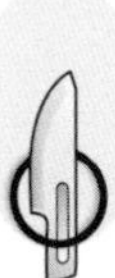

Circulating endothelial cells may be a novel marker of active ANCA-associated small-vessel vasculitis. The clinical use of this tool and the pathogenic mechanisms leading to these findings require further investigation.[82]

Treatment is with immunosuppressants.

Cutaneous vasculitis/ small-vessel vasculitis

The vessels primarily involved in small-vessel vasculitis are the postcapillary venules, although capillaries and arterioles may also be involved. When first described, small-vessel vasculitis was named hypersensitivity angiitis.[83] At one time, small-vessel vasculitis was thought to be identical to the microscopic form of PAN. However, the latter affects mainly small arteries and arterioles rather than venules. **Box 12.4** lists the clinical syndromes associated with cutaneous vasculitis.

Box 12.4 • Clinical syndromes of cutaneous vasculitis

Idiopathic cutaneous vasculitis
Necrotising vasculitis secondary to
Drugs, e.g. antibiotics, diuretics, NSAIDs, anticonvulsants
Infection, e.g. upper respiratory tract virus, *Streptococcus*, hepatitis B, HIV
Immunological disorders, e.g. connective tissue diseases
Cutaneous vasculitis as a manifestation of systemic disease
Connective tissue disease
Mixed cryoglobulinaemia
Allergic granulomatosis (Churg–Strauss syndrome)
Behçet's disease

HIV, human immunodeficiency virus; NSAIDs, non-steroidal anti-inflammatory drugs.

IDIOPATHIC CUTANEOUS VASCULITIS

This is the most common form of vasculitis in the skin.[84] It is usually manifest by palpable purpura most commonly occurring in the lower limb, often below the knee. The involvement of the lower limb tends to be symmetrical and is worsened by periods of sitting or standing. The lesions occur in crops, initially appearing as macular erythema and then progressing to purpura. Uncommonly, this type of vasculitis can present as urticaria and it can be distinguished from typical urticaria by the fact that the lesions persist for more than 24 hours. Biopsies of the lesion shows leucocytoclastic vasculitis with endothelial cell swelling, often necrosis as well as haemorrhage, fibrin deposition and infiltration with polymorphonuclear neutrophils.

NECROTISING VASCULITIS ASSOCIATED WITH INFECTIONS, DRUGS OR CTD

The aetiology of this form of vasculitis is presumed to be hypersensitivity to various factors, including infective agents and drugs, or underlying systemic disease. Nevertheless, in approximately half the cases no definitive precipitating agent can be found.[83] Infection is associated with cutaneous necrotising vasculitis in approximately 10% of cases. Most often these are viruses associated with the upper respiratory tract and cause vasculitis such as Henoch–Schönlein purpura, although bacterial organisms have also been found capable of inducing a hypersensitivity vasculitis. The most commonly implicated drugs are antibiotics, particularly penicillin and sulphonamides. Diuretics and non-steroidal anti-inflammatory drugs (NSAIDs) have also been linked to the condition. Leucocytoclastic vasculitis may also be associated with a number of immunological disorders with systemic manifestations; most commonly these are of the CTD type.

CUTANEOUS VASCULITIS AS A MANIFESTATION OF SYSTEMIC DISEASE

Small-vessel vasculitis affecting the skin may be a manifestation of underlying systemic disease. The most common diseases in this category are the CTDs, particularly systemic lupus erythematosus but also mixed cryoglobulinaemia. The clinical and histological appearances of this type of vasculitis are often indistinguishable from those of the lesions of idiopathic cutaneous vasculitis. It is of crucial importance to examine any patient with skin vasculitis in a thorough fashion, focusing on the potential for the presence of CTD.

Another systemic disease associated with cutaneous vasculitis is Churg–Strauss vasculitis. The most common type of skin manifestation appears mainly in the extremities and is maculopapular in appearance. It may be accompanied by vesicles and occasionally by bullae. Behçet's disease, which is characterised by oral and genital ulceration, may also present with a variety of non-specific skin changes including papules, vesicles, pyoderma and erythema nodosum-like lesions. Most patients with small-vessel vasculitis have disease limited to the skin.[83] Investigation of these patients should be aimed at confirming the diagnosis by biopsy and then elucidating potential aetiological agents or underlying systemic disorder.

Most patients with small-vessel vasculitis limited to the skin experience a single episode that is often short-lived and associated with minimal symptomatology. Therapy for these individuals may not be required or may be limited to the use of antihistamines or NSAIDs. However, for individuals with more severe or recurrent episodes, treatment with corticosteroids may have to be considered.

Conclusion

Vasculitis will present to the vascular clinician as skin ischaemia. The predilection of a number of vasculitic disorders for the lower limb may mimic large-vessel disease or emboli. The cornerstone of diagnosis is the finding of an acute-phase response, e.g. elevated ESR, plasma viscosity and CRP levels. Screening for autoantibodies may be helpful, but diagnosis is often only made by analysis of biopsy material and this should be considered in all cases of vasculitis, unless the tissue is too ischaemic to sustain wound healing.

Key points

- Raynaud's phenomenon should be classified appropriately into primary Raynaud's disease and secondary Raynaud's syndrome. Management includes general measures, drugs, sympathectomy and attention to any underlying disease.
- Vasculitis may present to the vascular clinician as skin ischaemia. Constitutional symptoms of fever, weight loss and fatigue are often clues to the diagnosis. Key investigations are ESR/plasma viscosity, CRP, autoantibodies and biopsy. Immunosuppression is the cornerstone of treatment of vasculitis.

REFERENCES

1. Raynaud MD. Asphyxre et de la gangrene symetriques des extremities. Paris, 1862. (Trans. Thomas Barlow, London, New Sydenham Society, 1988.)
2. Brotzu G, Falchi S, Mannu B et al. The importance of presynaptic beta receptors in Raynaud's disease. J Vasc Surg 1989; 9:767–71.
3. Baron M, Feiglin D, Hyland R et al. ^{67}Gallium lung scans in progressive systemic sclerosis. Arthritis Rheum 1983; 26:969–74.
4. Belch JJ, Land D, Park RH et al. Decreased oesophageal blood flow in patients with Raynaud's phenomenon. Br J Rheumatol 1988; 27:426–30.
5. Kahan A, Devaux JY, Amor B et al. Nifedipine and thallium-201 myocardial perfusion in progressive systemic sclerosis. N Engl J Med 1986; 314:1397–402.
6. de Trafford JC, Lafferty K, Potter CE et al. An epidemiological survey of Raynaud's phenomenon. Eur J Vasc Surg 1988; 2:167–70.
7. Olsen N, Nielsen SL. Prevalence of primary Raynaud phenomena in young females. Scand J Clin Lab Invest 1978; 38:761–4.
8. Porter JM, Bardana EJ Jr, Baur GM et al. The clinical significance of Raynaud's syndrome. Surgery 1976; 80:756–64.
9. Smyth AE, Hughes AE, Bruce IN et al. A case–control study of candidate vasoactive mediator genes in primary Raynaud's phenomenon. Rheumatology (Oxford) 1999; 38:1094–8.
10. Tan FK, Arnett FC. Genetic factors in the etiology of systemic sclerosis and Raynaud phenomenon. Curr Opin Rheumatol 2000; 12:511–19.
11. Porter JM, Rivers SP, Anderson CJ et al. Evaluation and management of patients with Raynaud's syndrome. Am J Surg 1981; 142:183–9.
12. Kallenberg CG, Wouda AA, The TH. Systemic involvement and immunologic findings in patients presenting with Raynaud's phenomenon. Am J Med 1980; 69:675–80.
13. Allen EV, Brown GE. Raynaud's disease: a critical review of minimal requisites for diagnosis. Am J Med Sci 1932; 183:187–200.
14. Taylor W. The hand–arm vibration syndrome: diagnosis, assessment and objective tests. A review. J R Soc Med 1993; 86:101–3.
15. Letz R, Cherniack MG, Gerr F et al. A cross sectional epidemiological survey of shipyard workers exposed to hand–arm vibration. Br J Ind Med 1992; 49:53–62.
16. Mirbod SM, Yoshida H, Nagata C et al. Hand–arm vibration syndrome and its prevalence in the present status of private forestry enterprises in Japan. Int Arch Occup Environ Health 1992; 64:93–9.
17. Koskimies K, Pyykko I, Starck J et al. Vibration syndrome among Finnish forest workers between 1972 and 1990. Int Arch Occup Environ Health 1992; 64:251–6.
18. Hedlund U. Raynaud's phenomenon of fingers and toes of miners exposed to local and whole-body vibration and cold. Int Arch Occup Environ Health 1989; 61:457–61.
19. Kennedy G, Khan F, McLaren M et al. Endothelial activation and response in patients with hand arm vibration syndrome. Eur J Clin Invest 1999; 29:577–81.
20. Taylor W, Pelmear PL. The hand–arm vibration syndrome: an update. Br J Ind Med 1990; 47:577–9.
21. Benefits Agency (Department of Social Security). If you have an industrial disease. NI 2 August 1995; p. 2–4.
22. Freedman RR, Sabharal SC, Desai N et al. Increased alpha-adrenergic responsiveness in idiopathic Raynaud's disease. Arthritis Rheum 1989; 32:61–5.
23. Olsen N, Petring OU. Vibration elicited vaso-constrictor reflex in Raynaud's phenomena. Br J Ind Med 1988; 45:415–19.
24. Carter SA, Dean E, Kroeger EA. Apparent finger systolic pressures during cooling in patients with Raynaud's syndrome. Circulation 1988; 77:988–96.
25. Lau CS, O'Dowd A, Belch JJ. White blood cell activation in Raynaud's phenomenon of systemic sclerosis and vibration induced white finger syndrome. Ann Rheum Dis 1992; 51:249–52.
26. Lau CS, Bridges AB, Muir A et al. Further evidence of increased polymorphonuclear cell activity in patients with Raynaud's phenomenon. Br J Rheumatol 1992; 31:375–80.
27. Belch JJ, Drury J, McLaughlin K et al. Abnormal biochemical and cellular parameters in the blood of patients with Raynaud's phenomenon. Scott Med J 1987; 32:12–14.
28. Belch JJ, Zoma AA, Richards IM et al. Vascular damage and factor-VIII-related antigen in the rheumatic diseases. Rheumatol Int 1987; 7:107–11.
29. Belch JJ, McLaren M, Anderson J et al. Increased prostacyclin metabolites and decreased red cell deformability in patients with systemic sclerosis and Raynaud's syndrome. Prostaglandins Leukot Med 1985; 18:401–2.
30. Belch JJ, O'Dowd A, Forbes CD et al. Platelet sensitivity to a prostacyclin analogue in systemic sclerosis. Br J Rheumatol 1985; 24:346–50.
31. Zamora MR, O'Brien RF, Rutherford RB et al. Serum endothelin-1 concentrations and cold provocation in primary Raynaud's phenomenon. Lancet 1990; 336:1144–7.
32. Kahaleh B, Fan PS, Matucci-Cerinic M et al. Study of endothelial dependent relaxation in scleroderma (abstract). Am Coll Rheum 1993; B233:S180.

33. Khan F, Belch JJ. Skin blood flow in patients with systemic sclerosis and Raynaud's phenomenon: effects of oral L-arginine supplementation. J Rheumatol 1999; 26:2389–94.

34. Nakamura H, Matsuzaki I, Hatta K et al. Blood endothelin-1 and cold-induced vasodilation in patients with primary Raynaud's phenomenon and workers with vibration-induced white finger. Int Angiol 2003; 22:243–9.

35. Kurozawa Y, Nasu Y. Circulating adhesion molecules in patients with vibration-induced white finger. Angiology 2000; 51:1003–6.

36. Lau CS. Haemostatic abnormalities in Raynaud's phenomenon and the potential for treatment with manipulation of the arachidonic acid pathway. MD thesis, University of Dundee, 1993.

37. Lafferty K, De Trafford JC, Potter C et al. Reflex vascular responses in the finger to contralateral thermal stimuli during the normal menstrual cycle: a hormonal basis to Raynaud's phenomenon? Clin Sci 1985; 68:639–45.

38. Cutolo M, Sulli A, Pizzorni C et al. Nailfold videocapillaroscopy assessment of microvascular damage in systemic sclerosis. J Rheumatol 2000; 27:155–60.

39. Malamet R, Wise RA, Ettinger WH et al. Nifedipine in the treatment of Raynaud's phenomenon. Evidence for inhibition of platelet activation. Am J Med 1985; 78:602–8.

40. Maricq HR, Jennings JR, Valter I et al. Evaluation of treatment efficacy of Raynaud phenomenon by digital blood pressure response to cooling. Raynaud's Treatment Study Investigators. Vasc Med 2000; 5:135–40.

41. La Civita L, Pitaro N, Rossi M et al. Amlodipine in the treatment of Raynaud's phenomenon. Br J Rheumatol 1993; 32:524–5.

42. Rhedda A, McCans J, Willan AR et al. A double blind placebo controlled crossover randomized trial of diltiazem in Raynaud's phenomenon. J Rheumatol 1985; 12:724–7.

43. Leppert J, Jonasson T, Nilsson H et al. The effect of isradipine, a new calcium-channel antagonist, in patients with primary Raynaud's phenomenon: a single-blind dose–response study. Cardiovasc Drugs Ther 1989; 3:397–401.

44. Saniabadi AR, Lowe GD, Belch JJ et al. The novel effect of a new prostacyclin analogue ZK36374 on the aggregation of human platelets in whole blood. Thromb Haemost 1983; 50:718–21.

45. Belch JJ, Capell HA, Cooke ED et al. Oral iloprost as a treatment for Raynaud's syndrome: a double blind multicentre placebo controlled study. Ann Rheum Dis 1995; 54:197–200.

46. Murai C, Sasaki T, Osaki H et al. Oral limaprost for Raynaud's phenomenon. Lancet 1989; ii:1218.

47. Vayssairat M. Preventive effect of an oral prostacyclin analog, beraprost sodium, on digital necrosis in systemic sclerosis. French Microcirculation Society Multicenter Group for the Study of Vascular Acrosyndromes. J Rheumatol 1999; 26:2173–8.

48. Rosenkranz S, Diet F, Karasch T et al. Sildenafil improved pulmonary hypertension and peripheral blood flow in a patient with scleroderma-associated lung fibrosis and the Raynaud phenomenon. Ann Intern Med 2003; 139:871–3.

49. Muir AH, Robb R, McLaren M et al. The use of Ginkgo biloba in Raynaud's disease: a double-blind placebo-controlled trial. Vasc Med 2002; 7:265–7.

An interesting pilot study needing confirmation in larger studies.

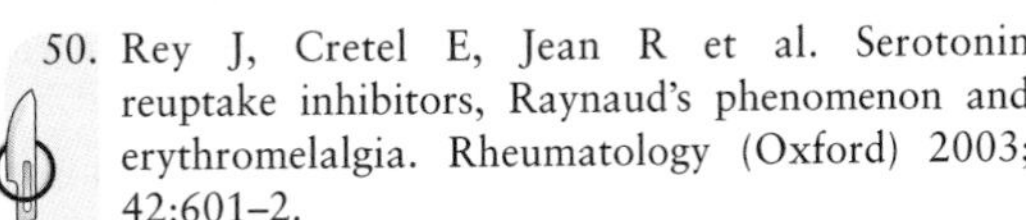

50. Rey J, Cretel E, Jean R et al. Serotonin reuptake inhibitors, Raynaud's phenomenon and erythromelalgia. Rheumatology (Oxford) 2003; 42:601–2.

51. Belch JJ. Raynaud's phenomenon: its relevance to scleroderma. Ann Rheum Dis 1991; 50(suppl. 4): 839–45.

52. Kallenberg CG. Early detection of connective tissue disease in patients with Raynaud's phenomenon. Rheum Dis Clin North Am 1990; 16:11–30.

53. Friedman EI, Taylor LM Jr, Porter JM. Late-onset Raynaud's syndrome: diagnostic and therapeutic considerations. Geriatrics 1988; 43:59–63, 67–70.

54. Duffy CM, Laxer RM, Lee P et al. Raynaud syndrome in childhood. J Pediatr 1989; 114:73–8.

55. Franceschini F, Calzavara-Pinton P, Valsecchi L et al. Chilblain lupus erythematosus is associated with antibodies to SSA/Ro. Adv Exp Med Biol 1999; 455:167–71.

56. Cardelli MB, Kleinsmith DM. Raynaud's phenomenon and disease. Med Clin North Am 1989; 73:1127–41.

57. Cupps TR, Fauci AS. The vasculitides. Philadelphia: WB Saunders, 1981.

58. Choe YH, Han BK, Koh EM et al. Takayasu's arteritis: assessment of disease activity with contrast-enhanced MR imaging. Am J Roentgenol 2000; 175:505–11.

59. Haynes BF, Allen NB, Fauci AS. Diagnostic and therapeutic approach to the patient with vasculitis. Med Clin North Am 1986; 70:355–68.

60. Giordano JM. Surgical treatment of Takayasu's arteritis. Int J Cardiol 2000; 75(suppl. 1): S123–S128.

61. Lie JT. The Canadian Rheumatism Association, 1991 Dunlop-Dottridge Lecture. Vasculitis, 1815 to 1991: classification and diagnostic specificity. J Rheumatol 1992; 19:83–9.

62. Stvrtinova V, Ambrozy E, Stvrtina S et al. 90 years of Buerger's disease: what has changed? Bratisl Lek Listy 1999; 100:123–8.

63. Bozkurt AK, Koksal C, Ercan M. The altered hemorheologic parameters in thromboangiitis obliterans: a new insight. Clin Appl Thromb Hemost 2004; 10:45–50.

64. Mills JL, Porter JM. Thromboangiitis obliterans (Buerger's disease). In: Churg A, Churg I (eds) Systemic vasculitides. New York, Tokyo: Igaku-Shoin, 1991; pp. 229–39.

65. Cupps TR, Fauci AS. Thromboangiitis obliterans (Buerger's disease, endarteritis obliterans). In: The vasculitides. Philadelphia: WB Saunders, 1981; pp. 133–6.

66. Fiessinger JN, Schafer M. Trial of iloprost versus aspirin treatment for critical limb ischaemia of thromboangiitis obliterans. The TAO Study. Lancet 1990; 335:555–7.

67. Rao JK, Allen NB. Polymyalgia rheumatica and giant cell arteritis. In: Belch JJF, Zurier RB (eds) Connective tissue diseases. London: Chapman & Hall Medical, 1995; pp. 249–70.

68. Machado EB, Gabriel SE, Beard CM et al. A population-based case–control study of temporal arteritis: evidence for an association between temporal arteritis and degenerative vascular disease? Int J Epidemiol 1989; 18:836–41.

69. Goodman BW, Jr. Temporal arteritis. Am J Med 1979; 67:839–52.

70. Sonnenblick M, Nesher G, Rosin A. Nonclassical organ involvement in temporal arteritis. Semin Arthritis Rheum 1989; 19:183–90.

71. Kyle V, Hazelman BL. Stopping steroids in polymyalgia rheumatica and giant cell arteritis. Br Med J 1990; 300:344–5.

72. Hoffman GS, Cid MC, Hellmann DB et al. A multicenter, randomized, double-blind, placebo-controlled trial of adjuvant methotrexate treatment for giant cell arteritis. Arthritis Rheum 2002; 46:1309–18.

73. Jover JA, Hernandez-Garcia C, Morado IC et al. Combined treatment of giant-cell arteritis with methotrexate and prednisone. a randomized, double-blind, placebo-controlled trial. Ann Intern Med 2001; 134:106–14.

74. Liozon E, Herrmann F, Ly K et al. Risk factors for visual loss in giant cell (temporal) arteritis: a prospective study of 174 patients. Am J Med 2001; 111:211–17.

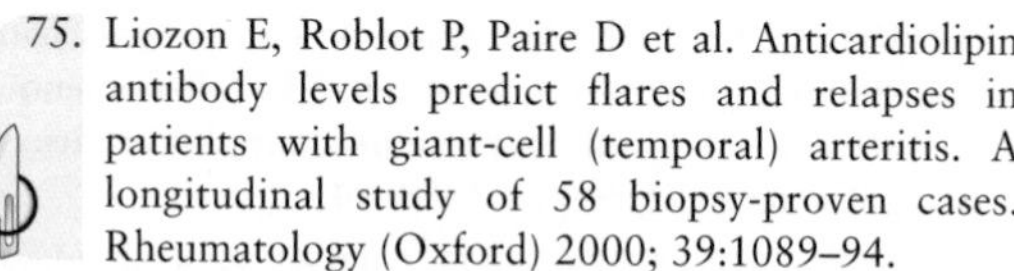

75. Liozon E, Roblot P, Paire D et al. Anticardiolipin antibody levels predict flares and relapses in patients with giant-cell (temporal) arteritis. A longitudinal study of 58 biopsy-proven cases. Rheumatology (Oxford) 2000; 39:1089–94.

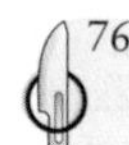

76. Weyand CM, Fulbright JW, Evans JM et al. Corticosteroid requirements in polymyalgia rheumatica. Arch Intern Med 1999; 159:577–584.

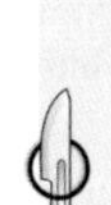

77. Hernandez-Rodriguez J, Segarra M, Vilardell C et al. Elevated production of interleukin-6 is associated with a lower incidence of disease-related ischemic events in patients with giant-cell arteritis: angiogenic activity of interleukin-6 as a potential protective mechanism. Circulation 2003; 107:2428–34.

A prospective pilot study that correlated increased IL-6 levels to in vitro angiogenic activity. Results need to be confirmed in larger studies.

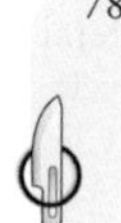

78. American College of Rheumatology Ad Hoc Committee on Glucocorticoid-induced Osteoporosis. Recommendations for the prevention and treatment of glucocorticoid-induced osteoporosis: 2001 update. Arthritis Rheum 2001; 44:1496–503.

79. McMahon BJ, Heyward WL, Templin DW et al. Hepatitis B-associated polyarteritis nodosa in Alaskan Eskimos: clinical and epidemiologic features and long-term follow-up. Hepatology 1989; 9:97–101.

80. Conn DL. Polyarteritis. Rheum Dis Clin North Am 1990; 16:341–62.

81. Langford CA, McCallum RM. Idiopathic vasculitis. In: Belch JJF, Zurier RB (eds) Connective tissue diseases. London: Chapman & Hall Medical, 1995; pp. 179–217.

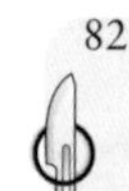

82. Woywodt A, Streiber F, de Groot K et al. Circulating endothelial cells as markers for ANCA-associated small-vessel vasculitis. Lancet 2003; 361:206–10.

This novel prospective case–control study may prove to be a landmark study. It is one of the few studies demonstrating a link between endothelial cells and vascular disease. Further work in this area will determine the clinical validity and usefulness of this measure. Patients with vasculitis had a dramatically raised endothelial cell count compared with healthy controls and the cell count reduced as the vasculitis was treated.

83. Swerlick RA, Lawley TJ. Cutaneous vasculitis: its relationship to systemic disease. Med Clin North Am 1989; 73:1221–35.

84. Sanchez NP, Van Hale HM, Su WP. Clinical and histopathologic spectrum of necrotizing vasculitis. Report of findings in 101 cases. Arch Dermatol 1985; 121:220–4.

CHAPTER

Thirteen

Peripheral and abdominal aortic aneurysms

Michael Murphy, Richard McWilliams and Peter L. Harris

DEFINITION OF AN ANEURYSM

Defining an aneurysm as a focal arterial dilatation based upon absolute measurements of diameter is problematical, given the natural increase in diameter with age, and variation between the sexes. For an elderly male, the upper limit of the normal range of abdominal aortic diameter is said to be 3 cm, whereas for a woman it is probably 2.5 cm or less. Therefore, the ratio between the maximum diameter of the aneurysmal artery and that of the non-dilated vessel is probably more meaningful. Thus, a good working definition of an aneurysm is a localised dilatation of an artery with an increase in diameter of 50% or more than that of the non-dilated adjacent vessel.[1] The fact that the risk of small aneurysms rupturing is higher in women, who have smaller arteries than men, adds credence to a definition based on diameter ratios rather than absolute measurements.[2]

PREVALENCE OF ARTERIAL ANEURYSMS

Large-scale population screening studies provide evidence about the true prevalence of abdominal aortic aneurysm (AAA).[3–6] The prevalence of this condition has increased dramatically over the last four decades and this trend appears to be continuing.[7] Age-standardised death rates from arterial aneurysms have apparently increased 20-fold during this period.[8]

Population screening studies undertaken in the UK indicate that the prevalence of AAA increases with age.[6,9] In men over the age of 65, the prevalence is approximately 7–8%.[9,10] The prevalence is six times higher in men than in women,[11] and in women the aneurysms tend to occur one decade later in their lives. In men, rupture of an AAA is the seventh most common cause of death in the UK.

There is considerably less information about the prevalence of peripheral aneurysms, although it is recognised that these frequently occur in association with AAAs. Approximately 25% of patients with AAA have coexisting femoral[12] or popliteal aneurysms. It is likely therefore that peripheral true aneurysms share a common aetiology with AAA and that changes in their prevalence match those of aortic aneurysms.

PATHOGENESIS OF AORTIC ANEURYSMS

In comparison with a non-aneurysmal artery, the wall of an aneurysm contains considerably less elastin, with fragmentation or complete disruption of the elastic lamina and a considerable increase in collagen. These changes within the connective tissue are associated with loss of smooth muscle cells within the media and widespread inflammatory infiltration.[13]

The loss of elastin from the wall of arterial aneurysms has been related to increased proteolytic activity.[14] Elevated levels of matrix metalloproteinases have been identified in the serum of patients with AAA and within the wall of the aneurysm itself.[14–18] The distribution of matrix metalloproteinases within the wall appears to be extremely heterogeneous, with relative 'hotspots'.[19] Prostaglandins and proteolytic enzymes released from infiltrating leucocytes may also contribute to elastolysis, and leucocytes also secrete growth factors that stimulate angiogenesis and chemotaxis within the wall.[20–23]

There is strong evidence to indicate a genetic basis for the pathogenesis of aneurysmal disease. Aneurysms occur in Marfan's syndrome and Ehlers–Danlos type 4 disease, both of which are inherited disorders. It has been recognised for many years that there is a subset of younger patients with aneurysms who lack the stigmata of these diseases, though there is a very strong familial association, and who have disorders of aortic connective tissue similar to that found in patients with Marfan's syndrome. The prevalence of AAA in the siblings of patients with a known aneurysm is approximately four times greater than that in individuals with no known family history of this condition. Two independent studies used segregation analysis to examine multigenerational aneurysm pedigrees and concluded that inheritance may be due to a single identifiable locus.[24,25] However, no single gene has yet been identified as causing arterial aneurysms.

Coggon et al.[26] demonstrated an inverse relationship between the decreasing prevalence of peripheral vascular disease and the increasing prevalence of aortic aneurysms. Most epidemiological evidence now suggests that atherosclerosis and arterial aneurysms arise from differing processes. Baxter et al.[27] have reported that extracellular matrix abnormalities are identifiable in non-aneurysmal arterial wall of patients with AAA.

In approximately 15% of AAAs the wall becomes densely thickened, often to a depth of 1 cm or more, due to the deposition of massive amounts of collagen and dense inflammatory infiltrate. Externally, this thickening gives rise to a white glistening appearance variously described as 'ivory' and 'sugar icing' aneurysms. This process involves the peritonealised surface of the aneurysm only and never extends beyond the limits of the aneurysm itself. The term 'inflammatory aneurysm' has been applied to lesions showing this appearance.[28] The 'fibrous' plaques may involve adjacent structures, particularly the duodenum and the ureters, resulting in ureteric obstruction. The histological appearance of the 'fibrous' plaques of inflammatory aneurysms is identical to that of retroperitoneal fibrosis, which may occur without an aneurysm. Both conditions display clinical, biochemical and immunological features of autoimmune disease.

Some arterial aneurysms clearly result from infections. Syphilitic aneurysms have been consigned to history and the most common infective organism is now *Salmonella typhi*.[29,30] Most *Salmonella* aneurysms occur in the aorta and typically develop some 6–8 weeks following symptoms of gastrointestinal infection. Mycotic aneurysms sometimes occur as a result of staphylococcal infections, particularly in association with subacute bacterial endocarditis. Aneurysms of infective aetiology appear to be a well-defined and discrete entity. However, culture of thrombus acquired from apparently non-infected aneurysms yields organisms in approximately one-third of cases[31] and, occasionally, typical fusiform AAAs are found to be grossly infected. This raises the possibility that infection may play a more significant role in the pathogenesis of arterial aneurysms than has previously been considered to be the case. Although *Chlamydia* has been isolated from atherosclerotic plaques responsible for occlusive arterial disease,[32,33] the organism has not been reported in association with aneurysms.

In summary, there is strong evidence to support a genetic predisposition to the development of aneurysmal disease but the exact pathogenesis of aneurysm remains speculative, with varying degrees of evidence to support atherosclerotic, proteolytic, autoimmune and infective mechanisms that may not be mutually exclusive.

INFRARENAL ABDOMINAL AORTIC ANEURYSMS

The majority of AAAs remain asymptomatic until the point of rupture. Approximately 75% are symptom-free when first diagnosed. Most of these are detected as an incidental finding during the course of investigation of unrelated symptoms, for example backache or urinary symptoms. Occasionally, patients do present with a pulsatile mass that they themselves have detected.

If an aneurysm should present with chronic abdominal pain with tenderness over the aneurysm and no evidence of circulatory collapse, an inflammatory aneurysm should be suspected. Peripheral embolisation is a rare mode of presentation of an AAA. However, this diagnosis should be suspected in a patient who presents with acute embolic arterial occlusion in the lower limb in the absence of a cardiac source of an embolus.

Rupture of an AAA is a sudden catastrophic event with severe abdominal and/or back pain with circulatory collapse. Frequently, rupture occurs into the retroperitoneal space and bleeding may be arrested by a combination of hypotension and tamponade within this space. Although transient and unstable, this circumstance does provide an opportunity for emergency life-saving surgery. Free rupture into the peritoneal cavity is rapidly fatal.

Approximately 75% of patients with ruptured aneurysms die before reaching hospital.

The clinical diagnosis of ruptured AAA is usually made on the basis of a classical triad of severe abdominal or back pain of sudden onset, hypovolaemic shock and a pulsatile abdominal mass. However, it is not always possible to palpate the aneurysm, particularly in obese hypotensive patients. The differential diagnosis in these patients includes massive myocardial infarction and acute pancreatitis. Rarely, an aortic aneurysm will rupture or erode into the inferior vena cava (**Fig. 13.1**).[34] Patients with an aorto-caval fistula develop high-output heart failure. A loud machinery murmur will usually be audible within the abdomen. Aorto-intestinal fistulas are more common following previous aortic repair with a prosthetic graft. Primary and secondary aorto-intestinal fistulas may present with sudden massive blood loss via the intestinal tract, but this dramatic event is often presaged by smaller 'sentinel' bleeds.

Population screening

Given that (i) the majority of AAAs remain asymptomatic until the point of rupture, (ii) 75% of patients with rupture die without reaching hospital and (iii) elective surgical treatment of AAA is effective, then population screening for AAA is an attractive proposition.

B-mode ultrasound scanning using portable equipment has been shown to be effective in detecting AAA and is inexpensive.[35,36] Studies undertaken in the UK in the late 1980s mostly concentrated on males over 60 years of age. In this population, it has been reported that 8% of patients have an aortic diameter in excess of 3 cm and 2.5% have an aneurysm greater than 4 cm.[9,37,38] It has been estimated that a single ultrasound scan in males of 65 years of age would detect 90% of aneurysms at risk of rupture.[39]

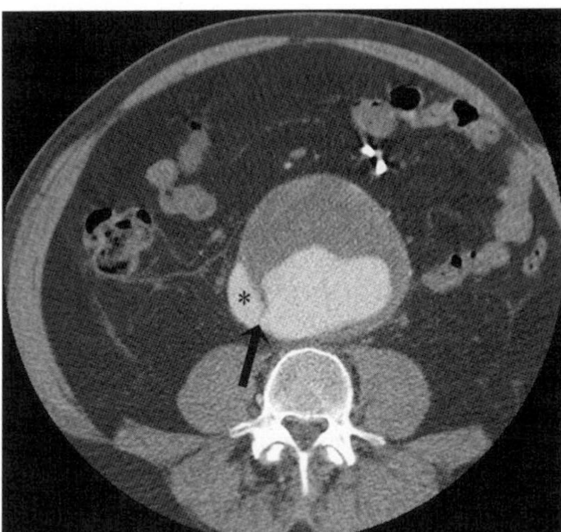

Figure 13.1 • Large abdominal aneurysm with fistulation (arrow) into the vena cava (asterisk).

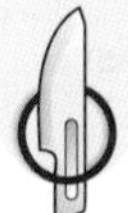

The recently published MASS trial has provided good statistical evidence to show that the prevalence of aneurysm-related death is reduced significantly in a screened male population aged 65–74 years, with a 53% reduction in those who attended for screening.[6] Because other causes of death overshadow those due to ruptured AAA, it has not been possible to demonstrate a statistically significant overall survival advantage for the screened population. Nevertheless, the case for extending population-based screening for AAA is convincing.

Interestingly, the detection of aneurysms in a screened population does not appear to affect quality of life adversely.

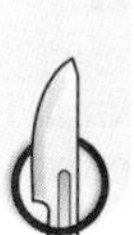

The MASS trial data shows that over 4 years the mean incremental cost-effectiveness ratio for screening was £28 400 per life-year gained, equivalent to approximately £36 000 per quality-adjusted life-year. It was estimated that this would fall to approximately £8000 per life-year gained at 10 years.[40]

Compared with existing screening programmes, for example for breast and cervical cancer, screening for AAA appears to be relatively cost-effective.

General management

The therapeutic strategy for a patient with an infrarenal AAA must be determined on an individual basis as the risks of treatment must be balanced against the risk of death from rupture of the aneurysm. However, a number of general principles apply to all patients. These are based on a knowledge of the average risks of surgery and death from rupture derived from a number of sources, most importantly the UK Small Aneurysm Trial and the ADAM trial undertaken in the USA, and from available natural history studies.[41,42]

Szilagyi et al.[43] established in the early 1970s that the risk of rupture of an aneurysm increases exponentially with its maximum diameter. Pooling of available data suggests that the 5-year rupture rates for aneurysms of diameters 5–5.9, 6–6.9 and over 7 cm are 25%, 35% and 75% respectively.

The small aneurysm trials have addressed the difficult dilemma of how to manage patients in whom the risk of surgery and the risk of rupture were both considered to be within the same order of magnitude.[41,42] The Medical Research Council-sponsored UK Small Aneurysm Trial randomised 1090 patients with asymptomatic AAAs of 4.0–5.5 cm diameter to either initial conservative management with ultrasound surveillance (527 patients) or immediate surgical intervention (563 patients). In the surveillance group, 321 patients eventually underwent surgery due to rapid expansion or growth of the diameter to above the 5.5-cm threshold. In the early surgery group, the 30-day operative mortality rate was 5.8%. There was no difference in survival between the two groups and it was concluded that the trial did not support a policy of early operative intervention for patients with AAAs of less than 5.5 cm diameter. The rupture rate for untreated small aneurysms in this trial was less than 2% per annum. However, the rate was relatively higher in females and this suggests that elective surgery may be indicated for smaller aneurysms in this group of patients. However, at present the data are insufficiently robust to support this conclusion convincingly. The results of the ADAM trial and the conclusions drawn were similar.

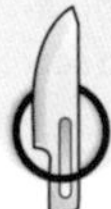

Surveillance of patients with small aneurysms

Following publication of the small aneurysm trials, it is recommended that patients with AAAs of less than 5.5 cm diameter should be managed initially conservatively with best medical therapy and regular surveillance by ultrasound scanning at 'safe' intervals.

Best medical therapy is largely focused on attention to blood pressure and smoking cessation. Attempts to lower blood pressure as a means of protecting against aneurysm expansion have concentrated on beta-blockers and specifically propranolol.[44] In addition to reducing the mean blood pressure, beta-blockers act specifically to lower the systolic peak and thereby the pulse pressure, which is thought to have additional potential advantages. Gadowski et al.[45] demonstrated that treatment with propranolol was associated with a significant reduction in the expansion rate of large AAAs.

However, another two clinical trials have recently reported disappointing results with propranolol treatment of aneurysms detected by screening.[46,47] Larger-scale randomised studies are necessary to evaluate the effectiveness of this and other pharmacotherapeutic agents for reducing the growth rate and risk of rupture of aortic aneurysms.

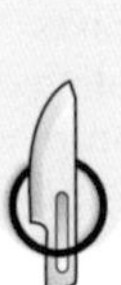

The optimum surveillance interval remains controversial, requiring a balance between cost and inconvenience on one side and safety on the other. It has recently been shown that an aneurysm with a diameter of less than 3 cm in a man aged 65 years of age or over is associated with minimal risk of eventual rupture[48] and thus there is probably no justification for continued ultrasound surveillance of lesions of this size. For larger aneurysms, there is no good information upon which to base a surveillance programme. However, drawing upon information available, screening intervals of 1 year for aneurysms of 3.5–4.4 cm and 6 months for those of 4.5–5.4 cm would appear to be appropriate.

Intervention

Currently available evidence supports elective surgical intervention for treatment of aneurysms of 5.5 cm diameter or greater subject to evaluation of the patients' general health and fitness for surgery.[41] Elective surgical intervention is also undertaken for patients whose aneurysms have expanded rapidly by more than 1 cm in a 12-month period and for those with symptomatic (i.e. painful) aneurysms.

The decision to intervene electively is followed by further detailed investigation in order to plan safe surgery and assess suitability for an endovascular approach.

INVESTIGATION OF THE PATIENT WITH A KNOWN AAA

The aims of evaluation of patients diagnosed with an AAA are threefold:

1. to identify those patients in whom the balance of risks favours operative intervention;
2. to reduce perioperative morbidity and mortality by identifying patients who may require further investigation or treatment of comorbidity prior to surgery;
3. to assess the anatomical suitability of the aneurysm for open or endovascular repair.

Accurate clinical assessment is imperative. It is recognised that perioperative mortality is related to the pre-existing physiological status of the patient,[49] and many clinical scoring systems, like the Goldman Cardiac Risk Index[50] and simpler revised forms such as that proposed by Lee,[51] can be used to predict operative risk.

The majority of deaths immediately following AAA repair are related to cardiac events and if pre-existing cardiac abnormalities are detected and treated prior to surgery, a substantial improvement in survival rates can potentially be achieved.[52] It has been suggested that expensive non-invasive tests for coronary artery disease are most useful in patients whose clinical features suggest moderate risk for cardiac complications and that they have limited impact in high-risk or low-risk patients.[53,54] Low-risk patients without any history or clinical evidence of cardiac disease do not necessarily require any investigations. Patients at moderate risk (e.g. history of cardiac impairment, age greater than 70 years, diabetic) should be investigated with non-invasive tests such as multiple gated acquisition technetium-99m radioisotope scanning[55] or dipyridamole–thallium scan.[56] Those patients with marked cardiac dysfunction will require further investigation by coronary angiography. Coronary revascularisation procedures may be required in up to 10% of patients, and there is evidence to show that this approach is effective in reducing the total perioperative mortality in this selected group.[57] The timing of coronary revascularisation procedures is a contentious issue, with some institutions advocating a combined synchronous approach at the time of AAA repair[58] whereas others prefer to perform coronary revascularisation prior to aneurysm surgery.[59–61] Convincing evidence to support either position is lacking, but if there is an endovascular option for coronary revascularisation then this is probably best carried out prior to surgical treatment of the aneurysm.

Respiratory complications are the most common form of morbidity after major abdominal surgery and occur after 25–50% of all such operations, including aortic aneurysm repair.[62] Pulmonary function testing, if requested selectively and interpreted correctly, can be useful for planning of the perioperative management of patients with lung disease.

The risk of perioperative renal failure is increased in those with pre-existing renal disease, diabetes or coexisting cardiac disease and in those aged over 60 years. Patients undergoing preoperative evaluation with computed tomography (CT) and selected for endovascular aneurysm repair (EVAR) require intravenous contrast, which is associated with renal failure in these high-risk patients. The probability of inducing renal failure can be reduced by limiting the use of non-steroidal anti-inflammatory agents, ensuring adequate hydration and diuresis before and after the contrast medium load, and potentially by using iso-osmolar contrast media.[63] In a few centres EVAR is performed using carbon dioxide angiography, which is not nephrotoxic.[64]

PREPROCEDURAL IMAGING

Ultrasound is useful for the detection and measurement of an AAA. Virtually all elective patients now undergo more detailed cross-sectional imaging with contrast-enhanced CT. With thin-slice acquisition of data, both spiral and multidetector row scanners provide excellent three-dimensional images from which to plan endovascular repair (**Fig. 13.2**). Given the wide availability and high quality of axial and three-dimensional reconstruction of CT imaging, aortography is rarely required preoperatively.

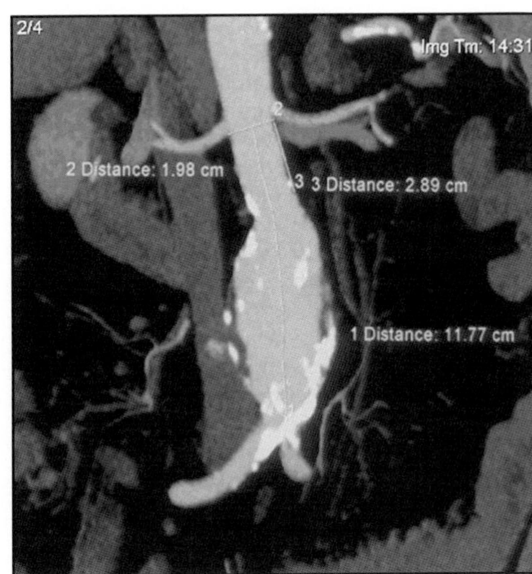

Figure 13.2 • CT reformatted image of infrarenal aneurysm with measurements.

Gadolinium-enhanced magnetic resonance imaging (MRI) is being used increasingly for assessment of patients prior to endovascular repair.[65,66]

ELECTIVE OPEN SURGICAL OPERATION

General anaesthesia is preferred, and is frequently combined with epidural anaesthesia for postoperative pain control. Epidural anaesthesia may be employed as the sole method, particularly in those patients with severe respiratory disease.

An antibiotic (e.g. 1.5 g cefuroxime) should be administered on induction of anaesthesia as prophylaxis against graft infection. Heparin 5000 units should be administered prior to the application of clamps.

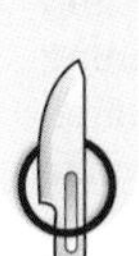

A trial conducted by the Joint Vascular Research Group of Great Britain and Ireland showed that while heparin does not have any influence on the risk of bleeding or thromboembolic complications, the incidence of perioperative myocardial infarction was reduced to 1.4% compared with 5.7% in patients who did not receive heparin.[67]

There is evidence to support the use of a beta-blocker, commencing 48 hours preoperatively and continued for several days after operation as a means of reducing the risk of perioperative cardiac complications including death.[68–70] Randomised trials are required to establish the efficacy of this treatment conclusively.

Although operative blood loss is minimal in most patients, excessive bleeding can occasionally be encountered either from back-bleeding lumbar arteries following opening of the sac or from the anastomotic suture lines. The use of a cell saver to preserve the patient's own red cells is a useful adjunct under these circumstances.[71] However, at least 4 units of crossmatched blood should be available at the start of the operation.

The aorta is a longitudinal midline structure and most operations for aortic aneurysm repair involve proximal and distal anastomoses within the abdomen. Therefore, the preferred incision is longitudinal and midline and the approach transperitoneal. Alternatives include a transverse incision with a transperitoneal approach, and an oblique left-sided abdominal incision with an extraperitoneal approach, both of which may be advantageous in selected patients. With a transperitoneal approach, the intestines should be retained within the abdominal cavity, being packed to the right side and held in place with a suitable self-retaining retractor. Drawing the intestines outside the abdomen is likely to result in prolonged postoperative ileus and is therefore to be discouraged.

The aneurysm is exposed by incising the posterior parietal peritoneum and carefully mobilising the duodenum to the right. The renal vein marks the upper limit of dissection for an infrarenal aneurysm. Inferiorly, both common iliac arteries are dissected in preparation for clamping, care being taken to avoid damage to the hypogastric plexus of nerves in sexually active males. It is not necessary to encircle either the aorta or the iliac arteries. Minimal dissection only is required to enable placement of clamps inserted from the front. Fabric grafts constructed from polyester (Dacron) or polytetrafluoroethylene (PTFE) may be used. Knitted Dacron grafts that have been 'presealed' with collagen or gelatin are particularly well suited for aortic aneurysm repair. Although ectatic dilatation of the common iliac arteries is commonly found in association with AAA, true iliac aneurysms are comparatively infrequent. Therefore, 60–70% of AAAs can be repaired using a simple tube graft anastomosed to the infrarenal neck proximally and to the aortic bifurcation distally. In the remaining 30–40% of cases, it is necessary to use a bifurcated graft with anastomoses either to the common iliac bifurcation or to the common femoral artery in the groin.

For repair of juxtarenal aneurysms, suprarenal clamping is essential. Under these circumstances, clamping of the supracoeliac aorta exposed through the lesser sac with separation of the fibres of the crura of the diaphragm is to be preferred, since this allows more explicit exposure of the orifices of the renal arteries and less risk also of renal embolisation than a clamp placed immediately above the renal arteries. A thoraco-abdominal approach with extraperitoneal exposure of the abdominal aorta is rarely necessary for juxtarenal aneurysms, but should be considered especially for obese patients in whom access is predicted to be problematical.

Inflammatory aneurysms pose specific technical problems for the surgeon.[72] The dense fibrous plaques incorporate adjacent structures, especially the duodenum, renal vein and ureters. Some surgeons prefer an intraperitoneal approach via an oblique left-sided abdominal or abdominothoracic incision for these aeurysms. If a standard midline incision is used, minimal dissection should be undertaken and this should be confined, as near as possible, to the midline in order to avoid damage to adherent structures. Ureterolysis is not recommended since the fibrous plaques resolve spontaneously once the aneurysm has been excluded. When ureteric obstruction with hydronephrosis is present, this should be relieved by insertion of JJ stents or, alternatively, by percutaneous nephrostomy preoperatively. If it can be avoided, no attempt should be made to mobilise the duodenum from the front of the aorta since to do so risks breaching the integrity of the duodenum with subsequent graft infection. It is preferable to incise the aorta to the left side of the duodenum, leaving it in place. If mobilisation of the duodenum is unavoidable, it may be possible to find a plane within the fibrous plaque itself, which can be developed by a combination of blunt and sharp dissection.[72] The inflammatory change does not extend beyond the limits of the aneurysm. Therefore, in the case of infrarenal aneurysms, the renal vein is often not involved. However, in juxtarenal aneurysms with incorporation of the renal vein within the inflammatory change, supracoeliac clamping is advised with minimal dissection of the neck of the aneurysm.

MINIMALLY INVASIVE ANEURYSM REPAIR

The advent of endovascular techniques has stimulated interest in developing other less invasive alternatives to conventional open surgery. These include shorter (6-cm) incisions and totally laparoscopic techniques.[73–75] Specially designed retractors and other instrumentation have been developed for these procedures. It is claimed that surgical trauma is reduced significantly, with benefits in terms of lower operative mortality and morbidity rates and more rapid recovery of the patients. However, to date, reliable comparative data are lacking.

EMERGENCY OPEN SURGICAL REPAIR

Successful emergency repair of ruptured aortic aneurysms depends mainly on surgical intervention being undertaken during a 'window of opportunity' when active bleeding is temporarily arrested by hypotension and tamponade of the haematoma by the posterior parietal peritoneum. In order to conserve this 'window of opportunity' for the time necessary, minimal resuscitation is required. In this context, the concept of permissive hypotension is important. Effective venous access lines should be established as quickly as possible. However, infusion of fluid should be kept to a minimum until surgical control of the bleeding has been obtained. A systolic blood pressure of 60–80 mmHg should be accepted prior to this being achieved.

The chances of survival after rupture of an AAA are extremely poor in patients who have suffered a cardiac arrest, in the very elderly and in those who remain persistently unconscious. A decision not to offer surgical intervention to such patients is justified. However, low or absent urinary output should not be considered a contraindication to surgery.

OUTCOMES FOLLOWING OPEN SURGICAL REPAIR

Elective open surgical repair of AAAs has been shown to be an effective procedure with good graft durability.

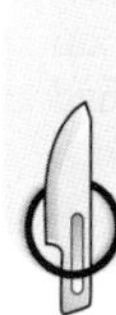

The Canadian Aneurysm Study demonstrated an in-hospital mortality rate of 4.7%, with a 5-year survival rate of 68%.[52,76] The UK Small Aneurysm Trial shows a 30-day mortality rate of 5.8% and the recent EVAR 1 trial a 30-day mortality rate of 4.7% in patients fit for surgery.[77]

Previous studies have demonstrated that patients with AAAs have a markedly decreased life expectancy in comparison with age- and sex-matched control populations. The 5-year survival of patients post surgery varies from 62 to 72% (compared with 83–90% in age- and sex-matched populations), with the majority of deaths due to coronary artery disease.[52,78,79] Quality-of-life studies have shown an improved perception of general health in the first 2 years after open repair in comparison with patients who are under surveillance.[80]

The UK Small Aneurysm Trial showed that only about 25% of patients with ruptured aneurysms make it to theatre for emergency repair.[41] Many series of unselected patients treated surgically for ruptured aneurysms report a perioperative mortality rate of approximately 50%.[81,82] A recent meta-analysis by Bown et al.[83] showed that there has been a progressive improvement in survival following surgery for ruptured AAAs over the last 40 years in the order of 3.5% per decade. However, this study also showed that the estimate of operative mortality rate remains high at approximately 41%.

The use of scoring systems in ruptured aneurysms has been proposed in order to assist rational selection of patients for surgical intervention according to their chances of survival.[84,85] However, these are not considered to be sufficiently reliable to predict individual outcomes at the present time and should therefore be used with caution.

ENDOVASCULAR REPAIR

The first case of endovascular repair of an AAA was reported by Parodi et al. in 1991.[86] Since then, this minimally invasive technique has become increasingly popular with physicians and patients. There are well-documented early benefits for EVAR and supportive evidence for this technique is available from large observational studies. National randomised trials to compare the results of endovascular and open repair of infrarenal AAAs are underway in the UK, the Netherlands, France and the USA. However, while the 30-day mortality results are very promising, there is not yet level 1 evidence in the form of long-term results to support the preferential use of the endovascular operation.

Devices

Endovascular repair is performed using a medical device that comprises metal and fabric, a stentgraft, of which there are numerous commercially available devices. Stentgrafts are available in tube, bifurcated and aorto-uni-iliac versions.

Aortic tube grafts have been used where the distal point of attachment is in the aorta just above the aortic bifurcation. These grafts have performed poorly, with a high incidence of intermediate-term failure owing to loss of seal in the distal aorta and are now rarely used.

Bifurcated stentgrafts are the most commonly used device (**Fig. 13.3**) and are either modular or single piece. Modular bifurcated stentgrafts are made from two or three separate components, which are assembled in vivo. The body and ipsilateral iliac limb are inserted via one femoral artery and the contralateral iliac limb is delivered from the other femoral artery to form an inverted Y graft similar to a surgical bifurcated graft. This design allows for numerous combinations of body and limb lengths and diameters in order to accommodate a range of aneurysm morphologies and vascular anatomy. However, there is an inherent risk of separation of the modular components with time. Single-piece bifurcated grafts are delivered via one common femoral artery, with the contralateral iliac limb being positioned using guidewires directed across the aortic bifurcation. The advantage of this system is that there are no modular components to disengage from each other and no risk of late failure of the repair from this cause. However, in com-

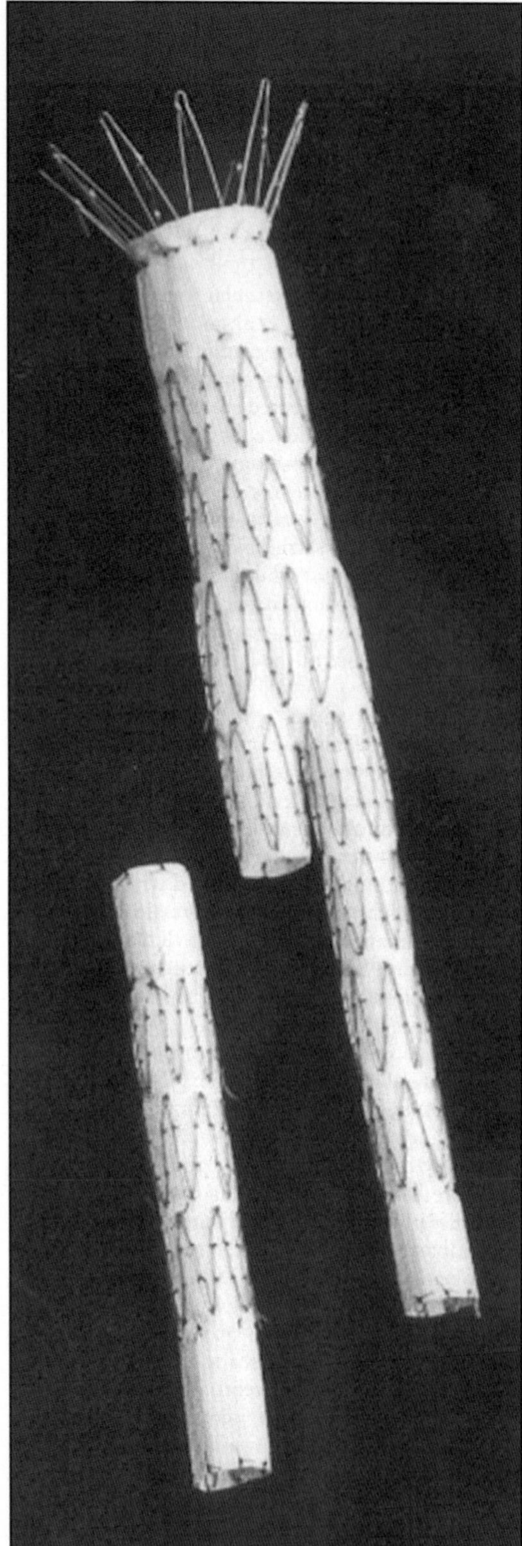

Figure 13.3 • Modular bifurcated device with limb extension.

parison with modular devices, single-piece bifurcated endografts can be more complicated to deploy and offer limited opportunities for 'customisation' in order to accommodate complex or irregular variations in vascular anatomy. The number and range of patients in whom they can be applied are therefore relatively limited.

The aorto-uni-iliac device is placed from the aorta proximally to one iliac artery distally. The other iliac artery is occluded with an endovascular occlusion device to prevent retrograde flow into the aneurysm and a surgical femoro-femoral crossover graft is performed to maintain flow into both legs.

Both fixation and seal of the endograft depend to some degree upon the radial force exerted by the internal metallic stent against the wall of the aorta. To optimise this force without risking excessive folding or pleating of the fabric, the upper 'fixation' stent of the endograft should be 'oversized' relative to the aortic diameter by 10–20%. Some devices have either barbs (**Fig. 13.4**) or suprarenal uncovered stents incorporated to resist subsequent distal migration of the device.

Endoleak and endotension

Endoleak is defined as persistent blood flow outside the graft and within the aneurysm sac.[87–91] Endoleak may be described as primary, from the time of EVAR, or secondary, referring to endoleak not seen at completion angiography but demonstrated on subsequent imaging. Endoleak has been classified according to the source of perigraft flow, with further subdivisions (**Box 13.1**).[91]

Endoleaks can be associated with aneurysm enlargement and eventual rupture.[92] This is most often seen in type I and III leaks that communicate directly with the aortic lumen, and secondary intervention is almost always necessary in these patients.

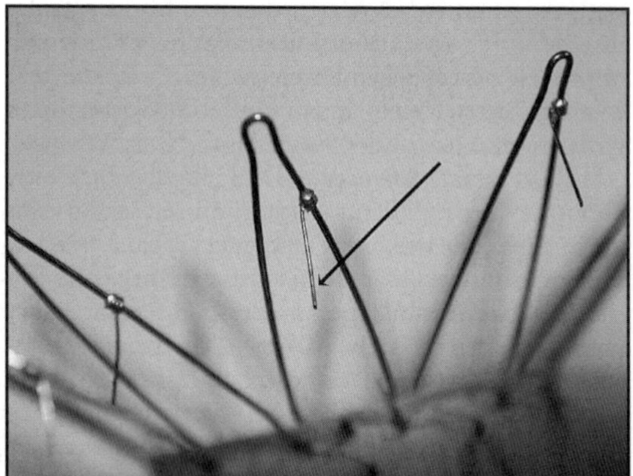

Figure 13.4 • Suprarenal bare metal stent with barbs (arrow).

Box 13.1 • Classification of endoleaks according to the source of perigraft flow

Type I: due to graft attachment site leaks	
A	Proximal end of endograft
B	Distal end of endograft
C	Iliac occluder
Type II: branch leaks (without attachment site connection)	
A	Simple or to-and-fro (from only one patent branch)
B	Complex or flow-through (with two or more patent branches)
Type III: graft defect	
A	Junctional leak or modular disconnection
B	Fabric disruption (midgraft hole): minor (<2 mm); major (2 mm or more)
Type IV: graft wall porosity (<30 days after graft placement)	

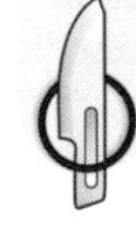

Of 4291 enrolled patients in the EUROSTAR registry in 2002, analysis of 34 patients with recorded rupture following EVAR showed that type I (**Fig. 13.5**) and type III endoleak and severe modes of structural disintegration of stentgrafts with or without migration were the most commonly documented findings at the time of rupture.[92]

Type II endoleaks are caused by retrograde flow into the sac from aortic side branches, usually the lumbar or inferior mesenteric arteries. There was a vogue for attempting preoperative embolisation of these side branches but this was not clinically effective.[93] Although rupture has been reported with type II leaks, it is now being recognised to be a more benign entity[94] and conservative management is probably appropriate unless the aneurysm sac is enlarging.

Persistent high pressure may exist within the 'excluded' aortic sac with or without evidence of an endoleak. Continued or renewed pressurisation of the aneurysm sac without a visible endoleak is referred to as 'endotension'.[95,96] This may lead to expansion of the aneurysm and a risk of rupture. Potential causes include endoleaks that are undetectable on imaging, microleaks through tiny suture holes in the fabric, transmission of pressure through thrombus that is 'sealing' an endoleak, or fluid accumulation in the sac by an osmotic process linked to degradation of intrasac thrombus (hygroma). There is anecdotal evidence that low-grade sepsis is another cause of sac enlargement without endoleak.

Migration of endovascular stentgrafts

Pulsatile blood flow and pressure on bifurcated stentgrafts generate a longitudinal distraction force in the range of 7–9 N and a sideways force on the curved limbs of 1.5 N.[97,98] These distraction forces may cause the proximal graft to migrate caudally or the iliac attachment to migrate superiorly. The end result of graft migration may be delayed type I endoleak with the risk of fatal rupture. Distraction

(a)

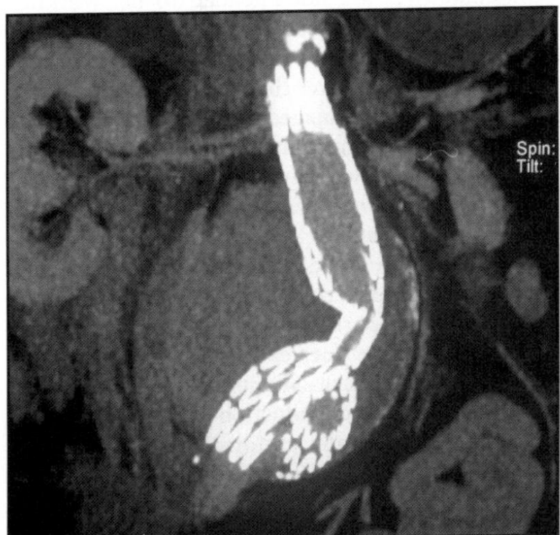

(b)

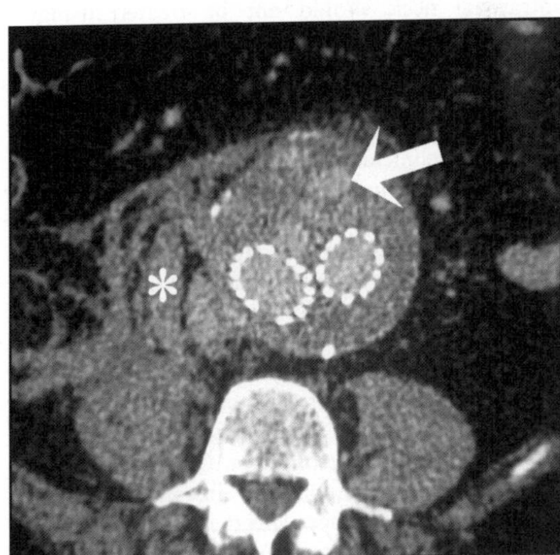

Figure 13.5 • **(a)** Proximal migration of the right iliac limb with **(b)** associated distal type I endoleak (arrow), with associated aortic rupture and retroperitoneal haematoma (asterisk).

forces also place stress on the overlap zones of modular grafts, which may incrementally distract causing type III endoleak, again with the risk of delayed rupture. Migration may also lead to graft distortion, which can predispose to graft thrombosis. Detection of migration postoperatively is usually an indication for secondary intervention.

Stent fractures

There have been reports of isolated stent fracture in almost all stentgrafts and this is an important obervation as it may result in loss of radial force in the sealing stent in the aortic neck and result in migration, endoleak and rupture. The fractured metallic ends may also result in fabric erosion or puncture with a resultant endoleak. All such observations should be reported to the manufacturers and regulatory authorities.

Anatomical requirements for EVAR

Not all infrarenal aneurysms are suitable for conventional endovascular stentgrafting and an understanding of the anatomical limitations is essential when planning the procedure and selecting an endograft.

A non-aneurysmal and relatively disease-free 'proximal neck' is an essential prerequisite for an effective seal and the avoidance of a proximal endoleak. The diameter should not exceed 30 mm and the length should be at least 15 mm. It should be free from mural thrombus and ideally be angulated not more than 60°. If an endograft with suprarenal fixation is to be used, some degree of 'conicality' of the neck can be accepted but the diameter should not increase by more than 3 mm for each 10 mm distance from the lowest renal artery. Aneurysms with an inadequate length of infrarenal neck should not be treated using a conventional endograft. New configurations of endograft incorporating 'fenestrations' or branches designed to permit a 'seal' at or above the level of the visceral arteries are in the process of development and clinical evaluation but require further assessment. Occlusive disease or extreme tortuosity in the iliac arteries may prevent passage of the introducer sheath of the stentgraft. Angioplasty prior to, or at the time of, endovascular repair may resolve this problem. Tortuous iliac arteries may straighten sufficiently following the introduction of stiff guidewires but, if not, limited surgical exposure and gentle downward traction on the external iliac and common femoral arteries will often be effective. Alternatively, a Dacron tube 'conduit' may be anastomosed to the common iliac artery to allow access of the introducer sheath. It is rare for iliac artery disease to render EVAR impossible but heavy calcification will prevent tortuous arteries from being straightened by any means and total iliac occlusion will also prevent access by this route. Under these circumstances, consideration might be given to the use of an aorto-uni-iliac device. Ectatic iliac arteries with diameters up to 22 mm can be treated with flared iliac extension limbs. If there is an aneurysm of the common iliac artery, the endovascular reconstruction may be extended into the external iliac artery. The internal iliac artery should be embolised beforehand to prevent endoleak from this source.

Endograft deployment

The ideal venue provides a sterile environment, high-quality imaging and facilities for open surgery if required for arterial access or rarely for fashioning an access conduit or for conversion to open repair. Radiation protection should not be forgotten for both the patient and staff. Unquestionably these aims are best realised in a dedicated endovascular theatre with fixed imaging.

Most devices range from 16 to 24 Fr and surgical exposure and control of the femoral artery is usual. However, an increasing number of centres now use percutaneous suture-mediated closure devices to enable an entirely percutaneous approach on both sides. Local, regional or general anaesthesia may be used, although a long procedure under local anaesthesia may be difficult for the patient.

Iodinated contrast media are normally used for imaging, although carbon dioxide angiography is a valuable alternative.[64] In centres where the facilities exist, intravascular ultrasound is a useful addition to conventional imaging techniques in order to guide optimal positioning of the device.[99,100]

After femoral access is achieved, a soft wire and catheter are placed into the suprarenal aorta and a stiff guidewire is introduced through the catheter. Stiff guidewires are not intended to be 'working' wires and it is not sensible to try to negotiate tortuous iliac vessels with them. The stentgraft body is introduced over the stiff guidewire and the renal arteries are imaged. The image intensifier should be angled to optimise the view of the renal arteries and this typically requires a small amount of craniocaudal and oblique tilt.

An imaging catheter is left alongside the graft body as the top stents are released in stages and short angiographic runs should be performed to ensure precise positioning relative to the renal arteries. Modular devices require cannulation in situ of the short leg or 'stump' of the main body of the device prior to introduction of the contralateral limb. This is generally performed by a retrograde approach from the contralateral femoral artery using angled catheters. Confirmation of successful cannulation is needed to avoid the error of inadvertently deploying the contralateral limb alongside rather than within the main graft.

The iliac limbs are deployed close to the internal iliac origins, which are defined using oblique projections. Substantial overlap at the modular connections is essential to avoid late disconnections.

Completion angiography is performed to determine whether the aneurysm has been excluded and to ensure that there has been no encroachment by the fabric of the graft on the orifices of the visceral or internal iliac arteries. Every effort must be made to resolve all primary graft-related (type I) endoleaks before the patient is allowed to leave the operating room.

Surveillance after EVAR

The modes of failure after endovascular grafting are well documented.[101] It is mandatory that all patients are recruited onto a programme of systematic postoperative surveillance with the aim of detecting causes of late rupture.

The principal concerns are graft-related endoleak, aneurysm enlargement and migration of stents at the aortic or iliac landing zones or at the modular connections. Options for the method of surveillance include ultrasound, CT, MRI and plain radiography.

CT is the standard employed in most centres. Undertaken as an arterial-phase contrast-enhanced scan, it can be used to detect graft-related (type I) and side branch-related (type II) endoleaks. It also permits precise measurement of aortic diameters and recognition of migration of the stentgraft in relation to fixed anatomical reference points such as the superior mesenteric artery, renal artery and hypogastric artery. It is generally necessary to report these studies by comparison with previous CT examinations.

It has been shown that ultrasound can be used to detect graft-related (type I) endoleaks reliably.[102,103] Ultrasound is less effective for the detection of type II endoleaks, but since it is known that type II endoleaks are not associated with a significant risk of adverse clinical events, this may be regarded as an acceptable limitation. Changes in the diameter of the aneurysm can be tracked by ultrasound but it is poor in the detection of migration.

Plain radiography using a standardised protocol[104] is an effective method for the detection of device migration. Stent fractures and separation of modular components are also relatively easy to identify. It is comparatively inexpensive and usefully complements ultrasound scanning. Used in combination these two methods represent a potentially acceptable alternative to CT for surveillance. MRI (**Fig. 13.6**) may be used where the device is made from compatible metals (i.e. nitinol).[105,106]

It is generally accepted that surveillance after EVAR should be lifelong. The surveillance intervals vary but typically include baseline imaging with CT and plain radiography at 1 month after EVAR.

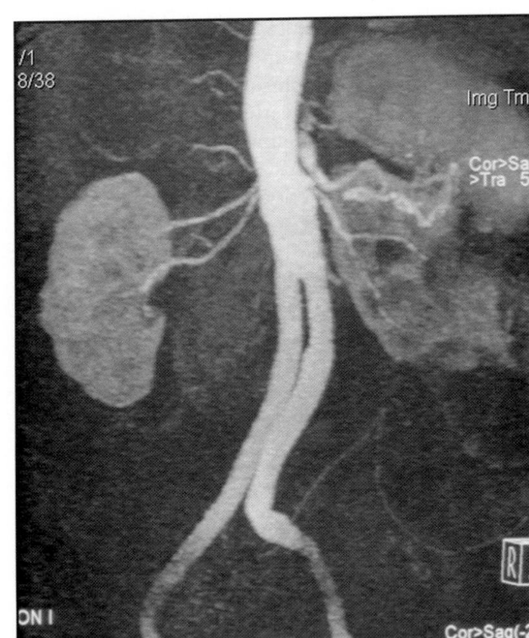

Figure 13.6 • Surveillance magnetic resonance aortogram after endovascular repair.

Most protocols include more frequent surveillance intervals during the first 2 years, with annual surveillance thereafter.

Outcomes after EVAR

In the last few years evidence from case series and observational studies, including large national and international registries,[107–109] has established that endovascular repair of AAAs can be undertaken with an operative mortality risk in the order of 2–3%,[110,111] even in high-risk patients. Intensive care facilities are rarely required and the duration of hospital stay and convalescence appear to be short compared with conventional open repair.[112]

There are a number of complications that occur more commonly after EVAR compared with the open technique. Ischaemic episodes are seen in up to 9% of patients[113] and these may involve the arterial supply of the limbs, colon, buttocks, kidneys and spinal cord, the commonest being limb ischaemia. The majority of limb ischaemic complications are readily amenable to endovascular or open surgical treatment. Renal failure after EVAR is associated with an increased rate of mortality;[114] the aetiology of the renal failure may relate to thrombus or cholesterol emboli or occlusion of the renal ostium by graft fabric or is secondary to the nephrotoxic effects of large volumes of iodinated contrast media. The introduction of iso-osmolar contrast media, carbon dioxide angiography and intravascular ultrasound and MRI for stentgraft evaluation, deployment and follow-up should help decrease the risks of nephrotoxicity. It is rare for the renal ostia to be inadvertently covered by graft fabric, and careful planning and deployment decrease the risk of this occurring. There was a worry that the introduction of suprarenal bare-stent fixation would lead to increased rates of renal failure especially in patients with pre-existing renal impairment; however, a recent study by Mehta et al.[115] showed no significant difference in renal failure in these cases.

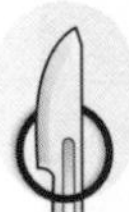

The initial results of the first randomised trial comparing EVAR with open surgical repair showed a significant difference in the 30-day mortality (1.7% vs. 4.7% respectively).[77]

While there is a clearly demonstrated early benefit, the longer-term results of this and other randomised trials such as the Dutch DREAM trial[116] will be crucial as data from registries such as EUROSTAR suggest further intervention will be required in up to 25% of EVAR patients and there remains a very small cumulative risk of rupture in the order of 0.26% per year with modern devices.[117,118]

The future of EVAR

The anatomical requirements for conventional endoluminal grafts exclude many patients, primarily because of an unsuitable infrarenal aortic neck. The transrenal and juxtarenal aorta can be used to create a 'neck' if holes or fenestrations are manufactured in the graft to precise preoperative plans (**Fig. 13.7**). The early data on the use of these devices are promising.[119–121]

Branched endografts have been used to preserve flow in hypogastric arteries and in the treatment of aortic arch and thoraco-abdominal aneurysms. Available evidence of efficacy is currently restricted to case reports and small case series.[122–124] Concerns about these devices include uncertainty regarding the long-term patency of stents in normal branch vessels, the increased number of modular connections and the possibility that the branches may kink if the aneurysm shrinks.

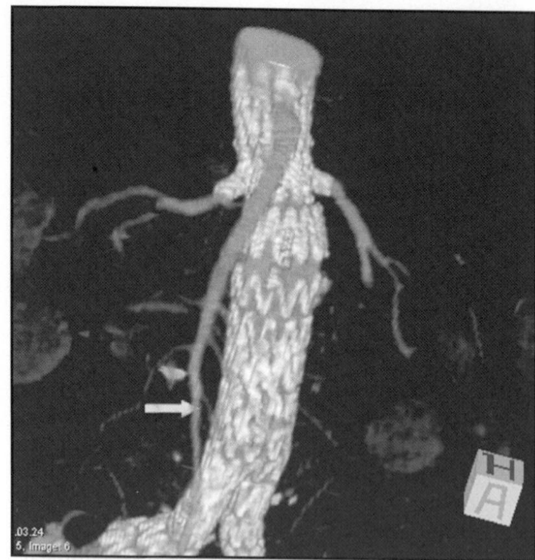

Figure 13.7 • Three-dimensional reconstructed CT image of juxtarenal aneurysm that has been treated with a fenestrated graft with bilateral renal artery stenting.

PERIPHERAL ANEURYSMS

Iliac aneurysms

Iliac aneurysms usually occur in association with aortic aneurysms. Isolated iliac aneurysms are comparatively unusual, the prevalence having been estimated to be less than 2% of that of aortoiliac aneurysms. Most iliac aneurysms affect either the common or internal iliac arteries. Aneurysmal disease of the external iliac artery is extremely rare.

The risk of rupture of iliac aneurysms has not been accurately quantified and the criteria for elective surgical intervention have not been clearly defined. Commonly accepted guidance is that elective open or endovascular intervention is indicated for asymptomatic iliac aneurysms greater than 3 cm in diameter. Symptomatic and ruptured aneurysms mandate immediate surgical intervention.

Common femoral aneurysms

True aneurysms of the common femoral artery are associated with AAAs in 25% of cases. In this situation, true aneurysms are considerably less common than false aneurysms developing at the site of anastomosis of an aorto-femoral graft. Their clinical presentation usually takes the form of a painless pulsatile swelling. Rupture can occur but is rare. Most patients seek treatment before the risk of rupture becomes appreciable.

Small femoral artery aneurysms can be managed expectantly with clinical assessment at intervals. Surgical treatment is indicated for symptoms and probably for most aneurysms of 3 cm or more in size. Usually, a short interposition or inlay tube graft anastomosed proximally at the level of the inguinal ligament and distal to the common femoral bifurcation is required. This is a relatively small operation with durable results.

Popliteal artery aneurysms

Popliteal aneurysms are the most commonly encountered peripheral aneurysm, accounting for more than 80% of all peripheral aneurysms. The ratio of popliteal aneurysms to AAAs is approximately 1:15. Half are bilateral and 40% are associated with AAAs.

Although rupture is rare, 50% of cases present with peripheral limb-threatening ischaemia. In common with aneurysms at all other sites, laminated thrombus develops within popliteal aneurysms. However, the fact that the popliteal artery is continually subjected to flexion and extension greatly increases the risk of disintegration and embolisation of this thrombus. In many patients, microembolisation of the peripheral circulation occurs silently prior to main vessel occlusion or thrombosis of the popliteal aneurysm itself. For this reason, the viability of the limb may be seriously threatened. Furthermore, compromise of the run-off circulation can impact adversely on the outcome from emergency bypass surgery. The bigger the aneurysm, the more likely there is to be thrombus. The presence of intraluminal thrombus is therefore a more important indication for elective surgical intervention than the size of the aneurysm. Any thrombus detected by ultrasound, CT or MRI constitutes an indication for elective treatment. In the absence of laminated thrombus, it is generally accepted that aneurysms with a diameter of 2 cm or greater warrant consideration for elective surgical repair.

Traditionally, popliteal aneurysms are treated by proximal and distal ligation and bypass using autologous vein undertaken via a medial approach. However, recent studies have identified persistent flow within the popliteal aneurysm in 30% of patients treated in this way.[125] Furthermore, there is a significant risk of continued expansion and even rupture due to pressurisation of the sac resulting from back-flow through geniculate branches. Therefore, a posterior approach and insertion of an inlay graft is to be preferred.

An acutely thrombosed popliteal aneurysm is a clinical emergency. Preoperative or on-table thrombolysis has been used to open up the run-off vessels and thereby facilitate bypass surgery. There is some low-level evidence to suggest that this approach may improve the chances of successful limb salvage.[126,127]

With the evolution of flexible endografts, endovascular repair is now a viable alternative to open surgery for the treatment of some popliteal aneurysms.[128]

Key points

- The prevalence of AAAs has increased dramatically over the last four decades and this trend appears to be continuing.
- The case for extending population-based screening for AAAs is convincing.
- The Small Aneurysm Trial did not support a policy of early operative intervention for patients with AAAs of less than 5.5 cm diameter.
- The UK EVAR 1 trial reported a significant difference in the 30-day mortality, with 1.7% mortality in the EVAR group compared with 4.7% in those allocated to open repair. Long-term results are needed before changes in clinical practice can be justified.

REFERENCES

1. Johnston KW, Rutherford RB, Tilson MD et al. Suggested standards for reporting on arterial aneurysms. Subcommittee on Reporting Standards for Arterial Aneurysms, Ad Hoc Committee on Reporting Standards, Society for Vascular Surgery and North American Chapter, International Society for Cardiovascular Surgery. J Vasc Surg 1991; 13:452–8.
2. Brown LC, Powell JT. Risk factors for aneurysm rupture in patients kept under ultrasound surveillance. UK Small Aneurysm Trial Participants. Ann Surg 1999; 230:289–96.
3. Collin J, Araujo L, Walton J, Lindsell D. Oxford screening programme for abdominal aortic aneurysm in men aged 65 to 74 years. Lancet 1988; ii:613–15.
4. Multicentre Aneurysm Screening Study. A comparative study of the prevalence of abdominal aortic aneurysms in the United Kingdom, Denmark, and Australia. J Med Screen 2001; 8:46–50.
5. Hak E, Balm R, Eikelboom BC, Akkersdijk GJ, van der GY. Abdominal aortic aneurysm screening: an epidemiological point of view. Eur J Vasc Endovasc Surg 1996; 11:270–8.
6. 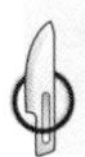 Ashton HA, Buxton MJ, Day NE et al. The Multicentre Aneurysm Screening Study (MASS) into the effect of abdominal aortic aneurysm screening on mortality in men: a randomised controlled trial. Lancet 2002; 360:1531–9.

UK multicentre population-based screening study of 67 800 men, aged 65–74 years, who were randomly allocated to be invited to attend for ultrasound assessment or not. The primary outcome measure was aneurysm-related death and there was a 42% risk reduction in the invited group.

7. Office of National Statistics United Kingdom: Statistics Online. http://www.statistics.gov.uk/
8. Fowkes FG, Macintyre CC, Ruckley CV. Increasing incidence of aortic aneurysms in England and Wales. Br Med J 1989; 298:33–5.
9. Lucarotti M, Shaw E, Poskitt K, Heather B. The Gloucestershire Aneurysm Screening Programme: the first 2 years' experience. Eur J Vasc Surg 1993; 7:397–401.
10. Norman PE, Jamrozik K, Lawrence-Brown M et al. Population based randomised controlled trial on impact of screening on mortality from abdominal aortic aneurysm. Br Med J 2004; 329:1259–62.
11. Vardulaki KA, Walker NM, Day NE et al. Quantifying the risks of hypertension, age, sex and smoking in patients with abdominal aortic aneurysm. Br J Surg 2000; 87:195–200.
12. Cutler BS, Darling RC. Surgical management of arteriosclerotic femoral aneurysms. Surgery 1973; 74:764–73.
13. Koch AE, Haines GK, Rizzo RJ et al. Human abdominal aortic aneurysms. Immunophenotypic analysis suggesting an immune-mediated response. Am J Pathol 1990; 137:1199–213.
14. McMillan WD, Pearce WH. Increased plasma levels of metalloproteinase-9 are associated with abdominal aortic aneurysms. J Vasc Surg 1999; 29:122–7.
15. Mao D, Lee JK, VanVickle SJ, Thompson RW. Expression of collagenase-3 (MMP-13) in human abdominal aortic aneurysms and vascular smooth muscle cells in culture. Biochem Biophys Res Commun 1999; 261:904–10.
16. Newman KM, Malon AM, Shin RD et al. Matrix metalloproteinases in abdominal aortic aneurysm: characterization, purification, and their possible sources. Connect Tissue Res 1994; 30:265–76.
17. Vine N, Powell JT. Metalloproteinases in degenerative aortic disease. Clin Sci 1991; 81:233–9.
18. Cohen JR, Sarfati I, Danna D, Wise L. Smooth muscle cell elastase, atherosclerosis, and abdominal aortic aneurysms. Ann Surg 1992; 216:327–30.
19. Vallabhaneni SR, Gilling-Smith GL, How TV et al. Heterogeneity of tensile strength and matrix metalloproteinase activity in the wall of abdominal aortic aneurysms. J Endovasc Ther 2004; 11:494–502.
20. Thompson MM, Jones L, Nasim A, Sayers RD, Bell PR. Angiogenesis in abdominal aortic aneurysms. Eur J Vasc Endovasc Surg 1996; 11:464–9.
21. Newman KM, Jean-Claude J, Li H et al. Cellular localization of matrix metalloproteinases in the abdominal aortic aneurysm wall. J Vasc Surg 1994; 20:814–20.
22. Szekanecz Z, Shah MR, Harlow LA, Pearce WH, Koch AE. Interleukin-8 and tumor necrosis factor-alpha are involved in human aortic endothelial cell migration. The possible role of these cytokines in human aortic aneurysmal blood vessel growth. Pathobiology 1994; 62:134–9.
23. Reilly JM, Miralles M, Wester WN, Sicard GA. Differential expression of prostaglandin E2 and interleukin-6 in occlusive and aneurysmal aortic disease. Surgery 1999; 126:624–7.
24. Majumder PP, St Jean PL, Ferrell RE, Webster MW, Steed DL. On the inheritance of abdominal aortic aneurysm. Am J Hum Genet 1991; 48:164–70.
25. Verloes A, Sakalihasan N, Koulischer L, Limet R. Aneurysms of the abdominal aorta: familial and genetic aspects in three hundred thirteen pedigrees. J Vasc Surg 1995; 21:646–55.
26. Coggon D, Winter P, Martyn C, Inskip H. Contrasting epidemiology of aortic aneurysm and peripheral vascular disease in England and Wales. Br Med J 1996; 312:948.
27. Baxter BT, Davis VA, Minion DJ et al. Abdominal aortic aneurysms are associated with altered matrix proteins of the nonaneurysmal aortic segments. J Vasc Surg 1994; 19:797–802.
28. Walker DI, Bloor K, Williams G, Gillie I. Inflammatory aneurysms of the abdominal aorta. Br J Surg 1972; 59:609–14.
29. Hsu RB, Tsay YG, Wang SS, Chu SH. Surgical treatment for primary infected aneurysm of the descending thoracic aorta, abdominal aorta, and iliac arteries. J Vasc Surg 2002; 36:746–50.
30. Hsu RB, Tsay YG, Wang SS, Chu SH. Management of aortic aneurysm infected with *Salmonella*. Br J Surg 2003; 90:1080–4.
31. Farkas JC, Fichelle JM, Laurian C et al. Long-term follow-up of positive cultures in 500 abdominal aortic aneurysms. Arch Surg 1993; 128:284–8.
32. Gutierrez J, Linares J, Fernandez F et al. Relationship between peripheral arterial occlusive disease and infection by *Chlamydophila pneumoniae*. [In Spanish] Med Clin (Barc) 2004; 123:561–6.
33. Linares-Palomino JP, Gutierrez J, Lopez-Espada C, de Dios LJ, Ros E, Maroto C. Genomic, serologic, and clinical case–control study of *Chlamydia pneumoniae* and peripheral artery occlusive disease. J Vasc Surg 2004; 40:359–66.
34. Hickey NC, Downing R, Hamer JD, Ashton F, Slaney G. Abdominal aortic aneurysms complicated by spontaneous iliocaval or duodenal fistulae. J Cardiovasc Surg (Torino) 1991; 32:181–5.
35. Lindholt JS, Vammen S, Juul S, Henneberg EW, Fasting H. The validity of ultrasonographic scanning

as screening method for abdominal aortic aneurysm. Eur J Vasc Endovasc Surg 1999; 17:472–5.

36. Collin J. Screening for abdominal aortic aneurysm. Br J Surg 1993; 80:1363–4.

37. Vardulaki KA, Prevost TC, Walker NM et al. Incidence among men of asymptomatic abdominal aortic aneurysms: estimates from 500 screen detected cases. J Med Screen 1999; 6:50–4.

38. Bengtsson H, Nilsson P, Bergqvist D. Natural history of abdominal aortic aneurysm detected by screening. Br J Surg 1993; 80:718–20.

39. Emerton ME, Shaw E, Poskitt K, Heather BP. Screening for abdominal aortic aneurysm: a single scan is enough. Br J Surg 1994; 81:1112–13.

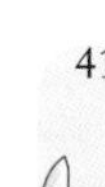

40. The Multicentre Aneurysm Screening Study Group. Multicentre aneurysm screening study (MASS): cost effectiveness analysis of screening for abdominal aortic aneurysms based on four year results fom randomised controlled trial. bmj.com 2002; 325:1135.

See reference 6. Cost-effectiveness analysis at 4 years showed that the cost per quality-adjusted life-year was £36 000. It is projected that this value will fall to £8000 per quality-adjusted life-year at 10 years, which is well below the funding threshold in the UK health service.

41. The UK Small Aneurysm Trial Participants. Mortality results for randomised controlled trial of early elective surgery or ultrasound surveillance for small abdominal aortic aneurysms. Lancet 1998; 352(9141):1649–55.

Multicentre randomised controlled trial of 1090 patients with asymptomatic aneurysms of diameter 4.0–5.5 cm were randomly allocated to early elective surgery or ultrasound surveillance. There was no significant survival advantage at 6 years for those undergoing surgical repair.

42. Lederle FA, Wilson SE, Johnson GR et al. Design of the abdominal aortic Aneurysm Detection and Management Study. ADAM VA Cooperative Study Group. J Vasc Surg 1994; 20:296–303.

43. Szilagyi DE, Elliott JP, Smith RF. Clinical fate of the patient with asymptomatic abdominal aortic aneurysm and unfit for surgical treatment. Arch Surg 1972; 104:600–6.

44. Leach SD, Toole AL, Stern H, DeNatale RW, Tilson MD. Effect of beta-adrenergic blockade on the growth rate of abdominal aortic aneurysms. Arch Surg 1988; 123:606–9.

45. Gadowski GR, Pilcher DB, Ricci MA. Abdominal aortic aneurysm expansion rate: effect of size and beta-adrenergic blockade. J Vasc Surg 1994; 19:727–31.

46. Lindholt JS, Henneberg EW, Juul S, Fasting H. Impaired results of a randomised double blinded clinical trial of propranolol versus placebo on the expansion rate of small abdominal aortic aneurysms. Int Angiol 1999; 18:52–7.

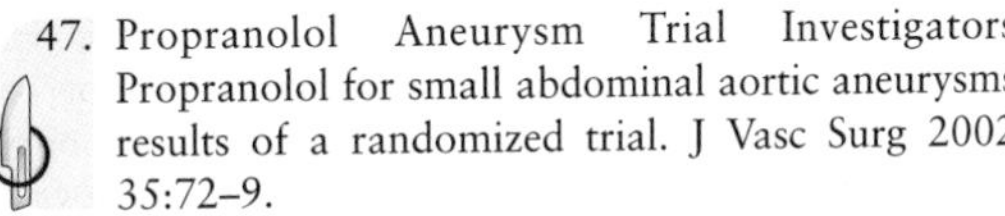

47. Propranolol Aneurysm Trial Investigators. Propranolol for small abdominal aortic aneurysms: results of a randomized trial. J Vasc Surg 2002; 35:72–9.

Two randomised trials (46, 47) showing that propranolol is not well tolerated by patients with diagnosed aneurysms and is ineffective in the prevention of aneurysm growth.

48. Couto E, Duffy SW, Ashton HA et al. Probabilities of progression of aortic aneurysms: estimates and implications for screening policy. J Med Screen 2002; 9:40–2.

49. Katz DJ, Stanley JC, Zelenock GB. Operative mortality rates for intact and ruptured abdominal aortic aneurysms in Michigan: an eleven-year statewide experience. J Vasc Surg 1994; 19:804–15.

50. Goldman L, Caldera DL, Nussbaum SR et al. Multifactorial index of cardiac risk in noncardiac surgical procedures. N Engl J Med 1977; 297:845–50.

51. Lee TH, Marcantonio ER, Mangione CM et al. Derivation and prospective validation of a simple index for prediction of cardiac risk of major noncardiac surgery. Circulation 1999; 100:1043–9.

52. Johnston KW. Nonruptured abdominal aortic aneurysm: six-year follow-up results from the multicenter prospective Canadian aneurysm study. Canadian Society for Vascular Surgery Aneurysm Study Group. J Vasc Surg 1994; 20:163–70.

Prospective analysis of 680 patients undergoing elective aneurysm surgery showed that cardiac-related death is the major perioperative risk and cardiac and cerebrovascular events are the major causes of death at 6 years.

53. Mangano DT, Goldman L. Preoperative assessment of patients with known or suspected coronary disease. N Engl J Med 1995; 333:1750–6.

54. Eagle KA, Froehlich JB. Reducing cardiovascular risk in patients undergoing noncardiac surgery. N Engl J Med 1996; 335:1761–3.

55. Karkos CD, Thomson GJ, Hughes R et al. Prediction of cardiac risk prior to elective abdominal aortic surgery: role of multiple gated acquisition scan. World J Surg 2003; 27:1085–92.

56. Klonaris CN, Bastounis EA, Xiromeritis NC, Balas PE. The predictive value of dipyridamole–thallium scintigraphy for cardiac risk assessment before major vascular surgery. Int Angiol 1998; 17:171–8.

57. Cambria RP, Brewster DC, Abbott WM et al. The impact of selective use of dipyridamole–thallium scans and surgical factors on the current morbidity of aortic surgery. J Vasc Surg 1992; 15:43–50.

58. Braunberger E, Combes MA, Meimoun P et al. Coronary bypass surgery on the beating heart and surgery of an abdominal aortic aneurysm. Immediately sequential surgical treatments. [In French] Arch Mal Coeur 2001; 94:291–4.

59. Brooks MJ, Mayet J, Glenville B, Foale R, Wolfe JH. Cardiac investigation and intervention prior to thoraco-abdominal aneurysm repair: coronary angiography in 35 patients. Eur J Vasc Endovasc Surg 2001; 21:437–44.

60. Nataf P, Gandjbakhch I, Pavie A et al. Value and results of coronary surgery before the repair of abdominal aortic aneurysm. [In French] Arch Mal Coeur 1990; 83:1547–51.

61. Nataf P, Gandjbakhch I, Pavie A et al. Surgical strategy in polyarterial disease. Value and results of combined surgery. [In French] Presse Med 1990; 19 (10):460–4.

62. Zibrak JD, O'Donnell CR, Marton K. Indications for pulmonary function testing. Ann Intern Med 1990; 112:763–71.

63. Aspelin P, Aubry P, Fransson SG et al. Nephrotoxic effects in high-risk patients undergoing angiography. N Engl J Med 2003; 348:491–9.

64. Bush RL, Lin PH, Bianco CC et al. Endovascular aortic aneurysm repair in patients with renal dysfunction or severe contrast allergy: utility of imaging modalities without iodinated contrast. Ann Vasc Surg 2002; 16:537–44.

65. Anbarasu A, Harris PL, McWilliams RG. The role of gadolinium-enhanced MR imaging in the preoperative evaluation of inflammatory abdominal aortic aneurysm. Eur Radiol 2002; 12(suppl. 3): S192–S195.

66. Thurnher SA, Dorffner R, Thurnher MM et al. Evaluation of abdominal aortic aneurysm for stent-graft placement: comparison of gadolinium-enhanced MR angiography versus helical CT angiography and digital subtraction angiography. Radiology 1997; 205:341–52.

67. Thompson JF, Mullee MA, Bell PR et al. Intraoperative heparinisation, blood loss and myocardial infarction during aortic aneurysm surgery: a Joint Vascular Research Group study. Eur J Vasc Endovasc Surg 1996; 12:86–90.

68. Fleisher LA, Corbett W, Berry C, Poldermans D. Cost-effectiveness of differing perioperative beta-blockade strategies in vascular surgery patients. J Cardiothorac Vasc Anesth 2004; 18:7–13.

69. Auerbach AD, Goldman L. Beta-blockers and reduction of cardiac events in noncardiac surgery: scientific review. JAMA 2002; 287:1435–44.

70. Auerbach AD, Goldman L. Beta-blockers and reduction of cardiac events in noncardiac surgery: clinical applications. JAMA 2002; 287:1445–7.

71. Goodnough LT, Monk TG, Sicard G et al. Intraoperative salvage in patients undergoing elective abdominal aortic aneurysm repair: an analysis of cost and benefit. J Vasc Surg 1996; 24:213–18.

72. Barr H, Cave-Bigley DJ, Harris PL. The management of inflammatory abdominal aortic aneurysms. J R Coll Surg Edinb 1985; 30:217–20.

73. Kolvenbach R, Schwierz E, Wasilljew S et al. Total laparoscopically and robotically assisted aortic aneurysm surgery: a critical evaluation. J Vasc Surg 2004; 39:771–6.

74. Kolvenbach R, Ceshire N, Pinter L et al. Laparoscopy-assisted aneurysm resection as a minimal invasive alternative in patients unsuitable for endovascular surgery. J Vasc Surg 2001; 34:216–21.

75. Silva L, Kolvenbach R, Pinter L. The feasibility of hand-assisted laparoscopic aortic bypass using a low transverse incision. Surg Endosc 2002; 16:173–6.

76. Johnston KW, Scobie TK. Multicenter prospective study of nonruptured abdominal aortic aneurysms. I. Population and operative management. J Vasc Surg 1988; 7:69–81.

Multicentre study of operative management of 666 patients with non-ruptured aneurysms of the abdominal aorta.

77. Greenhalgh RM, Brown LC, Kwong GP, Powell JT, Thompson SG. Comparison of endovascular aneurysm repair with open repair in patients with abdominal aortic aneurysm (EVAR trial 1), 30-day operative mortality results: randomised controlled trial. Lancet 2004; 364:843–8.

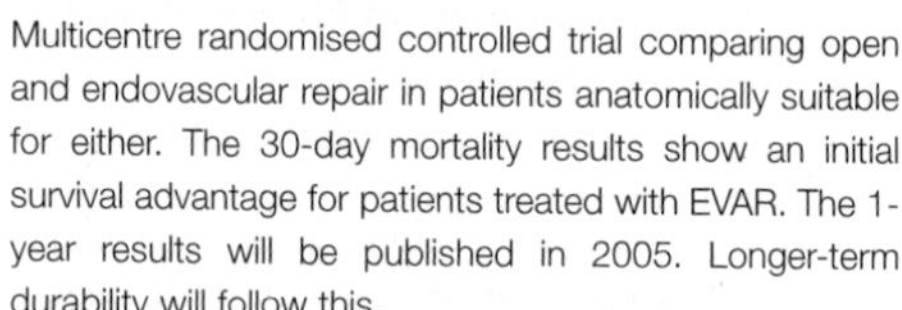
Multicentre randomised controlled trial comparing open and endovascular repair in patients anatomically suitable for either. The 30-day mortality results show an initial survival advantage for patients treated with EVAR. The 1-year results will be published in 2005. Longer-term durability will follow this.

78. Batt M, Staccini P, Pittaluga P et al. Late survival after abdominal aortic aneurysm repair. Eur J Vasc Endovasc Surg 1999; 17:338–42.

79. Hallett JW Jr, Naessens JM, Ballard DJ. Early and late outcome of surgical repair for small abdominal aortic aneurysms: a population-based analysis. J Vasc Surg 1993; 18:684–91.

80. Lederle FA, Johnson GR, Wilson SE et al. Quality of life, impotence, and activity level in a randomized trial of immediate repair versus surveillance of small abdominal aortic aneurysm. J Vasc Surg 2003; 38:745–52.

81. Markovic M, Davidovic L, Maksimovic Z et al. Ruptured abdominal aortic aneurysm. Predictors of survival in 229 consecutive surgical patients. Herz 2004; 29:123–9.

82. Hans SS, Huang RR. Results of 101 ruptured abdominal aortic aneurysm repairs from a single surgical practice. Arch Surg 2003; 138:898–901.

83. Bown MJ, Sutton AJ, Bell PR, Sayers RD. A meta-analysis of 50 years of ruptured abdominal aortic aneurysm repair. Br J Surg 2002; 89:714–30.

84. Boyle JR, Gibbs PJ, King D et al. Predicting outcome in ruptured abdominal aortic aneurysm: a prospective study of 100 consecutive cases. Eur J Vasc Endovasc Surg 2003; 26:607–11.

85. Neary WD, Crow P, Foy C et al. Comparison of POSSUM scoring and the Hardman Index in selection of patients for repair of ruptured abdominal aortic aneurysm. Br J Surg 2003; 90:421–5.

86. Parodi JC, Palmaz JC, Barone HD. Transfemoral intraluminal graft implantation for abdominal aortic aneurysms. Ann Vasc Surg 1991; 5:491–9.

87. White GH, Yu W, May J. Endoleak: a proposed new terminology to describe incomplete aneurysm exclusion by an endoluminal graft. J Endovasc Surg 1996; 3:124–5.

88. White GH, Yu W, May J, Chaufour X, Stephen MS. Endoleak as a complication of endoluminal grafting of abdominal aortic aneurysms: classification, incidence, diagnosis, and management. J Endovasc Surg 1997; 4:152–68.

89. White GH, May J, Waugh RC, Yu W. Type I and Type II endoleaks: a more useful classification for reporting results of endoluminal AAA repair. J Endovasc Surg 1998; 5:189–91.

90. White GH, May J, Waugh RC, Chaufour X, Yu W. Type III and type IV endoleak: toward a complete definition of blood flow in the sac after endoluminal AAA repair. J Endovasc Surg 1998; 5:305–9.

91. Veith FJ, Baum RA, Ohki T et al. Nature and significance of endoleaks and endotension: summary of opinions expressed at an international conference. J Vasc Surg 2002; 35:1029–35.

92. Fransen GA, Vallabhaneni SR Sr, van Marrewijk CJ et al. Rupture of infra-renal aortic aneurysm after endovascular repair: a series from EUROSTAR registry. Eur J Vasc Endovasc Surg 2003; 26:487–93.

Series of 34 patients from the EUROSTAR registry who ruptured following EVAR analysed to determine the risk factors for late rupture. See text.

93. Gould DA, McWilliams R, Edwards RD et al. Aortic side branch embolization before endovascular aneurysm repair: incidence of type II endoleak. J Vasc Intervent Radiol 2001; 12:337–41.

94. Resch T, Ivancev K, Lindh M et al. Persistent collateral perfusion of abdominal aortic aneurysm after endovascular repair does not lead to progressive change in aneurysm diameter. J Vasc Surg 1998; 28:242–9.

95. White GH, May J, Petrasek P et al. Endotension: an explanation for continued AAA growth after successful endoluminal repair. J Endovasc Surg 1999; 6:308–15.

96. Gilling-Smith G, Brennan J, Harris P et al. Endotension after endovascular aneurysm repair: definition, classification, and strategies for surveillance and intervention. J Endovasc Surg 1999; 6:305–7.

97. Mohan IV, Harris PL, van Marrewijk CJ, Laheij RJ, How TV. Factors and forces influencing stent-graft migration after endovascular aortic aneurysm repair. J Endovasc Ther 2002; 9:748–55.

98. Liffman K, Lawrence-Brown MM, Semmens JB et al. Analytical modeling and numerical simulation of forces in an endoluminal graft. J Endovasc Ther 2001; 8:358–71.

99. White RA, Donayre C, Kopchok G et al. Intravascular ultrasound: the ultimate tool for abdominal aortic aneurysm assessment and endovascular graft delivery. J Endovasc Surg 1997; 4:45–55.

100. Zanchetta M, Rigatelli G, Pedon L et al. Endovascular repair of complex aortic aneurysms: intravascular ultrasound guidance with an intracardiac probe. Cardiovasc Intervent Radiol 2003; 26:448–53.

101. Murphy MG, McWilliams RG. Postoperative radiology of endovascular abdominal aortic aneurysm repair. Semin Ultrasound CT MR 2004; 25:261–76.

102. McWilliams RG, Martin J, White D et al. Use of contrast-enhanced ultrasound in follow-up after endovascular aortic aneurysm repair. J Vasc Intervent Radiol 1999; 10:1107–14.

103. Sato DT, Goff CD, Gregory RT et al. Endoleak after aortic stent graft repair: diagnosis by color duplex ultrasound scan versus computed tomography scan. J Vasc Surg 1998; 28:657–63.

104. Murphy M, Hodgson R, Harris PL et al. Plain radiographic surveillance of abdominal aortic stent-grafts: the Liverpool/Perth protocol. J Endovasc Ther 2003; 10:911–12.

105. van der Laan MJ, Bartels LW, Bakker CJ, Viergever MA, Blankensteijn JD. Suitability of 7 aortic stent-graft models for MRI-based surveillance. J Endovasc Ther 2004; 11:366–71.

106. Hilfiker PR, Quick HH, Debatin JF. Plain and covered stent-grafts: in vitro evaluation of characteristics at three-dimensional MR angiography. Radiology 1999; 211:693–7.

107. Harris PL, Buth J, Mialhe C, Myhre HO, Norgren L. The need for clinical trials of endovascular abdominal aortic aneurysm stent-graft repair: The EUROSTAR Project. EUROpean collaborators on Stent-graft Techniques for abdominal aortic Aneurysm Repair. J Endovasc Surg 1997; 4:72–7.

108. Thomas SM, Gaines PA, Beard JD. Short-term (30-day) outcome of endovascular treatment of abdominal aortic aneurysm: results from the prospective Registry of Endovascular Treatment of Abdominal Aortic Aneurysm (RETA). Eur J Vasc Endovasc Surg 2001; 21:57–64.

109. Lifeline Registry: collaborative evaluation of endovascular aneurysm repair. J Vasc Surg 2001; 34:1139–46.

110. Vallabhaneni SR, Harris PL. Lessons learnt from the EUROSTAR registry on endovascular repair of abdominal aortic aneurysm repair. Eur J Radiol 2001; 39:34–41.

111. Thomas S, Beard JD. The RETA database: what have we learned? In: Wyatt M, Watkinson AF (eds) Endovascular intervention: current controversies. London: Tfm Publishers, 2004; pp. 37–45.

112. Adriaensen ME, Bosch JL, Halpern EF, Myriam Hunink MG, Gazelle GS. Elective endovascular versus open surgical repair of abdominal aortic aneurysms: systematic review of short-term results. Radiology 2002; 224:739–47.

113. Maldonado TS, Rockman CB, Riles E et al. Ischemic complications after endovascular abdominal aortic aneurysm repair. J Vasc Surg 2004; 40:703–9.

114. May J, White GH, Waugh R et al. Adverse events after endoluminal repair of abdominal aortic aneurysms: a comparison during two successive periods of time. J Vasc Surg 1999; 29:32–7.

115. Mehta M, Cayne N, Veith FJ et al. Relationship of proximal fixation to renal dysfunction in patients undergoing endovascular aneurysm repair. J Cardiovasc Surg (Torino) 2004; 45:367–74.

116. Prinssen M, Verhoeven EL, Buth J et al. A randomized trial comparing conventional and endovascular repair of abdominal aortic aneurysms. N Engl J Med 2004; 351:1607–18.

Multicentre randomised trial comparing open surgical and endovascular repair in 345 patients with 5 cm or larger AAA; 30-day mortality was 4.6% in the open repair group and 1.2% in the endovascular group.

117. van Marrewijk C, Buth J, Harris PL et al. Significance of endoleaks after endovascular repair of abdominal aortic aneurysms: the EUROSTAR experience. J Vasc Surg 2002; 35:461–73.

118. Torella F. Effect of improved endograft design on outcome of endovascular aneurysm repair. J Vasc Surg 2004; 40:216–21.

Analysis of patients after EVAR enrolled in the EUROSTAR registry. Patients treated with devices subsequently withdrawn were compared with patients receiving currently available grafts. The analysis showed that modern endografts are associated with improved results.

119. Anderson JL, Berce M, Hartley DE. Endoluminal aortic grafting with renal and superior mesenteric artery incorporation by graft fenestration. J Endovasc Ther 2001; 8:3–15.

120. Greenberg RK, Haulon S, O'Neill S, Lyden S, Ouriel K. Primary endovascular repair of juxtarenal aneurysms with fenestrated endovascular grafting. Eur J Vasc Endovasc Surg 2004; 27:484–91.

121. Verhoeven EL, Prins TR, Tielliu IF et al. Treatment of short-necked infrarenal aortic aneurysms with fenestrated stent-grafts: short-term results. Eur J Vasc Endovasc Surg 2004; 27:477–83.

122. Abraham CZ, Reilly LM, Schneider DB et al. A modular multi-branched system for endovascular repair of bilateral common iliac artery aneurysms. J Endovasc Ther 2003; 10:203–7.

123. Chuter TA, Gordon RL, Reilly LM, Pak LK, Messina LM. Multi-branched stent-graft for type III thoracoabdominal aortic aneurysm. J Vasc Intervent Radiol 2001; 12:391–2.

124. Tse LW, Steinmetz OK, Abraham CZ et al. Branched endovascular stent-graft for suprarenal aortic aneurysm: the future of aortic stent-grafting? Can J Surg 2004; 47:257–62.

125. Kirkpatrick UJ, McWilliams RG, Martin J et al. Late complications after ligation and bypass for popliteal aneurysm. Br J Surg 2004; 91:174–7.

126. Marty B, Wicky S, Ris HB et al. Success of thrombolysis as a predictor of outcome in acute thrombosis of popliteal aneurysms. J Vasc Surg 2002; 35:487–93.

127. Dorigo W, Pulli R, Turini F et al. Acute leg ischaemia from thrombosed popliteal artery aneurysms: role of preoperative thrombolysis. Eur J Vasc Endovasc Surg 2002; 23:251–4.

128. Gerasimidis T, Sfyroeras G, Papazoglou K et al. Endovascular treatment of popliteal artery aneurysms. Eur J Vasc Endovasc Surg 2003; 26:506–11.

CHAPTER

Fourteen

Thoracic and thoraco-abdominal aortic aneurysms, dissection and acute aortic syndrome

Peter R. Taylor and
Michael J.H.M. Jacobs

INTRODUCTION

This chapter is concerned with diseases of the descending thoracic aorta, principally dissection and aneurysms. The ascending aorta and the arch are currently the province of cardiothoracic surgeons, although this may change with the development of endovascular technology. Aneurysms of the ascending aorta and proximal arch are not discussed in this chapter and dissections affecting this aortic segment are only mentioned briefly. Acute aortic syndrome is a blanket term that has been introduced to include any acute pathology of the thoracic aorta irrespective of the aetiology. The common causes include acute dissection, transection and rupture of an aneurysm. Trauma, including aortic transection, is discussed in Chapter 10.

INCIDENCE

Aneurysms

The incidence of aneurysms of the descending thoracic aorta ranges between six and ten new aneurysms per 100 000 person-years.[1,2] The incidence is increasing, with a rise of 17% being recorded in England and Wales from 1974 to 1984.[3] The majority (80%) are degenerative in origin, although approximately 15% are related to aneurysmal dilatation of the false lumen of a chronic dissection. The remaining 5% are caused by Marfan's syndrome, infection, aortitis and previous aortic surgery. Aneurysms localised to the descending thoracic aorta and those affecting the distal arch should be classified separately from thoraco-abdominal aneurysms that affect the segment of abdominal aorta giving rise to the visceral vessels. Thoraco-abdominal aneurysms have been classified by Crawford into four types depending on their extent.[4]

- Type I affects the descending thoracic aorta and includes the proximal abdominal aorta with sparing of the infrarenal aorta.
- Type II is the most extensive and affects the whole of the descending thoracic aorta and abdominal aorta to the aortic bifurcation.
- Type III has a normal segment of proximal descending thoracic aorta and usually starts distal to T6.
- Type IV starts at the level of the diaphragm and affects the abdominal aorta with sparing of the thoracic aorta.

The aetiology of thoracic aneurysms remains unclear. Genetic studies have shown a high incidence of aneurysms in first-degree relatives of patients with thoracic aneurysms, and there is some evidence that aneurysms with a genetic basis grow faster than those occurring sporadically and may be inherited in an autosomal dominant fashion. The roles of inflammation and metalloproteinases, which have been studied extensively in the pathogenesis of infrarenal aortic aneurysms, have not yet been defined in thoracic aneurysmal disease.

Dissection

Aortic dissection affects around 10 per 100 000 of the population per year.[5] Deaths due to aortic dissection exceed those due to ruptured abdominal aortic aneurysm and 35% of cases are not diagnosed before death.[5,6] The mortality of aortic dissection exceeds 1% per hour in the first 48 hours.[6–10] Early death is more common with proximal dissections affecting the ascending aorta and arch compared with distal dissections involving the descending thoracic aorta.[11] If left untreated, 62–91% of patients will be dead in 1 week, and only 10% of proximal dissections and 40% of distal dissections will be alive at 1 year.[6–10] Patients with a proximal tear die from rupture into the pericardial cavity causing tamponade or from rupture into the mediastinum, pleura or abdomen. Early deaths from distal dissections are usually due to either rupture into the pleura or complications of branch vessel ischaemia. Branch vessel ischaemia complicates 30–50% of all dissections, resulting in myocardial ischaemia (3%), stroke (3–7%), paraplegia (3%), peripheral limb ischaemia (24%), visceral ischaemia (5%) and renal ischaemia (8%).[12]

Marfan's syndrome is one of the common inherited disorders of connective tissue, with a prevalence of 1 in 10 000. It is characterized by abnormalities of the cardiovascular system, musculoskeletal system and eyes. This is due to a defect in the gene producing fibrillin-1 (a component of elastin), which has been located on the long arm of chromosome 15.[13,14] The inheritance is autosomal dominant in 80%, while the remaining 20% are new mutations. Progressive dilatation of the aortic root causes rupture, dissection and aortic valve regurgitation. Dissection and aneurysm formation can also affect the arch and descending thoracic aorta. A second chromosomal locus on 3p24–25 has been identified with a Marfan-like condition associated with thoracic aortic aneurysms.

CLASSIFICATION OF DISSECTIONS

There are a number of systems used to classify aortic dissections. DeBakey classified them into three groups depending on the distribution of the dissected aorta, not the site of entry.

- Type 1 affects both ascending and descending aorta.
- Type 2 affects the ascending aorta only (often associated with Marfan's disease).
- Type 3 affects the aorta distal to the left subclavian artery (type 3a extending to the diaphragm and type 3b into the abdomen).

The Crawford classification divides them into proximal dissections, where the ascending aorta and arch are affected irrespective of the distal extent, and distal dissections, where the aorta distal to the left subclavian is involved with sparing of the proximal aorta. Again, the site of entry has no bearing on the classification. The Stanford classification separates them into type A, where the dissection affects the ascending aorta, and type B, where the ascending aorta is not affected. There is confusion as to how involvement of the arch aorta is classified and, once again, the classification takes no notice of the site of entry. In all classifications the dissection is considered to be acute if it presents within 14 days and chronic if longer than this. The European Society of Cardiologists has classified aortic dissection into five groups.[15]

- Type 1 is the traditional dissection with true and false lumens separated by a membrane (see **Fig. 14.7a**).
- Type 2 comprises intramural haemorrhage or haematoma associated with disruption of the media.
- Type 3 is a discrete or subtle dissection with a bulge at the tear site but no haematoma.
- Type 4 is rupture of a plaque or a penetrating ulcer (see **Fig. 14.6a**).
- Type 5 is either caused iatrogenically or is related to trauma.

This classification may be helpful in deciding which types are suitable for endovascular treatment. Those with a localised entry point, such as types 3, 4 and 5, are suitable for endovascular treatment. Type 2 may not have a clearly defined entry tear on imaging, and type 1 may have either single or multiple entry tears.

PRESENTATION

Aneurysm

Thoracic aneurysms are usually asymptomatic and are diagnosed on chest radiography performed for other reasons (**Fig. 14.1**). They may present with symptoms related to compression of surrounding structures. These include dysphagia from oesophageal compression, recurrent pneumonia due to pressure on the lung parenchyma and bronchioles, and chest or back pain from pressure on the thoracic vertebrae or adjacent ribs. They may cause shortness of breath, haemoptysis and, rarely, haematemesis. Aneurysms affecting the distal arch may cause stridor from compression of the trachea and can also affect the recurrent laryngeal nerve, causing a hoarse voice and bovine cough. Sudden chest pain can be caused by aneurysm expansion, localised rupture with a contained leak, or free rupture into the mediastinum or pleura. Rarely thoracic aneurysms may be the source of distal emboli.

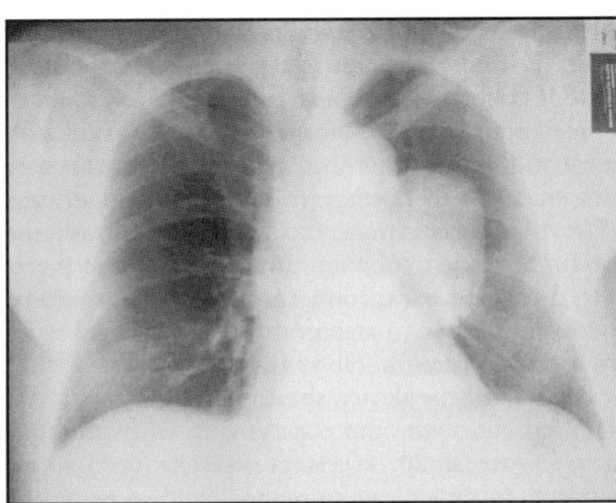

Figure 14.1 • Chest radiograph showing a thoracic aneurysm.

Dissection

The classic presentation of an acute type B dissection is a severe ripping interscapular pain. Proximal extension towards the heart may cause stroke, myocardial infarction, aortic valve regurgitation and finally cardiac tamponade. Distal extension may present with paraplegia, visceral and renal ischaemia and acute limb ischaemia. Chronic dissection may cause aneurysms associated with progressive dilatation of the false lumen, which occurs in 30–40% of patients.

Risk of rupture and timing of intervention

The prognosis of patients with thoracic aortic aneurysms is poor, with only 13–21% surviving for 5 years compared with 75% of age-matched controls.[1,16,17] The commonest cause of death is aortic rupture, which is usually fatal and accounts for half the deaths in these patients.[16,18] One series showed that 10% of patients with aneurysms less than 6 cm in diameter had ruptured and therefore advised 5 cm as the threshold for surgery.[18]

The risk of rupture appears to be higher for aneurysms related to dissection compared with degenerative aneurysms.[1,19] The overall median expansion of degenerative aneurysms is 1.4 mm/year, but increases with increasing aortic diameter in an exponential manner.[20] Intraluminal thrombus, previous stroke, smoking and peripheral vascular disease are important factors associated with aneurysm growth. Some authorities suggest that, given the relatively high risks involved in open surgery, the risk–benefit ratio only tilts in favour of surgery in aneurysms greater than 8 cm; those less than 5.5 cm can be safely observed and those between 5.5 and 7.5 cm can be closely observed.[21,22] The threshold for intervention in asymptomatic thoracic aneurysms in the USA is lower than that in the UK, which may explain their low 30-day mortality figures of 8–10%.[23–25] Reports from the UK have much higher mortality rates, ranging from 15 to 42% depending on the extent of the aneurysm in one series.[26] An audit of the majority of cardiothoracic centres in the UK showed a mortality of 28% for procedures on the descending thoracic aorta.[27] This is similar to a large study of 1542 patients identified from a discharge database in the USA, which showed an average mortality of 22%.[28] Saccular aneurysms have a higher risk of rupture and should be repaired at a smaller diameter than fusiform aneurysms. Symptomatic aneurysms should be repaired if the patient is fit enough, as the average length of time to rupture has been estimated to be 2 years.

INVESTIGATION

Aneurysm

High-quality multislice computed tomography (CT) is the investigation of choice for thoracic and thoraco-abdominal aneurysms (**Fig. 14.2**).[29–33] The proximal and distal extent of the aneurysm and its relation to the important branches should be clearly demonstrated. Magnetic resonance angiography (MRA) with gadolinium enhancement is a realistic alternative but is not as readily available as CT. Intra-arterial digital subtraction angiography (DSA) may be required as a secondary investigation. DSA may show ostial stenoses of branches more clearly and may help to clarify the length of any aneurysm (with a measuring catheter) if an endovascular approach is contemplated. Intravascular ultrasound has its proponents but is not widely used.[34,35] Assessment of renal function with the percentage contribution of each kidney by nuclear medicine scans can be useful. A full cardiac work-up is essential for open surgery and usually includes cardiac echocardiography and coronary angiography.

Dissection

Transoesophageal echocardiography, if available, is a quick investigation that can differentiate type A from type B dissections.[34] However, the usual first-line investigation is multislice CT, although MRA can also be used. High-quality imaging will correctly identify the true and false lumens, the extent of the dissection, any rupture, and the origins of the major branch vessels. The false lumen usually tracks around the convex border of the aortic knuckle, and where there is collapse of the true lumen due to high pressure within the false lumen, the false

(a)

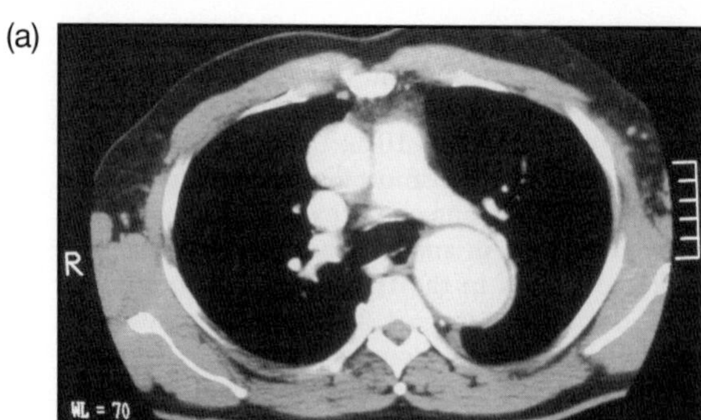

(b)

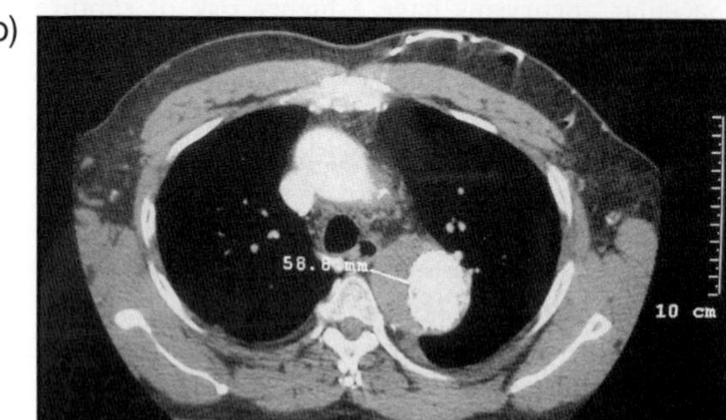

Figure 14.2 • **(a)** CT scan showing a large aneurysm of the descending thoracic aorta. **(b)** CT scan following successful endovascular repair showing a stentgraft containing all the intravenous contrast within its structure thereby excluding the aneurysm.

lumen will have a convex border bulging into the true lumen. Having correctly identified the lumen, it is then relatively easy to be confident about the correct placement of catheters in the true and false lumen. If the dissection extends to the iliac vessels, then the tear usually enters at the bifurcation of the aorta or the common iliac artery. Intravascular ultrasound is not readily available in many centres but can be very useful in distinguishing true from false lumens and also in the treatment of dissection.[36,37]

ANEURYSMS

Endovascular techniques

The proximal landing zone should be of a diameter suitable to accommodate the currently available devices and be at least 2 cm long. In patients with short aneurysm necks, it is possible to occlude the origin of the left subclavian artery thereby lengthening the proximal landing zone. This usually results in minimal symptoms, such as a cold hand and mild ischaemic pain on exercise, which resolve over a few weeks.[38] Rarely, this may cause paraplegia, which can be reversed with a cerebrospinal fluid (CSF) drain. There is also a theoretical risk of type II endoleaks and posterior circulation strokes. Some authorities recommend revascularisation with a carotid–subclavian transposition or bypass before placement of the stentgraft. Distal arch aneurysms (**Fig. 14.3**) may require the stentgraft to cover the origin of the left common carotid artery, and therefore a right-to-left carotid–carotid bypass should be performed prior to stentgraft deployment in order to maintain cerebral blood flow.

The size of the device sheath currently requires a femoral cut-down and occasionally when the iliac arteries are small, access grafts may need to be sutured to either the common iliac artery or the aorta. The procedure is usually performed under epidural anaesthesia, antibiotics are given routinely, and the patient's blood should be grouped and saved. A diagnostic catheter is placed from either the contralateral femoral artery using a simple percutaneous puncture, or from the brachial artery. The brachial approach enables a pigtail catheter to be curled around the origin of the left subclavian artery to mark its position at all times without the use of contrast. Marked tortuosity of the descending thoracic aorta is common and care must be taken when advancing the device into the optimum position. A stiff wire (e.g. Meier wire or Lunderquist) is used to straighten out tortuosity and allows deployment of the device around an angulated aneurysm. However, a through-and-through wire from the right brachial artery can be helpful in difficult cases. This should be used with a catheter to protect the origins of the vessels from damage due to a cheese-wire effect. The through-and-through wire should not be performed routinely since it traumatises the brachiocephalic artery and increases the risk of stroke. Where very accurate deployment of the proximal end is required, induction of asystole or reduction in blood pressure may be helpful but this is not required in the majority of cases. Thoracic aneurysms tend to be long and it is therefore common practice to trombone one stentgraft within another. With shrinkage of the aneurysm, there is a risk of dislocation of the tromboned stentgrafts within the aneurysm and therefore a considerable segment of overlap is required.

Following deployment of the stentgraft, conventional angiography is repeated to ensure that there are no endoleaks. Follow-up CT is performed at 30 days, 6 months, 1 year and then annually. This should be combined with formal chest radiography to check the integrity of the graft skeleton and its position. Some authorities suggest four-view chest radiography, with anteroposterior, lateral and right and left oblique views to adequately image the stents in order to exclude stent fractures.

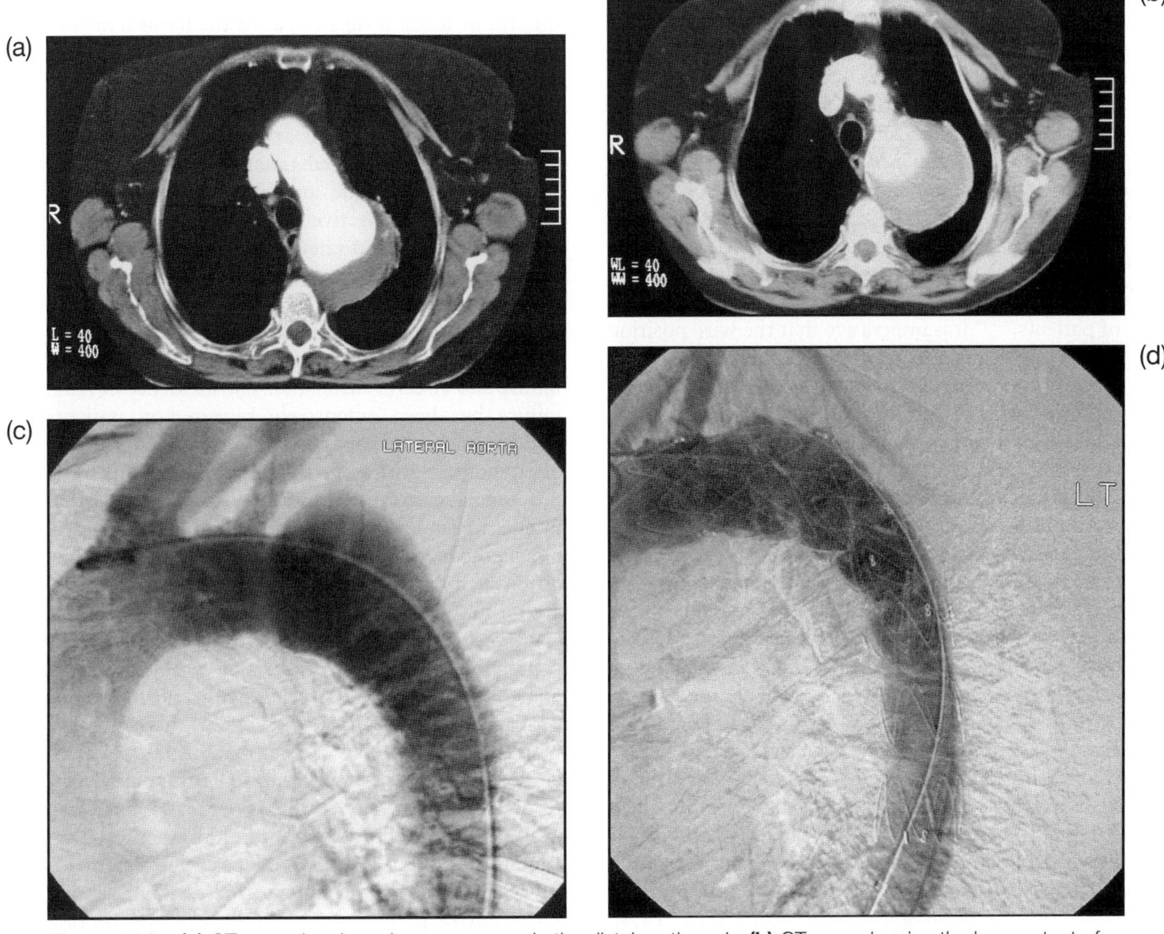

Figure 14.3 • **(a)** CT scan showing a large aneurysm in the distal aortic arch. **(b)** CT scan showing the large extent of the aneurysm on the superior aspect of the arch filled with thrombus. **(c)** Intra-arterial digital subtraction angiogram showing the aneurysm in relation to the arch vessels. **(d)** Intra-arterial digital subtraction angiogram after deployment of a stentgraft excluding the aneurysm.

RESULTS OF ENDOVASCULAR TECHNIQUES

The early results were published by Dake and colleagues from Stanford, California.[39,40] The initial 'first-generation' experience used custom-made stentgrafts, which comprised Gianturco-Z stents covered with an uncrimped woven polyester graft. A total of 144 patients were treated, 63% of whom were considered unsuitable for open surgical repair because of a combination of comorbid conditions. The operative mortality rate was 8% and major complications included stroke in 5%, paraplegia in 3%, myocardial infarction in 2% and respiratory insufficiency in 10%. The paraplegia rate increased to 11% in those who underwent simultaneous repair of an abdominal aortic aneurysm.[40] Primary success (isolation of the aneurysm) was achieved in 75% of patients, and this increased to 85% with secondary procedures. The median length of stay was 5 days.

Dake et al. subsequently used commercially made 'second-generation' stentgraft devices, namely the Thoracic Excluder (W.L. Gore & Associates).[39] This had a lower deployment profile, was extremely flexible and had rapid delivery compared with their custom-made version. The mean hospital stay decreased to 3 days and the early (30-day) mortality was reduced to 3.7% (1 of 27 patients). All patients were treated successfully and the complication rate was low, with only one myocardial infarction, no persistent paraplegia, impaired renal function in three patients and pulmonary impairment in eight. The low mortality of less than 10% has been confirmed by other centres using stentgrafts to treat thoracic aneurysms.[41–44] Endoluminal treatment of urgent and emergency cases, such as aneurysms that have leaked, can also be performed with relatively low morbidity and mortality.[45] Aneurysms related to previous coarctation repair can also be treated successfully with stentgrafts.[46] However, paraplegia and stroke affect about 5% of patients. Paraplegia can be reversed with CSF drainage if recognised early, which is an advantage of epidural or local anaesthesia compared with general.[42] One series used a CSF drain routinely for the first 24 hours and had the same rate of paraplegia seen with selective use.[44] Damage to iliac arteries due to the large size of the sheaths can occur in up to 10% of patients.[42,44] It is imperative that the wire position is not lost at the end of the procedure in case iliac artery rupture has occurred. Further endoluminal repair is possible with appropriate stentgrafts if the wire position is maintained. The alternative is open surgical repair.

Unfortunately, the Thoracic Excluder, manufactured from nitinol and polytetrafluoroethylene (PTFE), has recently been voluntarily withdrawn from the market for redesigning following reports of fractures in the nitinol frame in 10% of patients in the USA.[44] The commercially manufactured devices currently available in Europe include the Talent thoracic stent (Medtronic AVE), which consists of a nitinol frame covered with polyethylene, and Endofit (Endomed Inc.), which comprises a nitinol frame with a PTFE cover. The Talent can be difficult to deploy around the arch and its relatively short length is a drawback. This device is relatively inflexible so that it requires an adequate overlap when using more than one stentgraft to prevent them from separating in a tortuous aorta (**Fig. 14.4**). Mid-term follow-up of the Talent has also reported fractures of the metal stent.[44] The Endofit has poor column strength, which allows it to move distally during deployment. There have been reports of deaths from a kinked device and of stroke using the Endofit, and one device that collapsed had to be removed surgically.[47] Type I, II and III endoleaks have been reported during follow-up with thoracic devices, and continued surveillance for life is essential.[43,44,47]

The definitive stentgraft has not yet been manufactured, and further advances in thoracic stentgraft design are eagerly awaited. Branched stentgrafts are being developed to treat complex thoracic aortic aneurysms involving the aortic arch and visceral vessels.[48–50] Surgery is currently the optimum way of repairing thoraco-abdominal aneurysms.

Surgery

The majority of patients with descending thoracic and thoraco-abdominal aortic aneurysm (TAAA) have comorbid conditions associated with generalized atherosclerosis. The surgeon must therefore balance the risk of surgical repair against the natural history of this condition. Preoperative assessment of risk factors is essential, although proposed scoring systems have not been validated in prospective studies. Risk factors for death after extensive aortic surgery include impaired renal function, coronary artery disease, chronic lung disease and advanced age. The aim of elective surgery is to prevent the fatal complication of aneurysm rupture and is only of benefit if the gain in life expectancy exceeds the risk of the operation.

The major postoperative complications after thoracic and TAAA repair are paraplegia, renal failure and visceral ischaemia. The incidence of renal failure has been extensively reported in patients undergoing TAAA repair but to a much lesser extent after thoracic aortic aneurysm exclusion. The main difference between these operations is the potential ischaemic time during cross-clamping. In thoracic aortic aneurysms, clamp time depends on the time required for the proximal and distal anastomoses and, if necessary, for the reattachment of intercostal arteries. In TAAA repair, clamp time is significantly prolonged by the additional visceral and renal anastomoses. Renal failure is a significant risk factor for early and late postoperative mortality.[51,52]

Paraplegia remains one of the most devastating complications of thoracic and TAAA repair. Several techniques, such as left heart bypass[53] and CSF drainage,[54] have been shown to reduce neurological deficit, although the risk of paraplegia remains substantial. Ischaemic injury to the spinal cord is the result of permanent or temporary interruption in its blood supply. Permanent interruption is related to the variable and unpredictable anatomy of the arterial blood supply to the spinal cord, especially in a calcified aorta with plaques, mural thrombus or dissection, as well as to the extent of the aneurysm. One of the most important limitations during surgery is the inability to assess the adequacy of spinal cord blood flow. If a particular strategy fails to re-establish or restore spinal cord perfusion, this insufficiency will be detected only after the patient wakes up, when irreversible damage has already occurred. Adequacy of spinal cord blood flow can be assessed neurophysiologically with somatosensory evoked potentials (SSEPs) or motor evoked potentials (MEPs). The main disadvantages of SSEPs are the high incidence of false-negative and false-positive responses. This is because SSEPs assess conduction in the dorsal part of the spinal cord, whereas the motoneuronal system is located in the anterior horn. MEPs specifically reflect motor function and motor tract blood supply.[55,56] Paraplegia and temporary paraparesis has been reduced to 2–3% in extensive TAAA repair by the use of MEPs.[57]

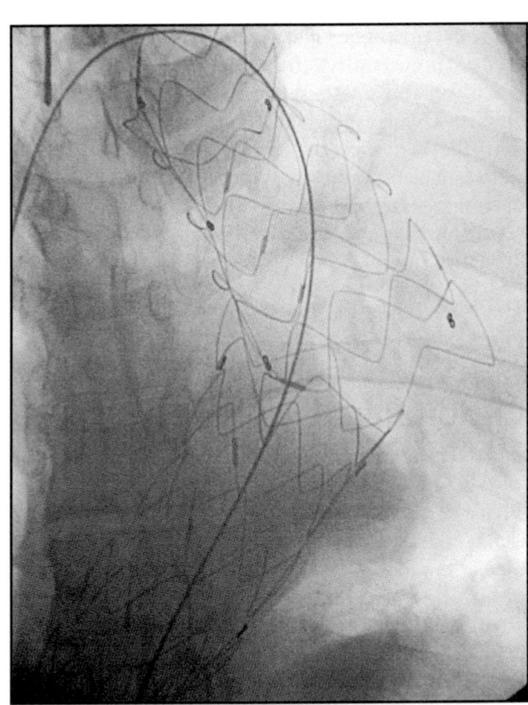

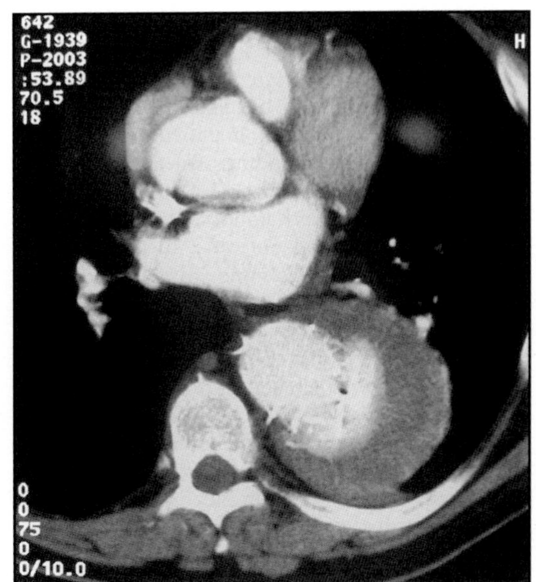

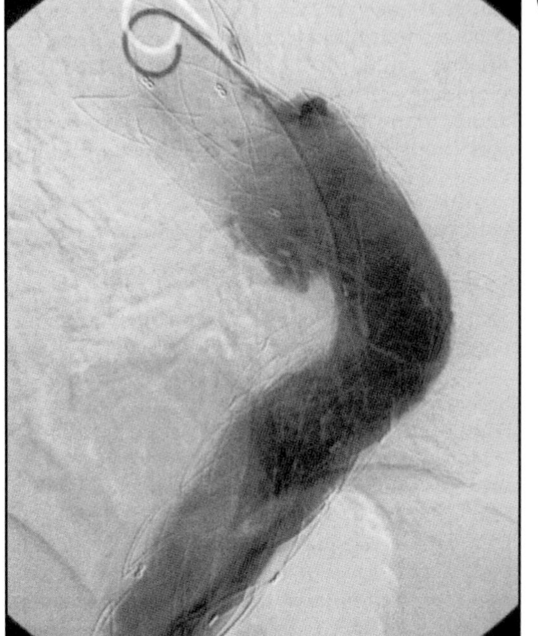

Figure 14.4 • **(a)** Dislocation of two Talent stentgrafts with separation causing a type III endoleak. **(b)** CT scan showing an endoleak associated with separation of the stentgrafts. **(c)** Repair with two further interposition Talent stentgrafts to bridge the gap.

The surgical protocol includes insertion of a catheter into the intrathecal space to drain CSF spontaneously if CSF pressure increases above 10 mmHg. Following intubation with a double-lumen endotracheal tube, patients are placed in the right lateral position on a vacuum beanbag. In TAAA repair, thoracotomy is usually performed in the sixth intercostal space and the incision extended to the abdomen. It is not necessary to completely transect the diaphragm, thereby reducing post-operative respiratory problems. The major part of the extracorporeal circulation system is heparin-coated, so therefore only limited heparinisation is required (0.5 mg/kg). Distal aortic perfusion (DAP) is established by cannulation of the left pulmonary vein or left atrium proximally and the femoral artery distally. Following aortic cross-clamping, DAP pressure is kept above 60 mmHg in order to maintain adequate MEPs and urine output.

In patients with type II, III and IV TAAA, the abdominal part of the procedure can be performed with selective perfusion of the coeliac, superior mesenteric and renal arteries.[58] Volume flow and pressure can be assessed during perfusion in order to guarantee adequate blood supply. During the aortic reconstruction, body temperature is allowed to fall spontaneously to between 31 and 34°C as measured by a rectal temperature probe. Following the proximal anastomosis and reattachment of intercostal arteries and visceral vessels, left heart bypass is used to rewarm the patient to 36°C.

Paraplegia following descending thoracic aneurysm repair occurs in 0–6% of patients. Obviously, the paraplegia rate significantly increases with the extent of the aortic repair, reaching 10–15% in type II aneurysms, despite DAP and CSF drainage. However, monitoring MEPs has significantly improved these results. Renal failure also depends on the extent of the procedure but specifically relates to preoperative renal function. In patients with normal kidney function undergoing an uncomplicated aneurysm resection of a thoracic aortic aneurysm, the clamp-and-sew technique without adjunctive procedures has a good outcome. In patients with renal insufficiency (creatinine >200 μmol/L), the clamp-and-sew technique, irrespective of the ischaemic clamp time, will lead to temporary or permanent renal failure. The incidence of gastrointestinal, hepatopancreatic and biliary ischaemia following extensive TAAA repair is small but probably underestimated. The immune responses of the visceral ischaemia–reperfusion injury and the subsequent impact on multiple organ failure are significant and can be limited by using DAP and selective organ perfusion. Respiratory failure is the most common complication after descending thoracic aortic repair. Independent predictors for respiratory failure, defined as ventilatory support exceeding 48 hours, are chronic pulmonary disease, history of smoking, and the development of cardiac and renal complications.[59] Patients who develop respiratory failure following thoracic aortic repair have a significantly higher mortality compared with those without postoperative pulmonary dysfunction.[60] Overall mortality following thoracic aortic aneurysm and TAAA repair can be estimated at 5% and 10–15% respectively. It should be emphasised that these figures are applicable to experienced centres, using adjunctive procedures. However, mortality rates are significantly higher in TAAA repair in inexperienced centres without the required infrastructure.

DISSECTION

Endoluminal repair

ACUTE DISSECTION

There are two mechanisms of branch vessel ischaemia:[61] static obstruction, where the aortic dissection extends into a branch vessel so compromising the lumen; and dynamic obstruction, where the aortic dissection flap moves across the origin of the branch vessel. Conventional stents can be placed within the true lumen to try to maintain patency of the true lumen (**Fig. 14.5**) or they can be placed in the occluded branch vessel to improve flow from either the true or false lumen. Where a branch vessel is ischaemic because of poor flow in

(a)

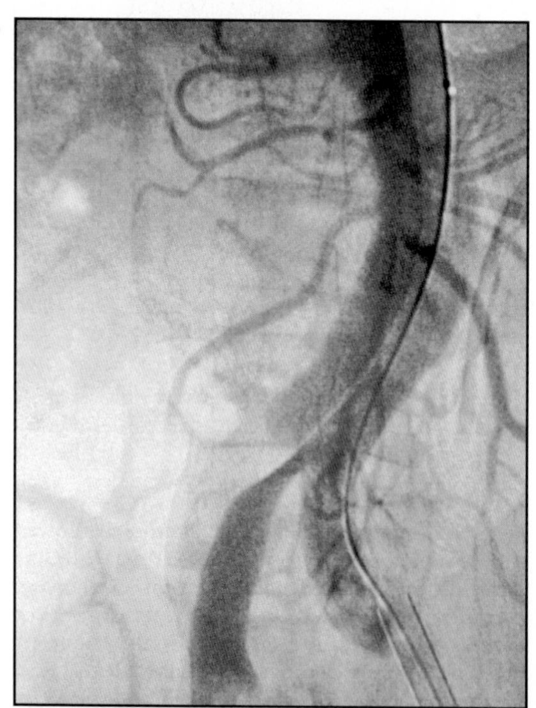

(b)

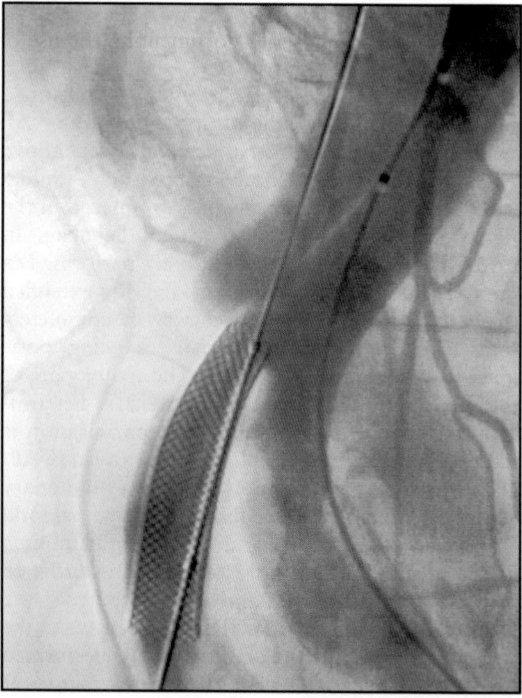

Figure 14.5 • **(a)** Static obstruction of the origin of the right common iliac artery by the false lumen. The large sheath in the left common iliac artery has been used to deploy a stentgraft across the primary tear. **(b)** The true lumen is dilated by the deployment of an uncovered stent.

one of the aortic lumens, a percutaneous fenestration may be performed. In this technique both true and false aortic lumens are catheterised and a stiff guidewire is passed across the dissection flap using either a balloon or an intravascular ultrasound catheter as the target. A large balloon then creates a tear in the flap and improves flow from one lumen to another. If there is persistent branch vessel occlusion, the origin of the branch vessels can be treated with conventional stents. If there is persistent aortic lumen collapse, stents may be used to hold open the lumen. Using such a technique in 40 patients, Slonim et al.[62] demonstrated successful flow to ischaemic regions in 93% of cases. The 30-day mortality rate of 25% was significantly lower than that following surgery but there was a high rate of late deaths due to rupture. Williams et al.[63] reported similar results, with successful revascularisation in 88% (21 of 24) and a mortality rate of 25% (6 of 24). Another small series of 41 patients reported successful revascularisation of side branches in 95%, with a mortality of 17%.[64]

More recently, several groups have advocated the concept of using stentgrafts to treat the primary entry tear (**Figs 14.6** and **14.7**). This decreases the pressure in the false lumen by obliterating flow into it and encouraging thrombosis. Thrombosis of the false lumen is associated with good long-term outcome.[65] Covering the primary tear can also be an effective treatment for dynamic and static obstruction of aortic side branches.

There are very few series documenting the use of this new technology to treat type B dissection.[66] The endpoints are 30-day or in-hospital mortality and thrombosis of the false lumen in the thorax, which may be complete or partial. Only three series give this information and all are small, treating less than 15 patients each.[67–69] The mortality ranges from 0 to 16% and the majority of patients achieve complete thrombosis of the false lumen. However, 7–21% of patients achieve only partial thrombosis of the false lumen. At present, there is no evidence as to how to treat patients who do not achieve complete thrombosis of the false lumen. The majority are treated expectantly, but in theory the use of bare stents may encourage thrombosis of the false lumen without occluding important intercostal, visceral or renal arteries. The fragility of the intimal flap in the acute stage militates against the use of bare stents, but they could be useful in the chronic phase of the dissection if the false lumen is not thrombosed. Balloon dilatation to fix the stentgraft to the aortic wall should not be used in acute dissection, as cases of conversion of type B to type A dissection have been reported with disastrous consequences. The length of aorta that should be covered is also currently not defined. Most authorities accept that covering the primary tear is all that should be done, but others advise covering the full length of the descending thoracic aorta. Clearly the latter would increase the incidence of paraplegia, and at present is not recommended.

(a)

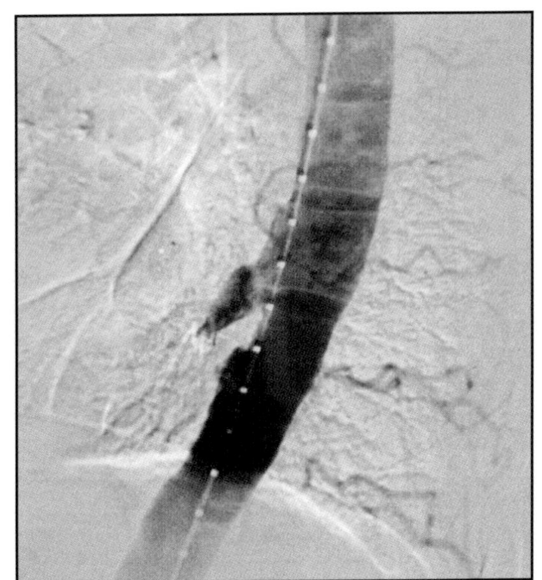

(b)

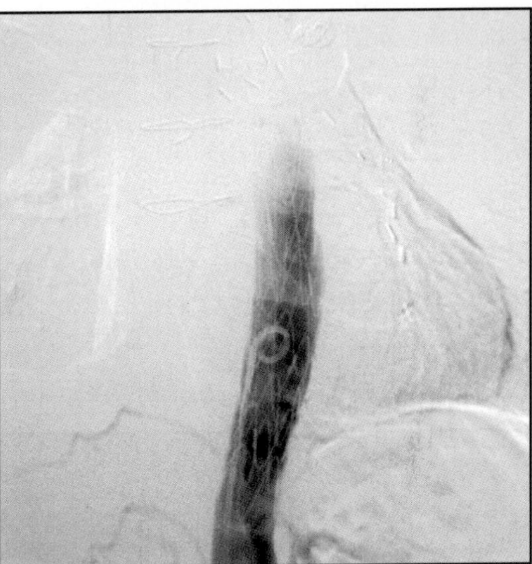

Figure 14.6 • **(a)** Intra-arterial digital subtraction angiogram showing a penetrating ulcer in the lower descending thoracic aorta, classified as type 4 dissection by the European Society of Cardiology. **(b)** Intra-arterial digital subtraction angiogram after stentgraft deployment showing exclusion of the ulcer.

It would appear that endovascular management of complicated type B dissections with branch vessel ischaemia is a highly useful therapeutic manoeuvre. Current data indicate that the preferred option is placement of a stentgraft across the primary tear.

(a)

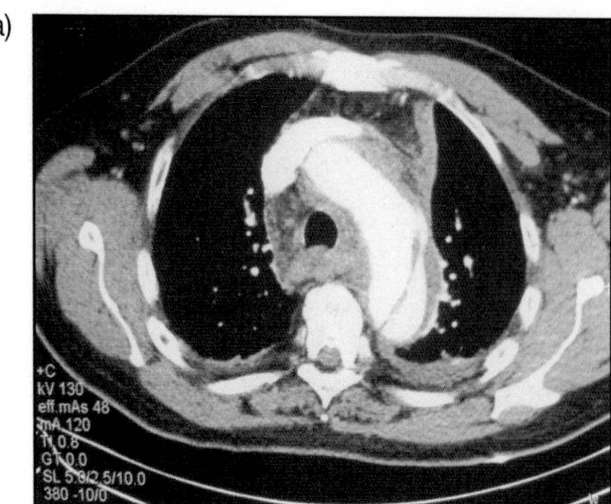

(b)

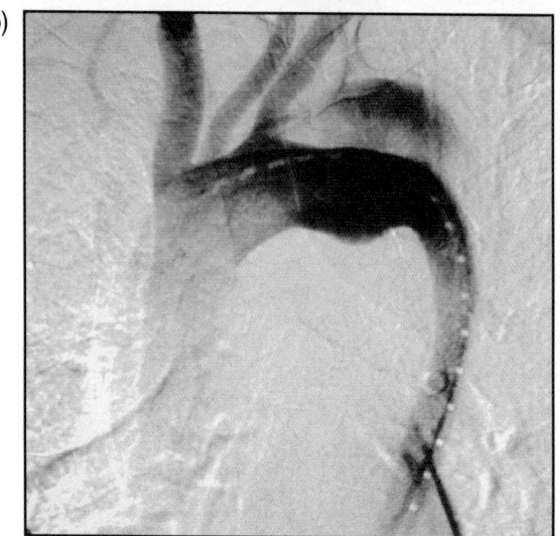

(c)

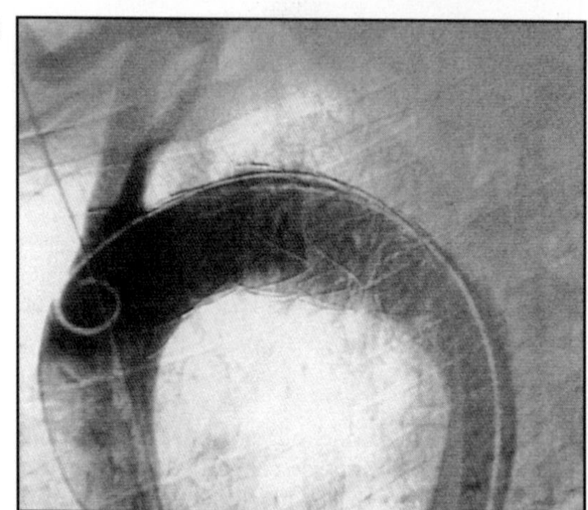

Figure 14.7 • **(a)** CT scan of an acute type B dissection showing marked periaortic haematoma with bilateral pleural effusions. **(b)** Intra-arterial digital subtraction angiogram showing the primary entry tear distal to the left subclavian artery. **(c)** Intra-arterial digital subtraction angiogram after stentgraft insertion showing exclusion of the false lumen.

Where there is relief of branch vessel ischaemia, no further intervention is required. If branch vessel ischaemia persists after a stentgraft is deployed across the primary tear, then peripheral stents should be used to maintain patency. Fenestration should be reserved for those cases where stentgrafting of the entry tear has failed or is not possible. These include residual false lumen encroachment upon the iliac vessels despite a technically successful stentgraft to the primary entry tear, and a dissection that only involves the aorta below the diaphragm.

Randomised trials need to be performed to identify the best treatment for acute dissection. These should comprise stentgraft versus best medical therapy for uncomplicated type B dissections, and surgery versus stentgraft for complicated type B dissection.

CHRONIC DISSECTION

Stentgrafts have been used to manage chronic type B dissections (**Fig. 14.8**). Nienaber et al.[68] treated 12 patients with a thoracic aortic diameter greater than 5.5 cm or continued expansion with pain and compared their results against a surgical group. There was no morbidity or mortality following endovascular repair of the chronic type B dissections and at 3 months all the false lumens had thrombosed. In the comparative surgical group there was a perioperative mortality of 8%, 25% had renal failure, 17% paraplegia and 25% a neurological deficit. There were no deaths in the endovascular group but 42% of the surgical group had died at 1 year. These early data are encouraging but long-term follow-up is required. A trial of surgery versus stentgrafting for aneurysms secondary to chronic dissection is required.

Surgery

Acute aortic dissection can occur at different ages and comprises several aetiologies, ranging from the young Marfan patient to the older, atherosclerotic, hypertensive patient. Furthermore, the clinical spectrum can vary from asymptomatic uncomplicated presentation to rupture with subsequent death. This heterogeneous population requires a selective approach.

Emergency surgery is indicated in patients with rupture, shock and haemodynamic instability. Ischaemia of visceral organs and kidneys, as well as spinal cord and lower limbs, requires immediate treatment. The surgical spectrum ranges from a limited fenestration to complete thoraco-abdominal aortic replacement. The extent of the disease, involvement of aneurysm and associated ischaemia determine the surgical strategy. The main problem in acute dissected aortas is the fragile nature of the aorta, when even cross-clamping can be fatal.

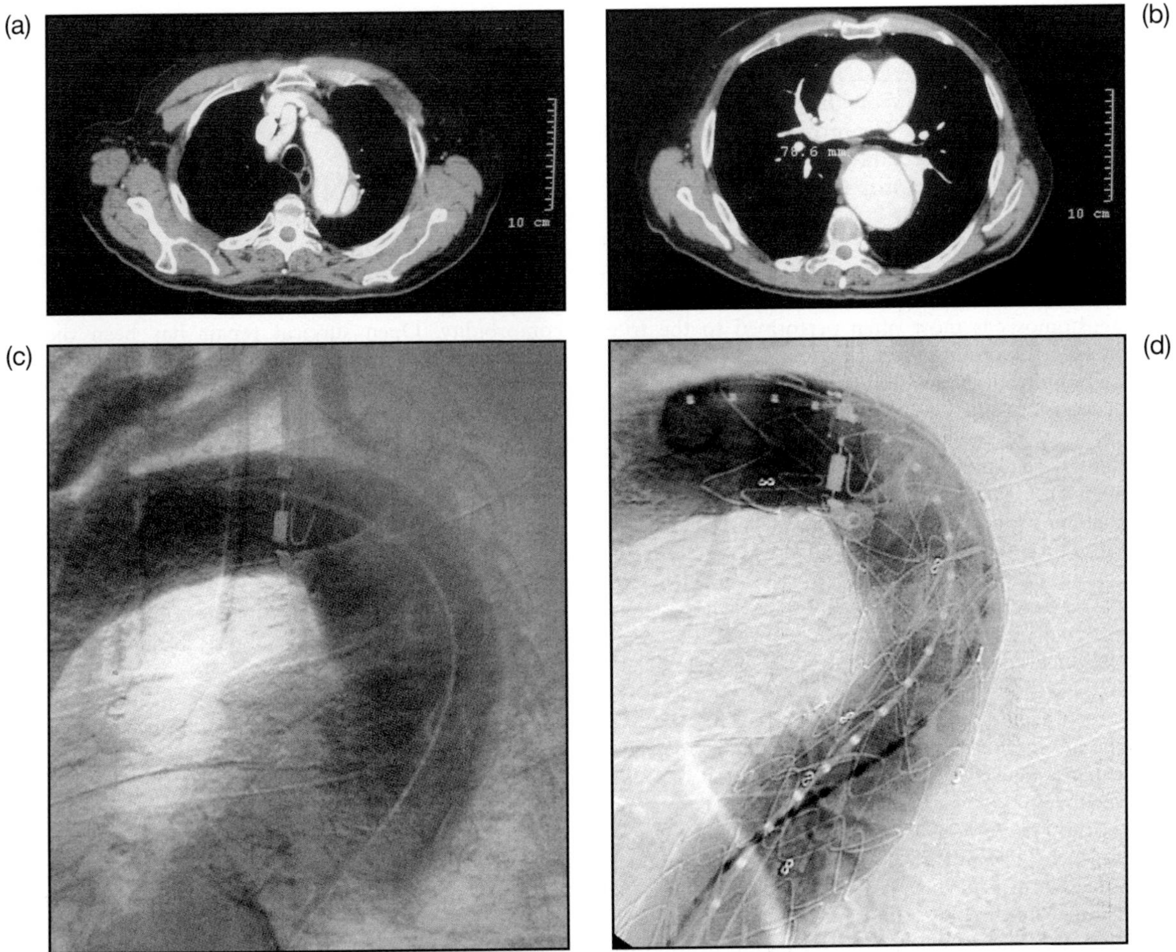

Figure 14.8 • **(a)** CT scan of a chronic type B dissection commencing in the distal arch. **(b)** CT scan showing an aneurysm of the more distal descending thoracic aorta. **(c)** Intra-arterial digital subtraction angiogram confirming the aneurysm in the descending thoracic aorta. **(d)** Intra-arterial digital subtraction angiogram after stentgraft deployment with exclusion of the aneurysm.

Limited procedures can end up in extensive reconstructions because of the parlous state of the aorta. The increase in cross-clamp times and the lack of collateral vessels result in death, paraplegia, renal failure and visceral infarction as compared with elective TAAA repair.[70]

Surgery for acute dissection has two primary objectives: replacement of the aortic segment at risk of rupture and relief of distal organ ischaemia. Because rupture is frequently located in the proximal half of the descending thoracic aorta, replacement can be limited to this portion. It is rare to replace the entire thoraco-abdominal aorta, although pre-existing aneurysmal disease and extensive ischaemia might require such a procedure.

Several techniques have been described, including thrombo-exclusion, tailored aortoplasty and local glue aortoplasty. The most recent and frequently reported procedures are prosthetic replacement of the thoracic aorta and aortic fenestration. The techniques of left heart bypass, selective organ perfusion and CSF drainage have contributed to better clinical results. Furthermore, improvements have been made in suture material, vascular clamps, impermeable grafts, tissue adhesives and haemostatic agents. Biological glue can be used to reinforce the proximal anastomosis but distal application is not recommended because conjoining the aortic layers might induce exclusion of important side branches.

The standard approach on the operating table is similar to elective TAAA repair, with the patient in the right lateral decubitus position and the left pelvis rotated posteriorly for access to the left femoral vessels. For limited thoracic aortic access, the fourth or fifth intercostal space is used; if a thoraco-abdominal approach is required, the sixth intercostal space is used. Following left heart bypass and aortic cross-clamping, a longitudinal aortotomy is made to show the intimal tear and the false and true lumens. The proximal anastomosis is performed at a dissection-free segment, reinforced with a circular Teflon strip if necessary. The level of the distal anastomosis can vary considerably and depends on many factors. The most limited scenario involves attachment a few centimetres distal to the proximal anastomosis. In acute dissection this anastomosis is most often performed to the true lumen, obliterating the false lumen. In chronic dissection distal fenestration is carried out by excising several centimetres of the dissected membrane, followed by reinforcement of the outer layer with subsequent end-to-end anastomosis. The main reason for this difference in surgical technique is to maintain blood flow to side branches originating from both the false and true lumen.

When the total descending thoracic aorta has to be replaced, the dissected membrane is completely resected, leaving a longitudinal rim at the non-dissected edges. Intercostal arteries are reattached if the aortic quality allows a safe anastomosis. A circumferential Teflon strip can be used to reinforce the anastomosis. Visceral, renal or limb ischaemia can be relieved by means of fenestration or open repair, although endovascular treatment is preferred as the first option because of its limited invasiveness. In most cases, infrarenal fenestration is effective in relieving a dynamic obstruction. The goal is to re-establish the same arterial pressures in the false and true lumens by creating a large re-entry in the infrarenal aorta. It should be noted that primary closure of the diseased aorta is not always feasible, and may require a small interposition graft. Lower limb ischaemia, in the absence of proximal ischaemic problems, is usually relieved by means of catheter fenestration or extra-anatomical bypass such as femoro-femoral or axillo-femoral bypass.

CONCLUSIONS

The incidence of aneurysms of the descending thoracic aorta is increasing. The prognosis for these patients is poor and they frequently have serious comorbidity. Open surgical repair has been the mainstay of treatment but is associated with significant mortality and morbidity. This can be reduced with adjuvant techniques such as DAP and drainage of CSF. Monitoring the function of the spinal cord has also improved outcome.

Acute dissection of the thoracic aorta is associated with high mortality. Dissections affecting the ascending aorta should be treated surgically. Type B dissections should be treated medically with effective hypotensive therapy. Intervention in type B dissection is reserved for those patients with complications.

Endoluminal techniques using stentgrafts for treating both aneurysms and the complications of dissection offer some real advantages in terms of reduced morbidity and mortality but their overall use is limited. Durability remains an important issue for stentgrafts and long-term follow-up is essential to prove their efficacy. Current endoluminal devices require significant improvements and future developments in branched and fenestrated stentgrafts will extend their role in the treatment of thoracic aortic disease. Clinical trials will eventually be required to gain level I evidence for their role.

Key points

- Acute dissection is classified according to the site of the primary tear. Type A affects the ascending thoracic aorta while type B usually affects the aorta distal to the left subclavian artery.
- The diagnosis can be made with transoesophageal echocardiography and/or multislice CT.
- Type A dissection is treated with surgical repair.
- Type B dissection is treated with hypotensive medication, and intervention is reserved for end-organ ischaemia, rupture and false aneurysm formation.
- The diameter at which intervention is justified for thoracic aneurysms remains contentious but lies between 5.5 and 7.5 cm. The risk–benefit equation for intervention should be assessed for each individual patient.
- Thoraco-abdominal aneurysms involve the origins of the visceral arteries and open surgery is the mainstay of treatment. Adjunctive techniques, such as DAP and CSF drainage, help to improve the outcome.
- Clinical trials are urgently required to assess the efficacy of endoluminal repair compared with surgery for both complicated type B dissection and aneurysms of the descending thoracic aorta.
- The development of stentgrafts for treating thoracic aortic disease is in its infancy. Improvements in design will increase their use and reliability. Branched devices may ultimately allow the treatment of type A dissections and thoraco-abdominal aneurysms.

REFERENCES

1. Bickerstaff LK, Pairolero PC, Hollier LH et al. Thoracic aortic aneurysms: a population-based study. Surgery 1982; 92:1103–8.
2. Clouse WD, Hallett JW Jr, Schaff HV et al. Improved prognosis of thoracic aortic aneurysms. JAMA 1998; 280:1926–9.
3. Fowkes FG, MacIntyre CC, Ruckley CV. Increasing incidence of aortic aneurysms in England and Wales. Br Med J 1989; 298:33–5.
4. Crawford ES. Thoracoabdominal and abdominal aortic aneurysm involving renal, superior mesenteric and celiac arteries. Ann Surg 1974; 179:763–72.
5. Svensson LG, Crawford ES. Aortic dissection and aortic aneurysm surgery: clinical observations, experimental investigations, and statistical analyses. Part II. Curr Probl Surg 1992; 29:913–1057.
6. Hirst AE Jr, Johns VJ Jr, Klime SE Sr. Dissecting aneurysm of the aorta: a review of 505 cases. Medicine (Baltimore) 1958; 37:217–79.
7. Roberts WC. Aortic dissection: anatomy, consequences and causes. Am Heart J 1981; 101:195–214.
8. Lindsay J Jr, Hurst JW. Clinical features and prognosis in dissecting aneurysms of the aorta: a re-appraisal. Circulation 1967; 35:880–8.
9. Anagnostopoulos CE, Prabhakar MJS, Vittle CE. Aortic dissections and dissecting aneurysms. Am J Cardiol 1972; 30:263–73.
10. Applebaum A, Karp RB, Kirklin JW. Ascending vs. descending aortic dissections. Ann Surg 1976; 183:296–300.
11. Doroghazi RM, Slater EE, DeSanctis RW et al. Long-term survival of patients with treated aortic dissection. J Am Coll Cardiol 1984; 3:1026–34.
12. Fann JI, Sarris GE, Mitchell SR et al. Treatment of patients with aortic dissection presenting with peripheral vascular complication. Ann Surg 1990; 212:705–13.
13. Dietz HC, Gutting GR, Pyeritz RE et al. Marfan syndrome caused by a recurrent de novo missense mutation in the fibrillin gene. Nature 1991; 352:337–9.
14. Kainulainen K, Pulkkinen L, Savolainen A et al. Location on chromosome 15 of the new gene defect causing Marfan syndrome. N Engl J Med 1990; 323:935–9.
15. Erbel R, Alfonso F, Boileau C et al. Diagnosis and management of aortic dissection. Eur Heart J 2001; 22:1642–81.
16. Pressler V, McNamara JJ. Aneurysms of the thoracic aorta. J Thorac Cardiovasc Surg 1985; 89:50–4.
17. Borst HG, Jurmann M, Bühner B, Laas J. Risk of replacement of descending aorta with a standardized left heart bypass technique. J Thorac Cardiovasc Surg 1994; 107:126–33.
18. Crawford ES, DeNatale RW. Thoracoabdominal aortic aneurysm: observation regarding the natural course of the disease. J Vasc Surg 1986; 3:578–82.

19. Griepp RB, Ergin MA, Galla JD et al. Natural history of descending thoracic and thoracoabdominal aneurysms. Ann Thorac Surg 1999; 67:1927–30.
20. Bonser RS, Pagano D, Lewis ME et al. Clinical and patho-anatomical factors affecting expansion of thoracic aortic aneurysms. Heart 2000; 84:277–83.
21. Pitt MPI, Bonser RS. The natural history of thoracic aortic aneurysm: an overview. J Cardiovasc Surg 1997; 12:270–8.
22. Elefteriades JA. Natural history of thoracic aortic aneurysms: indications for surgery and surgical versus nonsurgical risks. Ann Thorac Surg 2002; 74:S1877–S1880.
23. Svensson LG, Crawford ES, Hess KR et al. Experience with 1509 patients undergoing thoraco-abdominal aortic operations. J Vasc Surg 1993; 17:357–68.
24. Hollier LH, Money SR, Haslund TC et al. Risk of spinal cord dysfunction in patients undergoing thoracoabdominal aortic replacement. Am J Surg 1992; 164:210–13.
25. Safi HJ, Campbell MP, Miller CC III et al. Cerebral spinal fluid drainage and distal aortic perfusion decrease the incidence of neurological deficit: the results of 343 descending and thoracoabdominal aneurysm repairs. Eur J Vasc Endovasc Surg 1997; 14:118–24.
26. Gilling-Smith GL, Worswick L, Knight PF et al. Surgical repair of thoracoabdominal aortic aneurysms: 10 years' experience. Br J Surg 1995; 82:624–9.
27. Keogh BE, Kinsman R. National adult cardiac surgical database report 1998. Concord Services London: Society of Cardiothoracic Surgeons of Great Britain and Ireland, 1999.

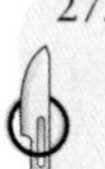

A registry of the results for operations including thoracic aneurysms undertaken by cardiothoracic units in the UK and Ireland.

28. Cowan JA Jr, Dimick JB, Henke PK et al. Surgical treatment of intact thoracoabdominal aortic aneurysms in the United States: hospital and surgeon volume-related outcomes. J Vasc Surg 2003; 37:1169–74.
29. Rubin GD, Walker PJ, Dake MD et al. Three-dimensional spiral computed tomographic angiography: an alternative imaging modality for the abdominal aorta and its branches. J Vasc Surg 1993; 18:656–65.
30. Balm R, Eikelboom BC, van Leeuwen MS et al. Spiral CT-angiography of the aorta. Eur J Vasc Surg 1994; 8:544–51.
31. Van Hoe L, Baert AL, Gryspeerdt S et al. Supra- and juxtarenal aneurysms of the abdominal aorta: preoperative assessment with thin-section spiral CT. Radiology 1996; 198:443–8.
32. Broeders I, Blankensteijn J, Olree M et al. Preoperative sizing of grafts for transfemoral endovascular aneurysm management: a prospective comparative study of spiral CT angiography, arteriography and conventional CT imaging. J Endovasc Surg 1997; 4:252–61.
33. Urban BA, Bluemke DA, Johnson KM, Fishman EK. Imaging of thoracic aortic disease. Cardiol Clin 1999; 17:659–82.
34. Vignon P, Spencer KT, Rambaud G et al. Differential transesophageal echocardiographic diagnosis between linear artifacts and intraluminal flap of aortic dissection or disruption. Chest 2001; 119:1778–90.
35. Rapezzi C, Rocchi G, Fattori R et al. Usefulness of transesophageal echocardiographic monitoring to improve the outcome of stent-graft treatment of thoracic aortic aneurysms. Am J Cardiol 2001; 87:315–19.
36. Buck T, Gorge G, Hunold P, Erbel R. Three-dimensional imaging in aortic disease by lighthouse transesophageal echocardiology using intravascular ultrasound catheters. Comparison to three-dimensional transesophageal echocardiology and three-dimensional intra-aortic ultrasound imaging. J Am Soc Echocardiogr 1998; 11:243–58.
37. Manninen HI, Rasanen H. Intravascular ultrasound in interventional radiology. Eur Radiol 2000; 10:1754–62.
38. Gorich J, Asquan Y, Seifarth H et al. Initial experience with intentional stent-graft coverage of the subclavian artery during endovascular thoracic aortic repairs. J Endovasc Ther 2002; 9(suppl. 2:II): 39–43.
39. Dake MD. Endovascular treatment for thoracic aortic aneurysms. In: Branchereau A, Jacobs M (eds) Surgical and endovascular treatment of aortic aneurysms. Armonk, NY: Futura, 2000; pp. 27–33.
40. Dake MD, Miller DC, Mitchell RS et al. The 'first generation' of endovascular stent-grafts for patients with aneurysms of the descending thoracic aorta. J Thorac Cardiovasc Surg 1998; 116:689–704.
41. Orend KH, Scharrer-Pamler R, Kapfer X et al. Endovascular treatment in diseases of the descending thoracic aorta: 6-year results of a single center. J Vasc Surg 2003; 37:91–9.
42. Bell RE, Taylor PR, Aukett M, Sabharwal T, Reidy JF. Mid-term results for second-generation thoracic stent grafts. Br J Surg 2003; 90:811–17.
43. Criado FJ, Clark NS, Barnatan MF. Stent graft repair in the aortic arch and descending thoracic aorta: a 4-year experience. J Vasc Surg 2002; 36:1121–8.
44. Ellozy SH, Carroccio A, Minor M et al. Challenges of endovascular tube graft repair of thoracic aortic aneurysm: midterm follow-up and lessons learned. J Vasc Surg 2003; 38:676–83.
45. Bell RE, Taylor PR, Aukett M, Sabharwal T, Reidy JF. Results of urgent and emergency thoracic

procedures treated by endoluminal repair. Eur J Vasc Endovasc Surg 2003; 25:527–31.

46. Bell RE, Taylor PR, Aukett M et al. Endoluminal repair of aneurysms associated with coarctation. Ann Thorac Surg 2003; 75:530–3.

47. Melissano G, Tshomba Y, Civilini E, Chiesa R. Disappointing results with a new commercially available thoracic endograft. J Vasc Surg 2004; 39:124–30.

48. Chuter TA, Gordon RL, Reilly LM et al. Multi-branched stent-graft for type III thoracoabdominal aneurysm. J Vasc Intervent Radiol 2001; 12:391–2.

49. Inoue K, Hosokawa H, Iwase T et al. Aortic arch reconstruction by transluminally placed endovascular branched stent graft. Circulation 1999; 100(suppl. 19):316–321.

50. Chuter TAM, Schneider DB, Reilly LM, Lobo EP, Messina LM. Modular branched stent graft for endovascular repair of aortic arch aneurysm and dissection. J Vasc Surg 2003; 38:859–63.

51. Safi HJ, Harlin SA, Miller CC et al. Predictive factors for acute renal failure in thoracic and thoracoabdominal aortic aneurysm surgery. J Vasc Surg 1996; 24:338–45.

52. Cambria RP, Davison JK, Zanetti S, L'Italien G, Atamian S. Thoracoabdominal aneurysm repair: perspectives over a decade with the clamp-and-sew technique. Ann Surg 1997; 226:294–303.

53. Coselli JS, LeMaire SA. Left heart bypass reduces paraplegia rates after thoracoabdominal aortic aneurysm repair. Ann Thorac Surg 1999; 67:1931–4.

54. Safi HJ, Hess KR, Randel M et al. Cerebrospinal fluid drainage and distal aortic perfusion: reducing neurologic complications in repair of thoracoabdominal aortic aneurysm types I and II. J Vasc Surg 1996; 23:223–8.

55. Jacobs MJ, Elenbaas TW, Schurink GW, Mess WH, Mochtar B. Assessment of spinal cord integrity during thoracoabdominal aortic aneurysm repair. Ann Thorac Surg 2002; 74:S1864–S1866.

56. Jacobs MJ, Meylaerts SA, de Haan P, de Mol BA, Kalkman CJ. Assessment of spinal cord ischemia by means of evoked potential monitoring during thoracoabdominal aortic surgery. Semin Vasc Surg 2000; 13:299–307.

57. Jacobs MJ, de Mol BA, Elenbaas T et al. Spinal cord blood supply in patients with thoracoabdominal aortic aneurysms. J Vasc Surg 2002; 35:30–7.

58. Jacobs MJ, Eijsman L, Meylaerts SA et al. Reduced renal failure following thoracoabdominal aortic aneurysm repair by selective perfusion. Eur J Cardiothorac Surg 1998; 14:201–5.

59. Svensson LG, Hess KR, Coselli JS, Safi HJ, Crawford ES. A prospective study of respiratory failure after high-risk surgery on the thoracoabdominal aorta. J Vasc Surg 1991; 14:271–82.

60. Money SR, Rice K, Crockett D et al. Risk of respiratory failure after repair of thoraco-abdominal aortic aneurysms. Am J Surg 1994; 168:152–5.

61. Williams DM, Do YL, Hamilton BH et al. The dissected aorta. Part III. Anatomy and radiological diagnosis of branch vessel compromise. Radiology 1997; 203:37–44.

62. Slonim SM, Miller DC, Mitchell RS et al. Percutaneous balloon fenestration and stenting for life threatening ischemic complications in patients with acute aortic dissection. J Thorac Cardiovasc Surg 1999; 117:1118–27.

63. Williams DM, Lee DY, Hamilton BH et al. The dissected aorta: percutaneous treatment of ischaemic complications. Principles and results. J Vasc Intervent Radiol 1997; 8:605–25.

64. Gaxotte VD, Haulon S, Willoteaux S et al. Endovascular treatment in complications of aortic dissection: retrospective study on 52 patients. Cardiovasc Intervent Radiol 2002; 25(suppl. 2): S157.

65. Bernard Y, Zimmermann H, Chocron S et al. False lumen patency as a predictor of late outcome in aortic dissection. Am J Cardiol 2001; 87:1378–82.

66. Bell RE, Taylor PR. Endovascular treatment of aortic type B dissection. In: Branchereau A, Jacobs M (eds) Vascular emergencies. New York: Futura, Blackwell Publishing 2003; pp. 99–106.

67. Dake MD, Kato NK, Mitchell RS et al. Endovascular stent-graft placement for the treatment of acute aortic dissection. N Engl J Med 1999; 340:1546–52.

68. Nienaber CA, Fattori R, Lund G et al. Non-surgical reconstruction of thoracic aortic dissection by stent-graft placement. N Engl J Med 1999; 340:1539–45.

69. Lonn L, Delle M, Lepore V et al. Endograft therapy of the thoracic aorta in aortic dissections. Cardiovasc Intervent Radiol 2002; 25(suppl. 2):S158.

70. Hagan PG, Nienaber CA, Isselbacher EM et al. The International Registry of Acute Aortic Dissection (IRAD): new insights into an old disease. JAMA 2000; 283:897–903.

CHAPTER

Fifteen

Renal and intestinal vascular disease

Jonathan G. Moss, Philip A. Kalra, Trevor Cleveland and George Hamilton

RENAL ARTERY DISEASE

Renal artery stenosis is an anatomical description of a lesion that may lead to a variety of pathophysiological disease processes or that may simply be silent throughout life. The pathological entity in the vast majority of patients in the Western world is atherosclerosis and the term 'atherosclerotic renovascular disease' has been coined. The remainder are a rare group of disparate arteritides that have little in common with their atherosclerotic counterpart. This small group are distinct and dealt with briefly and separately in this chapter.

ARTERITIS

The arteritides make up a rare group of disparate disorders of which the most common is fibromuscular disease.[1] This in itself consists of five different types. In general, a younger group of patients is affected than the group with atherosclerosis, with a female predominance. Some undoubtedly go through life undetected but the commonest presentation is hypertension. It is always worth imaging the renal arteries in these young patients as fibromuscular disease in particular responds well to percutaneous transluminal angioplasty (PTA), with good clinical results.[2] Fibromuscular disease has been reported to progress in up to one-third of patients, but this almost never leads to occlusion and loss of renal function is exceptional. Although an abdominal bruit may be present, the diagnosis will usually require conventional digital subtraction angiography. Selective angiographic views may be necessary to detect subtle branch lesions. Although magnetic resonance angiography (MRA) can detect fibromuscular disease in the proximal vessels, it is less sensitive for detecting the second- and third-order branches where fibromuscular disease can be located. The results of PTA are good, with 10-year cumulative patency rates of 87% and up to 50% of patients cured of their hypertension, the remainder having a reduced drug burden and improved blood pressure control.[1,2]

Takayasu's arteritis is a non-specific inflammatory disease that mainly affects large arteries such as the aorta and its main branches including the renal artery. It is the most common cause of renovascular hypertension in India and China, in contrast to Western countries. The majority of patients can be managed medically on corticosteroids, with monitoring of disease activity using the erythrocyte sedimentation rate (ESR). In the chronic inactive stage, PTA can produce a reasonable blood pressure response.[3]

ATHEROSCLEROTIC RENAL VASCULAR DISEASE

Definition and pathology

By far the most common cause of renovascular disease is atheromatous narrowing of the renal arteries. Lesions are usually 'ostial' (90%), occurring within 1 cm of the origin of the renal artery,[4] and atheromatous disease of the aorta is very frequently responsible. Because occlusion of the renal artery is present in up to 50% of patients, the condition is best described as atherosclerotic renovascular disease (ARVD) rather than as renal artery stenosis (RAS). Disease may be unilateral or bilateral and multiple atheromatous lesions are recognised. Exactly what degree of angiographic luminal narrowing is representative of significant RAS is controversial; some authors suggest greater than 75% of the diameter, others greater than 50%. Experiments in the dog have demonstrated a significant pressure gradient across a RAS of 60%,[5] but in humans even RAS lesions of less than 50% can be associated with gradients of 15 mmHg.[6] Risk factors for the development of ARVD are the same as for atheroma elsewhere.

Epidemiology and clinical features

ARVD is very common and is a disease of ageing. A post-mortem study from over three decades ago showed the incidental finding of significant ARVD (defined as RAS >50%) in over 40% of patients aged over 75 years,[7] irrespective of their cause of death. Many patients are likely to have 'clinically silent' ARVD so that it is not possible to estimate the true prevalence of the condition in the general population. However, using a definition of RAS as greater than 60% luminal narrowing (determined by Doppler ultrasound), Hansen et al.[8] showed that 6.8% of 834 community-based individuals aged over 65 years had significant (and incidental) ARVD.

Presentation

ARVD should be considered as part of a diffuse vascular disease process rather than as a solitary disease affecting the renal circulation. Extrarenal vascular comorbidities should not be forgotten during the assessment of patients with ARVD as these may be the major contributors to the poor outcome of these patients. However, it is the patient with ARVD and renal failure that has led to the greatest interest in this common condition.

HYPERTENSION AND ARVD

ARVD is found in 2–5% of all cases of hypertension[9] but, as discussed later, it is likely that the hypertension precedes the development of ARVD in many cases and that the latter is incidental to the pathophysiology of the hypertension. In the Cooperative Study of Renovascular Hypertension, older age, shorter duration of hypertension, accelerated hypertension, grade III or IV retinopathy, and the presence of coronary, peripheral or cerebrovascular disease or an abdominal bruit were the clinical findings significantly associated with a renovascular aetiology, when comparing patients to those with essential hypertension.[10] Some investigators suggest that the coexistence of hypertension and renovascular disease equates to renovascular hypertension, but the most rigorous definition of the latter necessitates demonstration of a cure or considerable improvement in hypertension following revascularisation.

ARVD AND CHRONIC RENAL FAILURE

Patients with chronic renal failure and ARVD are common and most are found to have associated hypertension, which may be of paramount importance in the pathogenesis of the chronic renal failure. The prevalence of ARVD in patients with end-stage renal failure is at least 15%, and may reach over 25% in the elderly.[11] Current thinking suggests that ARVD is an association, rather than the cause, of the majority of these cases of chronic renal failure and end-stage renal failure, which has important implications for treatment.

ARVD AND ACUTE RENAL FAILURE

Patients with ARVD can present with acute renal failure when there is bilateral renal artery occlusion, cholesterol atheroembolisation, damage from iodinated radiographic contrast agents during angiography, or with injudicious use of angiotensin-converting enzyme (ACE) inhibitors (or angiotensin II receptor blockers). The avoidance of renal artery occlusion has underpinned the historical rationale for revascularisation in patients with tight RAS lesions (see below).

Cholesterol embolisation is probably commoner than currently recognised, but it should be suspected when acute renal failure is seen in patients with severe aortic atheroma who undergo aortic surgical or angiographic procedures, thrombolysis or anticoagulation. The progression of renal dysfunction is variable but end-stage renal failure is not inevitable, especially where anticoagulants can be withdrawn and statins administered. Associated clinical features include purpuric skin rash or livedo reticularis, proteinuria and eosinophilia.

Cases of ACE inhibitor (or angiotensin II receptor blocker)-related uraemia have been reported ever since the introduction of these agents in the early 1980s, and the incidence (about 3% of all acute uraemic admissions) does not appear to be declining. Acute renal failure occurs when such agents are given to patients with RAS in whom glomerular perfusion is critically dependent upon angiotensin II. However, it is not only patients with ARVD who are at risk; two-thirds of those with ACE inhibitor-related uraemia will have normal renal vasculature on angiography but low cardiac output states such that further renal haemodynamic stress supervenes during intercurrent illness. Nevertheless, recovery of renal function should be expected when agents are withdrawn.

ARVD AND CORONARY HEART DISEASE

When abdominal aortography is performed at the time of coronary angiography, up to 15% of patients can be expected to have significant RAS (>50% luminal narrowing), with a similar proportion having insignificant RAS.[12,13]

ARVD AND CARDIAC DYSFUNCTION

'Flash' pulmonary oedema (sudden-onset left heart failure in patients with no previous cardiac history and well-preserved echocardiographic function) is a well-documented manifestation of ARVD, affecting over 10% of these patients. Patients with bilateral disease are at increased risk of this condition, which is currently one of the few widely accepted indications for renal artery revascularisation.[14] There is also a high prevalence of ARVD in patients with congestive cardiac failure, with over one-third of elderly patients likely to have RAS.[15]

ARVD AND AORTIC ANEURYSM/ PERIPHERAL VASCULAR DISEASE

ARVD is present in 33–44% of patients with peripheral vascular disease and 38% of those with an abdominal aortic aneurysm.[16,17]

CEREBROVASCULAR DISEASE AND ITS RELATIONSHIP TO ARVD

In an autopsy series of 346 cases of brain infarcts, RAS (>75% luminal narrowing) was found in 10.4% and carotid artery stenosis in 33.6% of subjects. Patients with carotid stenosis were more likely to have ARVD than those without carotid artery disease.[18] Conversely, carotid disease is more likely to occur in patients with significant ARVD. In a prospective study of 60 patients, the prevalence of carotid disease was 46% in patients with RAS but only 12% in patients without RAS.[19]

CLINICAL POINTERS TO THE DIAGNOSIS OF ARVD

- Hypertension
- Renal insufficiency
- Other vascular disease
- ACE-induced renal insufficiency
- Unexplained pulmonary oedema
- Vascular bruits

Specific clinical features include ACE inhibitor-related renal dysfunction or unexplained pulmonary oedema. However, the presence of femoral, renal or aortic bruits and the coexistence of severe extra-renal vascular disease are the main clinical pointers to ARVD.[20] Hypertension may be absent in patients with chronic cardiac dysfunction. In hypertensive patients without chronic renal failure, increased vigilance for RAS is advised in cases with severe (often mainly systolic) hypertension, especially when unresponsive to three or more antihypertensive agents and with evidence of widespread vascular disease.[10]

Natural history of RAS lesions

Invasive[21] and non-invasive studies[22] have demonstrated a rapid rate of progression of high-grade RAS lesions to renal artery occlusion (e.g. 11% of RAS lesions >60% over 2 years), with consequent loss of functioning renal mass. However, a more recent study has suggested a lower rate of RAS progression and that other factors, such as hypertension, may be more important than renal artery occlusion in determining progression to renal atrophy.[23]

Most studies have demonstrated unpredictable renal functional outcome after revascularisation, irrespective of the technique used.[24,25] Hence, the majority of patients with severe RAS lesions manifest no improvement in renal function, and some show progressive renal functional decline despite restoration of renal artery patency.

Pathogenesis of chronic renal dysfunction in ARVD

LACK OF RELATIONSHIP BETWEEN SEVERITY OF RAS AND RENAL DYSFUNCTION

There is no doubt that in some patients with ARVD a drop in renal perfusion, associated with a tight stenosis in the main renal artery, will result in impaired renal function simply due to a hydraulic effect, but this is likely to be the case in a minority of patients. However, studies in large cohorts of patients with ARVD have shown a lack of relationship between the severity of ARVD lesions and the degree of renal dysfunction.[26–28]

IMPORTANCE OF HYPERTENSIVE INTRARENAL INJURY IN ARVD

In an ultrasound study of 122 patients with ARVD that examined the incidence of, and risk factors for, renal atrophy (defined as reduction in renal length of 1 cm or more), systolic hypertension (systolic blood pressure >180 mmHg) was strongly and independently associated with high risk for renal atrophy.[23] As renal atrophy was linked with deteriorating renal function, it is clear that hypertensive damage to the kidney contributed significantly to the renal dysfunction in these patients. Few would argue that stringent control of blood pressure in patients with ARVD is now a fundamental therapeutic intervention.

RELEVANCE OF PROTEINURIA

Proteinuria appears to be a key marker of renal histopathological damage in patients with ARVD, and there is a clear relationship between lower baseline glomerular filtration rate and increased degree of proteinuria.[26] More recently, a prospective study has demonstrated that increased proteinuria at ARVD diagnosis was the chief predictor of future deteriorating function,[29] just as it is in a variety of other diseases of the renal parenchyma (e.g. chronic glomerulonephritis).

RENAL HISTOPATHOLOGICAL DAMAGE IN PATIENTS WITH ARVD

The term 'ischaemic nephropathy' has been used to describe the intrarenal damage in ARVD,[30] although other investigators prefer to call this 'atherosclerotic nephropathy', recognising that ischaemic injury is not a major feature in many patients. Other than hypertensive damage, cholesterol atheroembolism, intrarenal vascular disease and focal segmental or global sclerosing glomerular lesions have been shown to contribute to renal parenchymal injury.

Definite indications for renal revascularisation

Despite the lack of an adequate evidence base, most clinicians would agree that revascularisation is indicated for significant RAS in patients with:

- recurrent flash pulmonary oedema;
- severe hypertension resistant to all medical therapy;
- ACE inhibitor-related uraemia who require ACE inhibitors or angiotensin II blockers (e.g. for cardiac failure);
- dialysis-dependent renal failure (in such patients there is probably little to be lost and much, potentially, to be gained by intervention);
- deteriorating renal function associated with bilateral RAS (or RAS in a solitary kidney).

Treatment options and results

MEDICAL TREATMENT

The majority of patients with ARVD are unlikely to benefit from renal revascularisation, but optimal medical therapy is appropriate for all patients with ARVD. Although there is no evidence base to guide best medical management, it is clear that attention should be directed to limiting progression of atheromatous disease and to vigorous control of blood pressure. Patients should be advised to stop smoking, and antidiabetic therapy should be optimised where appropriate. All patients should be considered for the following medications.

- Antiplatelet agents (e.g. aspirin).
- Statins: the target total cholesterol should be less than 5 mmol/L. If cholesterol is already lower than this at presentation, then current evidence would suggest that the patient should still receive statin therapy.
- Antihypertensive therapy: patients may require combinations of several antihypertensive drugs to effect blood pressure control (target <140/80 mmHg, or 125/75 mmHg in those with significant proteinuria). Surprisingly, both ACE inhibitors and angiotensin II receptor blockers are optimal antihypertensive choices for patients with ARVD, especially if they have evidence of chronic parenchymal disease, with proteinuria. Clearly, careful monitoring of renal function is indicated, especially in patients with significant bilateral RAS or RAS affecting a solitary kidney.

ENDOVASCULAR TREATMENT

Renal stenting has become the initial technique of choice to revascularise an atherosclerotic RAS and has effectively replaced PTA and surgery as first-line treatment in the vast majority of patients. There have been many technological advances since the first renal PTA reported by Gruntzig et al.[31] in 1978, particularly the use of stents.[32]

Work-up before stenting

Three-dimensional gadolinium-enhanced MRA has all but replaced other methods of renal artery imaging[33] and should be available as a preoperative vascular map (**Fig. 15.1a,b**). The angle of origin of the renal arteries varies widely and is different for each side.[34] Using this information allows the fluoroscopic C-arm to be accurately angled to match the image on MRA and allows the stent to be placed accurately, completely covering the renal ostium and protruding into the aorta by 1–3 mm. Additionally, if the renal artery is steeply angled caudally, then access from a brachial or radial approach may be preferable.[35] The length of each kidney is also available from MRA (**Fig. 15.1a**) and in general 8 cm is used as a cut-off point below which revascularisation is unlikely to be of benefit (due to severe parenchymal disease).

(a)
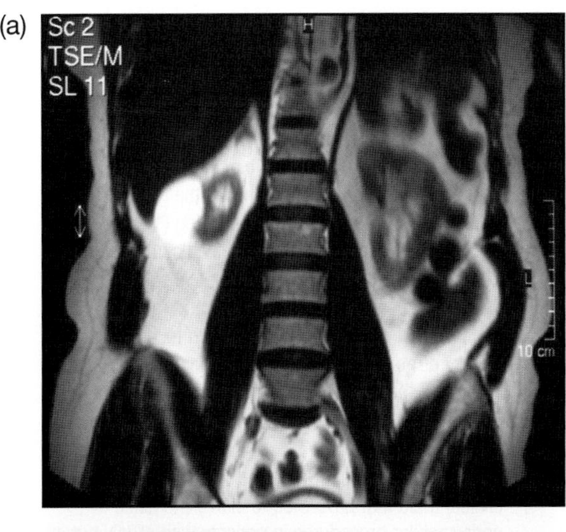

(b)
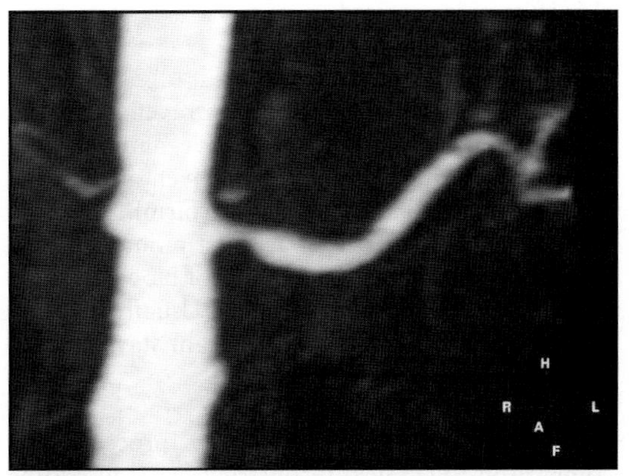

(c)
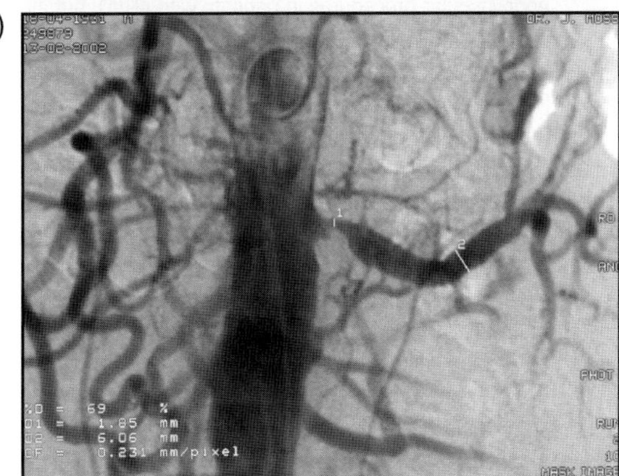

(d)
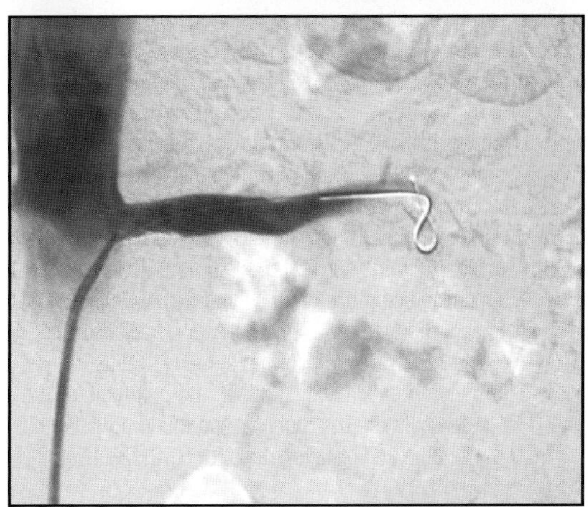

Figure 15.1 • **(a)** Magnetic resonance scan shows a small right kidney containing a cyst. **(b)** Magnetic resonance angiogram demonstrates an ostial stenosis of the left renal artery and an occluded right renal artery. **(c)** Conventional angiography at the time of treatment confirms these findings. **(d)** A stent has been placed at the ostium of the left renal artery.

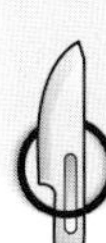

Patients should be hydrated with intravenous fluids 12 hours before stenting. This will reduce the incidence of contrast-induced nephropathy.[36] There is some evidence that giving *N*-acetylcysteine also reduces the incidence of contrast-induced nephropathy, although the results of randomised controlled trials have been conflicting.[37] All patients should be on aspirin (or clopidogrel if contraindicated).

Procedure (Fig. 15.1c,d)

It should be borne in mind that iodinated contrast is nephrotoxic when there is pre-existing renal impairment, particularly so if the patient is diabetic. Therefore all attempts should be made to minimise the dose of iodinated contrast. It is perfectly feasible to perform the procedure using carbon dioxide as the sole contrast agent since it has no known nephrotoxicity. There is now evidence that the newer iso-osmolar contrast agents (iodixanol, Amersham UK) are less toxic than conventional non-ionic agents and these should be used if iodinated contrast cannot be avoided.[38] Assuming a femoral approach (which is suitable for 90% of cases), a 7 Fr renal double-curve guiding catheter is introduced into the abdominal aorta. The renal artery is best selected with a reverse-curve type catheter (Sos Omni, E-Z-EM Ltd, UK) using a soft-tipped wire to cross the lesion. Vasodilators (glyceryl trinitrate) are given through the catheter to prevent spasm. The lesion is then predilated using a 3-mm PTA balloon and the stent placed over the same wire. Careful imaging is important at this stage, with the C-arm correctly angulated to ensure that the entire renal ostium is covered. Failure to do so leads to almost inevitable restenosis. A balloon-expandable stent is much easier to deploy accurately than a self-expanding one in this location, and as the disease is very focal only a short stent (15–19 mm) is required.

Post procedure

Patients should continue with intravenous fluids for a further 12 hours and receive another dose of *N*-acetylcysteine if this was given before the procedure. Antiplatelet therapy (aspirin) should be continued for life. Patients are best monitored in a renal unit where close observation of blood pressure and renal function can be made. Usually patients can be discharged after one overnight stay.

Complications

Although often seen as a minor procedure in comparison to surgical reconstruction, it would be naive to assume that an endovascular procedure is risk-free. The literature quotes complication rates ranging from 0 to 66% for renal PTA/stenting.[39]

In the single randomised controlled trial comparing surgery with PTA,[40] the major complication rate following PTA was 17% versus 31% following surgery, with minor complications in 48% of the PTA group versus 7% in the surgical group. The Dutch randomised controlled trial comparing PTA with stenting reported a 39% complication rate following PTA and a 43% rate following stenting,[41] most of these complications being minor and groin related. A meta-analysis of 24 publications found no difference between the complication rates for PTA (13%) versus stenting (11%).[42]

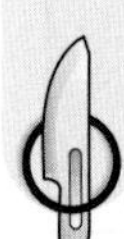

Many complications can be avoided by good technique, and the use of small platform systems, adequate hydration, closure devices and pre-stent imaging have all made a contribution. Perforation of the renal artery is a rare but dreaded complication that can usually be treated either by simple balloon tamponade or stent graft. Surgical salvage is rarely required and often is too late to save a kidney due to the relatively short warm ischaemia time. Deterioration in renal function (usually temporary) is one of the commonest complications. It is usually due to the effects of iodinated contrast and appears in the first 24–48 hours. Efforts to minimise this have been discussed above but once it does occur supportive treatment usually suffices. Cholesterol embolisation is perhaps the most significant complication and can be silent and under-appreciated. The onset is insidious (over 1–3 weeks) and may be associated with an elevated ESR, eosinophilia and the typical livedo reticularis skin rash. The prognosis is guarded and little can be done beyond general supportive measures. Attempts to minimise cholesterol embolisation include small platform systems, but the future lies in the use of protection devices as developed for the carotid artery. Preliminary results are encouraging, although a dedicated system still needs to be developed to meet the special challenges of the renal artery anatomy.[43,44]

Results of renal angioplasty and stenting

A recent meta-analysis[42] compared the results of PTA (10 articles, 644 patients) with stenting (14 articles, 678 patients). None were randomised controlled trials. Stent placement had a higher technical success rate and lower restenosis rate than PTA and the complication rate was similar for both techniques. The cure rate for hypertension was higher (20% vs. 10%) and the improvement rate for renal function was lower (30% vs. 38%) after stent placement compared with PTA.

At the present time there are only four published clinical trials that have tried to clarify the place of endovascular procedures in patients with ARVD, but all involved only relatively small patient numbers. Hence, Van Jaarsveld et al.[45] randomised 106 patients with RAS of greater than 50% and significant hypertension (but only mild–moderate renal impairment; creatinine <200 μmol/L) to angioplasty or medical therapy. No differences were noted in the primary endpoint of blood pressure control, or in renal function. The other two trials incorporated similar design but contained only 49 and 55 patients.[46,47] There are two published meta-analyses of the above trials.[48,49] Both come to the same conclusion, namely that the effect of PTA on hypertension is at best modest and that none of these small trials were powered to detect changes in renal function. A moderate but clinically worthwhile benefit could not be excluded and further large-scale randomised trials are required. Two such trials (ASTRAL and STAR) are currently recruiting patients. Finally, a single randomised controlled trial has compared PTA with stenting in 85 patients with ostial lesions.[41] The technical success rate of stents was superior to PTA (88% vs. 55%) and the primary 6-month patency likewise superior (75% vs. 29%). The trial was stopped following an interim analysis of the data. The clinical outcomes in the two groups were similar, although the study was not powered to detect differences in blood pressure or renal function. Very few radiologists would now use PTA alone for ostial atherosclerotic RAS.

The restenosis rate following renal stenting is approximately 15% assessed by follow-up angiography at 6–12 months.[41] Treatment of restenosis is problematic and there is no consensus.

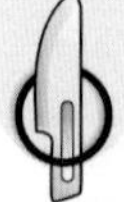

SURGICAL TREATMENT

There is a range of surgical options available to treat renal artery disease (**Box 15.1**). The decision to proceed to surgery, and the type of surgery to be performed, is dependent on several factors. These include whether one or both kidneys are involved,

Box 15.1 • Surgical revascularisation

Aortic graft and renal bypass
Aortorenal bypass
Aortorenal endarterectomy
Extra-anatomical bypass
Extracorporeal bench surgery

Table 15.1 • Reported results of surgical revascularisation

Benjamin et al. (1996)[52] Dean (1997)[53]	Treatment of hypertension (cure or improvement)	63–91%
Benjamin et al. (1996)[52] Reilly et al. (1996)[54]	Treatment of renal failure (cure or improvement)	33–91%
Steinbach et al. (1997)[55] Darling et al. (1995)[56]	Primary patency rates	93–97%
Weibull et al. (1993)[40] Novick et al. (1987)[57]	Restenosis rate	3–4%
Darling et al. (1995)[56]	Morbidity	6–43%
Reilly et al. (1996)[54] Steinbach et al. (1997)[55] Cambria et al. (1996)[58]	Mortality	2–8%

the amount of renal parenchymal loss or fibrosis that has occurred, the condition of the native aorta, and the cardiorespiratory fitness of the patient if aortic cross-clamping and direct aortic surgery is planned. Between 20 and 40% of patients undergoing aortic surgery will have concomitant RAS, and some 70% undergoing surgery for RAS will also have aortic disease.[50] The site of the lesion is also important, and if extra-anatomical bypass is considered, the condition of the other visceral vessels must be optimal. In patients with renal artery occlusion, renal biopsy (performed either preoperatively or perioperatively) can indicate whether the kidney is viable and functionally salvageable on the basis of collateral vessels. The presence of extensive glomerular hyalinisation usually precludes revascularisation. However, this procedure is not without risk of bleeding and even the loss of a kidney.[51]

In the past, hypertension control was the main indication for surgery but this has now been superseded by the need to preserve renal function. Reported results of surgical revascularisation are shown in **Table 15.1**. The incidence of late bypass graft stenosis is approximately 10% over 5–10 years.[59] In a retrospective study of 222 patients from 1974 to 1987, with a mean follow-up of 7.4 years, operative mortality was 2.2%, hypertension was improved in 72.4% and renal function was preserved in 71.3%. The 5-year survival was comparable with an age-matched population, whereas the 10-year survival was decreased (53% vs. 77%) due to cardiovascular comorbidity.[55] Despite the perception that surgical revascularisation is a high-risk option, the quoted mortality and morbidity have set the standards against which other treatment modalities can be compared. In a study of 397 patients treated for atherosclerotic RAS,[60] renal revascularisation was preferred to nephrectomy in selected hypertensive patients when a normal distal artery was demonstrated. However, surgical patients are a selected group because a significant proportion of these patients are not suitable for such intervention.

Nephrectomy is the oldest surgical procedure used to treat renovascular hypertension. It remains the option of choice for a shrunken (i.e. <8 cm) kidney where there is a normal contralateral kidney and renal artery. Nephrectomy may often be required as part of a procedure of revascularisation of a viable kidney on the other side. In this situation measurement of renal vein renin levels is of value, with nephrectomy being indicated when the ratio of renal vein renins is greater than 1.5.

Simultaneous aortic replacement and renal revascularisation is associated with much higher mortality rates than renal revascularisation alone and should only be undertaken where there is a significant abdominal aortic aneurysm or aortic occlusive disease requiring treatment. There is no evidence, as yet, about whether a staged approach to combined aortic and renal disease is of any benefit. If the results of stent angioplasty for RAS prove to be durable, then this would be an attractive option to perform before undertaking the vascular or endovascular repair of the aneurysm. In combined procedures there are two surgical options for renal revascularisation: endarterectomy and bypass grafting. Most commonly, a 6–8 mm limb of Dacron and PTFE is sutured onto the aortic graft and then an end-to-end renal anastomosis is made. Where bilateral RAS is present, an inverted bifurcated Dacron graft is preferred. Alternatively, in the presence of ostial disease it is possible to clamp above the renal arteries with reasonable safety and to perform a 'blind' endarterectomy from within the aortic lumen before the proximal anastomosis is fashioned.

Transaortic renal endarterectomy is an attractive surgical option where the aorta does not need to be replaced. The disadvantage of this approach is that it requires extensive dissection of the visceral aorta and complete aortic cross-clamping, with its attendant problems of left ventricular strain and distal embolisation. The endarterectomy can be achieved either with a transverse incision across the aorta at the level of the renal arteries or by using a trapdoor anterolateral incision, which has the added benefit of allowing access to the origin of the superior mesenteric and coeliac arteries. Most commonly, transaortic renal endarterectomy is performed using a partial aortic clamping technique, with an incision made from the aorta across the origin of the renal artery, careful endarterectomy and inspection of the end point, and patch closure of first one side and then the other (**Fig. 15.2**). In experienced hands, 5-year patencies in the order of 90% can be achieved for renal artery endarterectomy.[61]

In many of the patients the problem is one of renal failure due to RAS where the aorta does not require replacement. In these patients the option of an extra-anatomical bypass graft is attractive, avoiding any aortic dissection or cross-clamping and with access obtained via a simple subcostal incision. Providing there is no significant stenosis on the coeliac axis, revascularisation is achieved by use of either the hepatic or the splenic artery as the inflow site (**Fig. 15.3**). The right kidney can be revascularised from the common hepatic artery. In up to 50% of cases this can be via the gastroduodenal branch, providing it is of sufficient calibre and length to be anastomosed end to end onto the renal artery; where this is not possible, an interposition saphenous vein graft can be used. The key to success in this procedure is full mobilisation of the inferior vena cava, the right renal vein and often also the left renal vein. On the left side, the splenic artery is dissected from its midpoint from the pancreas. Taking care to divide the multiple small branches, careful proximal dissection is performed sufficient to provide enough length to reach the divided renal artery for an end-to-end anastomosis. The spleen does not need to be removed since there is sufficient blood supply from splenic collaterals and the short gastric arteries. The iliac artery as an inflow vessel is rarely possible because in most patients with atherosclerotic RAS it is diffusely diseased. Rarely, in the presence of severe coeliac and aorto-iliac disease a widely patent superior mesenteric artery can be used. A recent review from the Cleveland Clinic documented 175 extra-anatomical revascularisations over a 12-year period.[62] This was achieved with an operative mortality rate of 2.9%. Postoperative arterial thrombosis in the bypass occurred in 4%. Renal function was improved in 40% and stabilised in 40%. Hypertension was improved or cured in three-quarters of the series.

Direct aorto-renal bypass is a simple technique using long saphenous vein, PTFE, Dacron or rarely the internal iliac artery. The choice of inflow site will depend very much on the condition of the infrarenal aorta, which is to be preferred if it is sufficiently free of disease. If not, the supracoeliac aorta is usually suitable and can be approached via a 'rooftop' abdominal incision with mobilisation and reflection of the oesophagus to the patient's left and the left lobe of the liver to the patient's right. Alternatively, the thoracic aorta can be used as the inflow site and a bypass graft passed through the aortic hiatus to reach the renal arteries. Where more than one renal or visceral artery has to be revascularised simultaneously, a bifurcated Dacron graft will provide two limbs for subsequent anasto-

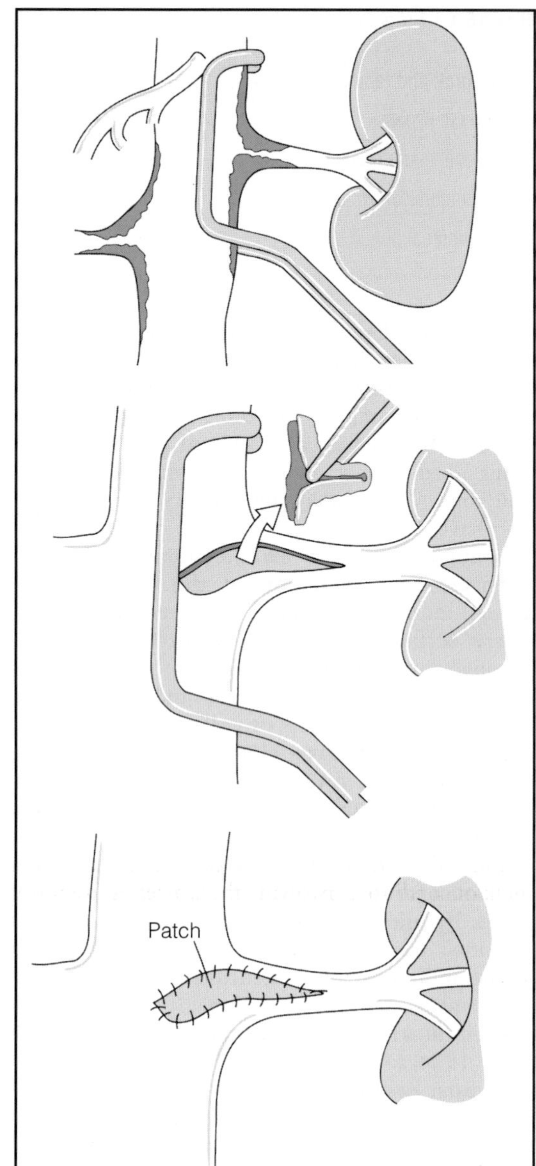

Figure 15.2 • Transaortic renal endarterectomy with patch closure.

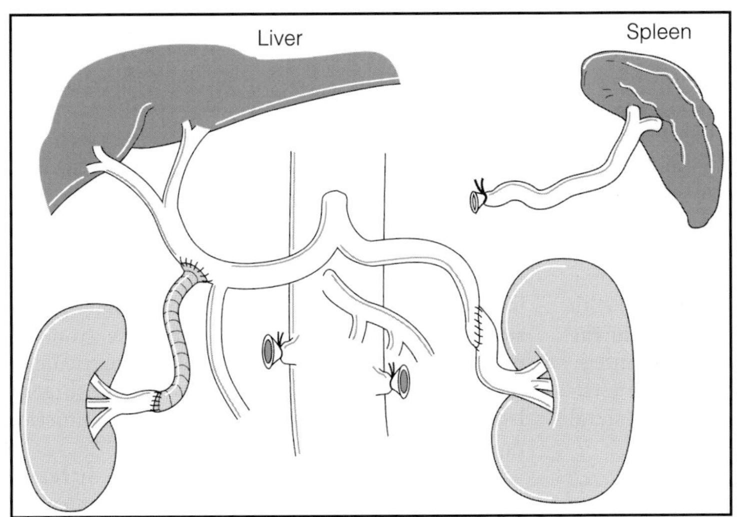

Figure 15.3 • Extra-anatomical renal revascularisation from the hepatic or splenic arteries.

mosis onto stenosed vessels. Results of revascularisation are similar irrespective of the graft material used. Where vein has been used, however, graft dilatation in the long term is a specific problem but not usually to the extent of requiring further corrective surgery.

Because multiple small anastomoses need to be made, extracorporeal or bench surgery is required for patients with disease in the branch renal arteries. Fibrous dysplasia, renal aneurysm, arteriovenous fistulas, dissection, atheroma and arteritis form the bulk of conditions involving these arteries. Removal of the kidney, cooling and preservation exactly as in a renal transplant harvest procedure will allow multiple microvascular anastomoses to be performed in safety before autotransplantation of the reconstructed kidney back onto the iliac vessels. The internal iliac artery with its multiple small branches is ideal for direct end-to-end anastomosis onto the small branch renal vessels. Alternatively, prefashioned branch saphenous vein grafts or occasionally the inferior epigastric artery can be used. The Cleveland Clinic has the largest reported series of autotransplantation, with excellent and durable results in these difficult cases.[63]

In conclusion, surgery in the young fit patient may be a better, more cost-effective option than angioplasty, especially in the light of a long-term restenosis rate following surgery of 3–4%.[41,57]

Choice of treatment

Insufficient controlled evidence exists to compare results of the various treatments. Clearly, all patients should receive best medical treatment. There have been no trials comparing stenting with surgery. Although it is unlikely that the patency rates of any endovascular technique will match those of surgical reconstruction, the advantage of stenting is its minimally invasive nature. A rare indication for surgery is stent technical failure, which most commonly occurs when attempting to treat complete occlusions. It seems reasonable to use stenting as the primary mode for revascularisation, reserving surgery for failures. A team approach to management based on nephrology, interventional radiology and vascular surgery is essential to maximise the therapeutic potential for each individual patient.

INTESTINAL ISCHAEMIA

Gut ischaemia is an uncommon condition that presents particular problems of diagnosis and management. The various syndromes of intestinal ischaemia are broadly classified as acute or chronic, both of which are serious conditions associated with poor outcome. Mesenteric arterial embolism and thrombosis, mesenteric venous thrombosis, non-occlusive mesenteric ischaemia and iatrogenic bowel ischaemia are acute syndromes. Intestinal and mesenteric angina and the median arcuate ligament compression syndrome constitute chronic syndromes.

PATHOPHYSIOLOGY

Certain aspects of the mesenteric anatomy merit elaboration. The arterial circulation to the gut is characterised by extensive collaterals that provide multiple sources of blood inflow. As a result, despite the high prevalence of arteriosclerotic disease of the three main visceral vessels, mesenteric ischaemia is uncommon. Certain collateral patterns are well recognised depending on the extent of arterial blockage, which invariably occurs at the origin of the major vessels (**Fig. 15.4**). Where stenosis or blockage affects either the coeliac or superior mesenteric artery (SMA), the gastroduodenal and pancreatico-duodenal arteries provide the main collateral circulation. The main collateral channels between the superior and inferior mesenteric arteries occur in the splenic flexure region between the middle and left colic arteries. The marginal artery of Drummond and the arch of Riolan (an ascending branch of the left colic artery anastomosing with branches of the SMA) enlarge significantly in the presence of either superior or inferior mesenteric artery occlusion. In the presence of inferior mesenteric artery occlusion, a further important collateral circulation is that between the internal iliac artery via the superior haemorrhoidal arteries to the left colic artery. Thus blood can be channelled between the upper and lower intestinal circulations. In addition, lesser collaterals develop between the systemic and visceral circulations in areas such as the diaphragm.

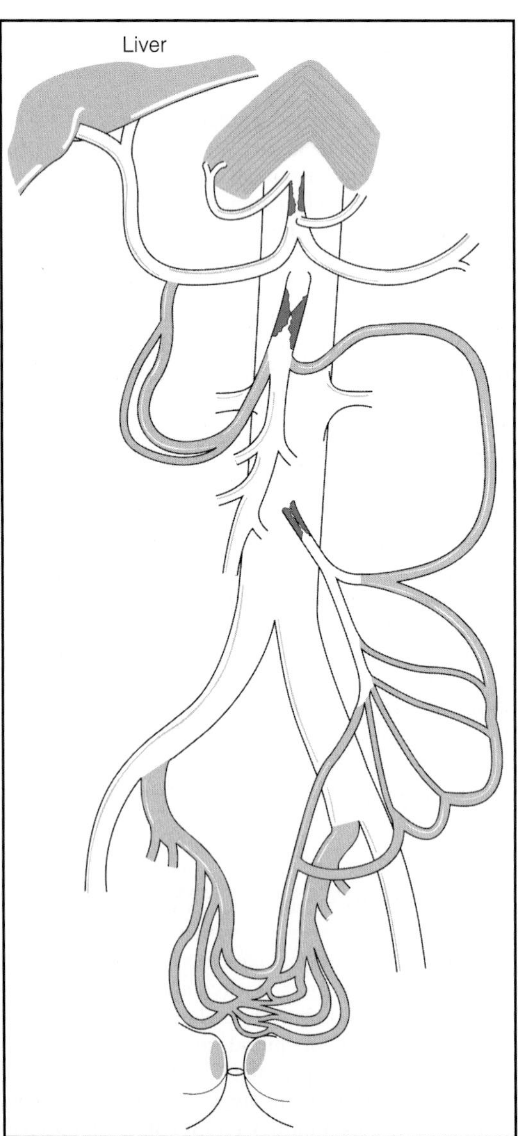

Figure 15.4 • Collateral circulation of the intestine.

Because of the richness of this collateral circulation, symptomatic intestinal ischaemia will usually present when at least two of the three main intestinal branches are either blocked or have severe stenosis. However, symptoms can arise from an isolated stenosis affecting the SMA, particularly where there has been previous abdominal surgery. Isolated stenosis of either the coeliac or inferior mesenteric artery rarely gives problems.[64]

After eating, intestinal blood flow increases significantly depending on the size and content of the meal (postprandial hyperaemia).[65] Coeliac artery flow barely changes with meals of all types. Major changes occur in the SMA, with a significant increase seen 2–30 minutes after eating, becoming maximal after 90 minutes and lasting up to 4–6 hours. This response is stimulated by the presence of food in the stomach and foregut, the earliest response being to carbohydrates but the most prolonged resulting from a mixed meal of carbohydrate, protein and fat. Thus, blood flow increases dramatically to the small bowel and pancreas. Blood flow to the mucosa is disproportionately large, in excess of 75% of the total, despite comprising less than half of the mass of the small bowel.

After a meal the process of digestion, consisting of active absorption of food together with increased bowel muscular activity, requires increased oxygen consumption by the gut.[66] In the presence of severe intestinal ischaemia, significant induction of anaerobic metabolism will result in the production of metabolites that cause pain in a similar manner to that seen in ischaemia in other vascular beds. However, an alternative hypothesis suggests that where there is significant mesenteric artery disease, a steal from the gastric circulation takes place resulting in diminished gastric blood flow. This causes increased acid production, transient peptic inflammation or ulceration and thus pain.[67] However, the lack of effect of histamine H_2 antagonists or proton pump inhibitors on chronic intestinal ischaemic pain makes this mechanism unlikely to be important.

All causes of acute intestinal ischaemia result in prolonged hypoxia with persistent severe pain out of proportion to the clinical findings. Associated with these acute syndromes of severe gut ischaemia are early development of acidosis, hyperamylasaemia and leucocytosis. A further component of intestinal ischaemia is ischaemic damage to the mucosa, resulting in loss of the mucosal barrier. This allows translocation of bacteria, endotoxins and cytokines, with major systemic effects such as septicaemia and multiorgan failure. Less commonly recognised is a reperfusion syndrome that may give similar effects. In this situation, release of free radicals after successful reperfusion causes an inflammatory response with release of many cytokines, activated leucocytes and inflammatory mediators.[68,69] This causes local mucosal and hepatic inflammation and systemic effects leading to multiorgan failure after revascularisation of both acute and, to a lesser extent, chronic intestinal bowel ischaemia.[70]

CLINICAL SYNDROMES

Clinical presentation, diagnosis and treatment are best considered according to the individual clinical syndromes of intestinal ischaemia.

Acute arterial intestinal ischaemia

This is the most common presentation, accounting for about 50% of all cases of intestinal ischaemia. Between 1980 and 1990, approximately 2000–2500 deaths per annum were attributed to intestinal ischaemia.[71,72] The cause is usually embolisation of organised thrombus into the SMA. There is usually atrial fibrillation or other arrhythmia or, less commonly, a mural thrombus from an acute myocardial infarction. A history of previous embolic events is common. More rarely, iatrogenic cholesterol embolisation from interventional radiological manoeuvres, paradoxical embolism or atrial myxoma may be the source. The SMA is by far the most common site of occlusion, although coeliac embolisation does occur. Females are more often affected than males (ratio 2:1), with a median age of 70 years.

There is a history of constant severe epigastric or periumbilical pain of sudden onset frequently followed by copious vomiting and explosive diarrhoea. Typically the patient was previously well. The abdominal signs are often lacking or non-specific, with distension, absent or normal bowel sounds but without any signs of peritonism. This combination of symptoms and signs is a typical feature, referred to as severe abdominal pain out of all proportion to the clinical findings. Peritonism, or blood in the stool or vomitus, indicates severe advanced intestinal ischaemia with likely infarction. Unfortunately, the early lack of signs may result in a delayed diagnosis until such time as the ischaemia is so advanced as to cause peritonism. This explains the poor survival rate, with historical reports from 1967 to 1990 showing an average mortality of 78% (range 44–100%).[73] SMA thrombosis may occur as the result of progression of SMA stenosis that had not previously been diagnosed or treated. Often in these patients there is a history of intestinal angina with severe weight loss. Mortality from SMA thrombosis is higher because the thrombosis takes place at the origin of the artery. In embolism, the occlusion may be distal to the origin of the pancreatico-duodenal and middle colic branches, which allows some blood flow to the small intestine to be maintained.

DIAGNOSIS

Diagnosis depends on a high index of suspicion in the appropriate clinical setting. Features of cardiac disease or widespread arteriosclerosis (40% have evidence of peripheral vascular disease) should be sought. Worthwhile investigations include the white cell count, which may be markedly elevated, serum amylase or inorganic phosphate, which may be elevated in about half of the patients, and blood gases to assess for metabolic acidosis. Plain radiographs of the abdomen may reveal non-specific small bowel dilatation.

Mesenteric angiography will confirm the diagnosis but at the cost of delay in treatment. If there are clear abdominal signs of peritonism, angiography is not indicated, with urgent laparotomy the best course of action. In patients who have pain but minimal abdominal signs, catheter angiography (or MRA) is indicated with views of the visceral aorta and its branches. In SMA embolism, the proximal artery may be clearly visualised.

Duplex scanning is impaired by the increased intestinal gas that is frequently present in this condition. MRA will reliably demonstrate the proximal mesenteric vessels but, at present, imaging of more distal branches is not good. As noted above, the identification of ischaemic and infarcted bowel preoperatively is difficult, and MRA may potentially be helpful but to date has little clinical utility.

TREATMENT

In all cases the patient is initially resuscitated, given broad-spectrum intravenous antibiotics and fully heparinised. Interventional radiological treatment such as angioplasty and intra-arterial mesenteric thrombolytic therapy are attractive options that may be considered at the time of radiological diagnosis. However, even in successful revascularisation, the likelihood of a portion of the bowel having frank necrosis is high. As yet, in acute intestinal ischaemia, the twin goals of revascularisation and resection of non-viable bowel can only be achieved by surgical means. This form of treatment has improved results, although mortality is still high; in a retrospective analysis of 92 patients mortality was 21%.[74]

After rapid resuscitation, laparotomy is performed as soon as possible since this represents a true surgical emergency. The first step is an assessment of the degree and extent of bowel viability. Free, foul-smelling peritoneal fluid is a sign of advanced necrosis. Ischaemic bowel has a characteristic appearance, with loss of its normal sheen, dull grey colour and a non-peristaltic/flabby tone. Infarcted bowel is purplish black in colour, often friable and perforated. The presence of proximal mesenteric artery pulsation will suggest that embolism has taken place, whereas complete absence of pulsation in the SMA from its origin will indicate thrombosis.

In many cases the bowel ischaemia will be so extensive and advanced that no surgical revascularisation is undertaken and palliative care is given. Where there is hope of sufficient bowel viability, revascularisation should take place before any resection is considered. After successful revascularisation, previously precarious segments of intestine may have become viable and resection of clearly ischaemic bowel can then take place. Revascularisation can be achieved by embolectomy or reconstruction.

SMA embolectomy

The proximal portion of the SMA is dissected free as it emerges from the pancreatic neck into the base of the mesentery. Approximately 3–4 cm of artery is cleared, taking care not to damage the branches. If the patient is not already fully anticoagulated, 5000 units of heparin are given intravenously. A transverse arteriotomy is made and a 3 or 4 Fr gauge embolectomy catheter is passed proximally and distally to clear the embolism and re-establish vigorous pulsatile flow. If proximal flow cannot be established, thrombosis of a superior mesenteric stenosis is likely and reconstructive surgery will be required.

SMA reconstruction

Revascularisation can be performed using either bypass grafting from the aorta to the patent SMA or by aortic reimplantation of the healthy portion of the SMA. In the presence of perforated bowel or frank ischaemia requiring bowel resection, prosthetic grafts must not be used. Reversed saphenous vein aorto-mesenteric grafting or direct SMA reimplantation are the procedures of choice in this situation (**Fig. 15.5**). In the emergency situation, single-vessel revascularisation is usually adequate despite the current opinion, which favours multiple-vessel revascularisation.

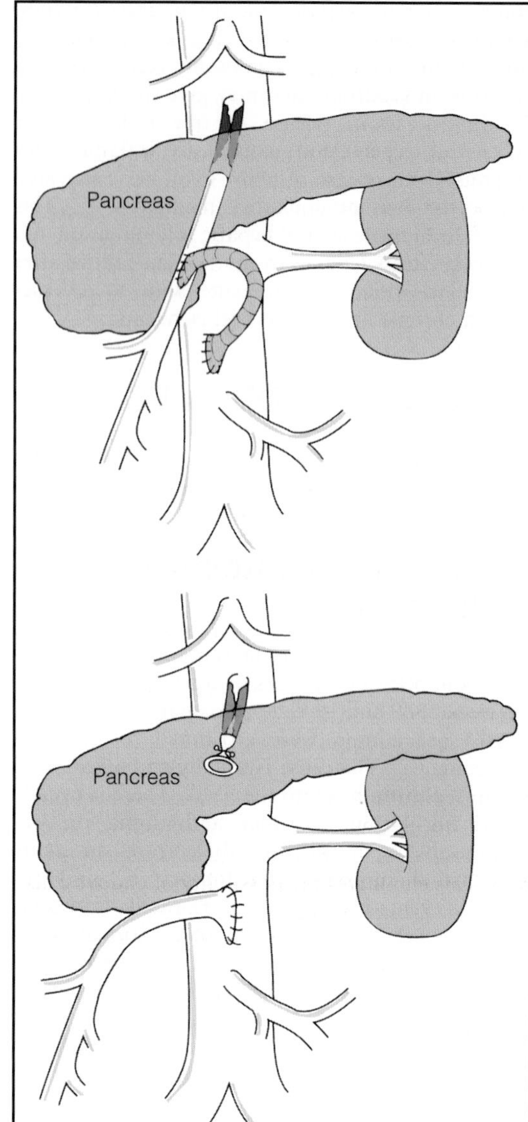

Figure 15.5 • Revascularisation of the superior mesenteric artery.

Assessment of intestinal viability

Determination of which portions of bowel are non-viable can be difficult, particularly where infarction is extensive, and decisions about how much to resect can be crucially important to the long-term outcome. Clinical assessment by detecting pulsation in the arcades, colour of the bowel, peristalsis and bleeding from cut edges is most commonly used. The Doppler probe can be used to detect blood flow in the intestinal wall in addition to flow in the arcade vessels. A further, more cumbersome method is the use of fluorescein (10–15 mL/kg injected intravenously) and subsequent inspection with a Wood's lamp. Lack of rapid fluorescence is diagnostic of non-viable bowel. Other methods of assessing perfusion, such as pulse oximetry and laser Doppler flowmetry, may be of value.[75,76] A combination of clinical assessment and use of the Doppler probe is usually sufficient. Ischaemic bowel is resected with the aim of preservation of as much bowel as possible; several segmental resections with multiple anastomoses may be required.

The postoperative management of patients who have undergone extensive bowel resection is important. If both ileum and colon are resected, fluid losses (especially potassium) need to be carefully monitored; in addition, total parenteral nutrition may be started early in the postoperative period.

Contemporary practice, particularly where a short gut syndrome may be created, is to leave all marginally viable intestine after revascularisation. A second laparotomy 24–48 hours after the initial procedure is therefore mandatory to assess the viability of these marginally perfused parts of the bowel and to check the intestinal anastomoses. If there is still doubt, further laparotomies are planned until the viable status of the remaining bowel is established. Such patients require intensive care with optimisation of cardiac and respiratory status, particularly where reperfusion multiorgan failure has supervened. Parenteral nutrition may be required for some time if there is short gut syndrome.

Endovascular treatment

As noted above, patients with acute bowel ischaemia frequently present with established bowel infarction. This eliminates the possibility of endovascular management, as an emergency laparotomy is indicated with bowel resection. In the less urgent situation, when angiography has been performed, this usually shows localised arterial thrombus or an embolus. There may be roles for intra-arterial thrombolysis and percutaneous aspiration thrombectomy, with or without balloon angioplasty or adjunctive stenting. However, reports of such activity are sparse.[77] Even in seemingly favourable circumstances, the extent of intestinal ischaemia cannot be accurately predicted from physical examination or any laboratory or diagnostic test. As a result, although thrombolytic and endovascular therapy may be successful in restoring the arterial supply to the ischaemic bowel, many patients with acute intestinal ischaemia will have at least some area of bowel that is irreversibly damaged.

Mesenteric venous thrombosis

Mesenteric venous thrombosis is rare, accounting for 5–15% of all acute mesenteric ischaemia. It is either primary (where no cause is recognised) or secondary. Secondary mesenteric venous thrombosis may follow hypercoagulable states, portal venous stasis and hypertension, intra-abdominal infection and inflammation, oral contraceptive use (accounting for 4–5% of all cases), intra-abdominal malignancy or splenectomy.

The clinical presentation is usually less acute than with arterial occlusion, with severe but vague abdominal pain, and little in the way of any abdominal findings except tenderness, distension and decreased bowel sounds. The pain tends to be vague, colicky and slowly progressive with localisation over the involved segment. The pain is usually out of proportion to the physical findings. Faecal occult blood is present in more than 50% of patients. The temperature in 25–50% of patients is greater than 38°C and in 20% there is tachycardia.[78] Frank peritonitis is seen only when transmural infarction or perforation has occurred. Diagnosis of mesenteric venous thrombosis is frequently delayed due to the absence of specific symptoms, signs or laboratory findings. Plain abdominal radiographs may reveal distended small bowel with wall oedema (thumbprinting) or gas in the bowel wall or portal vein. Contrast-enhanced computed tomography can reveal the extent of thrombus, show air in the mesenteric vein or portal system and reveal collateral flow. Duplex ultrasound may help to exclude biliary disease and detect free peritoneal fluid, although its use may be limited in the presence of bowel gas. Magnetic resonance imaging may be helpful in patients allergic to iodinated contrast medium.

If an early diagnosis of mesenteric venous thrombosis is made, with no evidence of peritonitis or intestinal infarction, aggressive intravenous fluid resuscitation, nasogastric decompression and full anticoagulation is required.

Unfortunately, the diagnosis is most commonly made at laparotomy or autopsy. At laparotomy, blood-stained free peritoneal fluid may be found. Affected bowel is cyanotic, oedematous and feels rubbery. There are mesenteric arterial pulsations but the veins contain clots that extrude when cut. Infarction is most common in the mid-small bowel. Full anticoagulation must be established rapidly. Infarcted bowel should be resected, with liberal margins, and primary anastomosis performed (if perfusion of the remaining bowel is found to be adequate). Long-term anticoagulation is important because of the high recurrence rate. Second-look laparotomy is planned when there is doubtful viability. Thrombectomy has poor results with a high recurrence rate and is rarely indicated.

Thrombolytic therapy given either intra-arterially or into the superior mesenteric vein has been reported[79] and may offer an alternative treatment modality if the diagnosis is made early.

Investigation of the underlying prothrombotic disorder together with prolonged anticoagulation with warfarin improves survival. However, the perioperative mortality of this disease remains high at 27%, with a high recurrence rate and long-term survival related to the underlying disease.[80]

Non-occlusive mesenteric ischaemia

This syndrome develops in severe systemic illness in association with cardiorespiratory shock and multi-organ failure. Typically, these are patients on the intensive care unit with congestive cardiac failure or severe cardiac dysfunction. Most commonly there is shock, either cardiogenic or secondary to septicaemia. The pathophysiology is of mesenteric vasoconstriction in response to both normovolaemic and hypovolaemic shock, usually aggravated by use of inotropic agents. Abdominal pain is the commonest symptom, occurring in 75%, but in the unconscious patient abdominal distension, gastrointestinal bleeding, leucocytosis or fever may be the presentation. The diagnosis is made with a high index of clinical suspicion and can be confirmed by angiography. This will show intestinal arterial vasospasm and exclude a significant arterial lesion. Treatment depends on optimising cardiac output, treating underlying conditions such as sepsis and, where possible, removing adverse pharmacological agents such as the inotropes. In severe cases, intra-mesenteric arterial infusion of papaverine at a dose of 30–60 mg/hour is beneficial. Glucagon (2–4 mg/hour) will increase splanchnic blood flow and has the advantage of being given intravenously.[81] However, mortality in this condition remains high at 70–80% despite these therapies.

Iatrogenic bowel ischaemia

This condition can occur after interventional radiological procedures, usually in an aorta that has widespread arteriosclerosis. Embolisation is usually widespread, involving the kidneys, pelvis and lower limbs in addition to the viscera, and carries a high mortality. The correct treatment is unknown but full anticoagulation, appropriate resuscitation and infusion of prostacyclin or its analogues, or prostaglandin E_1, are recommended.

Left colon ischaemia can occur after aortic reconstruction where either the direct or collateral blood supply has been interrupted. This problem arises much more commonly after aneurysm repair with ligation of a patent inferior mesenteric artery, with an accepted incidence of about 2% (range 0.2–10%) being quoted in the literature. There is an associated overall mortality of 40–50% in this condition. However, where ischaemia involves the full bowel wall thickness, mortality approaches 90%.[82,83] Prospective studies using routine postoperative colonoscopy have shown that significant ischaemia complicates about 4% of aortic occlusive reconstructions and 7.4% of aneurysm resections, with an overall incidence of 12% when ruptured aneurysms were included.[84]

Diagnosis can be difficult in the immediate postoperative period and is mainly from raised clinical awareness. Any patient with watery diarrhoea, bloody or non-bloody, should undergo urgent bedside colonoscopy. Left-sided peritonism may be a presentation but this can be difficult to detect in the early postoperative abdomen. A leucocytosis greater than 20 000/mm^3, severe metabolic acidosis, fever and shock should alert the surgeon to the possibility of severe colonic ischaemia. Outcome relates to the severity of bowel ischaemia. In experienced hands where mild to moderate ischaemia is suspected, treatment may be supportive with broad-spectrum antibiotics and complete bowel rest without the need for surgery. Any sign of worsening ischaemia, as evidenced by deteriorating clinical condition or colonoscopic appearance, mandates urgent laparotomy.

A Hartmann's procedure is usually required and primary anastomosis is contraindicated. The aortic graft and its limbs must be protected from contamination during the procedure using swabs soaked in antiseptic. If necessary, at the end of the procedure exposed grafts should be covered by a well-perfused omental pedicle flap.

Most cases of colonic ischaemia can be avoided by careful technique at the time of the primary aortic procedure. The inferior mesenteric artery should be ligated close to the aortic wall or preferably its orifice suture ligated from within the sac. The sigmoid colon and rectum must be inspected after completion of the aortic procedure and the inferior mesenteric artery reimplanted if necessary. The objective assessment of colonic perfusion is difficult, but Doppler assessment of arterial blood flow and intraluminal rectosigmoidal pH tonometry are the most useful techniques.[85]

Chronic intestinal ischaemia syndromes

MEDIAN ARCUATE LIGAMENT COMPRESSION SYNDROME

There is considerable scepticism regarding the clinical importance of this syndrome. Typical symptoms are of pain after eating, often not as severe as in mesenteric angina, epigastric cramping, bloating and moderate weight loss. The diagnosis is made at visceral angiography, usually performed at the end of exhaustive investigation of these symptoms.

Usually the coeliac artery or occasionally the SMA is shown to be severely stenosed at its origin, often with poststenotic dilatation.

Compression occurs when the fibres of the aortic hiatus press on these vessels due to either a low diaphragmatic insertion or a high origin of the visceral vessels. This cause of intestinal ischaemia is understandable where both the coeliac artery and SMA are involved but less so in the more common presentation of isolated coeliac artery compression.[86] Possibly the syndrome develops where there is a poorly developed collateral circulation between the coeliac and superior mesenteric visceral beds, with pain being gastric in origin. Treatment is by division of the tough crural fibres usually without the need for arterial reconstruction. The debate regarding the clinical importance of this syndrome is compounded by the observation of recurrence after surgical treatment.[87]

CHRONIC ARTERIAL INTESTINAL ISCHAEMIA

Despite the 10–25% of severe visceral disease documented in autopsy and angiographic studies, the clinical syndrome of intestinal ischaemia remains rare.[64,88] In those unfortunate patients in whom this diagnosis is not suspected, there is inevitable progression with profound weight loss and in many cases eventual bowel infarction and death.

Diagnosis

The clinical hallmark of this condition is mesenteric or visceral angina. This presents as food fear, where severe epigastric or mid-abdominal pain develops some 30–40 minutes after eating. Eating smaller meals, vomiting and avoidance of food altogether will relieve the pain and results in profound weight loss. The typical patient is a female, heavy smoker who has been extensively investigated for the possibility of an occult malignancy or psychiatric food disorder. General examination may reveal widespread arterial disease and abdominal bruits.

Imaging

Once a presumptive diagnosis of chronic mesenteric ischaemia has been made, it will be noted that the majority of patients are thin. These circumstances are well suited to investigation of the mesenteric artery origins by duplex ultrasound. Excellent views of the abdominal aorta and its major branches can usually be obtained with high-resolution ultrasound probes (5–10 MHz) and the mesenteric vessel origins can be relatively easily insonated with Doppler and colour flow imaging. Colour flow imaging facilitates the detection of mesenteric vascular stenoses by detecting a reduction in the functional lumen size, increased flow velocities and turbulence in blood flow in the region of the stenosis. This will identify an area of abnormality, which then must be investigated further using pulsed Doppler and spectral analysis. The peak systolic velocities measured can be compared against standard criteria. These data would indicate that an SMA peak systolic velocity of greater than 275 cm/s and a coeliac artery peak systolic velocity of greater than 200 cm/s appear to be good predictors of a 70% stenosis of the SMA and coeliac artery respectively.[89] Although duplex is useful for screening patients with possible mesenteric ischaemia, it may not be possible to obtain good views in the presence of intra-abdominal gas.

MRA, particularly contrast-enhanced MRA, has shown promise at producing highly detailed images of the proximal mesenteric vasculature. To date there are no studies that have validated MRA against the gold standard of catheter angiography.

If a patient has symptoms suggestive of chronic intestinal ischaemia, duplex ultrasound and/or magnetic resonance scan may help to plan angiography, as this may be performed as a prelude to endovascular intervention. Care must be taken when diagnosing stenoses of the coeliac artery to ensure that coeliac axis compression is not mistaken for fixed arterial stenosis. Reversible coeliac axis compression can be demonstrated angiographically and by duplex scanning in a number of asymptomatic individuals during different phases of respiration.

Treatment

Revascularisation should only be considered in symptomatic patients where there is reasonable confidence in the diagnosis of chronic intestinal ischaemia. These patients are severely and chronically malnourished and therefore a period of parenteral nutrition is to be recommended (ideally for 10–14 days) if surgical intervention is considered. Options for revascularisation include endovascular and open surgical techniques.

Endovascular technique During the treatment period, it is recommended that patients have combination antiplatelet therapy (e.g. aspirin and clopidogrel). Arterial access is obtained and once this has been secured, heparin is routinely administered to ensure anticoagulation during the period of catheter manipulation. There does not appear to be any need to maintain anticoagulation beyond this period.

A flush aortogram is performed and the target lesion identified. The ostium of the mesenteric vessel is identified, a guidewire manipulated across the stenosis and the decision of primary angioplasty or stenting is made. The literature mostly describes the use of short balloon-mounted stents, allowing as short a stent as possible to cover the lesion (**Figs 15.6** and **15.7**).

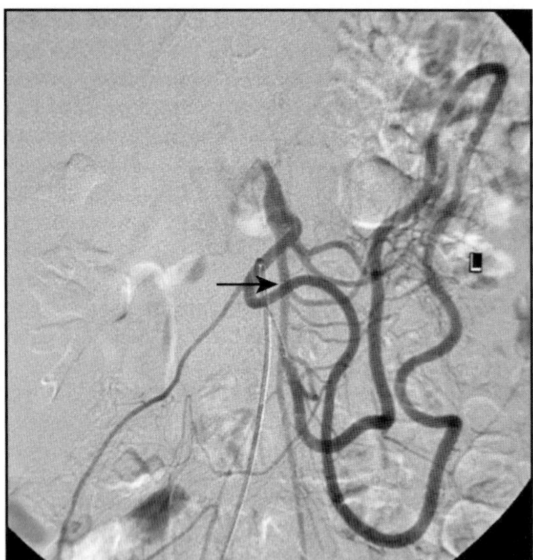

Figure 15.6 • Inferior mesenteric artery contrast injection, with filling of the superior mesenteric artery (arrow) via the wandering artery.

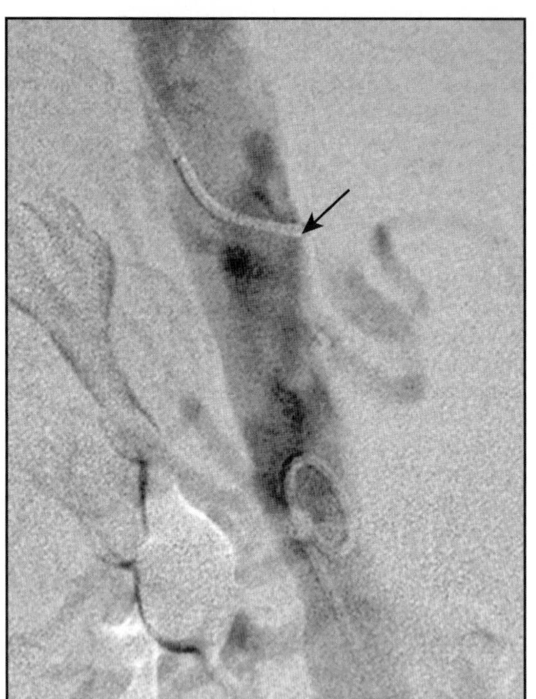

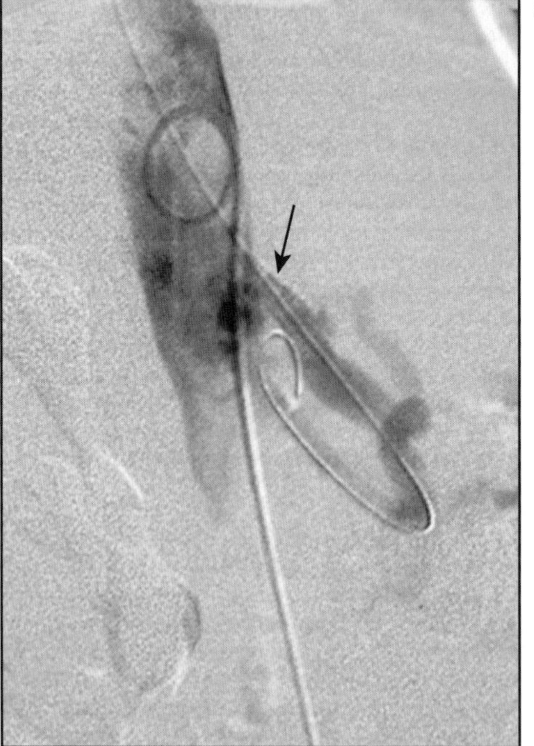

Figure 15.7 • **(a)** Angiogram showing tight coeliac artery stenosis (arrow); **(b)** following stenting of the stenosis (arrow).

Surgical revascularisation There is no clear evidence of superiority of any specific method, with reimplantation, bypass grafting and endarterectomy being the main procedures. Multiple-vessel rather than single-vessel revascularisation is currently recommended, although there is no objective basis for this policy.[90,91] Recent intestinal blood flow studies confirming the importance of the SMA in postprandial blood flow support the hypothesis that this is the most important vessel to reconstruct. Solitary mesenteric revascularisation in the emergency situation has had good long-term results, indicating preferential use of SMA revascularisation in all symptomatic patients unless there is diffuse disease of the mesenteric artery.[73]

Endarterectomy of the visceral arterial origins is performed with control of the suprarenal and infrarenal aorta, a major intervention with risk of severe left ventricular strain and visceral ischaemia. The aorta can be opened through either an anterior incision or a posterolateral trapdoor incision. Endarterectomy has excellent results in the hands of its proponents, although bypass surgery is more generally employed. Dacron or PTFE is the conduit of choice, with long saphenous vein being used in the presence of peritoneal infection. The infrarenal aorta, if suitable, can be used as the technically most simple inflow site. If both the coeliac artery and SMA are being revascularised, a bifurcated graft is anastomosed onto the anterior aortic wall, taking care to avoid kinking. The coeliac limb is passed

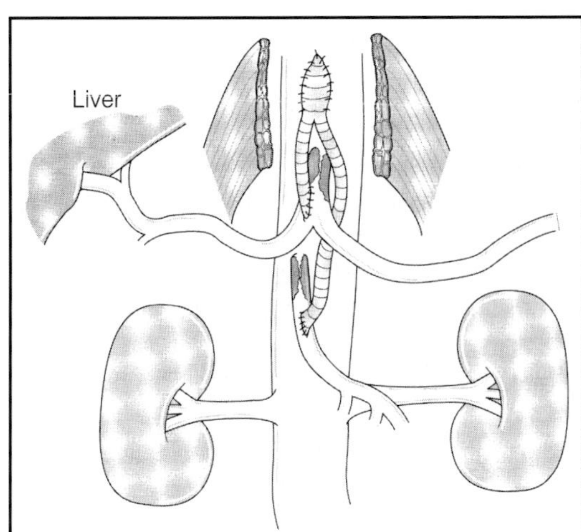

Figure 15.8 • The supracoeliac approach to intestinal bypass.

behind the neck of the pancreas and anastomosed onto the coeliac trunk at a suitable site. Alternatively, the supracoeliac aorta can be used as the inflow site (**Fig. 15.8**). This site is usually healthier than the infrarenal aorta and, with partial cross-clamping, hepatic and visceral ischaemia is avoided. This approach gives a better configuration between graft limbs and vessels. The grafts must be carefully excluded using retroperitoneal tissues and, if necessary, an omental flap.

If solitary SMA revascularisation is to be performed and the infrarenal aorta is healthy, the most simple procedure is direct reimplantation of this artery. Again, great care must be taken to avoid a configuration that will result in kinking.

At the end of the procedure the adequacy of flow in the reconstructed circulation must be verified using the hand-held Doppler, interrogating both the main visceral trunks and the arteries of the distal arcades.

Good postoperative care is of major importance in ensuring the success of reconstruction. Patients should be nursed in either the high-dependency unit or intensive care unit until the danger of a revascularisation syndrome has passed. Prolonged parenteral nutrition may be necessary because of delayed return of normal gut function due to reperfusion injury. Also, these patients have a long-standing fear of food and the process of returning to a normal diet may take several weeks.

Results of treatment

The endovascular option for treating this condition is attractive as the open operations are a major undertaking in a group of patients who are almost exclusively elderly and in whom there is significant comorbidity. In addition, the nature of chronic mesenteric ischaemia dictates that such patients have been chronically undernourished and are frequently relatively dehydrated and lacking in metabolic reserves. In such circumstances subjecting these patients to a major surgical procedure, with its associated catabolic consequences, makes little sense if this can be avoided.

Endovascular procedures have been used since 1980, and since then a number of reports have been published. The results were reviewed in 2003,[92] and showed an average complication rate of 7.5%, with primary patency of 60% on intention to treat. This success was improved to 70% by subsequent interventions.

The introduction of metallic endovascular stents could make a significant difference to the treatment of mesenteric vascular disease. Following the model of renal artery stenting, it would be expected that the majority of lesions causing chronic mesenteric ischaemia and amenable to endovascular treatment would be more easily managed by stenting than balloon angioplasty alone.

For surgical revascularisation, mortalities of 5–10% are reported in the literature but in poor-risk patients this will inevitably be higher. However, long-term patency rates are excellent, with patency and clinical success rates of 85–96% being recorded.[93]

Key points

Renal disease

- Angioplasty (PTA) is the procedure of choice for non-atheromatous lesions.
- The improvement of blood pressure control in non-atheromatous lesions is good to excellent following PTA.
- ARVD usually presents with hypertension, chronic renal failure, acute renal failure or pulmonary oedema. However, it is often asymptomatic and should not be forgotten in patients with extrarenal vascular disease.
- Stents have a higher technical success and patency rate compared with PTA in atheromatous ostial lesions.
- Surgery gives the lowest restenosis rates but should be reserved for stent failures or young fit patients.
- Improvement of blood pressure control in atheromatous lesions following PTA is marginal but may reduce the drug burden.
- Results in atheromatous patients with renal insufficiency following PTA are variable with no consensus.

Intestinal ischaemia

- Intestinal ischaemia is a rare condition that presents a major diagnostic and management challenge to the vascular specialist.
- Acute intestinal ischaemia remains a surgical emergency that should be treated by laparotomy, revascularisation and then resection of dead bowel, in most cases.
- Chronic intestinal ischaemia may be treated by surgical or endovascular methods. Endovascular techniques should be considered in poor-risk symptomatic patients and merit further objective assessment.

REFERENCES

1. Tegtmeyer CJ, Matsumoto AH, Angle JF. Percutaneous transluminal angioplasty in fibrous dysplasia and children. In: Novick A, Scoble J, Hamilton G (eds) Renal vascular disease. London: WB Saunders, 1996; pp. 363–83.
2. Tegtmeyer CJ, Selby JB, Hartwell et al. Results and complications of angioplasty in fibromuscular disease. Circulation 1991; 83(suppl.):I155.
3. Tyagi S, Singh B, Kaul UA et al. Balloon angioplasty for renovascular hypertension in Takayasu's arteritis. Am Heart J 1993; 125:1386–93.
4. Kaatee R, Beek FJA, Verschuyl EJ et al. Atherosclerotic renal artery stenosis: ostial or truncal. Radiology 1996; 199:637.
5. Hanovici H, Zinicda N. Experimental renal artery stenosis. Diagnostic significance of arterial haemodynamics. J Cardiovasc Surg 1962; 3:259–62.
6. Wasser MN, Weatenberg J, van der Hulst VP et al. Haemodynamic significance of renal artery stenosis: digital subtraction angiography versus systolically gated three dimensional phase contrast MR angiography. Radiology 1997; 202:333–8.
7. Schwartz CJ, White TA. Stenosis of the renal artery: an unselected necropsy study. Br Med J 1964; 2:1415–21.
8. Hansen KJ, Edwards MS, Craven TE et al. Prevalence of renovascular disease in the elderly: a population-based study. J Vasc Surg 2002; 36:443–51.
9. Rudnick KV, Sackell DL, Hirst S, Holmes C. Hypertension in family practice. Can Med Assoc J 1997; 117:492–7.
10. Maxwell MH, Bleifer KH, Franklin SS, Varady PD. Cooperative study of renovascular hypertension: demographic analysis of the study. JAMA 1972; 220:1195–204.
11. Herrara AH, Davidson RA. Renovascular disease in older adults. Clin Geriatr Med 1998; 14:237–53.
12. Harding MB, Smith LR, Himmelstein SI et al. Renal artery stenosis: prevalence and associated risk factors in patients undergoing routine cardiac catheterization. J Am Soc Nephrol 1992; 2:1608–16.
13. Crowley JJ, Santos RM, Peter RH et al. Progression of renal artery stenosis in patients undergoing cardiac catheterisation. Am Heart J 1998; 136:913–18.

14. Conlon PJ, O'Riordan E, Kalra PA. New insights into the epidemiologic and clinical manifestations of atherosclerotic renovascular disease. Am J Kidney Dis 2000; 35:573–87.
15. MacDowall P, Kalra PA, O'Donoghue DJ et al. Risk of morbidity from renovascular disease in elderly patients with congestive cardiac failure. Lancet 1998; 352:13–16.
16. Missouris CG, Buckenham T, Cappuccio FP, MacGregor GA. Renal artery stenosis: a common and important problem in patients with peripheral vascular disease. Am J Med 1994; 96:10–14.
17. Olin JW, Melia M, Young JR, Graor RA, Risius B. Prevalence of atherosclerotic renal artery stenosis in patients with atherosclerosis elsewhere. Am J Med 1990; 88(1N):46N–51N.
18. Kuroda S, Nishida N, Uzu T et al. Prevalence of renal artery stenosis in autopsy patients with stroke. Stroke 2000; 31:61–5.
19. Louie J, Isaacson JA, Zierler RE, Bergelin RO, Strandness DE Jr. Prevalence of carotid and lower extremity arterial disease in patients with renal artery stenosis. Am J Hypertens 1994; 7:436–9.
20. Shurrab AE, Mamtora H, O'Donoghue D, Waldek S, Kalra PA. Increasing the diagnostic yield of renal angiography for the diagnosis of atheromatous renovascular disease. Br J Radiol 2001; 74:213–18.
21. Schreiber MF, Pohl MA, Novick AC. The natural history of atherosclerotic and fibrous renal artery disease. Urol Clin North Am 1984; 11:383–92.
22. Zierler RE, Bergelin RO, Isaacson JA, Strandness DE Jr. Natural history of atherosclerotic renal artery stenosis: a prospective study with duplex ultrasonography. J Vasc Surg 1994; 19:250–8.
23. Caps MT, Zierler RE, Polissar NL et al. Risk of atrophy in kidneys with atherosclerotic renal artery stenosis. Kidney Int 1998; 53:735–42.
24. Middleton JP. Ischemic disease of the kidney: how and why to consider revascularisation. J Nephrol 1998; 11:123–36.
25. Textor SC. Revascularisation in atherosclerotic renal artery disease. Kidney Int 1998; 53:799–811.
26. Suresh M, Laboi P, Mamtora H, Kalra PA. Relationship of renal dysfunction to proximal arterial disease severity in atherosclerotic renovascular disease. Nephrol Dial Transplant 2000; 15:631–6.
27. Cheung CM, Wright JR, Shurrab AE et al. Epidemiology of renal dysfunction and patient outcome in atherosclerotic renal artery occlusion. J Am Soc Nephrol 2002; 13:149–57.
28. Farmer CKT, Reidy J, Kalra PA, Cook GJR, Scoble JE. Individual kidney function before and after renal angioplasty. Lancet 1998; 352:288–9.
29. Wright JR, Shurrab AE, Cheung C et al. A prospective study of the determinants of renal functional outcome and mortality in atherosclerotic renovascular disease. Am J Kidney Dis 2002; 39:1153–61.
30. Jacobson HR. Nephrology forum. Ischemic renal disease: an overlooked clinical entity. Kidney Int 1998; 34:729–43.
31. Gruentzig A, Vetter W, Meier B et al. Treatment of renovascular hypertension with percutaneous transluminal dilatation of a renal artery stenosis. Lancet 1978; 1(8068):801.
32. Cicuto KP, McLean GK, Oleaga JA et al. Renal artery stenosis: anatomical classification for percutaneous transluminal angioplasty. Am J Roentgenol 1981; 137:599–601.

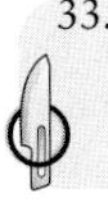

33. Tan KT, Van Beek EJR, Brown PWG et al. Magnetic resonance angiography for the diagnosis of renal artery stenosis. A meta-analysis. Clin Radiol 2002; 57:617–24.

Gadolinium-enhanced MRA may replace angiography in most patients with suspected RAS. Sensitivity is 97%, specificity 93%. It is non-invasive, avoids ionising radiation and uses a non-nephrotoxic contrast agent.

34. Verschuyl E-J, Kaatee R, Beek FJA et al. Renal artery origins: best angiographic projection angles. Radiology 1997; 205:115–20.
35. Kessel DO, Robertson I, Taylor EJ et al. Renal stenting from the radial artery: a novel approach. Cardiovasc Intervent Radiol 2003; 26:146–9.
36. Solomon R, Werner C, Mann D, D`Elia J, Silva P. Effects of saline, mannitol and furosemide on acute decreases in renal function induced by radiocontrast agents. N Engl J Med 1994; 331:1416–20.
37. Tepel M, van der Giet M, Schwarzfeld C et al. Prevention of radiographic contrast agent induced reductions in renal function by acetylcysteine. N Engl J Med 2000; 343:180–4.
38. Aspelin P, Aubry P, Fransson S et al. Nephrotoxic effects in high risk patients undergoing angiography. N Engl J Med 2003; 348:491–9.

Nephropathy induced by contrast medium may be less likely to develop in high-risk patients when iodixanol is used rather than a low-osmolar, non-ionic contrast medium.

39. Beek FJA, Kaatee R, Beutler JJ et al. Complications during renal artery stent placement for atherosclerotic ostial stenosis. Cardiovasc Intervent Radiol 1997; 20:184–90.
40. Weibull H, Bergqvist D, Bergentz S-E et al. Percutaneous transluminal renal angioplasty versus surgical reconstruction of atherosclerotic renal artery stenosis: a prospective randomised study. J Vasc Surg 1993; 18:841–52.
41. Van de ven PJG, Kaatee R, Beutler JJ et al. Arterial stenting and balloon angioplasty in ostial atherosclerotic renovascular disease: a randomised trial. Lancet 1999; 353:282–6.

This trial showed convincing superiority of stenting over angioplasty regarding technical success and primary patency.

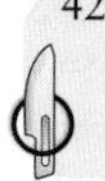

42. Leertouwer TC, Gussenhoven EJ, Bosch JL et al. Stent placement for renal arterial stenosis: where do we stand? A meta-analysis. Radiology 2000; 216:78–85.

Renal stenting is technically superior and clinically comparable to renal angioplasty alone.

43. Henry M, Klonaris C, Henry I et al. Protected renal stenting with the PercuSurge Guardwire device: a pilot study. J Endovasc Ther 2001; 8:227–37.

44. Holden A, Hill A. Renal angioplasty and stenting with distal protection of the main renal artery in ischaemic nephropathy: early experience. J Vasc Surg 2003; 38:962–8.

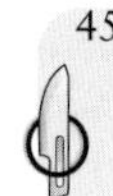

45. Van Jaarsveld BC, Krijnen P, Pieterman H et al. The effects of balloon angioplasty on hypertension in atherosclerotic renal artery stenosis. N Engl J Med 2000; 342:1007–14.

Largest randomised controlled trial (106 patients). In patients with hypertension and atherosclerotic RAS, angioplasty has little advantage over drug therapy alone.

46. Plouin P-F, Chatellier G, Darne B et al. Blood pressure outcome of angioplasty in atherosclerotic renal artery stenosis. Hypertension 1998; 31:823–9.

In unilateral atherosclerotic RAS, angioplasty is a drug-sparing procedure that involves some morbidity. Previous uncontrolled studies have overestimated its effect on hypertension.

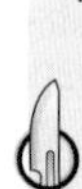

47. Webster J, Marshall F, Abdalla M et al. Randomised comparison of percutaneous angioplasty vs continued medical therapy for hypertensive patients with atheromatous renal artery stenosis. J Hum Hypertens 1998; 12:329–35.

Angioplasty results in a modest improvement in systolic blood pressure compared with drug therapy alone. This benefit was confined to bilateral disease. No patient was cured and renal function did not improve. Angioplasty was associated with significant morbidity.

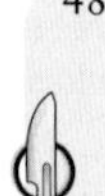

48. Ives N, Wheatley K, Stowe RL et al. Continuing uncertainty about the value of percutaneous revascularisation in atherosclerotic renovascular disease: a meta-analysis of randomised trials. Nephrol Dial Transplant 2003;18: 298–304.

Reported trials are too small to determine reliably the role of angioplasty in ARVD. Trials do exclude a large improvement in hypertension or renal function but are too small to exclude a clinically worthwhile benefit.

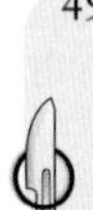

49. Nordmann AJ, Woo K, Parkes R et al. Balloon angioplasty or medical therapy for hypertensive patients with atherosclerotic renal artery stenosis? A meta-analysis of randomised controlled trials. Am J Med 2003; 114:44–50.

Angioplasty has a modest but significant effect on blood pressure and should be considered in poorly controlled hypertension in atherosclerotic patients. There is no evidence to support its use in improving or preserving renal function.

50. Brewster DC, Retana A, Waltman AC, Darling RC. Angiography in the management of aneurysms to the abdominal aorta. Its value and safety. N Engl J Med 1975; 292:822–5.

51. Novick AC. Patient selection for intervention to preserve renal function in ischaemic renal disease. In: Novick AC, Scoble J, Hamilton G (eds) Renal vascular disease. London: WB Saunders, 1996; pp. 323–38.

52. Benjamin ME, Hansen KJ, Craven TE et al. Combined aortic and renal artery surgery. A contemporary experience. Ann Surg 1996; 223:555–65.

53. Dean RH. Surgical reconstruction of atherosclerotic renal artery disease. In: Branchereau A, Jacobs M (eds) Long term results of arterial interventions. Armonk, NY: Futura, 1997; pp. 205–16.

54. Reilly JM, Rubin BG, Thompson RW et al. Revascularization of the solitary kidney: a challenging problem in a high risk population. Surgery 1996; 120:732–6.

55. Steinbach F, Novick AC, Campbell S, Dykstra D. Long-term survival after surgical revascularization for atherosclerotic renal artery disease. J Urol 1997; 158:38–41.

56. Darling RC III, Shah DM, Chang BB, Leather RP. Does concomitant aortic bypass and renal artery revascularization using the retroperitoneal approach increase perioperative risk? Cardiovasc Surg 1995; 3:421–3.

57. Novick AC, Ziegelbaum M, Vidt DG et al. Trends in surgical revascularization for renal artery disease. Ten years' experience. JAMA 1987; 257:498–501.

58. Cambria RP, Brewster DC, L'Italien G et al. Renal artery reconstruction for the preservation of renal function. J Vasc Surg 1996; 24:371–82.

59. Reilly JM, Rubin BG, Thompson RW et al. Long-term effectiveness of extraanatomic renal artery revascularization. Surgery 1994; 116:784–90.

60. Oskin TC, Hansen KJ, Deitch JS et al. Chronic renal artery occlusion: nephrectomy versus revascularization. J Vasc Surg 1999; 29:140–9.

61. Bergentz SE, Weibull H, Novick AC. Long-term patency after reconstructive surgery and PTA for renal artery stenosis. In: Greenhalgh RM, Hollier L (eds) The maintenance or arterial reconstruction. London: WB Saunders, 1991; pp. 384–96.

62. Fergany A, Kolettis P, Novick AC. The contemporary role of extra-anatomical surgical renal revascularization in patients with atherosclerotic renal artery disease. J Urol 1995; 153:1798–801.

63. Novick AC. Extracorporeal microvascular reconstruction and autotransplantation for branch renal artery disease. In: Novick AC, Scoble J, Hamilton G (eds) Renal vascular disease. London: WB Saunders, 1996; pp. 497–511.

64. Moneta GL, Lee RW. The management of visceral ischaemic syndromes. In: Rutherford RB (ed.) Vascular surgery, 4th edn. Philadelphia: WB Saunders, 1995; pp. 1267–77.

65. Moneta GL, Taylor DC, Helton WS et al. Duplex ultrasound measurement of postprandial intestinal blood flow: effect of meal composition. Gastroenterology 1988; 95:1294–301.

66. Chou CC. Relationship between intestinal blood flow and motility. Annu Rev Physiol 1982; 44:29–42.

67. Poole JW, Sammartano RJ, Boley SJ. Hemodynamic basis of the pain of chronic mesenteric ischemia. Am J Surg 1987; 153:171–6.

68. Granger DN, Hollwarth ME, Parks DA. Ischemia–reperfusion injury: role of oxygen-derived free radicals. Acta Physiol Scand Suppl 1986; 548:47–63.

69. Grisham MB, Hernandez LA, Granger DN. Xanthine oxidase and neutrophil infiltration in intestinal ischemia. Am J Physiol 1986; 251:G567–G574.

70. Harward TR, Brooks DL, Flynn TC, Seeger JM. Multiple organ dysfunction after mesenteric artery revascularization. J Vasc Surg 1993; 18:459–67.

71. Office of Population Censuses and Surveys. Mortality statistics: causes. 1980. London: HMSO, 1982.

72. Office of Population Censuses and Surveys. Mortality statistics: causes. 1990. London: HMSO, 1991.

73. Taylor LM, Porter JM. Treatment of acute intestinal ischaemia caused by arterial occlusions. In: Rutherford RB (ed.) Vascular surgery, 4th edn. Philadelphia: WB Saunders, 1995; pp. 1278–83.

74. Levy PJ, Krausz MM, Manny J. Acute mesenteric ischemia: improved results. A retrospective analysis of ninety-two patients. Surgery 1990; 107:372–80.

75. DeNobile J, Guzzetta P, Patterson K. Pulse oximetry as a means of assessing bowel viability. J Surg Res 1990; 48:21–3.

76. Oohata Y, Mibu R, Hotokezaka M et al. Comparison of blood flow assessment between laser Doppler velocimetry and the hydrogen gas clearance method in ischemic intestine in dogs. Am J Surg 1990; 160:511–14.

77. Loomer DC, Johnson SP, Diffin DC, DeMaioribus CA. Superior mesenteric artery stent placement in a patient with acute mesenteric ischaemia. J Vasc Intervent Radiol 1999; 10:29–32.

78. Hassan HA, Raufman JP. Mesenteric venous thrombosis. South Med J 1999; 92:558–62.

79. Train JS, Ross H, Weiss JD et al. Mesenteric venous thrombosis: successful treatment by intraarterial lytic therapy. J Vasc Intervent Radiol 1998; 9:461–4.

80. Rhee RY, Gloviczki P, Mendonca CT et al. Mesenteric venous thrombosis: still a lethal disease in the 1990s. J Vasc Surg 1994; 20:688–97.

81. Zelenock GB. Visceral occlusive disease. In: Greenfield LJ (ed.) Surgery: scientific principles and practice. Philadelphia: JB Lippincott, 1993; pp. 1619–23.

82. Farkas JC, Calvo-Verjat N, Laurian C et al. Acute colorectal ischemia after aortic surgery: pathophysiology and prognostic criteria. Ann Vasc Surg 1992; 6:111–18.

83. Tollefson DF, Ernst CB. Colon ischemia following aortic reconstruction. Ann Vasc Surg 1991; 5:485–9.

84. Ernst CB, Hagihara PF, Daughtery ME et al. Ischemic colitis incidence following abdominal aortic reconstruction: a prospective study. Surgery 1976; 80:417–21.

85. Fiddian-Green RG, Amelin PM, Herrmann JB et al. Prediction of the development of sigmoid ischemia on the day of aortic operations. Indirect measurements of intramural pH in the colon. Arch Surg 1986; 121:654–60.

86. Bech F, Loesberg A, Rosenblum J, Glagov S, Gewertz BL. Median arcuate ligament compression syndrome in monozygotic twins. J Vasc Surg 1994; 19:934–8.

87. Geelkerken RH, van Bockel JH, de Roos WK, Hermans J. Coeliac artery compression syndrome: the effect of decompression. Br J Surg 1990; 77:807–9.

88. Croft RJ, Menon GP, Marston A. Does 'intestinal angina' exist? A critical study of obstructed visceral arteries. Br J Surg 1981; 68:316–18.

89. Moneta GL, Yeager RA, Dalman R et al. Duplex ultrasound criteria for the diagnosis of splanchnic artery stenosis or occlusion. J Vasc Surg 1991; 14:511.

90. Cunningham CG, Reilly LM, Rapp JH et al. Chronic visceral ischemia. Three decades of progress. Ann Surg 1991; 214:276–87.

91. McAfee MK, Cherry KJ Jr, Naessens JM et al. Influence of complete revascularization on chronic mesenteric ischemia. Am J Surg 1992; 164:220–4.

92. Cleveland TJ, Nawaz S, Gaines PA. Mesenteric arterial ischaemia: diagnosis and therapeutic options. Vasc Med 2002; 7:311–21.

93. Taylor LM, Porter JM. Treatment of chronic visceral ischemia. In: Rutherford RB (ed.) Vascular surgery, 4th edn. Philadelphia: WB Saunders, 1995; pp. 1301–11.

CHAPTER

Sixteen

Extracranial cerebrovascular disease

A. Ross Naylor and
Peter A. Gaines

INTRODUCTION

Stroke is the third commonest cause of death after coronary disease and cancer and is the principal cause of neurological disability.[1] It is defined as an acute loss of focal cerebral function (occasionally global in coma or subarachnoid haemorrhage) with symptoms exceeding 24 hours (or leading to death), with no apparent cause other than that of a vascular origin. A transient ischaemic attack (TIA) has the same definition but a time scale of less than 24 hours. In the UK, the annual incidence of stroke is 2 per 1000 and 125 000 patients will suffer their first stroke each year.[2] Half of all strokes affect patients over 75 years of age, while only 25% occur in patients under the age of 65 years.[1] Stroke patients use 10% of hospital bed-days and 5% of annual healthcare expenditure.[3] Although stroke mortality has diminished by up to 20%, attributed to improved survival rather than a decline in incidence,[4] the overall incidence of stroke could increase by 30% by 2033 because of the ageing population.[5] Community studies suggest that about 36 000 patients will suffer a TIA each year, giving an annual UK incidence of about 0.5 per 1000.[6] The incidence of TIA increases with age, from 0.9 per 1000 for those aged 55–64 years to 2.6 per 1000 for those aged 75–84 years.[6]

AETIOLOGY AND RISK FACTORS

About 80% of strokes are ischaemic and 20% are haemorrhagic (intracerebral/subarachnoid); about 80% of all ischaemic strokes affect the carotid territory. Risk factors include increasing age, smoking, hypertension (50%), ischaemic heart disease (38%), cardioembolic source (20%), previous TIA (15%), diabetes (10%), peripheral vascular disease, high plasma fibrinogen and hypercholesterolaemia.[7] The principal causes of ischaemic infarction are detailed in **Box 16.1**.

Large-vessel thromboembolism

The commonest single cause of ischaemic stroke is thromboembolism of the internal carotid artery (ICA) and/or middle cerebral artery (MCA). Intracranial occlusive disease alone is rarely responsible,[6] while pure haemodynamic strokes account for less than 2% of all strokes.[8] Stenoses develop at the

Box 16.1 • Aetiology of carotid territory infarction

Thromboembolism of internal carotid artery/middle cerebral artery (50%)
Small-vessel disease (25%)
Cardiogenic brain embolism (15%)
Haematological disease (5%)
Non-atheromatous disease (5%)

From Dennis MS, Bamford JM, Sandercock PAG, Warlow CP. Incidence of transient ischaemic attacks in Oxfordshire, England. Stroke 1989; 20:333–9, with permission.

origin of the ICA (**Fig. 16.1**) because of a complex region of haemodynamic phenomena comprising low shear stress, flow stasis and flow separation that predisposes to atherosclerotic plaque formation, particularly on the posterolateral wall. Should the plaque undergo acute change (rupture, ulceration, intraplaque haemorrhage), the inner core of thrombogenic subendothelial collagen is exposed and predisposes towards the formation of thrombus and the onset of symptoms. The phenomenon of 'TIA clustering' can be explained because of the transient phasic nature of this thrombus, which tends to be present for a few weeks and then resolves.[9] There is much interest as to why the plaque should undergo acute disruption. Is this a local or systemic phenomenon? Understanding this key phase may enable pharmacological intervention in the future. Research suggests that the concentration, production and expression of the enzyme matrix metalloproteinase-9 is significantly higher in unstable plaques or in plaques retrieved from patients with recent-onset symptoms.[10] Evidence supporting a 'systemic trigger' comes from a reanalysis of data from the European Carotid Surgery Trial (ECST). Patients with evidence of plaque irregularity prior to endarterectomy were significantly more likely to have suffered a myocardial infarction in the past and were then significantly more likely to suffer a myocardial infarction or sudden cardiac death in the future.[11]

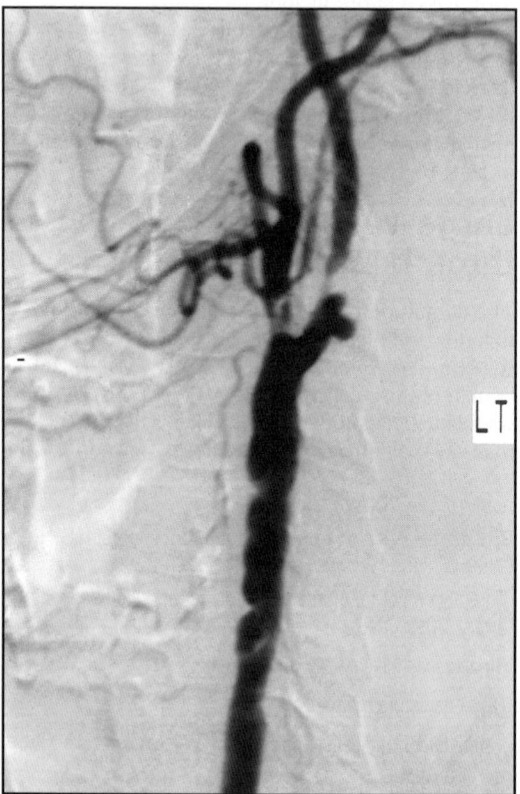

Figure 16.1 • Intra-arterial digital subtraction angiogram showing diffuse disease in the common carotid artery and severe stenoses at the origins of both the internal and external carotid arteries. There is also deep ulceration in the internal carotid artery plaque.

Small-vessel disease

Occlusion of the penetrating cerebral (end) arterioles produces lacunar infarcts, so named after the cavity or hole that remains after macrophages have removed the infarcted tissue. Autopsy studies suggest that the underlying occlusive process follows fibrinoid necrosis (associated with hypertensive encephalopathy), lipohyalinosis and microatheroma (associated with chronic hypertension) or microcalcinosis (associated with diabetes). The most common sites for lacunar infarction include the basal ganglia, thalamus and internal capsule.

Cardiogenic brain embolism

Important sources of cardiogenic brain embolism include ventricular mural thrombus (post-myocardial infarction, cardiomyopathy), left atrial thrombus (atrial fibrillation) and valvular lesions (vegetations, prostheses, calcified annulus, endocarditis).

Haematological disorders

Conditions such as myeloma, sickle-cell disease, polycythaemia, the oral contraceptive pill and related prothrombotic disorders may predispose towards stroke.

Non-atheromatous disease

Non-atheromatous conditions are rare but important causes of ischaemic stroke and include collagen vascular disorders (systemic lupus erythematosus, polyarteritis nodosa), arteritis, migraine, tumours, carotid dissection and fibromuscular dysplasia. The section below on non-atheromatous disease covers these conditions in more detail.

PRESENTATION

Asymptomatic carotid disease

This is usually discovered as a consequence of detecting a cervical bruit, as an incidental finding in the ICA contralateral to that under duplex investigation. Overall, 4% of patients over 45 years old will have a bruit,[12,13] rising to 12% in patients over 60 years old.[14] However, only 25–50% of symptomatic patients will have an audible bruit[13] and there is no evidence that either the presence or absence of a bruit or the quality of the bruit correlates with the degree of stenosis.[13,15] In particular, 30% of patients with a symptomatic ICA stenosis of 70–90% will not have a bruit, increasing to 60% for those with a 90–99% stenosis.[16] Paradoxically, up to 30% of patients with an ICA occlusion will still have an audible bruit. The latter observations are important as many general practitioners base the decision to refer patients to hospital on whether a bruit is present.[17] If no bruit is present at the time of examination, 1% of patients over the age of 65 years will develop a bruit each year thereafter.[18] The commonest reasons for a false-positive bruit (i.e. not due to ICA disease) are systolic cardiac murmurs, haemodynamic causes and bruits arising from the vertebral and external carotid arteries.[13,15]

Symptomatic carotid disease

The Oxfordshire Community Stroke Project (OCSP) has shown that clinical classification at the bedside reliably predicts outcome, vascular pathology and computed tomography (CT)/autopsy findings following ischaemic stroke.[19,20]

1. Patients classified as having total anterior circulation infarction (TACI) present with the triad of (i) hemisensory/motor deficit affecting face, arm and leg, (ii) homonymous hemianopia and (iii) higher cortical dysfunction (e.g. dysphasia, visuospatial neglect). Patients with TACI have the largest infarction volumes, occlusion of either the extracranial ICA or intracranial MCA mainstem, and a 30-day mortality of 37%. Only 7% are alive and independent at 1 year.[19,20]
2. Patients classified as having partial anterior circulation infarction (PACI) present with one or two components of the TACI triad, have focal infarcts on CT and rarely have evidence of major vessel occlusion. The 30-day mortality is 13%, and 71% are alive and independent at 1 year.[19,20]
3. Patients classified as having posterior circulation infarction (POCI) present with vertebrobasilar symptoms and have infarcts localised to the posterior circulation territory. The 30-day mortality rate is 7%, and 80% are independent by 30 days.[19]
4. Patients classified as having lacunar infarction (LACI) present with symptoms and signs that in pathological studies are associated with disease of the deep perforating arteries (pure motor stroke, pure sensory stroke, sensorimotor stroke and ataxic hemiparesis). Patients with lacunar infarction never have evidence of higher cortical dysfunction and major vessel occlusion is not a feature.[19,20]

The OCSP classification allows for prognosis and underlying vascular pathology to be predicted but requires knowledge of what constitutes an anterior circulation (or carotid) territory symptom as opposed to a posterior circulation (vertebrobasilar) territory symptom. Such a differentiation is very important now that the ECST and North American Symptomatic Carotid Endarterectomy Trial (NASCET) have identified the role of carotid surgery in symptomatic patients.[21,22]

Typical carotid territory symptoms are hemimotor/sensory signs, amaurosis fugax and higher cortical dysfunction (**Box 16.2**). Amaurosis fugax is a transient monocular visual loss that develops over a few seconds and usually clears within a few minutes. Failure to resolve within 24 hours is analogous to a stroke. A clear-cut history of amaurosis fugax in the absence of a carotid or cardiac source of embolisation should prompt referral to an ophthalmologist to exclude anterior ischaemic optic neuropathy (microvascular disease of the posterior ciliary arteries), which causes acute ischaemia of the optic nerve head.[23]

The differential diagnosis of carotid territory events includes epilepsy, tumour, giant aneurysm, hypoglycaemia and migraine. It is not usually possible to differentiate embolic from haemodynamic events, although where TIAs are precipitated by a heavy

Box 16.2 • Carotid and vertebrobasilar features

Typical carotid territory symptoms
Hemimotor/hemisensory signs
Monocular visual loss (amaurosis fugax)
Higher cortical dysfunction (dysphasia, visuospatial neglect, etc.)
Typical vertebrobasilar symptoms
Bilateral blindness
Problems with gait and stance
Hemilateral or bilateral motor/sensory signs
Dysarthria
Homonymous hemianopia
Diplopia, vertigo and nystagmus (provided it is not the only symptom)

meal, hot bath or exercise, a haemodynamically critical ICA stenosis should be suspected.

Vertebrobasilar symptoms include bilateral blindness, problems with gait and stance, hemilateral/bilateral motor or sensory impairment (10% have hemisensory/motor signs), dysarthria, homonymous hemianopia, nystagmus, dizziness, diplopia and vertigo (provided the latter three are not isolated). Historically, most clinicians have been taught to regard dizziness associated with neck movement as evidence suggestive of vertebrobasilar ischaemia, the rationale being that neck rotation 'nips' the vertebral arteries within the upper cervical transverse processes. In fact, colour transcranial imaging of the vertebral arteries during neck movements in these patients almost always shows no change in flow (direction or volume). These patients are more likely to have inner ear pathology and this should be excluded before a patient is labelled as having suffered vertebrobasilar events.

The term 'non-hemispheric' is ascribed to patients with isolated syncope (blackout, drop attack), presyncope (faintness), isolated dizziness, isolated double vision (diplopia) and isolated vertigo. These should never be considered carotid or vertebrobasilar in origin unless other more typical symptoms are present and it is important to exclude a cardiac or inner ear pathology.

NON-ATHEROMATOUS DISEASES

Kinking and coiling

Kinks and coils of the carotid arteries occur in up to 20% of patients undergoing carotid angiography[24] and a tortuous carotid artery lying superficial in the neck can easily be mistaken for an aneurysm. Intimal fibroplasia (a subtype of fibromuscular dysplasia) is associated with coiling/kinking of the distal ICA. The clinical significance of kinking is debatable, although embolisation may occur from coexistent atheromatous disease. However, it is important to correct for severe kinking immediately beyond the endarterectomy zone because this may predispose to postoperative thrombosis. More distal coils and kinks can be left alone but care should be taken when inserting a shunt to minimise the risks of intimal injury.

Fibromuscular dysplasia

Fibromuscular dysplasia is a rare disorder of unknown aetiology (affecting <1% of all carotid angiograms) that primarily affects the renal (majority) and carotid arteries in young women up to middle age. Fibromuscular dysplasia is classified into four subtypes: intimal fibroplasia (see above), medial fibroplasia, medial hyperplasia and perimedial dysplasia.[25] The commonest is medial fibroplasia, which is characterised by alternating segments of stenotic webs and dilatation and/or aneurysm formation (**Fig. 16.2**), typically in the mid-section of the ICA. In up to 60% of patients, fibromuscular dysplasia is bilateral. Patients may be asymptomatic or symptomatic (TIA, stroke, rupture, dissection, false aneurysm). Although management

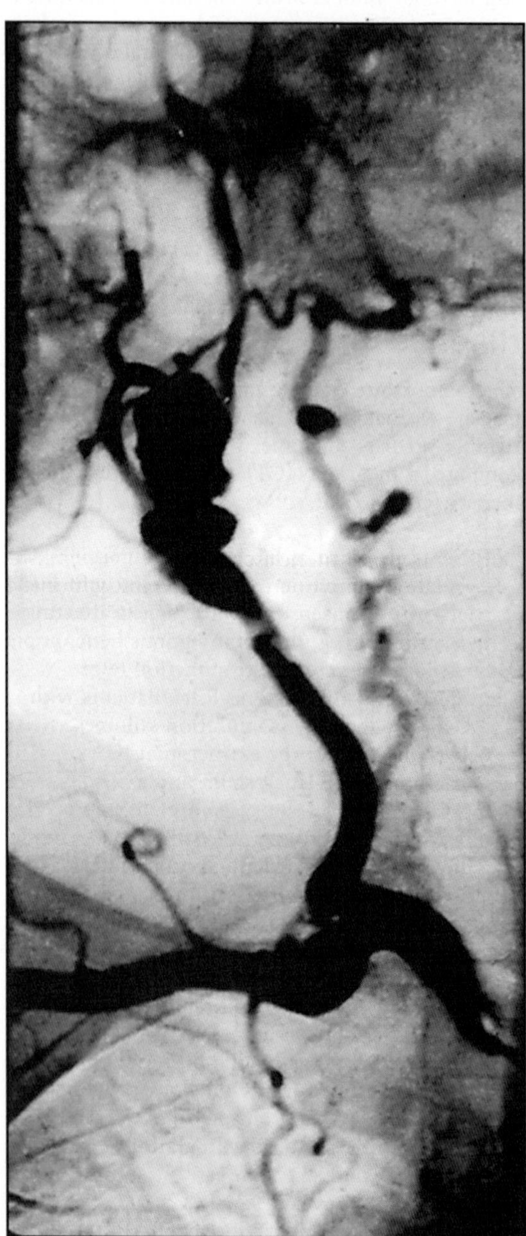

Figure 16.2 • Example of fibromuscular dysplasia causing early aneurysm formation in the carotid artery.

tends to be conservative in asymptomatic individuals, they should be maintained under regular clinical/duplex surveillance. Once symptomatic, the patient should be treated (i.e. the same policy as for symptomatic atherosclerotic disease), with options including resection and interposition bypass, open graduated internal dilatation or percutaneous angioplasty.

Arteritis

The inflammatory process in Takayasu's arteritis is transmural and granulomatous and ultimately leads to occlusion through fibrosis. Takayasu's arteritis predominantly affects young females (female to male ratio 7:1) and the initial presentation may be a relatively innocuous systemic illness comprising malaise, fever and arthralgia/myalgia. In the acute phase, there is a granulomatous vasculitis with medial disruption followed by transmural fibrosis during the chronic stage. Occasionally, focal aneurysms may form as a consequence of disruption of the internal elastic lamina and media. Neurological symptoms develop as a consequence of vascular occlusion or via renovascular hypertension. Type I Takayasu's arteritis (aortic arch and arch arteries) occurs in 8% of cases and presents with cerebral vascular and ocular symptoms. Type III Takayasu's arteritis (arch vessels plus abdominal aorta and its branches) accounts for 65% of cases and is characterised by stroke, renovascular hypertension and mesenteric ischaemia.[26] The mainstay of management is corticosteroid therapy, with cyclophosphamide and methotrexate as alternatives. Surgery should be avoided in the acute phase. Neither endarterectomy nor angioplasty is an option in Takayasu's arteritis of the carotid vessels (because of the long segments of fibrotic disease involvement) and if surgical intervention is required, then bypass is the preferred option. If surgery is required, it is imperative that the inflow is taken from the ascending aorta as opposed to the subclavian artery as the latter may be involved in the disease process.

Giant cell arteritis is another chronic granulomatous arteritis that primarily affects the older female population (female to male ratio 4:1). It is a systemic disorder and can affect any large artery, although the branches of the carotid artery tend to predominate with bilateral symmetrical involvement. The intracranial vessels are unaffected. The commonest presentation is generalised malaise in association with headache and myalgic pains. Jaw claudication is present in up to 50%, while 50% will develop pain over the temporal artery. Stroke is a rare presentation, the commonest being transient or permanent blindness. The ocular features (blindness, corneal ulcers and cataracts) can occur up to 6 months after the initial presentation. Treatment is primarily corticosteroid therapy, to which giant cell arteritis is sensitive (see Chapter 10).

Carotid aneurysm

Extracranial carotid aneurysm is rare (**Fig. 16.3**) and accounts for less than 4% of all peripheral aneurysms.[24] The currently accepted definition is a diameter exceeding 150% of the diameter of the common carotid artery (CCA) or twice the diameter of the distal ICA. The commonest single cause has traditionally been considered to be atherosclerosis, but carotid aneurysm (as with aortic aneurysm) may be due to abnormalities in matrix metalloproteinase metabolism. Less common aetiologies including trauma, carotid dissection and fibromuscular dysplasia should be considered. Clinical presentation includes discovery of a pulsatile swelling (with or without pain), thrombosis, dissection, rupture or embolisation. Treatment consists of exclusion and either primary anastomosis or interposition vein

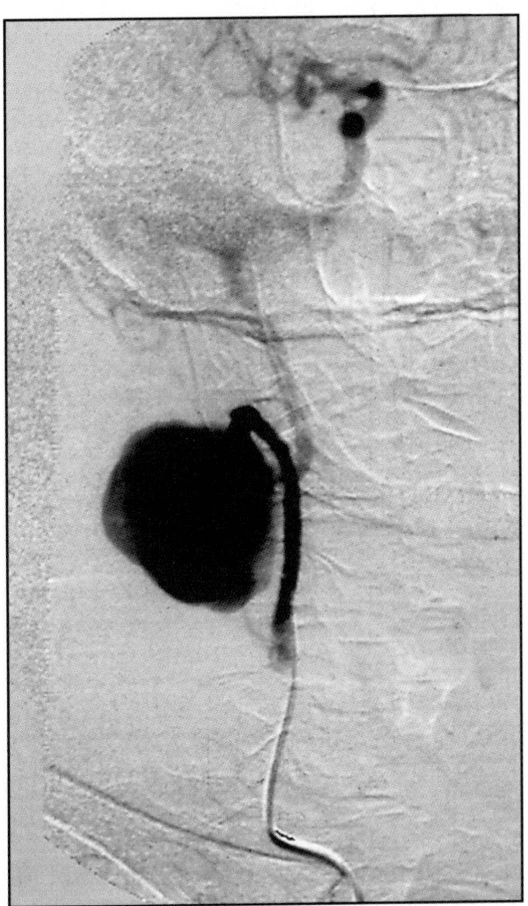

Figure 16.3 • Internal carotid artery aneurysm.

bypass, although endovascular intervention may become the treatment of choice in patients with aneurysms affecting the very distal aspects of the ICA.

Carotid dissection

Carotid dissection is responsible for 2% of all strokes, rising to 20% in young adults. One-fifth of trauma patients with an unexplained neurological deficit will have a dissection and 25% will be bilateral. Dissection can be spontaneous (e.g. fibromuscular dysplasia), can follow iatrogenic dissection (e.g. angioplasty), can be part of a central dissection (e.g. dissecting thoracic aorta) (**Fig. 16.4**) or can follow blunt trauma (e.g. direct crushing, forced hyperextension or forced rotation with crushing of the ICA between the mastoid process and the transverse process of C2). Carotid dissections are classed as type I if there is irregularity but no significant stenosis on angiography, type II if there is a stenosis greater than 70% and/or a 50% dilatation, or type III if dissections show a characteristic 'flame'-shaped occlusion about 2–3 cm distal to the bifurcation (**Fig. 16.5**). This characteristic appearance is due to compression of the true lumen by thrombus in the false channel.

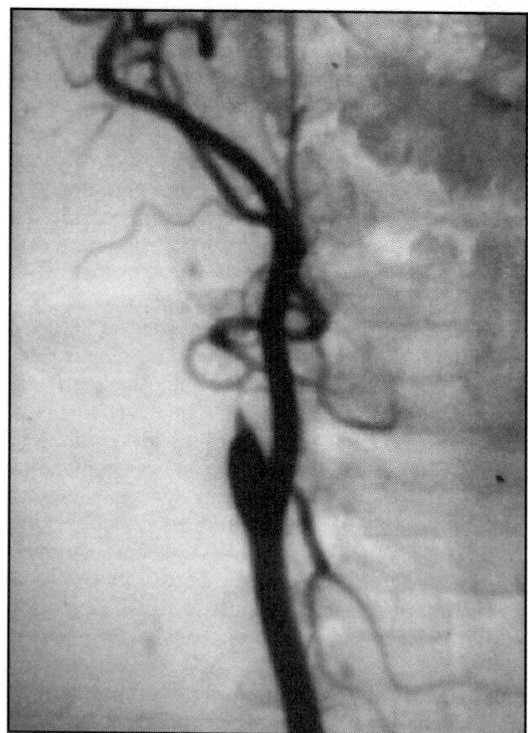

Figure 16.5 • Type III dissection of the internal carotid artery. The dissection starts 2–3 cm above the bifurcation. Blood in the false lumen has compressed the true lumen, giving rise to the characteristic 'flame'-shaped occlusion.

The commonest presentation following dissection is ipsilateral head/neck pain (70%) that precedes the onset of neurological symptoms. Between 50 and 75% of patients with a spontaneous dissection will present with TIA or stroke (usually embolic as opposed to thrombotic), pulsatile tinnitus, syncope, ocular signs or cranial nerve palsies (III, IV, VI, VII, IX, X, XII), which are usually due to mechanical compression from mural haematoma or stretching. Up to 60% of patients with spontaneous dissection will have ocular signs,[27] comprising oculosympathetic paresis (due to small-vessel occlusion and/or segmental ischaemia of the periadventitial sympathetic nerve plexus), amaurosis fugax (which can be aggravated by sitting or standing), hemianopia, ischaemic optic neuropathy and painful Horner's syndrome. The latter is probably due to segmental ischaemia of the postganglionic fibres distal to the superior cervical ganglion and may persist in 50%. The recognition of ocular symptoms in patients with dissection is important as up to 25% will suffer a stroke within 1 week.

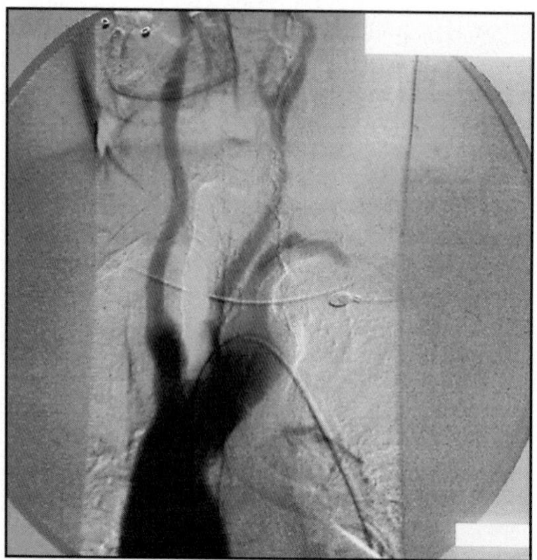

Figure 16.4 • Dissection flap extending from the aortic arch up into the left internal carotid artery.

Following duplex scanning, patients suspected of having a dissection should undergo intra-arterial digital subtraction angiography (DSA) or magnetic resonance angiography (MRA). This typically shows the dissection to start some 2–3 cm beyond the origin of the ICA. The distal limit is variable (but may be as high as the petrous segment) with varying combinations of stenosis, aneurysmal dilatation, intimal flaps and complete occlusion in the intervening segment. The majority are usually managed conservatively (systemic heparinisation followed by warfarinisation), with the aim being to reduce the incidence of thrombosis and embolism. Surgery tends to be reserved for complex trauma cases (usually type II) but may be indicated in patients with recurrent cerebral events despite medical therapy. Patients with type I dissections should be managed conservatively. Overall, carotid dissection carries a 20% mortality and a 30% rate of persisting disability.

Carotid body tumour

The carotid body is a discrete structure within the adventitia of the posterior aspect of the carotid bifurcation and is responsible for the monitoring of blood gases and pH. Despite its small size it has a greater blood supply than the brain.[28] A carotid body tumour is derived from cells originating from the neural crest ectoderm (chemoreceptor cells), is typically located within the space between the internal and external carotid arteries, and consists pathologically of nests of neoplastic epithelioid chief cells. As the tumour enlarges, the bifurcation splays and the patient becomes aware of a neck swelling. Alternative presentations include overlying pain, local invasion/compression causing hoarseness, cranial nerve palsies and Horner's syndrome. Carotid body tumour rarely presents with cerebral ischaemia but patients may present with a hormonally mediated syndrome comprising flushing, dizziness, arrhythmias and hypertension.[29] Diagnosis requires awareness (all too often the neck has been inadvertently explored) supplemented by angiography, CT/magnetic resonance imaging (MRI) (**Fig. 16.6**) or radionuclide imaging as appropriate. Overall, 5% of carotid body tumours are bilateral; metachronous tumours may subsequently appear; and 5% are locally and 5% systemically malignant. Treatment consists of surgical excision, although a more conservative approach might be adopted in elderly patients with small asymptomatic tumours.[29] The role of preoperative embolisation remains controversial but may reduce the risk of intraoperative haemorrhage.

The differential diagnosis for carotid body tumour includes glomus vagale and glomus jugulare tumours. The glomus vagale tumour is a paraganglionoma arising from chemoreceptor cells within the vagus nerve. It can be differentiated from a carotid body tumour because the bifurcation is not splayed. Instead, the tumour mass usually causes deviation of the ICA *above* the bifurcation (**Fig. 16.7**). It is preferable to have considered a glomus vagale tumour in the differential diagnosis preoperatively, as resection inevitably leads to swallowing problems and hoarseness and the patient should be warned of this.

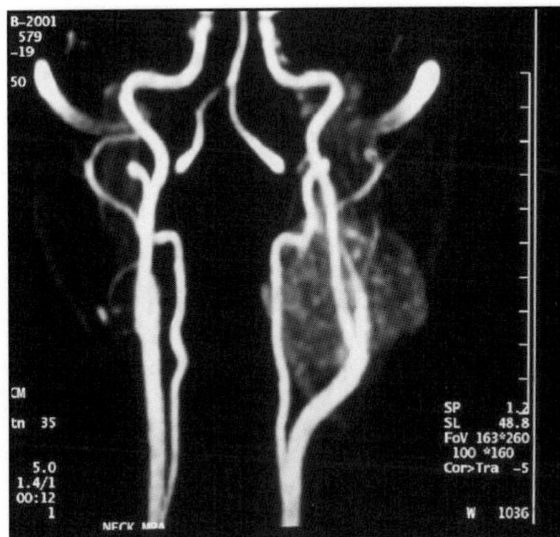

Figure 16.6 • Magnetic resonance angiogram of a carotid body tumour. The vascular tumour lies inside the carotid bifurcation and causes characteristic splaying of the internal and external carotid arteries.

INVESTIGATION

Duplex ultrasonography

Duplex combines B-mode (real-time) imaging with waveform analysis using pulsed-wave Doppler. Doppler waveform analysis is obtained by placing an electronic cursor within the insonated arterial lumen (imaged in B-mode) and the waveform is then displayed graphically (**Fig. 16.8**) as velocity (vertical axis) against time (horizontal axis). Older systems were limited by only being able to image in black and white but the advent of colour flow imaging has made duplex more versatile. The colour of each pixel reflects the mean velocity. It is conventional for red to represent flow towards the probe, whereas blue indicates flow away from the probe. In practice, the operator uses colour flow to identify the appropriate artery and areas of turbulence and then incorporates waveform analysis to accurately quantify flow velocity and degree of stenosis. Duplex is invaluable for screening neck masses (nodes, tortuous carotid vessels, true aneurysms, carotid body tumours). Its main role, however, is the investigation of carotid and vertebral artery occlusive disease. The vertebral arteries are visualised in 93% of patients, but the proximal one-third remains difficult to image clearly. However, despite being able to identify more than 95% of lesions responsible for carotid territory symptoms, worries about the comparability of angiography with duplex have previously restricted the application of duplex as a diagnostic modality in its

(a)

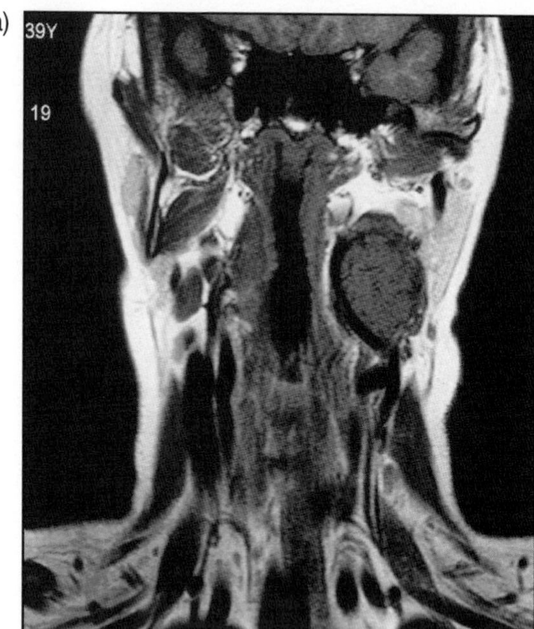

(b)

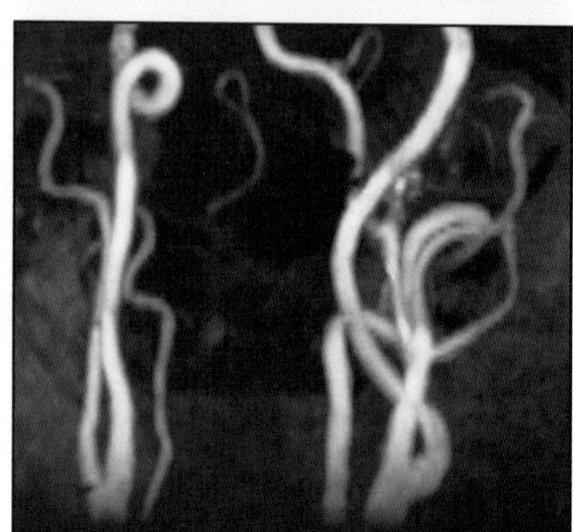

Figure 16.7 • **(a)** Magnetic resonance image of mass in left side of neck. Differential diagnosis was either carotid body tumour or glomus vagale. **(b)** Magnetic resonance angiogram shows no splaying of the left carotid bifurcation, but the mass causes significant displacement of the upper internal carotid artery indicating that this is most likely a glomus vagale tumour.

own right. However, current evidence suggests that reliance on duplex does not compromise operability or safety.[34]

Direct comparison between duplex and angiography must take into account operator experience, type of equipment, use of either the ECST or NASCET angiographic criteria (see later), and the presence or absence of colour flow technology. Moreover, it should be borne in mind that neither duplex nor MRA can ever be better than intra-arterial DSA if the latter is used as the 'gold standard'. The original Strandness criteria (**Table 16.1**) have now been revised to take into account the ECST and NASCET disease subgroups (**Table 16.2**). Each unit should develop its own internally validated criteria. In Leicester, UK, a combination of B-mode imaging together with peak systolic velocity (PSV) greater than 250 cm/s and end-diastolic velocity greater than 120 cm/s and/or a ratio of PSV (ICA) to PSV (CCA) greater than 4.0 is used to diagnose an ICA stenosis in excess of 70%. Angiography is currently reserved for patients in whom it is impossible to image either above or below the plaque or in whom a subtotal occlusion is suspected. Using these criteria, it is possible to reduce the angiography rate to less than 5%.[34]

Table 16.1 • Strandness criteria for categorising stenoses

Stenosis (%)	PSV (cm/s)	EDV (cm/s)	Spectral analysis
0	<125		Normal
1–15	<125		No flow reversal in bulb
16–49	<125		Spectral broadening during systole
50–79	>125		Marked spectral broadening
80–99	>125	>140	Marked spectral broadening
Occlusion	–	–	No flow

PSV, peak systolic velocity; EDV, end-diastolic velocity. Reprinted from Ultrasound Med Biol. Langlois Y, Roederer GO, Chan ATW et al. Evaluating carotid artery disease: 1983; 9:51–63, with permission from World Federation of Ultrasound in Medicine and Biology.

However, one of the main problems with duplex remains the differentiation of subocclusion from complete occlusion. Complete occlusions are diagnosed on the basis of no detectable flow and other supporting features, such as diastolic flow in the CCA approaching zero, increased velocity in the external carotid artery (ECA) and a 'thump' at the stump of the ICA. Using these criteria Kirsch et al.[35] showed a 97% positive predictive value for diagnosing occlusion, but the problem with false negatives remains and many units still recommend verification with angiography. However, the need to aggressively investigate patients with subocclusion (or the string sign) has recently been called into question.

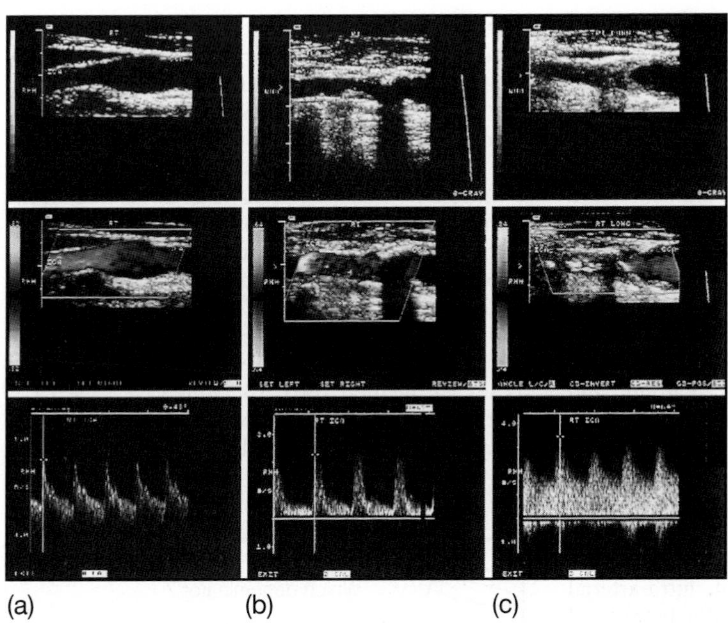

(a) (b) (c)

Figure 16.8 • Grey-scale images and corresponding colour flow images and Doppler waveforms from **(a)** normal internal carotid artery, **(b)** 50% stenosis of the internal carotid artery (note acoustic shadowing due to calcified plaque) and **(c)** 90% stenosis of the internal carotid artery (note increased flow velocity and turbulence).

Table 16.2 • Correlative duplex and angiographic criteria

Stenosis (%)	Criteria	Accuracy (%)	Sensitivity (%)	Specificity (%)	PPV (%)	NPV (%)
30+	PSV >120*	89	77	98	96	86
50+	PSV >130	97	97	97	93	99
	PSV >125, EDV <140	89	96	85	81	97
70+	PSV >210	93	89	94	75	78
	PSV >265	86	90	85	73	95
	PSV >270	88	96	86		
	PSV >325	88	83	91	80	92
	EDV >100	80	77	85	89	96
	EDV >110	93	91	93		
	PSV >210, EDV >100	95	81	98	89	70
	PSV >270, EDV >110	93	96	91		
	ICA:CCA PSV ratio <4		50			
	ICA:CCA PSV ratio >4	88	91	87	76	96

*PSV and EDV values are cm/s.
CCA, common carotid artery; EDV, end-diastolic velocity; ICA, internal carotid artery; NPV, negative predictive value; PPV, positive predictive value; PSV, peak systolic velocity.
Data from Faught et al.,[31] Moneta et al.[32] and Neale et al.[33]

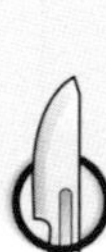

This is because secondary analyses of the ECST and NASCET databases indicate that while carotid endarterectomy confers a 26% absolute risk reduction (ARR) in stroke at 1 year in a symptomatic patient with 90–94% stenosis and no string sign, the equivalent ARR reduction in patients with subocclusion/string sign is only 4%.[36,37]

Duplex is also the only currently available method for evaluating plaque morphology. The simple Gray-Weale classification[38] ascribes plaques to subgroups according to whether they are echolucent (type 1), predominantly echolucent (type 2), predominantly echogenic (type 3) or echogenic (type 4). Unfortunately, correlation with histology and clinical risk remains variable[39] and newer methods such as automated plaque evaluation may prove more reliable in the future.[40]

Angiographic assessment

Angiographic assessment of the extracranial carotid arteries is now almost universally performed using digital subtraction techniques (see **Fig. 16.1**). The extracranial cerebral arteries are conventionally approached via a percutaneous femoral puncture under local anaesthesia and then selectively cannulated after preliminary arch views have identified their origins and basic anatomy and excluded common origins, etc. Images are obtained in at least two planes, followed by biplanar imaging of the intracranial circulation. The advantages of DSA include high contrast resolution, instantaneous acquisition, retrieval of real-time images, use of less contrast agent and avoidance of the need for selective catheterisation. In general, intra-arterial DSA is preferable to intravenous DSA because of the poor image quality associated with the latter.

However, carotid angiography is invasive and carries a small but important risk of stroke.[41–45] The risk varies according to the indication and disease severity. When all patients undergoing cerebral angiography are considered, 0.5% will suffer neurological complications (0.09% permanent, 0.45% temporary). This increases to 3.7% if only symptomatic patients are considered (0.5–3.2% temporary, 0.3–1.6% permanent). However, if duplex is used to screen out symptomatic patients with an ICA stenosis of less than 50%, the angiographic risk increases to 5% transient and 4% permanent.[45] Awareness of the risk of stroke during angiography has led to revisions in technique. Stroke is probably caused by the manipulation of catheters within a diseased aortic arch or carotid arteries. With the significant improvement in imaging modalities, the assessment of carotid disease is now commonly undertaken using only a pigtail catheter in the aorta (arch angiography) so as to avoid selective catheterisation. Accordingly, more recently published series suggest that the risk of stroke following angiography may now be as low as 0.5%.[46]

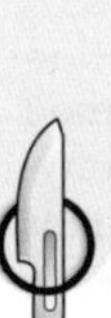

The risk of neurological complications decreases with seniority and experience and increases with the degree of stenosis[45] and in patients presenting with stroke/cerebral infarction. It should be borne in mind that angiographic stroke accounted for more than 50% of the perioperative surgical complications in the Asymptomatic Carotid Atherosclerosis Study (ACAS).[47]

There are currently two controversies concerning carotid angiography. The first relates to the optimal method for determining the degree of stenosis, whereas the second concerns observer variability. There are currently three methods of determining the degree of stenosis, each measuring the luminal diameter at the point of maximum stenosis (**Fig. 16.9**). In the ECST method, the denominator is the estimated normal arterial diameter at the level of the stenosis. In the NASCET method, the denominator is the diameter of a segment of disease-free ICA above the stenosis. The third method uses a segment of disease-free proximal CCA as the denominator.[47] Stenoses measured using the ECST method generate higher grades than those generated using the NASCET method (**Box 16.3**); however, the CCA method is probably the most reproducible.[48] With regard to observer variability in the diagnosis of

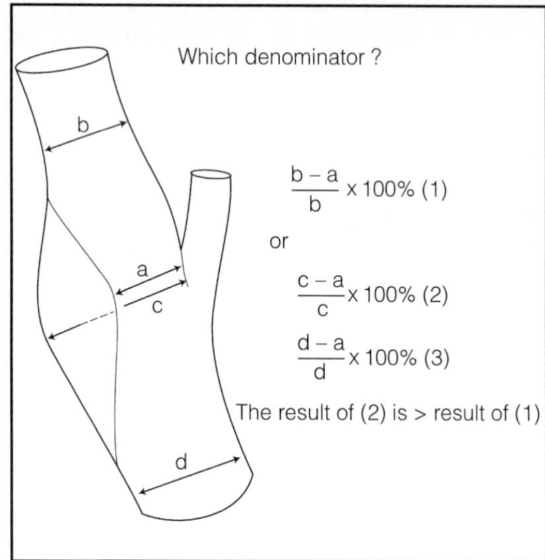

Figure 16.9 • Degree of internal carotid artery stenosis as measured by NASCET method (1), ECST method (2) and common carotid artery method (3).

Box 16.3 • Carotid stenoses: correlation between measurements using the ECST and NASCET methods

NASCET stenosis (%)	ECST stenosis (%)
30	65
40	70
50	75
60	80
70	85
80	90
90	95

ICA stenosis, Rothwell et al.[48] demonstrated intraobserver agreements of 96% for stenoses greater than 0%, 90% for stenoses over 50%, and 97% for total occlusion. Interobserver agreement was 93%, 85% and 97% for the same arteriograms and disease severity subgroups, respectively. However, as soon as the stenosis groups are subdivided further, the level of agreement deteriorates so that for diagnostic groups of 0%, 1–9%, 10–49%, 50–99% and 100%, intraobserver agreement falls to 83% whereas interobserver agreement falls to 75%.

MRA and CT angiography

MRA offers an attractive alternative to catheter-based studies because it is non-invasive and does not involve potentially nephrotoxic iodine-based contrast agents or the use of ionising radiation. The arteries are visualised either by using blood flow as the contrast agent (typically the 'time-of-flight' technique) or by introducing gadolinium intravenously (gadolinium MRA). Time of flight requires that the blood flow is at 90° to the imaging plane and these techniques are therefore usually limited to the neck. Gadolinium MRA is not so dependent on the orientation of the vessel in the imaging plane and therefore the field of view can be extended to the arch of aorta and intracranial vessels.

Although many of the studies comparing MRA with catheter angiography are of small size or poor construction, a few are worthy of mention. One recent study compared 71 carotid bifurcations in 39 symptomatic patients and compared the result with ultrasound and DSA.[49] For the detection of surgical lesions, gadolinium MRA was found to have a sensitivity of 95% and a specificity of 79%, with 10% false-positive and 2.5% false-negative rates. Ultrasound had similar accuracy. However, if ultrasound and gadolinium MRA were concordant (80% of cases), then all 70% stenoses were correctly identified and there were only 8.4% false-positive results. These false positives were 60–65% stenoses, which may well be worthy of treatment. A second study in 50 patients found that MRA misclassified 24% of surgically amenable lesions (ultrasound misclassified 36%), but when MRA and ultrasound were concordant (48% of lesions) there was 100% sensitivity and only 17% of lesions were misclassified.[50] No advantage was found for gadolinium MRA over non-contrast MRA. If MRA is to be used to non-invasively image the carotid arteries, current data would suggest that this is best done in conjunction with ultrasound. There are no studies describing the accuracy of MRA in assessing arch disease.

Multislice CT angiography permits the rapid acquisition of large amounts of cross-sectional data that can be reformatted in any plane. Contrast-enhanced multislice CT is used routinely to assess aneurysm but very few studies have assessed its use in carotid disease. A recent publication has suggested that CT angiography was unreliable in differentiating low-grade and high-grade stenoses of the carotid bifurcation.[51]

MANAGEMENT

'Best medical management'

All patients with extracranial cerebrovascular disease benefit from optimisation of risk factors, antiplatelet therapy and the exclusion of important comorbidity. Everyone should undergo chest radiography and ECG to exclude occult cardiac pathology, and baseline blood tests to exclude diabetes, arteritis, polycythaemia, anaemia, thrombocytosis, sickle cell disease and hyperlipidaemia.

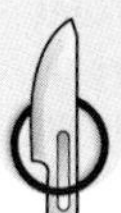

Angina therapy must be optimised, as the principal cause of late death is cardiac. Atrial fibrillation must be treated appropriately. Blood pressure should be maintained below 160/90 mmHg, although some would reasonably argue that 140/85 mmHg is a better target. Systematic overviews of published trials indicate that reducing the diastolic blood pressure by 5 mmHg lowers the relative risk of stroke by 35%, while the relative risk of myocardial infarction will fall by 25%.[52] However, evidence suggests that only 60% of patients with known hypertension will be receiving treatment prior to suffering their first stroke and only half of these will have a documented diastolic blood pressure below 90 mmHg.[53] Two studies (HOPE and PROGRESS) have evaluated the role of angiotensin-converting enzyme (ACE) inhibitors in reducing cardiovascular risk.[54,55]

PROGRESS randomised 6105 patients with a past history of stroke/TIA to 4 mg perindopril versus placebo. Perindopril conferred a relative risk reduction (RRR) of 28% in stroke at 4 years with no difference in benefit between hypertensive and non-hypertensive individuals.[54] HOPE randomised 9297 patients with 'vascular disease' but no impaired ejection fraction or heart failure to 10 mg ramipril versus placebo. Ramipril conferred a 22% reduction in any major vascular event and a 32% RRR in stroke.[55] At present there is no consensus among stroke physicians as to whether all patients with stroke/TIA should receive ACE inhibition. However, it should be considered as a new component of 'best medical therapy'. The most interesting observation from these studies was that clinical benefit was probably unrelated to blood pressure reduction, which was relatively modest in the two studies.

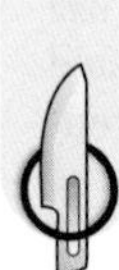

In the past, statin therapy was reserved for patients with symptomatic cerebral *and* coronary artery disease. However, publication of the British Heart Protection Study[56] has clearly shown that any patient presenting with a stroke or TIA benefits from statin therapy.

Table 16.3 summarises the principal results from this study, which randomised more than 20 000 patients with angina, stroke/TIA, diabetes or claudication to receive either 40 mg simvastatin or placebo daily. Note that patients randomised to statin therapy had an average 25% RRR in any major coronary event, any stroke and the need for revascularisation at 5 years. This significant benefit was irrespective of age, gender or presenting cholesterol level. The latter observation is of particular interest as it suggests that simvastatin's mode of action is probably not just cholesterol lowering but may be more specifically related to its ability to inhibit matrix metalloproteinases and so stabilise the plaque.

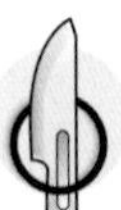

Aspirin is currently the first-line antiplatelet agent and meta-analyses suggest that it will reduce the long-term risk of stroke by 25%.[57]

However, there remains controversy regarding the optimal dose and the role of newer alternatives. The NASCET study suggested that patients receiving high-dose aspirin (650–1300 mg) had a lower perioperative risk than patients taking 0–325 mg aspirin daily.[22] This was an unplanned non-randomised analysis, and a randomised trial of 2849 patients undergoing carotid endarterectomy (CEA) subsequently showed that the risks of stroke, myocardial infarction and death within 30 days and 90 days of CEA were lower in patients receiving 80–325 mg as opposed to 650–1300 mg.[58] This would therefore suggest greater evidence for low-dose aspirin, while reducing the incidence of adverse effects associated with larger doses.

Dipyridamole, ticlopidine and clopidogrel are ADP inhibitors (aspirin is a cyclooxygenase pathway inhibitor).

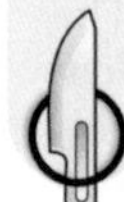

Although dipyridamole is a weak ADP inhibitor, randomised trials suggest that the combination of aspirin plus dipyridamole confers a significant reduction in late stroke risk as compared with either agent alone.[59] The latest NICE guidelines recommend aspirin and dipyridamole therapy in patients with stroke/TIA. Ticlopidine is a more potent ADP inhibitor but is limited by adverse effects including neutropenia, which requires careful haematological monitoring. Clopidogrel has been shown to significantly reduce the risk of ischaemic stroke, myocardial infarction or vascular death as compared with aspirin therapy alone (ARR 0.51%, RRR 8.7%, $P = 0.043$) in a randomised trial comprising 19 000 patients.[60]

However, the risk of ischaemic stroke alone was not reduced and clopidogrel has not been adopted into widespread clinical practice because of its significant cost. However, it is the second-line agent in patients who are unable to take aspirin.

Symptomatic carotid artery disease

CEA was introduced in 1954 by Eastcott et al.[61] and as awareness of the relationship between extracranial carotid disease and ischaemic stroke developed, the annual number of operations performed worldwide increased dramatically. However, by the early 1980s there was increasing awareness of the paradox that the very operation

Table 16.3 • Summary of findings from the British Heart Protection Study on the role of statin therapy in reducing cardiovascular events

	Simvastatin* **(*N* = 10 269)**	**Placebo (*N* = 10 267)**	**5-year ARR (%)**	**5-year RRR (%)**
Stroke	444 (4.3%)	585 (5.7%)	1.4	24.6
Major coronary event	898 (8.7%)	1212 (11.8%)	3.1	26.3
Revascularisation	939 (9.1%)	1205 (11.7%)	2.6	22.2
Any major vascular event	2033 (19.8%)	2585 (25.2%)	5.4	24.2

*Patients randomised to 40 mg simvastatin daily. Follow-up period 5 years.
ARR, absolute risk reduction; RRR, relative risk reduction.
From Heart Protection Study Collaborative Group. MRC/BHF Heart Protection Study of cholesterol lowering with simvastatin in 20536 high-risk individuals: a randomised placebo controlled trial. Elsevier (The Lancet 2002; 360:7–22), with permission.

that was undertaken to prevent stroke in the long term could itself cause a stroke in the perioperative period in a small but significant number of patients. Concern grew sufficiently[62,63] that two international trials (ECST and NASCET) were commenced. The question to be answered was simple: does CEA plus best medical therapy confer any additional benefit in terms of long-term stroke reduction over and above that achieved by best medical therapy alone in patients with carotid territory symptoms and an appropriate mild (0–30%), moderate (31–69%) or severe (70–99%) carotid stenosis?

Table 16.4 summarises the 30-day operative risk for death, death and disabling stroke, and death and any stroke in the ECST and NASCET. In these studies, the surgeons were only allowed to participate after review of their preceding 'track record'. The operative mortality rate varied from 0.6 to 1.5%. The risk of death and/or disabling stroke at 30 days was 2.1–3.7%, whereas the risk of death and/or any stroke was 4.6–7.9%. **Table 16.5** summarises the long-term risk of ipsilateral stroke (including the perioperative risk) from ECST and NASCET. The apparent transatlantic discrepancies are explained by the differing methods of quantifying stenosis (see **Fig. 16.9** and **Box 16.3**).

The data suggest that CEA is not indicated in symptomatic patients with a stenosis of less than 70% (ECST) or less than 50% (NASCET). The only possible exception might be the patient with repeated cerebral ischaemic events despite optimal medical

Table 16.4 • The 30-day risk following carotid endarterectomy in the ECST and NASCET

	ECST			NASCET	
	<30% (*N* = 138)	30–69% (*N* = 913)	70–99% (*N* = 750)	30–69% (*N* = 1087)	70–99% (*N* = 328)
Operative mortality	1.5%	1.1%	0.9%	1.2%	0.6%
Death with or without disabling stroke	2.3%	3.8%	3.7%	2.8%	2.1%
Death with or without any stroke	4.6%	7.9%	7.5%	6.7%	5.8%

From Naylor AR, Rothwell PM, Bell PRF. Overview of the principal results and secondary analyses from the European and the North American randomised trials of carotid endarterectomy. Eur J Vasc Endovasc Surg 2003; 26:115–29, with permission[64].

Table 16.5 • Long-term incidence of ipsilateral stroke (including perioperative stroke or death) in ECST and NASCET

Stenosis	Surgical risk (%)	Medical risk (%)	ARR (%)	RRR (%)	NNT	Strokes prevented per 1000 CEAs
ECST						
<30%	9.8 at 5 years	3.9 at 5 years	–5.9	n/a	n/a	n/a
30–49%	10.2 at 5 years	8.2 at 5 years	–2.0	n/a	n/a	n/a
50–69%	15.0 at 5 years	12.1 at 5 years	–2.9	n/a	n/a	n/a
70–99%	10.5 at 5 years	19.0 at 5 years	+8.5	45	12	83 at 5 years
NASCET						
30–49%	14.9 at 5 years	18.7 at 5 years	+3.8	20	26	38 at 5 years
50–69%	15.7 at 3 years	22.2 at 3 years	+6.5	29	15	67 at 3 years
70–99%	8.9 at 3 years	28.3 at 3 years	+19.4	69	5	200 at 3 years

ARR, absolute risk reduction; CEA, carotid endarterectomy; n/a, not applicable; NNT, number of CEAs to prevent one ipsilateral stroke; RRR, relative risk reduction.
From Naylor AR, Rothwell PM, Bell PRF. Overview of the principal results and secondary analyses from the European and the North American randomised trials of carotid endarterectomy. Eur J Vasc Endovasc Surg 2003; 26:115–29, with permission[64].

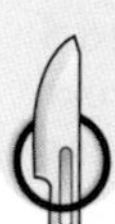

therapy. However, for patients with a severe (70–99%) stenosis, the conclusions of both ECST and NASCET were remarkably similar (**Table 16.5**). CEA plus best medical therapy conferred a sixfold to tenfold reduction in the long-term risk of stroke as compared with best medical therapy alone.[21,22] If all operative risk could be eliminated, CEA could reduce the long-term risk of stroke by 75%.

If one assumes that all surgeons carry out CEA with a 7.5% operative risk (based on the ECST data), then each surgeon must carry out 12 CEAs to prevent one long-term ipsilateral ischaemic stroke; this falls to nine if the operative risk is 2%.[64] However, the net effect on overall stroke reduction for the population at large would be less than 1%.[65] This compares with treating 67 patients with aspirin to prevent one stroke (3% overall stroke reduction), 44 patients with antihypertensive therapy (2% stroke reduction) and 30 with anticoagulants for atrial fibrillation (5% stroke reduction).

Following publication of the ECST and NASCET data, there has been growing concern that the results may not be generalisable into routine clinical practice. At present, 93% of CEAs in the USA are performed in non-NASCET hospitals, with a mortality that is significantly higher than in NASCET.[66,67] Accordingly, surgeons must quote their own results rather than simply justifying practice on the basis of the ECST and NASCET results.

ECST and NASCET have now published 48 papers over a 12-year period. Most of these have been secondary analyses that have increased our knowledge about the role of carotid surgery in patients with symptomatic

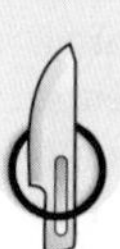

cerebral vascular disease.[64] One of the most important discoveries[68,69] has been the recognition that the benefit of CEA probably persists for longer than the conventional threshold of 6 months in patients with the more severe degrees of stenosis (**Fig. 16.10**).

For patients with a 70–79% stenosis who were treated medically, the annual stroke risk did not exceed 6% for each of the first 3 years. For those with an 80–89% stenosis, the annual stroke risk in medically treated patients was 11% in the first year and 6% in the second year. The respective risks for patients with a 90–99% stenosis were 18% and 14%. Thus it would seem appropriate to offer CEA in symptomatic patients with a 70–79% (ECST) stenosis for up to 6 months after the most recent event, while up to 12 months after the most recent event might now be permitted in patients with an 80–99% stenosis provided the operative risk remained below 7%.

However, it should be clear that approximately 70% of patients with a 70–99% stenosis will remain asymptomatic over 3 years on best medical therapy alone. A reanalysis of the ECST and NASCET data suggests that some patient subgroups are more likely to suffer a late stroke on best medical therapy.[64] These data should probably not be used to exclude patients from treatment, but rather to identify the very high-risk patient for expedited investigation and treatment (**Box 16.4**). Predictors of the greatest risk of stroke (only three CEAs or less required to prevent one stroke[64]) include:

- patients aged over 75 years (ARR conferred by CEA is 28% at 2 years);

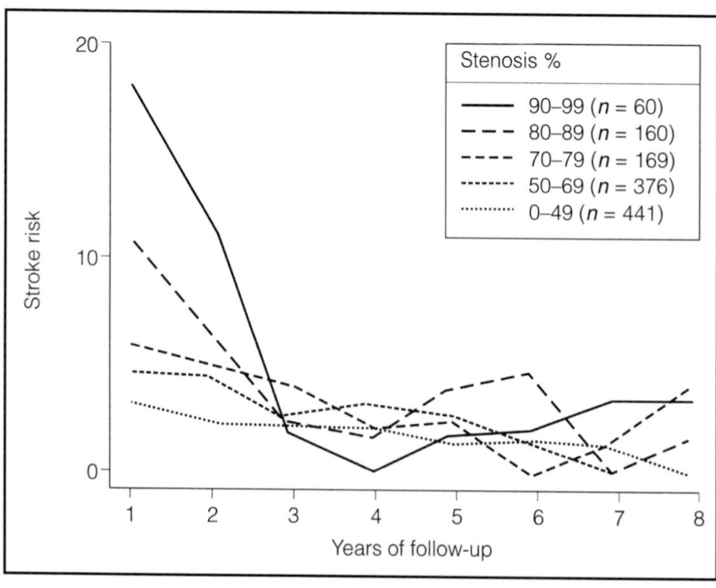

Figure 16.10 • Annual risk of stroke in medically treated patients in the ECST relative to the degree of stenosis. From European Carotid Surgery Trialists' Collaborative Group. Randomised trial of endarterectomy for recently symptomatic carotid stenosis: final results of the MRC European Carotid Surgery Trial (ECST). Elsevier (The Lancet 1998; 351:1379–87), with permission.

Box 16.4 • Which patients with symptomatic 70–99% stenoses are at higher risk of suffering a stroke on 'best medical therapy'?

Clinical predictors
Male versus female gender
Increasing age
Hemispheric vs. ocular symptoms
Cortical vs. lacunar stroke
Recurring cerebral events for more than 6 months
Symptoms within the last 2 months
Increasing comorbidity
Imaging predictors
Irregular vs. smooth plaques
Incrementally more severe stenoses apart from subocclusion/string sign
Contralateral occlusion
Tandem intracranial disease
No recruitment of intracranial collaterals

Adapted from Naylor AR, Rothwell PM, Bell PRF. Overview of the principal results and secondary analyses from the European and the North American randomised trials of carotid endarterectomy. Eur J Vasc Endovasc Surg 2003; 26:115–29, with permission[64].

- more than seven concurrent risk factors (ARR 30% at 2 years);
- recurrent events for more than 6 months (ARR 30% at 2 years);
- no intracranial collateral recruitment (ARR 31% at 2 years);
- greater than 85% stenosis with tandem intracranial disease (ARR 37% at 3 years);
- contralateral occlusion (ARR 47% at 2 years);
- 95% stenosis plus plaque ulceration (ARR 54% at 2 years).

Asymptomatic carotid artery disease

Between 5 and 10% of the population aged over 65 years will have an asymptomatic ICA stenosis of more than 50%,[70] increasing to 12% in those with peripheral vascular disease and 25% in patients with hypertension.[71,72] The management of asymptomatic carotid artery disease remains extremely controversial. Trials of intervention in asymptomatic disease include the Mayo Clinic Trial (MACE), the CASANOVA trial, the Veterans' Administration Trial, ACAS and, more recently, ACST.[47,73–76]

The MACE trial was prematurely stopped after recruiting 71 patients because of an excess risk of perioperative myocardial infarction in patients undergoing CEA.[73] CASANOVA excluded patients with a stenosis greater than 90% and was ultimately abandoned (despite showing some benefit in favour of surgery) after the steering committee concluded that at least 2000 patients would be required to complete the study.[74] The Veterans' Administration Trial ran for 9 years and excluded women, but did demonstrate a 50% RRR of stroke from 24.8% in the medical group to 12.8% in the surgical group.[75]

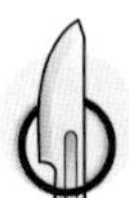

The principal results from the two most important studies (ACAS and ACST) are summarised in **Table 16.6**.

ACAS demonstrated a 53% RRR from 11.0% in medically treated patients to 5.1% in surgically treated patients, based on a projected life-table analysis to 5 years.[47] However, ACAS did attract considerable criticism. Concerns primarily related to the facts that the 30-day death/stroke rate was 2.3% (of which 1.2% was due to angiographic stroke) and not considered generalisable into routine practice, the 5-year risk was projected (median follow-up was only 2.7 years), there was no apparent benefit in women, CEA did not prevent disabling stroke,

Table 16.6 • Long-term risk of any stroke (including perioperative stroke or death) in ACAS and ACST*

Stenosis	Surgical risk (%)	Medical risk (%)	ARR (%)	RRR (%)	NNT	Strokes prevented per 1000 CEAs
ACAS 60–99%	5.1 at 5 years	11.0 at 5 years	+5.9	53	17	59 at 5 years
ACST 60–99%	6.4 at 5 years	11.7 at 5 years	+5.3	45	19	53 at 5 years

*Note that ACST and ACAS reported the long-term risk of any stroke or operative death as opposed to the ipsilateral stroke data for the symptomatic trials presented in **Table 16.5**.
ARR, absolute risk reduction; CEA, carotid endarterectomy; NNT, number of CEAs to prevent one ipsilateral stroke; RRR, relative risk reduction.

there was an *inverse* relationship between late stroke risk and stenosis severity in medically treated patients, and no data were forthcoming on the influence of concurrent risk factors.

ACST randomised 3120 patients with asymptomatic 60–99% carotid stenoses.[76] **Table 16.6** summarises the principal results. The 5-year risk of stroke in patients randomised to best medical therapy was 11.8%. This compares with 6.4% for patients randomised to immediate CEA (and includes the 2.8% operative risk). This equates to a 5.3% ARR at 5 years (RRR 45%). Further analysis shows that CEA was performed with a low operative risk (2.8%), maximum benefit was observed in patients aged under 75 years, CEA conferred the maximum benefit in males. There is still some debate about the magnitude of benefit in females. Significant benefit was observed irrespective of whether the stenosis was 60–79% or 80–99%. Most importantly, however, ACST showed that immediate CEA significantly reduced the risk of disabling/fatal stroke.

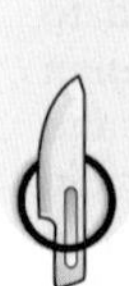

ACAS and ACST have therefore shown that CEA confers a small but significant benefit over deferred endarterectomy in asymptomatic patients. The key for the future will be to identify the high-risk patient subgroups that will gain most benefit so as to optimise resources and minimise unnecessary risk.[77]

However, critics of the use of CEA in asymptomatic disease should be aware of interesting data emerging from the Asymptomatic Carotid Stenosis Study Group.[78] This collaboration has analysed natural history data from patients recruited into the major symptomatic trials regarding the risk of ischaemic stroke ipsilateral to (i) the symptomatic severe stenosis and (ii) a contralateral asymptomatic severe carotid stenosis. At 3 years, the incidence of stroke was significantly higher ipsilateral to the symptomatic artery (21% vs. 8%). However, by 8 years there was no significant difference in stroke risk relative to the original symptom status of the artery (25% vs. 20%). This suggests that the risk of stroke ipsilateral to an asymptomatic carotid stenosis increases linearly and therefore CEA could certainly have an important role in younger patients.

CEA and synchronous coronary bypass

The role of prophylactic CEA in patients undergoing coronary artery bypass grafting (CABG) with an asymptomatic carotid stenosis remains an enduring controversy. However, there is less controversy regarding CABG patients who also have a symptomatic carotid stenosis, and many centres perform a combined CEA plus CABG in this situation.

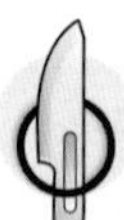

In a recent meta-analysis of 190 449 patients undergoing CABG,[79] the risk of stroke was 1.7% (95% CI 1.5–1.9).

Most (62%) occurred after more than 24 hours had elapsed and the overall mortality rate following post-CABG stroke was 23%. The meta-analysis was specifically interested in the role of carotid artery disease in the pathophysiology of post-CABG stroke and observed that three 'carotid' factors were significantly predictive: carotid bruit, a prior history of stroke or TIA, and the presence of a severe carotid stenosis or occlusion. The stroke risk in 4674 duplex-screened patients undergoing CABG was 1.8% in patients with no significant carotid disease (<50%), rising to 3.2% in patients with a unilateral 50–99% stenosis, 5.2% in those with bilateral 50–99% stenoses and 7–11% in patients with carotid occlusion.[79]

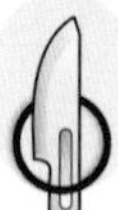

However, a number of factors emerged from the meta-analysis to suggest that carotid disease (alone) was not the principal cause of post-CABG stroke.

1. Most strokes occurred after 24 hours had elapsed. This is the exact opposite of what was observed in NASCET and ECST.[64]
2. Half of stroke victims had no ipsilateral carotid stenosis greater than 50%.
3. Although the risk of stroke increased with severity of the stenosis (see above), 85% of strokes occurring in the 4674 duplex-screened patients were not associated with any significant carotid artery disease.
4. At least 60% of stroke victims had areas of ischaemic infarction at autopsy or on CT with no ipsilateral carotid disease.

It is now generally held that while carotid disease is an important predictor for post-CABG stroke, the single most important cause is probably atheroembolism from the aortic arch.

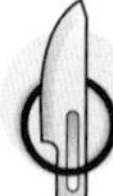

Two further meta-analyses have examined the results of staged and synchronous CEA in 8972 patients undergoing CABG.[80,81]

The principal findings are summarised in **Table 16.7**. In its simplest interpretation, mortality was highest following synchronous procedures, stroke was highest during reverse-staged procedures (CABG–CEA), while myocardial infarction was most prevalent after a staged CEA–CABG operation. However, when the cumulative cardiovascular risk was calculated, 11.5% (95% CI 8.9–14) of synchronous patients either died or suffered a non-fatal stroke or myocardial infarction. This compares

Table 16.7 • Operative risk following staged, reverse-staged or synchronous carotid endarterectomy (CEA) in patients undergoing coronary artery bypass grafting (CABG)

	N	Stroke (%)	Myocardial infarction (%)	Death (%)
Synchronous CEA and CABG	7863	4.6	3.6	4.6
CEA then staged CABG	917	2.7	6.5	3.9
CABG then staged CEA	302	6.3	0.9	2.0

Adapted from Naylor AR, Cuffe R, Rothwell PM, Bell PRF. A systematic review of outcomes following staged and synchronous carotid endarterectomy and coronary artery bypass. Eur J Vasc Endovasc Surg 2003; 25:380–9, with permission.

with 9.4% (95% CI 6.4–12.4) for patients undergoing either of the staged strategies. There was no statistically significant difference between the two groups. Clearly, both strategies carry a not insignificant cardiovascular risk.

Despite a plethora of publications in the world literature, the main problem in determining what advice to give patients remains an almost complete absence of high-quality natural history studies. This is because the few patients found to have severe carotid disease are not subjected to prophylactic CEA. Accordingly, most of the available conclusions have had to be made on a cohort with 50–99% stenoses, despite the majority under study probably having stenoses of only 50–70%.

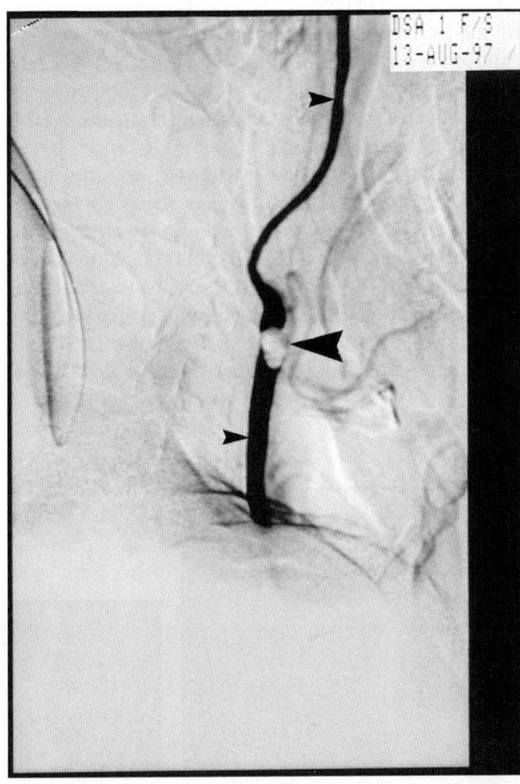

Figure 16.11 • Intra-arterial digital subtraction angiogram of large luminal thrombus (large arrow) overlying a distal common carotid stenosis in a patient with crescendo transient ischaemic attacks.

Emergency CEA

In the 1960s, emergency CEA for acute stroke was associated with major mortality and morbidity, mainly due to haemorrhagic transformation of ischaemic infarction.[82,83] This led not only to the abandonment of this strategy but also to the recommendation that any patient suffering a stroke should wait at least 6 weeks before undergoing CEA in order to allow the area of infarction to stabilise. At present, emergency CEA (i.e. immediate) should be reserved for patients who suffer a thrombotic stroke in the early postoperative period after CEA or following angiography/angioplasty. Urgent CEA (within 24 hours) is recommended in patients with stroke in evolution, stuttering hemiplegia or crescendo TIAs, especially if there is evidence of a critical or unstable carotid lesion (**Fig. 16.11**).

Early CEA (within 2–4 weeks) is being increasingly recommended in stroke patients who make a rapid recovery from their neurological deficit so as to reduce the 20% risk of recurrent stroke during the first 6-week period.[84] Although the latter strategy is not currently mainstream practice, evidence from a recent meta-analysis suggests that early CEA does not increase the operative risk.[85]

Extracranial–intracranial bypass

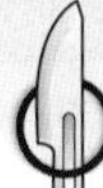

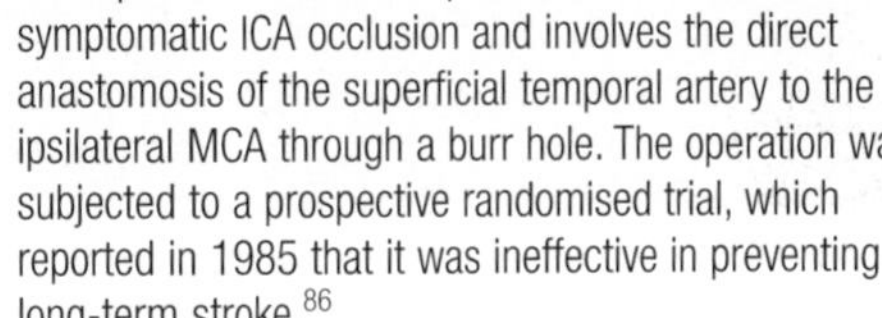

This operation was developed for the treatment of symptomatic ICA occlusion and involves the direct anastomosis of the superficial temporal artery to the ipsilateral MCA through a burr hole. The operation was subjected to a prospective randomised trial, which reported in 1985 that it was ineffective in preventing long-term stroke.[86]

However, the conclusions of this trial have been the subject of critical debate[87] and largely revolve around: (i) too broad entry criteria; (ii) worries about the methods of randomisation; (iii) the unusually large number of patients operated upon outwith the trial; and (iv) that no physiological variables (e.g. assessment of haemodynamic reserve) were employed to identify those at maximum risk. In short, the trial has virtually ended this operation and it is no longer covered by Medicare in the USA.

Vertebral artery reconstruction

The vertebrobasilar territory is affected in 15–25% of all ischaemic strokes but there have been no randomised trials similar to ECST or NASCET to guide optimal practice. In contrast to the primarily embolic aetiology of carotid territory stroke, vertebrobasilar events tend to be haemodynamic. In the UK, a policy of revascularisation for asymptomatic vertebral artery disease has never been considered normal practice. However, patients presenting with classical vertebrobasilar TIAs may be considered for surgery or angioplasty, although most vascular surgeons in the UK have little experience of these procedures. At the Leicester Royal Infirmary, only four reconstructions have been performed in the last 8 years for symptomatic vertebral artery disease (excluding treatment of patients with subclavian steal). The role of surgery in patients with 'non-hemispheric' symptoms (see earlier) remains controversial. However, if such symptoms were present and the patient's brain was reliant on a solitary diseased vertebral artery, the case for revascularisation becomes more compelling.

For patients with symptomatic lesions at the origin of the vertebral artery, surgical options include short vein bypass or transposition of the vertebral artery onto the CCA. However, angioplasty with or without stenting is now assuming an increasing role in this situation (**Fig. 16.12**). The latter may also have an important role in patients with more distal disease as surgical access to the upper two-thirds of the vertebral artery is difficult. An occlusion or severe stenosis at the origin of the subclavian artery may result in reversed flow down the ipsilateral vertebral artery to perfuse the arm (subclavian steal). Arm exercise may therefore result in vertebrobasilar ischaemia. The classical symptoms include forearm claudication, although coexistent vertebrobasilar symptoms are less common. In practice, we would only recommend intervention in patients with symptomatic lesions, especially the dominant arm, as both surgery and endovascular intervention carry a small risk of procedural stroke.

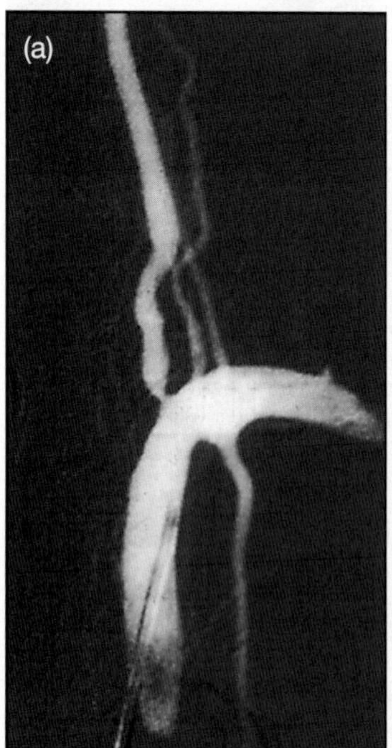

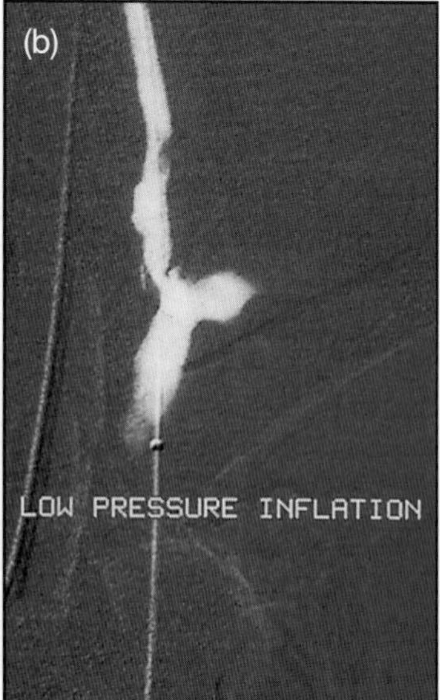

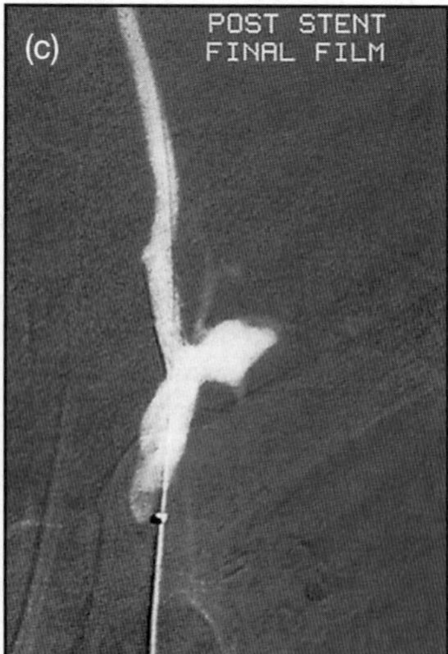

Figure 16.12 • Vertebral artery origin stenosis **(a)** treated by angioplasty and stenting. After angioplasty **(b)** there was a significant resistant stenosis treated by a Palmaz stent **(c)**.

CAROTID ENDARTERECTOMY

Anaesthesia

CEA can be performed under local or general anaesthesia. Local anaesthesia (superficial and deep cervical plexus blockade supplemented by local infiltration) has been used during CEA since the 1960s. CEA under regional anaesthesia is currently the only method for accurately predicting who needs a shunt, but it will not prevent complications due to thromboembolism (which is the principal cause of intraoperative stroke). Regional anaesthesia requires the patient to remain relatively still for long periods of time, swallowing makes fine dissection and reconstruction more complex, and urgent intubation is significantly more difficult.

In one of the few randomised trials there was no significant difference in mortality or neurological morbidity but there were significantly higher blood pressure and plasma noradrenaline (norepinephrine) levels when CEA was performed under local anaesthesia.[88] The advantages of general anaesthesia include patient compliance, reduced catecholamine levels and reduced cerebral metabolic requirements. The Cochrane Collaboration has recently performed a further meta-analysis of seven randomised studies (554 operations) and 41 non-randomised studies of CEA under regional anaesthesia (25 622 CEAs). The randomised trials showed no significant difference in the incidence of perioperative stroke, myocardial infarction or death, while the non-randomised trials showed significant reductions in stroke, myocardial infarction and pulmonary complications in patients receiving regional anaesthesia.[89]

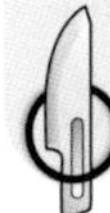

A further randomised trial is currently underway in the UK.

Surgical technique

CEA is usually performed under light general anaesthesia using loupe magnification with the extended head turned away from the side of operation and placed on a rubber ring. An incision is made over the anterior border of sternomastoid and dissection is continued down to the carotid bifurcation, which is exposed after division of the common facial vein. The carotid vessels are controlled with slings, although many surgeons prefer not to sling the ICA because of the potential for dislodging thrombus. Some surgeons infiltrate the carotid sinus with 1% lidocaine (lignocaine) to prevent reflex hypotension and bradycardia. Four randomised trials have addressed this question and none have found any evidence of benefit regarding this practice.[90]

The distal ICA must be mobilised 1 cm beyond the upper limit of the plaque and this can be facilitated by ligation and division of the small tethering vessels accompanying the hypoglossal nerve and/or division of digastric. If surgeons are worried about the need to proceed high into the neck, access can be facilitated preoperatively by nasolaryngeal intubation or temporomandibular subluxation although in reality this is rarely required. The latter manoeuvre has not been necessary in more than 1200 CEAs in Leicester. However, if the surgeon considers that this strategy may be needed, then maxillofacial colleagues must be contacted in advance of the procedure.

The principal cranial nerves (hypoglossal, vagus) must be identified and preserved. With high dissections, the glossopharyngeal nerve is at particular risk of injury. Any patient who has undergone a contralateral CEA or previous thyroidectomy must undergo a preoperative check of recurrent laryngeal and hypoglossal nerve function as bilateral injuries of either can be fatal.

Following systemic heparinisation (5000 units), soft clamps are applied to the distal ICA, CCA and ECA. A longitudinal arteriotomy is made from the distal CCA across the plaque and into the ICA beyond the stenosis. If a shunt is to be deployed it is inserted now (**Fig. 16.13**). The endarterectomy plane is entered using a Watson–Cheyne dissector and it is conventional to divide the plaque first at the CCA aspect and then carefully mobilise it up into the ICA where it is cut transversely using micro-scissors to avoid leaving a flap. The distal aspect usually feathers off smoothly but can be tacked down with interrupted fine prolene sutures. There is no systematic evidence that intimal tacking sutures influence outcome. All loose intimal fragments are removed in a radial, as opposed to axial, direction. An alternative technique to that described is the 'eversion' endarterectomy method. Here the origin of the ICA is transected and reimplanted after eversion endarterectomy of the ICA and conventional endarterectomy of the CCA and ECA.

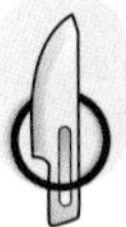

However, there is no evidence from systematic reviews that eversion endarterectomy confers any benefit over traditional endarterectomy provided the arteriotomy is closed with a patch.[90]

The arteriotomy is closed primarily with a running suture (6/0 prolene) or as a patch angioplasty (prosthetic, long saphenous vein). Flow is restored first up the ECA and then the ICA. After the procedure, the patient is woken and checked for any neurological deficit before being transferred to theatre recovery or the high-dependency unit for further monitoring.

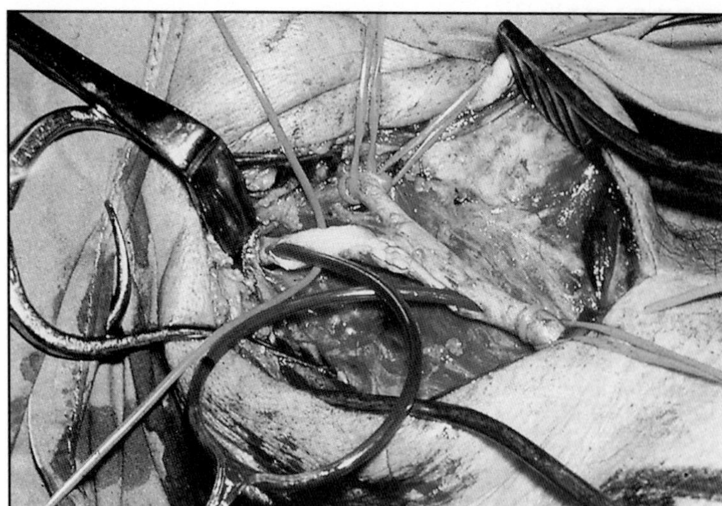

Figure 16.13 • Carotid endarterectomy. The carotid bifurcation has been exposed and the vessels controlled with slings. A longitudinal arteriotomy has been performed and the stenosis at the origin of the internal carotid artery can be seen. A Pruitt–Inahara shunt has been inserted to maintain cerebral perfusion during the procedure.

There is no evidence that reversal of anticoagulation with protamine is beneficial and it may increase the risk of postoperative thrombosis.[90] However, all patients should receive long-term antiplatelet therapy.[91] There is no evidence that anticoagulation reduces the risk of restenosis or late stroke.

PATCH ANGIOPLASTY OR PRIMARY CLOSURE?

The rationale underlying patch angioplasty is that it will reduce the risk of early postoperative thrombosis and late restenosis. Early carotid thrombosis complicates 2–3% of CEAs and is a major cause of perioperative stroke. Recurrent stenosis affects about 13% of patients but very few develop symptoms.[92] Critics of patching argue that it increases clamp or shunt times by 15–20 minutes, that a vein patch is susceptible to rupture, while a prosthetic patch is susceptible to infection.

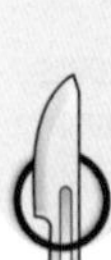

Seven randomised trials have been performed and the Cochrane Collaboration has performed an overview of the available data.[93] The meta-analysis suggests that a policy of routine patching is preferable to a policy of routine primary closure, with a threefold reduction in the risk of perioperative stroke, thrombosis and late restenosis.

If applied to future carotid practice, routine patching could prevent 28 strokes per 1000 operations within 30 days of surgery and a further 28 strokes during follow-up. No randomised trial has compared routine patching with selective patching and there is no systematic evidence that patch type (PTFE, Dacron, vein) influences stroke rate, mortality or arterial restenosis.[94]

SHUNT DEPLOYMENT

A temporary shunt may be used never, selectively or routinely and again there is no consensus among surgeons. Supporters of shunting argue that its routine use allows time for a more thorough endarterectomy, facilitates safer training of young surgeons and ensures familiarity with shunt insertion, which is useful when a difficult situation arises. Those who do not use shunts claim that there is an increased risk of intimal injury and embolisation and that the shunt physically interferes with the procedure. As a consequence, many deploy a shunt selectively on the basis of intraoperative monitoring.

The most commonly used shunts are the Javid shunt (which permits higher flow rates) and the double-ballooned Pruitt–Inahara shunt, which is more flexible.[95]

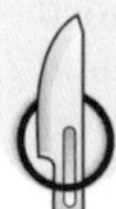

Few randomised studies are available to guide surgeons but a recent overview of the available data suggests that routine shunting does not alter outcome.[96] However, the Cochrane meta-analysis must be interpreted in the knowledge that in one of the biggest contributory studies, patients randomised to no shunt were then shunted if EEG abnormalities occurred during clamping.[97]

Perioperative monitoring

The aim of monitoring is to correct and/or prevent cerebral ischaemia before permanent neurological injury occurs. The simplest assessment of intracranial flow is a subjective assessment of ICA backflow or ICA stump pressure, but this may bear little relation to intracranial blood flow in the presence of circle of Willis anomalies or stenoses.

(a)

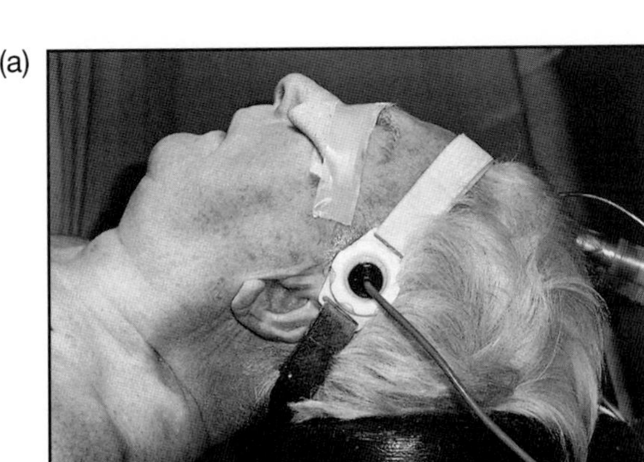

(b)

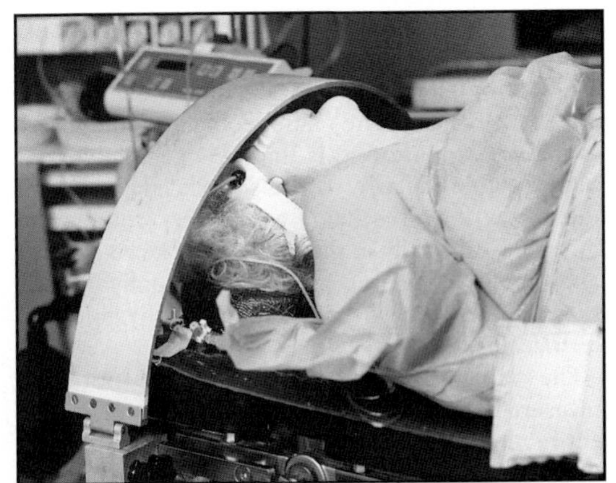

Figure 16.14 • Theatre set-up for transcranial Doppler monitoring. The 2-MHz probe is focused onto the middle cerebral artery and held in place with an elasticated band **(a)**. The probe is then protected from dislodgement by a semicircular metal head guard **(b)**.

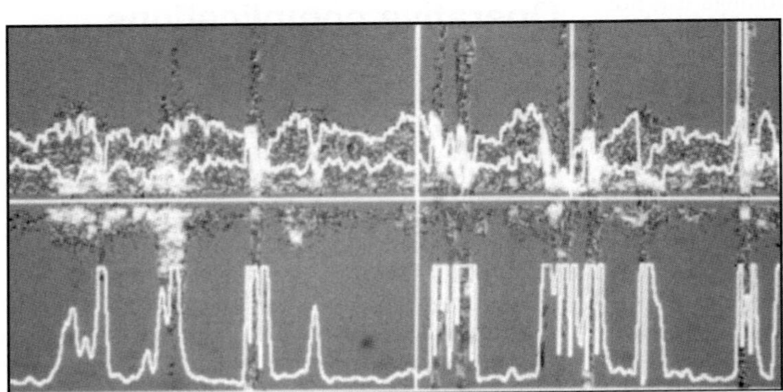

Figure 16.15 • Transcranial Doppler signal from the middle cerebral artery showing multiple embolic signals at the time of mobilising the internal carotid artery. A cluster of emboli have been detected, suggesting the presence of an unstable carotid plaque with friable overlying thrombus. The surgeon can either alter the dissection technique or clamp the internal carotid artery early.

Transcranial Doppler (TCD) is probably the most versatile and practical of the available monitoring methods (**Fig. 16.14**) and uses a low-frequency (2 MHz) pulsed-wave ultrasound beam directed through the thin temporal bone. This permits insonation of the basal cerebral vessels comprising the circle of Willis and especially the MCA, which receives 80% of ICA inflow. The quality of the signal depends on the thickness of the cranium and an inaccessible window may be present in about 10% of patients. TCD can anticipate the requirement and urgency for shunting, can diagnose intraoperative embolisation (**Fig. 16.15**) thereby permitting early ICA clamping in patients with unstable plaques,[39] and is invaluable in ensuring optimal shunt function.

Cerebral perfusion can be measured after bolus administration of intra-arterial xenon using the washout method, although this technique is rarely employed in the UK. An alternative is near-infrared spectroscopy, which depends on the absorption of near-infrared light, transmitted through the skull into the cerebral hemispheres, by the chromophores oxyhaemoglobin, deoxyhaemoglobin and oxidised cytochrome. Changes in cerebral haemoglobin oxygenation have been shown to correlate with MCA flow velocity;[98] however, the main disadvantages of near-infrared spectroscopy are extracranial contamination (despite subtraction methods) and cost.

Neurological activity can be evaluated directly by performing CEA under local anaesthesia (see earlier). This is a very sensitive method of detecting clamp ischaemia and is the 'gold standard' for determining who needs a shunt. However, it will not prevent thromboembolic complications. Neurological activity can be evaluated indirectly by EEG or sensory-evoked potential measurement. The principle underlying use of the EEG is that once perfusion falls below 18 mL/100 g brain per minute there is loss of high-frequency activity, whereas below 15 mL/100 g brain per minute the EEG becomes isoelectric.[99] However, one must remain aware that just because the EEG is flat does not mean that a neurological injury is inevitable, as this only tends to occur once perfusion falls below

10 mL/100 g brain per minute.[99] Thus loss of EEG function is used as a warning that insertion of a shunt or elevation of systemic blood pressure may be beneficial. The main problem with conventional EEG monitoring is that it is generally oversensitive (particularly to the superficial surface of the cortex) and the data can be very complex to interpret (especially in the presence of a pre-existing abnormality). Centres using EEG usually require the support of experienced neurophysiological technicians.

The advantage of sensory-evoked potential measurement is that it reflects the function of the entire afferent pathway from the peripheral nerves (usually the median nerve) to the somatosensory cortex. Ischaemia is associated with reduction in the amplitude of the primary cortical wave and prolongation of central conduction time. As with EEG, this information can then be used to modify surgical and anaesthetic practice, although it is not widely employed in the UK.[100]

Quality control assessment

Although most vascular surgeons undertake some form of quality-control assessment following peripheral reconstruction, the same does not apply after CEA. This is despite the fact that most neurological complications follow inadvertent technical error. The role of quality control is to identify incomplete endarterectomy, distal intimal flaps, adherent luminal thrombus, residual stenoses and wall irregularities such as intimal corrugations or kinking. However, the most important is exclusion of residual thrombus.[101] Current quality-control techniques include on-line TCD, on-table angiography, B-mode or colour duplex ultrasound, continuous-wave Doppler and angioscopy. On-line TCD ensures optimal shunt function and is the only method capable of diagnosing on-table carotid thrombosis and early postoperative occlusion. Angiography (which must be biplanar) has demonstrated that up to 26% of patients may have some degree of technical abnormality, although not all needed correction.[102] The principal advantage of angiography is that it provides easily interpretable anatomical data but requires ionising radiation and can only be performed after restoration of flow (i.e. any thrombus could be swept distally). Black and white B-mode probes tend to be too big and the image is compromised by difficulties in imaging through prosthetic patches and air in the deeper tissue planes. However, the newer colour duplex probes are smaller and more accessible because of the development of L-shaped probes, but inevitably the equipment is required in theatre (with a technician) when it might be needed elsewhere. Continuous-wave Doppler is occasionally used as a completion assessment on the basis that a residual stenosis will cause spectral abnormalities and velocities in excess of 125 cm/s.[103]

At the Leicester Royal Infirmary we now have experience of completion angioscopy in over 1200 patients. At the outset we used a multifibre angioscope but replaced this with a hysteroscope, as the former was too fragile. The principal advantage over all other quality-control techniques is that it can be performed prior to restoration of flow. Its main role is to identify the 4% with residual luminal thrombus (derived from bleeding from the vasa vasorum onto the highly thrombogenic endarterectomy surface) and the 3% with large intimal flaps. Since introducing this technique, our intraoperative stroke rate has fallen from 4% to 0.2% and it has contributed significantly towards an overall 60% reduction in the 30-day risk in our institution.[101]

Operative complications

MEDICAL PROBLEMS

In NASCET, 10% of the surgical patients suffered a medical complication within 30 days of operation. This compares with 3.2% of patients randomised to best medical therapy in the same time period. Of the 142 medical complications in CEA patients in NASCET,[104] 70% were of short duration and hospital stay was only prolonged in 38 patients (2.7%). Only five surgical patients (0.3%) suffered severe medical complications. Cardiovascular problems predominated, including myocardial infarction (1%), arrhythmia (1.5%), congestive cardiac failure (1%), severe hypertension (1.4%) and severe hypotension (1.7%). In the ECST, only four surgical patients suffered a myocardial infarction in the perioperative period and two suffered a pulmonary embolism.[64]

CRANIAL NERVE INJURIES

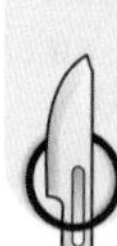

The potential for cranial nerve injury is rarely discussed before CEA but is an important source of perioperative morbidity. In a detailed review, Forsell et al.[105] have shown that up to 50% of patients will suffer some degree of cranial nerve injury and in up to 2.5% the injury is bilateral.

In the NASCET, the incidence of injury to the mandibular branch of the facial nerve was 2.2%, to the vagus 2.5%, to the spinal accessory nerve 0.2% and to the hypoglossal 3.7%. The overall rate of cranial nerve injury was 8.6%,[106] although 92% of these were classed as minor. Interestingly, there was no reference to any glossopharyngeal nerve injury, which is more common following high carotid dissections. It should be noted that these were clinical diagnoses. Studies using indirect laryngoscopy or video fluoroscopy reveal a much higher incidence of occult cranial nerve injury.[105] In the ECST, 6.4% of CEA patients suffered a cranial nerve injury.[64] In only nine patients was the injury permanent.

WOUND COMPLICATIONS

In the NASCET, a total of 132 patients (9.3%) developed wound complications following CEA, of which 76 (58%) were deemed minor, 52 (39%) moderate, while only 4 (3%) were classed as severe.[106] Early vein patch rupture occurs after less than 1% of CEAs and is more common if the vein is harvested from the ankle. The incidence of rupture from saphenous vein taken from the groin is very rare. Late patch infection complicates less than 1% of all endarterectomies and can be very difficult to manage.[107] The basic rule should be that no abscess overlying a CEA wound is incised before the patient has been seen by a vascular surgeon. If an infection is suspected, the CCA must be controlled well below the original incision. The prosthetic patch should be removed and replaced, where possible with a saphenous vein patch. If this is not possible, a reversed vein graft should be considered. Distal ligation should only be considered if some form of monitoring (e.g. TCD) suggests that collateral flow is satisfactory.[107]

PERIOPERATIVE STROKE

Neurological events are classed as intraoperative if the patient recovers from anaesthesia with a new deficit and postoperative if the event occurs some time later. In historical series, intraoperative stroke predominated[108] and was more likely to affect patients with a combination of cerebral infarction and partial or total haemodynamic compromise.[109] This suggests that high-risk patients are more vulnerable to otherwise minor changes in perfusion pressure or emboli, so that the margin for technical error is reduced or possibly non-existent.[100] Following introduction of a policy of completion angioscopy, the rate of intraoperative stroke in Leicester fell from 4% to 0.2% in our series of 1200 CEAs.

The commonest causes of postoperative stroke are ICA thrombosis (especially in the first six postoperative hours) and haemorrhage. Evidence suggests that most thromboembolic events follow inadvertent technical error and steps should be taken to identify these intraoperatively. Intracerebral haemorrhage and the hyperperfusion syndrome complicate 1–2% of CEAs and are more common in patients with severe bilateral extracranial disease in association with impaired cerebral vascular reserve, defective autoregulation and poor collateral flow patterns.[110] It is important that emergency medical units recognise the importance of early treatment in the CEA patient who presents with seizures, usually 5–7 days after surgery. These patients have a high risk of suffering intracranial haemorrhage and the mainstay of management is control of seizures and aggressive control of blood pressure.[111]

The strategy for managing perioperative events depends on (i) timing (intraoperative or postoperative), (ii) whether it is due to thrombosis, embolism or haemorrhage and (iii) the severity of the neurological deficit. In general, the more extensive the deficit, the more likely it is that the ICA or MCA has occluded.[20] For those without access to TCD ultrasound and duplex, the surgeon will have to assume that any neurological deficit occurring following recovery from anaesthesia or in the first 24 hours is thromboembolic. In this situation, the patient will have to be re-explored to exclude technical error and ongoing embolisation. Although re-exploration will not benefit patients with focal embolism or haemodynamic stroke, this cannot currently be avoided.

However, for those with access to TCD and duplex, decision-making can be made easier. The immediate priority is to identify patients with ICA thrombosis, as they require immediate exploration. Provided flow is restored within 1 hour, good neurological recovery can be expected. The pathognomonic TCD features of ICA occlusion include flow reversal in the ipsilateral anterior cerebral artery, enhanced flow in the ipsilateral posterior cerebral artery and, most importantly, flow velocities in the ipsilateral MCA that mimic those observed during carotid clamping. However, it would be preferable to prevent a thrombosis from happening in the first place. Evidence from three continents has now conclusively shown that thrombosis is preceded by 1–2 hours of increasing embolisation, which can be diagnosed using TCD,[112–117] and that 50–60% of patients with sustained embolisation will progress to a thrombotic stroke.[112–118] At the Leicester Royal Infirmary, we administer dextran 40 to the 5% of patients with high rates of embolisation (>25 emboli in any 10-minute period). Since this protocol was implemented in October 1995, more than 900 CEAs have been performed and no patient has suffered a stroke due to carotid thrombosis. This represents a major change to previous practice, where 2–3% of patients suffered a stroke due to carotid thrombosis in the first six postoperative hours.

Long-term follow-up and restenosis

The final results from the ECST show that the average annual risk of late ipsilateral stroke after CEA is 1–2%.[68] The risk of stroke in the contralateral, non-operated ICA territory is 1.4% per annum.[119] Meta-analyses indicate that the average annual risk of recurrent stenosis (50–100%) is 1.5–4.5%,[120,121] although the risk is probably highest in the first 12 months.[121] Accordingly, a number of surgeons have recommended serial clinical and duplex ultrasound surveillance with the intention of performing a repeat CEA in patients with recurrent stenoses greater than 70%, particularly following publication of the ACAS data.[47] However, there is little if any evidence to support this practice. A recent review suggests that the risk of late ipsilateral stroke in patients with recurrent stenoses greater than 50% is about 2% per annum, falling to 1% per annum in those with no recurrent disease or a stenosis below 50%.[122] Moreover, 11–20% of treated patients will develop a second recurrent stenosis after either repeat CEA or carotid angioplasty.[122] In ACAS, the risk of late stroke was unrelated to the presence of a recurrent stenosis and only one patient (0.15%) suffered a stroke and had a severe recurrent stenosis.[123] Thus there seems to be little clinical or cost-based evidence for recommending a policy of long-term surveillance. Patients can be safely discharged at 6 weeks and told to report back should they develop any further symptoms. The only exception to this practice is patients who have undergone carotid vein bypass graft as they have a 20% chance of recurrent stenosis within 3 years.[124] Our policy would be to survey these patients with duplex and thereafter treat any severe recurrent lesions with angioplasty.

ENDOVASCULAR TREATMENT OF CAROTID DISEASE

Over the last 10 years, increasing attention has been given to the management of carotid disease using endovascular techniques (**Fig. 16.16a**). The techniques to manage occlusive disease are still evolving and the data are maturing. While there is some experience in managing carotid dissections and extracranial aneurysms, these techniques are simple extensions of those used elsewhere throughout the vascular tree. This section focuses particularly on the endovascular management of symptomatic carotid atherosclerosis.

Technique

All patients should already be on best medical therapy (see earlier) prior to intervention. All patients should be reviewed by a clinician experienced in

(a)

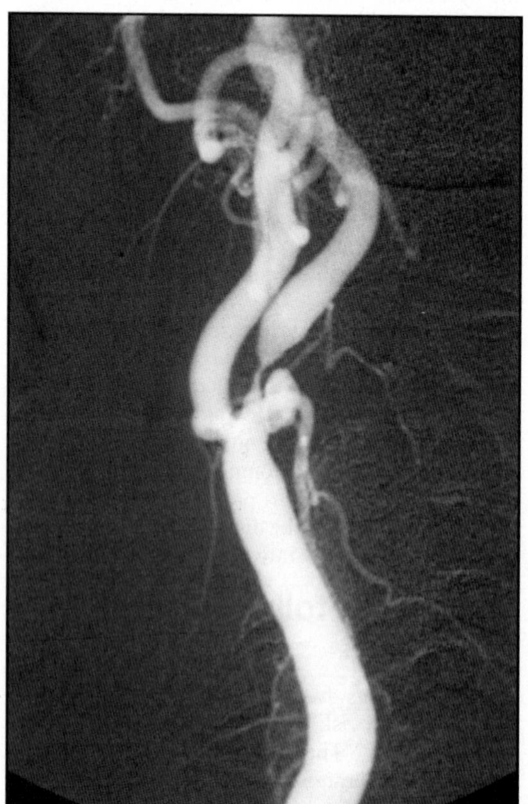

(b)

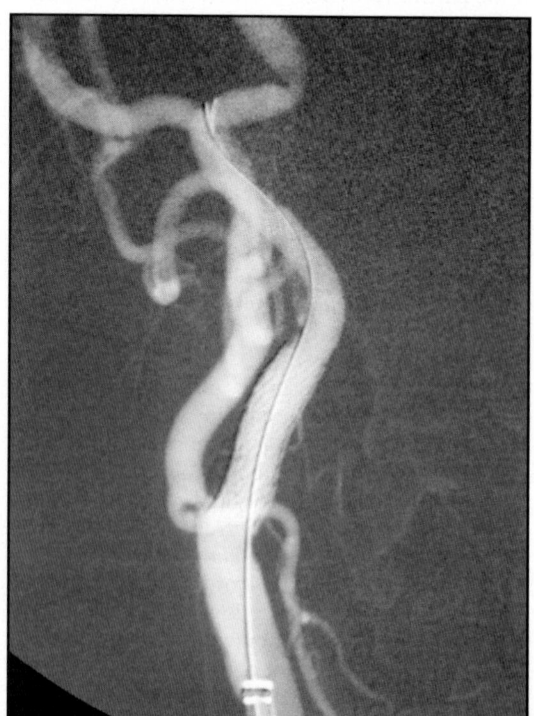

Figure 16.16 • Severe stenosis at the origin of the internal carotid artery **(a)** and following treatment with angioplasty and stenting **(b)**.

stroke medicine. At the Sheffield Vascular Institute, it is our practice, since MRA has not yet been validated, to routinely perform arch angiography on all patients on a separate occasion to the treatment episode so that arch origin disease and adverse anatomy can be excluded. This also allows patients to be offered either carotid artery stenting (CAS) or CEA on an informed basis through discussion with our surgical colleagues.

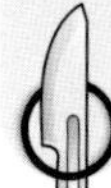

It is now routine practice in most units for dual antiplatelet therapy to be commenced prior to carotid stent placement. A randomised trial from the Sheffield unit[143] of aspirin plus clopidogrel versus aspirin plus 24-hour anticoagulation in patients undergoing CAS showed a significant and dramatic benefit in procedural adverse events and stent patency in favour of dual antiplatelet therapy. We would recommend the addition of clopidogrel 75 mg per day for 2 weeks prior to intervention, continuing for at least 4 weeks after stent placement.

The basic technique continues to undergo modification but basically is as follows.

- Femoral access is obtained in the usual manner. Direct carotid puncture has been advocated but probably involves a higher risk of puncture-site haematoma.
- Heparin 7500 units is administered, with repeated boluses to maintain an activated clotting time greater than 200 seconds.
- Selective catheterisation of the CCA using the usual catheter shapes (Headhunter 1, Sidewinder, Vitek).
- Placement of a stiff wire into the ECA.
- Over this stiff wire a suitable guiding catheter or long sheath is placed, with the tip 2–3 cm below the carotid bifurcation. The size of the guiding catheter or sheath is dependent on the diameter of the stent delivery system and currently we require a 6 Fr sheath or 8 Fr guiding catheter.
- The sizes of the internal and common carotid arteries are measured. The size of the ICA will determine the size of the protection device. As almost all stents are deployed from common to internal carotid artery, the size of the CCA will determine the diameter of the stent.
- Atropine (0.6–1.2 mg) or glycopyrrolate 0.6 mg is delivered into the CCA to block the carotid sinus baroreceptors.
- The ICA stenosis is crossed with the cerebral protection device (filter or occlusion balloon), which is then deployed. The lesion should be crossed only once and there should be no movement of the guidewire once the tip has been placed below the base of skull.
- Stent delivery systems are now down to 5 Fr. In a number of stenoses it may be possible to cross the lesion withought predilatation. However, the severity of the stenosis on a single plane can be deceptive and it is therefore our practice to predilate all lesions to 3 mm. Inflation times are necessarily short.
- The stent is delivered to the diseased segment.
- The stent is postdilated to ensure good apposition against the arterial wall and diseased segment. It is probably not necessary to aggressively dilate, and many practitioners now are happy to leave some residual stenosis rather than overdilate the lesion (**Fig. 16.16b**).
- A check arteriogram is performed to ensure there has been no cerebral embolisation and the system is then withdrawn.
- A closure device is used to close the femoral puncture.

If the reverse-flow type of cerebral protection is used, then this is deployed instead of the guiding catheter or long sheath and a conventional 014 wire is used to cross the lesion.

Case selection

Sensible case selection is an absolute requirement for safe practice. Contraindications to a carotid stent are an occluded ICA or visible thrombus. A difficult origin of the brachiocephalic artery from the ascending aorta or of the left CCA from the brachiocephalic artery may make selective catheterisation difficult or impossible. Because of problems with access, any severe tortuosity of the brachiocephalic artery or CCA is a relative contraindication to endovascular treatment. Tortuosity of the ICA above the stenosis may prevent use of a cerebral protection system other than reverse flow. This same tortuosity may be turned into a kink or occlusion by a stent. In all these situations, thought should be given to CEA.

Cerebral protection devices

The most sinister complication of stent placement is plaque embolisation. Three strategies have been proposed in order to limit embolisation.

1. Distal balloon occlusion: Theron used a distal protection balloon placed in the ICA above the carotid stenosis prior to stent placement, and commercial variations on distal balloon protection are now available. Although the basic principle is simple, there are a number of disadvantages. Angulated lesions may be difficult to cross, the balloon can inflict damage on the arterial wall, up to 10% of patients are

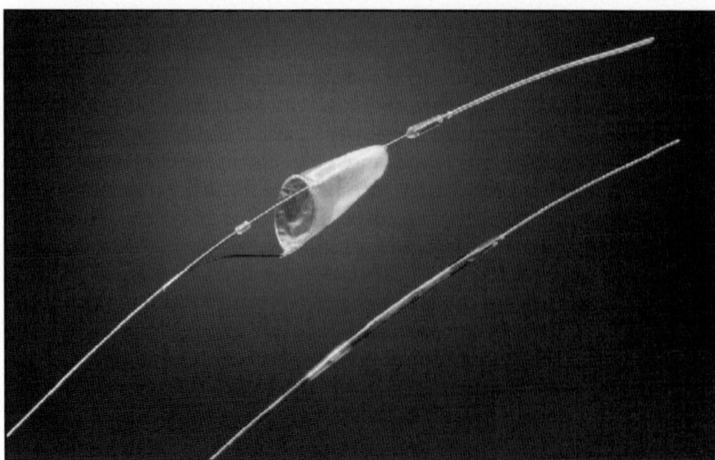

Figure 16.17 • Cerebral protection device incorporating a filter (Filterwire EZ, Boston Scientific Corporation).

intolerant of ICA occlusion, and the stenosis cannot be imaged while the ICA is occluded.

2. Distal filters: a growing number of such devices are being developed. They all basically require that the lesion be crossed with a constrained filter that is then deployed above the stenosis. The filter prevents the majority of emboli passing to the brain during manipulation of the stenosis, and is retrieved following final dilatation of the stent. All emboli are probably not removed and they do tend to cause spasm of the ICA (**Fig. 16.17**, see also Plate 13, facing p. 116).
3. A third variation involves the production of reverse flow within the ICA prior to any intervention. This is achieved by occluding flow in the CCA using a balloon on the guide-catheter and also in the ECA using a separate balloon occlusion system. The side arm of the guide-catheter is then connected percutaneously to the common femoral vein, effectively producing reverse flow through an arteriovenous fistula.

Do cerebral protection systems make a difference to the outcome of CAS? There are, as yet, no randomised trials. The world registry,[125,126] a systematic review of the literature[127] and data from individual units[128,129] suggest that these devices confer benefit by reducing stroke and death.

Results

Over the last two decades there have been many publications, of varying quality, on the use of CAS. Five randomised trials have been reported, of which three have been peer reviewed.

1. The first was very small and was stopped after only 17 patients because of a high stroke rate in the carotid stent group.[130]
2. CAVATAS[131] randomised 504 patients to endovascular therapy (251 patients) or endarterectomy (253 patients). Within the endovascular limb, the majority of patients (74%) were treated with angioplasty alone using large wires (0.035 inch, 0.89 mm) and balloons (5 Fr) that would no longer be thought suitable. At 30 days the overall stroke and death rate was 10% for CAS and 9.9% for CEA (not statistically different). There was a difference in non-embolic complications, with significantly more patients in the surgical limb suffering cranial nerve palsy or haematoma. Follow-up to 3 years did not show any difference in outcome (death and ipsilateral stroke). A recent review of stroke prevention out to 8 years (unpublished data) still shows identical stroke prevention.
3. A third trial,[132] as yet only published as an abstract, was stopped by the commercial sponsors after 219 patients were randomised to CAS or CEA. The 30-day periprocedural stroke and death rate was 12.1% for CAS and 4.5% for CEA ($P = 0.49$).
4. The Lexington Trial[133] randomised 104 symptomatic patients between CAS and CEA. There was no difference in the periprocedural complication rate, no strokes occurred in either arm of the trial and there was no difference in restenosis at 1 year.

The SAPPHIRE trial[134] has recently been completed; 334 patients with a symptomatic stenosis of 50% or more or with an asymptomatic stenosis of 80% or more were randomised between CEA or endovascular therapy using the Cordis Angioguard cerebral protection device and the PRECISE stent. Patients were considered to be at high risk for surgery and a registry was kept of patients fulfilling the entry criteria but not randomised. Only 30% of patients were symptomatic and 25% had surgical restenosis as the indication for treatment, indicating that although the patients were at high risk for surgery they were not at high risk for stroke. The 30-day endpoint was combined stroke, death and myocardial infarction, while the 1-year endpoint combined the 30-day endpoint with death and ipsilateral stroke at 1 year. At 30 days there was a significant difference ($P = 0.047$) in favour of CAS in the combined endpoint (5.8% CAS, 12.6% CEA) largely due to the excess myocardial infarction rate. At 1 year there was a significant difference in the combined endpoint favouring CAS, whether data were analysed as intention-to-treat or as treatment received. There was less clinically driven reintervention in the stent group ($P = 0.06$). However, of concern was the fact that CEA and CAS carried a 5.4% risk of death/stroke at 30 days in patients with asymptomatic carotid disease. At these levels of risk, there is no evidence that either treatment strategy is indicated in neurologically asymptomatic patients.

A recent Cochrane meta-analysis of these five trials shows no difference at 30 days between the two therapies (odds ratio 0.99, 95% CI 0.66–1.48).[135] The wide confidence interval justifies further trials in this area.

Restenosis

The exact restenosis rate of CAS is difficult to define. Although the rate of restenosis (≥70% narrowing) in CAVATAS[131] was reported to be high at 1 year (18.5% CAS vs 5.2% CEA), this was not reflected in an increased risk of stroke at 1 year. Other groups report lower rates of restenosis and, within CAVATAS, only 26% of patients received a stent. To further confuse the issue, it is recognised that ultrasound is not reliable in determining the severity of restenosis within a stented carotid artery and it should be noted that the clinically driven reintervention rate within SAPPHIRE was higher in the surgical group.

Stents for surgically high-risk patients

The SAPPHIRE trial data on high-risk patients are presented above. Among clinicians who may not be entirely convinced as to the overall data on patients with symptomatic atherosclerosis, proposed indications for carotid stenting include CEA restenosis, radiotherapy-induced lesions and high ICA stenoses. The data to support this are limited. These indications accounted for 38% of patients in the SAPPHIRE trial, but not all were symptomatic (see above). Small studies[136–141] have suggested that CAS is at least as safe as CEA but does not carry the burden of cranial nerve injury.

Conclusion

The science and practice of CAS is still evolving. Supported by the SAPPHIRE trial, it is possible that CAS for patients at high surgical risk for CEA will become the preferred treatment option. In units where there are experienced operators and audit showing outcomes equivalent to CEA, then CAS for symptomatic atherosclerosis can be considered a suitable alternative to CEA.[142] However, high-quality high-volume data are still required and recruitment to the large number of randomised trials currently underway is to be encouraged.

Key points

- Best medical therapy is indicated in all patients and includes risk factor prevention. It should not be delegated to junior team members. Best medical therapy depends on rapid access to cerebrovascular clinics and is not an alternative to consideration for carotid surgery.
- The beneficial role of CEA is supported by level I evidence in selected asymptomatic and symptomatic patients. It is dependent on being performed early with a low operative risk, and requires surgeons to quote their operative risk rather than trial data.
- Carotid stenting is emerging as an alternative to CEA and is being evaluated in a number of randomised trials. It cannot be justified in units with an excessive interventional risk, and requires interventionists to quote their procedural risk rather than trial data.

REFERENCES

1. Warlow CP. Disorders of the cerebral circulation. In: Walton J (ed.) Brain's diseases of the nervous system. Oxford: Oxford University Press, 1993; pp. 197–210.
2. Bamford J, Sandercock P, Dennid M, Burn J, Warlow CP. A prospective study of acute cerebrovascular disease in the community. The Oxfordshire Community Stroke Project 1981–1986. (I) Methodology, demography and incident cases of first ever stroke. J Neurol Neurosurg Psychiatry 1988; 51:1373–1380.
3. Dunbabin D, Sandercock P. Stroke prevention. Hosp Update 1992; July:540–5.

4. Modan B, Wagener DK. Some epidemiological aspects of stroke: mortality/morbidity trends, age, sex, race, socio-economic status. Stroke 1992; 23:1230–6.

5. Malmgren R, Bamford J, Warlow CP, Sandercock PAG, Slattery JM. Projecting the number of patients with first ever strokes and patients newly handicapped by stroke in England and Wales. Br Med J 1989; 298:656–60.

6. Dennis MS, Bamford JM, Sandercock PAG, Warlow CP. Incidence of transient ischaemic attacks in Oxfordshire, England. Stroke 1989; 20:333–9.

7. Sandercock PAG, Warlow CP, Jones LN, Starkey IR. Predisposing factors for cerebral infarction: the Oxfordshire Community Stroke Project. Br Med J 1989; 298:75–80.

8. Ringelstein EB, Sievers C, Echer S, Schneider PA, Otis SM. Non-invasive assessment of CO_2 induced cerebral vasomotor response in normal individuals and patients with internal carotid artery occlusions. Stroke 1988; 19:963–9.

9. Harrison MJG, Marshall J. The finding of thrombus at carotid endarterectomy and its relationship to the timing of surgery. Br J Surg 1977; 64:511–12.

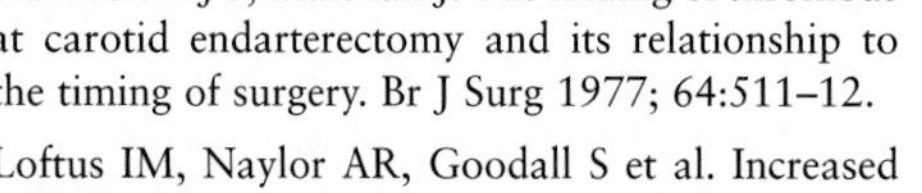

10. Loftus IM, Naylor AR, Goodall S et al. Increased MMP-9 activity in unstable carotid plaques: a potential role in acute plaque disruption. Stroke 2000; 31:40–7.

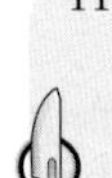

11. Rothwell PM, Villagra R, Gibson R, Donders RCJM, Warlow CP on behalf of the ECST Collaborative Group. Evidence of a chronic systemic cause of instability of atherosclerotic plaques. Lancet 2000; 355:19–24.

Supporting evidence that a systemic factor may trigger acute plaque disruption in the coronary and extracranial circulation.

12. Sandok BA, Whisnant JP, Furlan AJ, Mickell JL. Carotid artery bruits: prevalence survey and differential diagnosis. Mayo Clin Proc 1982; 57:227–30.

13. Khairi HS, Crowson MC. Carotid bruit: does it matter? Br J Hosp Med 1995; 53:426–7.

14. Hammond JH, Eisinger RP. Carotid bruits in 1000 normal subjects. Arch Intern Med 1962; 109:563–5.

15. Sauve JS, Laupacis A, Ostbye T, Feagan B, Sackett DL. Does this patient have a clinically important carotid bruit? JAMA 1993; 270:2843–5.

16. Sauve JS, Thorpe KE, Sackett DL et al. Can bruits distinguish high-grade from moderate symptomatic carotid stenosis? Ann Intern Med 1994; 120:633–7.

17. Bridgewater B, Naylor AR, Ratliff DA, Bell PRF. Benefits of carotid endarterectomy in symptomatic carotid artery disease: the message is not getting through. Br J Surg 1993; 80:722.

18. Wolf PA, Kannel WB, Sorlie P, McNamara P. Asymptomatic carotid bruit and risk of stroke: the Framingham Study. JAMA 1981; 245:1442–5.

19. Bamford J, Sandercock P, Dennis M, Burn J, Warlow C. A prospective study of acute cerebrovascular disease in the community. The Oxfordshire Community Stroke Project 1981–1986. (II) Incidence, case fatality rates and overall outcome at one year of cerebral infarction, primary intracerebral and subarachnoid haemorrhage. J Neurol Neurosurg Psychiatry 1990; 53:16–22.

20. Naylor AR, Sandercock PAG, Sellar RJ, Warlow CP. Patterns of vascular pathology in acute first-ever cerebral infarction. Scott Med J 1993; 38:41–4.

21. European Carotid Surgery Trialists Collaborative Group. MRC European Carotid Surgery Trial: interim results for symptomatic patients with severe (70–99%) or with mild (0–29%) carotid stenosis. Lancet 1991; 337:1235–41.

First level I evidence from Europe that CEA has a role in selected symptomatic patients with 70–99% carotid stenosis.

22. North American Symptomatic Carotid Endarterectomy Trial Collaborators. Beneficial effect of carotid endarterectomy in symptomatic patients with high grade stenosis. N Engl J Med 1991; 325:445–53.

First level I evidence from North America that CEA has a role in selected symptomatic patients with 70–99% carotid stenosis.

23. Amaurosis Fugax Study Group. Current management of amaurosis fugax. Stroke 1990; 1:201–8.

Systematic review of pathophysiology, prognosis and management of amaurosis fugax.

24. Lie JT. Pathology of occlusive disease of the extracranial arteries. In: Meyer FB (ed.) Sundt's occlusive cerebrovascular disease. Philadelphia: WB Saunders, 1994; pp. 25–44.

25. Stanley JC, Gewertz BL, Bove EL, Sottiurai V, Fry WJ. Arterial fibrodysplasia: histologic character and current aetiological concepts. Arch Surg 1975; 110:561–6.

26. Lupi-Herrerra E, Sanchez-Torres G, Marcustiamer J et al. Takayasu arteritis: clinical study of 107 cases. Am Heart J 1977; 93:94–103.

27. Biousse V, Touboul P-J, D'Anglejan-Chatillon J et al. Ophthalmological manifestations of internal carotid artery dissection. Am J Ophthalmol 1998; 126:565–77.

28. Nelson WR. Carotid body tumours. Surgery 1962; 51:326–35.

29. Barros D'Sa AB. Chemodectoma. In: Bell PRF, Jamieson CW, Ruckley CV (eds) Surgical management of vascular disease. London: WB Saunders, 1992; pp. 721–37.

30. Langlois Y, Roederer GO, Chan ATW et al. Evaluating carotid artery disease. Ultrasound Med Biol 1983; 9:51–63.

31. Faught WE, Mattos MA, van Bemmelen PS et al. Colour flow duplex scanning of carotid arteries: new velocity criteria based on receiver operator characteristic analysis for threshold stenoses used in the symptomatic and asymptomatic carotid trials. J Vasc Surg 1994; 19:818–28.

32. Moneta GL, Edwards M, Chitwood RW et al. Correlation of North American Symptomatic Carotid Endarterectomy Trial (NASCET) angiographic definition of 70–99% internal carotid artery stenosis with Duplex scanning. J Vasc Surg 1993; 17:152–9.

33. Neale ML, Chambers JL, Kelly AT. Reappraisal of Duplex criteria to assess significant carotid stenosis with special reference to reports from NASCET and ECST. J Vasc Surg 1994; 20:642–9.

34. Loftus IM, McCarthy MJ, Pau H et al. Carotid endarterectomy without angiography does not compromise operative outcome. Eur J Vasc Endovasc Surg 1998; 16:489–93.

35. Kirsch JD, Wagner LR, James WE et al. Carotid artery occlusion: positive predictive value of duplex sonography compared with arteriography. J Vasc Surg 1994; 19:642–9.

36. Morgenstern LB, Fox AJ, Sharpe BL et al. for the NASCET trial. The risks and benefits of carotid endarterectomy in patients with near occlusion of the carotid artery. Neurology 1997; 48:911–15.

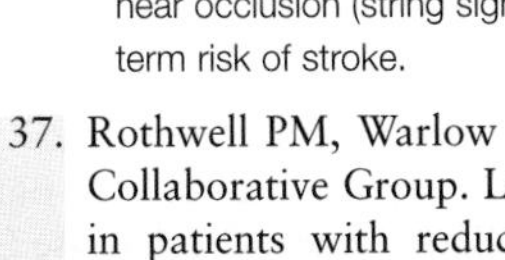

Subgroup analysis from NASCET database showing that near occlusion (string sign) is associated with a low long-term risk of stroke.

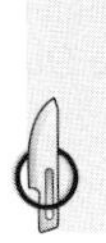
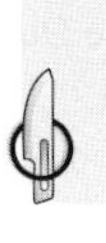

37. Rothwell PM, Warlow CP on behalf of the ECST Collaborative Group. Low risk of ischaemic stroke in patients with reduced internal carotid artery lumen diameter distal to severe symptomatic carotid stenosis: cerebral protection due to low post-stenotic flow. Stroke 2000; 31:622–30.

Subgroup analysis from ECST database showing that near occlusion (string sign) is associated with a low long-term risk of stroke.

38. Gray-Weale AC. Carotid artery atheroma: comparison of pre-operative B-mode ultrasound appearance with carotid endarterectomy specimen pathology. J Cardiovasc Surg 1988; 29:676–81.

39. Gaunt ME, Brown L, Hartshorne T et al. Unstable carotid plaques: pre-operative identification and association with intra-operative embolisation detected by transcranial Doppler. Eur J Vasc Endovasc Surg 1996; 11:78–82.

40. El-Barghouty N, Nicolaides A, Bahal V, Geroulakos G, Androulakis A. The identification of the high risk carotid plaque. Eur J Vasc Endovasc Surg 1996; 11:470–8.

41. Hankey JG, Warlow CP, Molyneux AJ. Complications of cerebral angiography for patients with mild carotid territory ischaemia being considered for carotid endarterectomy. J Neurol Neurosurg Psychiatry 1990; 53:542–8.

42. Heiserman JE, Dean BL, Hodak JA. Neurological complications of cerebral angiography. Am J Neuroradiol 1994; 15:1401–7.

43. Warnock NG, Bergvall U, Powell T. Complications of intra-arterial digital subtraction angiography in patients investigated for cerebral vascular disease. Br J Radiol 1993; 66:855–8.

44. Grzyska U, Freitag J, Zeumer H. Selective cerebral intra-arterial DSA: complication rate and control of risk factors. Neuroradiology 1990; 32:296–9.

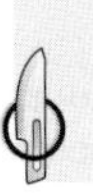

45. Davies KN, Humphrey PR. Complications of cerebral angiography in patients with symptomatic carotid territory ischaemia screened by carotid ultrasound. J Neurol Neurosurg Psychiatry 1993; 56:967–72.

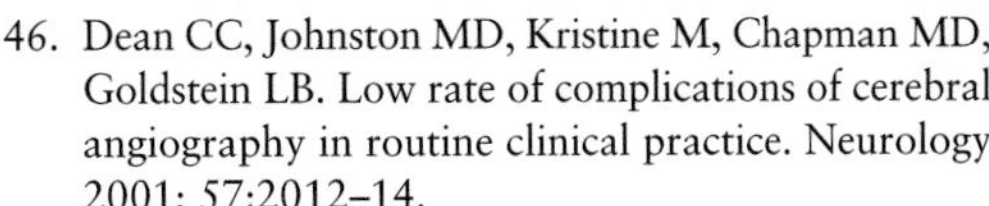

46. Dean CC, Johnston MD, Kristine M, Chapman MD, Goldstein LB. Low rate of complications of cerebral angiography in routine clinical practice. Neurology 2001; 57:2012–14.

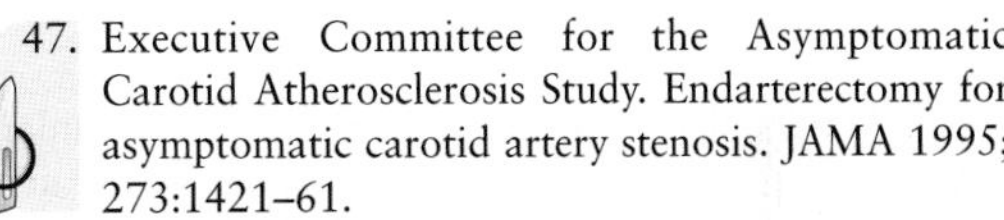

47. Executive Committee for the Asymptomatic Carotid Atherosclerosis Study. Endarterectomy for asymptomatic carotid artery stenosis. JAMA 1995; 273:1421–61.

First level I evidence from North America that CEA reduces long-term stroke risk in asymptomatic patients with a 60–99% stenosis.

48. Rothwell PM, Gibson RJ, Slattery J, Warlow CP for the ECST Collaborators Group. Prognostic value and reproducibility of measurements of carotid stenosis: a comparison of three methods on 1001 angiograms. Stroke 1994; 25:2440–4.

Subgroup analysis of the reproducibility and correlation between three methods of measuring carotid stenosis.

49. Borisch I, Horn M, Butz B et al. Preoperative evaluation of carotid artery stenosis: comparison of contrast-enhanced MR angiography and duplex sonography with digital subtraction angiography. Am J Neuroradiol 2003; 24:1117–22.

50. Johnston DCC, Eastwood JD, Nguyen T, Goldstein LB. Contrast-enhanced magnetic resonance angiography of carotid arteries. Utility in routine clinical practise. Stroke 2002; 33:2834–8.

51. Anderson GB, Ashforth R, Steinke DE, Ferdinandy R, Findlay JM. CT angiography for the detection and characterization of carotid artery bifurcation disease. Stroke 2000; 31:2168–74.

52. MacMahon S. Antihypertensive drug treatment: the potential, expected and observed effects on vascular disease. J Hypertens Suppl 1990; 8:S239–S244.

Systematic review showing that sustained reduction in blood pressure reduces the long-term risk of stroke.

53. Kalra L, Perez I, Melbourn A. Stroke risk management: changes in mainstream practice. Stroke 1998; 29:53–7.

54. PROGRESS Collaborative Group. Randomised trial of a perindopril-based blood-pressure-lowering regimen among 6105 individuals with previous stroke or transient ischaemic attack. Lancet 2001; 358:1033–41.

Low-dose ACE inhibition (perindopril) reduces cardiovascular risk.

55. The Heart Outcome Prevention Evaluation Study Investigators. Effects of an angiotensin-converting enzyme inhibitor, ramipril, on cardiovascular events in high-risk patients. N Engl J Med 2000; 342:145–53.

Low-dose ACE inhibition (ramipril) reduces cardiovascular risk.

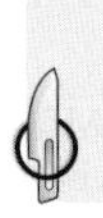
56. Heart Protection Study Collaborative Group. MRC/BHF Heart Protection Study of cholesterol lowering with simvastatin in 20536 high-risk individuals: a randomised placebo controlled trial. Lancet 2002; 360:7–22.

Randomised controlled trial showing level I evidence that statin therapy significantly reduces late cardiovascular risk.

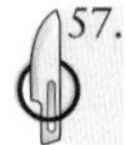
57. Antiplatelet Trialists Collaboration. Secondary prevention of vascular disease by prolonged antiplatelet treatment. Br Med J 1988; 296:320–31.

Systematic review of randomised controlled trials showing that antiplatelet therapy significantly reduces cardiovascular risk.

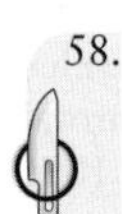
58. Taylor DW, Barnett HJM, Haynes RB et al. Low dose and high dose acetylsalicylic acid for patients undergoing carotid endarterectomy: a randomised trial. Lancet 1999; 353:2179–84.

Randomised controlled trial showing that low-dose aspirin is as effective as high-dose aspirin in preventing perioperative complications after CEA.

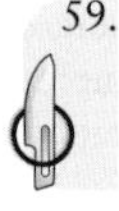
59. Diener H, Cunha L, Forbes C et al. European Stroke Prevention Study (ESPS) 2. Dipyridamole and acetylsalicylic acid in the secondary prevention of stroke. J Neurol Sci 1996; 143:1–13.

Despite showing that dual antiplatelet therapy was more effective than aspirin alone in preventing stroke, this randomised controlled trial has not really altered management.

60. CAPRIE Steering Committee. A randomised blinded trial of clopidogrel versus aspirin in patients at risk of ischaemic events. Lancet 1996; 348:1329–39.

Clopidogrel was more effective than aspirin in preventing composite vascular endpoint but the ARR was <1.0%.

61. Eastcott HHG, Pickering GW, Robb CG. Reconstruction of internal carotid artery in a patient with intermittent attacks of hemiplegia. Lancet 1954; ii:994–6.

62. Warlow CP. Carotid endarterectomy: does it work? Stroke 1984; 15:1068–76.

63. Barnett HJM, Walton JN, Plum F. Carotid endarterectomy: an expression of concern. Stroke 1984; 15:941–3.

64. Naylor AR, Rothwell PM, Bell PRF. Overview of the principal results and secondary analyses from the European and the North American randomised trials of carotid endarterectomy. Eur J Vasc Endovasc Surg 2003; 26:115–29.

Systematic review of 48 publications from the ECST and NASCET.

65. Warlow CP, Davenport RJ. The management of transient ischaemic attacks. Prescriber J 1996; 36:1–8.

66. Wennberg DE, Lucas FL, Birkmeyer JD, Bredenberg CE, Fisher ES. Variation in carotid endarterectomy mortality in the Medicare population. JAMA 1998; 279:1278–81.

67. Karp HR, Flanders D, Shipp CC, Taylor B, Martin D. Carotid endarterectomy among Medicare beneficiaries: a statewide evaluation of appropriateness and outcome. Stroke 1998; 29:46–52.

68. European Carotid Surgery Trialists' Collaborative Group. Randomised trial of endarterectomy for recently symptomatic carotid stenosis: final results of the MRC European Carotid Surgery Trial (ECST). Lancet 1998; 351:1379–87.

Update of the 1991 paper for all patients in the ECST.

69. Barnett HJM, Taylor DW, Eliaszíw M et al. Benefit of carotid endarterectomy in patients with symptomatic moderate or severe stenosis. N Engl J Med 1998; 339:1415–25.

Update of the 1991 paper for all patients in the NASCET.

70. Ricci S, Flamini F, Coloni MG. Prevalence of internal carotid artery stenosis in subjects older than 49 years: a population study. Cerebrovasc Dis 1991; 1:16–19.

71. Klop RBJ, Eikelboom BC, Taks ACJM. Screening of the internal carotid arteries in patients with peripheral vascular disease by colour-flow Duplex scanning. Eur J Vasc Surg 1991; 5:41–5.

72. Sutton-Turrell KC, Alcorn HG, Wolfson SK, Kelsey SF, Kuller LH. Prediction of carotid stenosis in older adults with and without isolated systolic hypertension. Stroke 1987; 18:817–22.

73. Mayo Asymptomatic Carotid Endarterectomy Study Group. Effectiveness of CEA for asymptomatic carotid stenosis: design of a clinical trial. Mayo Clin Proc 1989; 64:897–904.

Early randomised controlled trial comparing CEA with best medical therapy in patients with asymptomatic carotid disease. Did not influence practice.

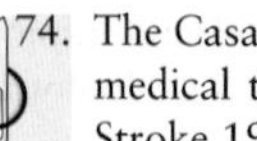
74. The Casanova Study Group. Carotid surgery versus medical therapy in asymptomatic carotid stenosis. Stroke 1991; 22:1229–35.

Early randomised controlled trial comparing CEA with best medical therapy in patients with asymptomatic carotid disease. Did not influence practice.

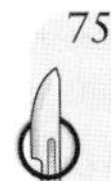
75. Hobson RW, Weiss DG, Fields WS and the VA Co-operative Study Group. Efficacy of carotid endarterectomy for asymptomatic carotid stenosis. N Engl J Med 1993; 328:221–7.

Early randomised controlled trial comparing CEA with best medical therapy in patients with asymptomatic carotid disease. Did not influence practice.

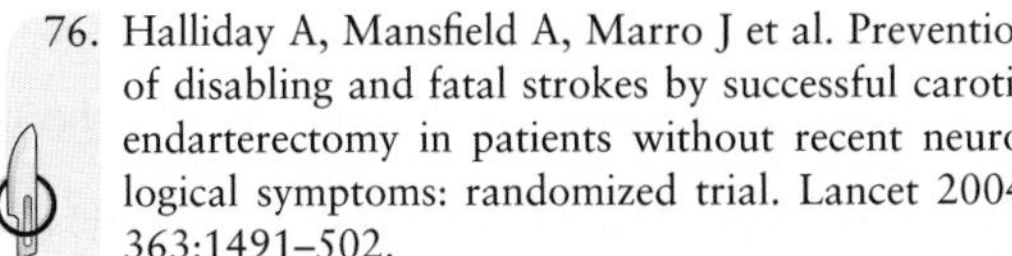
76. Halliday A, Mansfield A, Marro J et al. Prevention of disabling and fatal strokes by successful carotid endarterectomy in patients without recent neurological symptoms: randomized trial. Lancet 2004; 363:1491–502.

Level I evidence from European randomised controlled trial confirming benefit of immediate CEA over deferred CEA in patients with asymptomatic carotid artery disease.

77. Hankey GJ. Asymptomatic carotid stenosis: how should it be managed? Med J Aust 1995; 163:197–200.

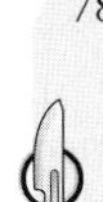
78. Rothwell PM, Gutnikov S. Differences in time course of risk of ischaemic stroke distal to symptomatic and asymptomatic carotid stenoses: the Asymptomatic Carotid Stenosis Study. Stroke 2000; 31:284.

Only published as an abstract showing that while risk of stroke for asymptomatic stenoses at 3 years was significantly lower than that for symptomatic stenoses, the difference was non-significant at 8 years. The inference is that the risk of stroke ipsilateral to an asymptomatic stenosis increases linearly with time.

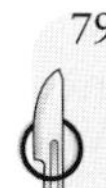
79. Naylor AR, Mehta Z, Rothwell PM, Bell PRF. Stroke during coronary artery bypass surgery: a critical review of the role of carotid artery disease. Eur J Vasc Endovasc Surg 2002; 23:283–94.

Systematic review of evidence supporting/refuting claim that carotid disease is an important cause of stroke following coronary bypass.

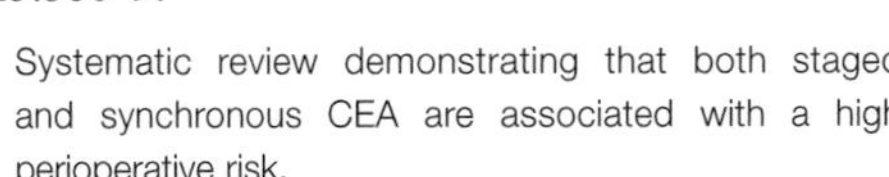
80. Naylor AR, Cuffe R, Rothwell PM, Bell PRF. A systematic review of outcomes following staged and synchronous carotid endarterectomy and coronary artery bypass. Eur J Vasc Endovasc Surg 2003; 25:380–9.

Systematic review demonstrating that both staged and synchronous CEA are associated with a high perioperative risk.

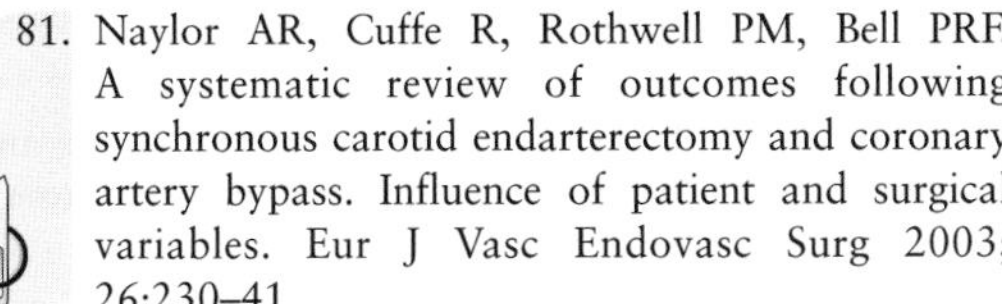
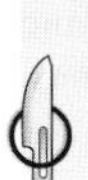
81. Naylor AR, Cuffe R, Rothwell PM, Bell PRF. A systematic review of outcomes following synchronous carotid endarterectomy and coronary artery bypass. Influence of patient and surgical variables. Eur J Vasc Endovasc Surg 2003; 26:230–41.

Factors influencing the operative risk following synchronous CEA and CABG. Increasing experience was not associated with a reduction in risk.

82. Blaisdell WF, Clauss RH, Goldbraith JG, Imparato AM, Wylie EJ. Joint study of extracranial arterial occlusion: a review of surgical considerations. JAMA 1979; 209:1889–95.

83. Wylie EJ, Hein MF, Adams JE. Intracranial haemorrhage following surgical revascularization for treatment of acute strokes. J Neurosurg 1964; 2:212–15.

84. Allenberg J, Eckstein HH. When should I operate after completed stroke? In: Naylor AR, Mackey W (eds) Carotid artery surgery: a problem based approach. London: Harcourt, 2000; pp. 36–41.

85. Mead GE, O'Neill PA, McCollum CN. Is there a role for carotid surgery in acute stroke? Eur J Vasc Endovasc Surg 1997; 13:112–21.

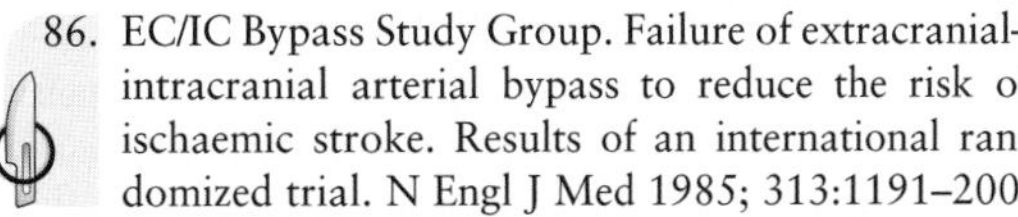
86. EC/IC Bypass Study Group. Failure of extracranial–intracranial arterial bypass to reduce the risk of ischaemic stroke. Results of an international randomized trial. N Engl J Med 1985; 313:1191–200.

Much-criticised randomised controlled trial showing that extracranial–intracranial bypass did not reduce stroke risk.

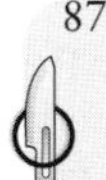
87. Sundt TM. Was the international randomized trial of extracranial–intracranial arterial bypass representative of the population at risk? N Engl J Med 1987; 316:814–16.

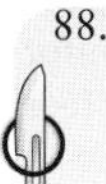
88. Forsell C, Takolander R, Bergqvist D, Johansson A. Local versus general anaesthesia in carotid surgery: a prospective randomised study. Eur J Vasc Surg 1989; 3:503–9.

One of the few randomised trials comparing general with local anaesthesia.

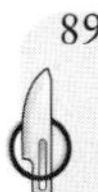
89. Rerkasem K, Bond R, Rothwell PM. Local versus general anaesthesia for carotid endarterectomy. Cochrane Database Systematic Review 2004(2) CD 000126.

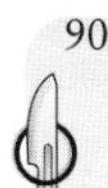
90. Naylor AR. Surgical controversies. In: Chaturverdi S, Rothwell P (eds) Carotid artery stenosis: current and emerging treatments. XXXX: Marcel Dekker, 2003; pp. 000–000.

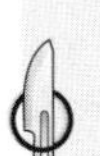
91. Kretschmer G, Bischof G, Pratschner T et al. Antiplatelet or anticoagulant therapy after carotid endarterectomy: results of a trial and an analysis supported by post-data matching. In: Greenhalgh RM, Hollier LH (eds) Surgery for stroke. London: WB Saunders, 1993; pp. 319–27.

One of the few randomised trials that have been undertaken regarding optimal medical therapy following carotid surgery. This trial showed no evidence that anticoagulation offered any benefit over antiplatelet therapy.

92. Naylor AR, John T, Howlett J et al. Surveillance imaging of the operated artery does not alter clinical outcome following carotid endarterectomy. Br J Surg 1996; 83:522–6.

93. Counsell C, Salinas R, Warlow CP, Naylor AR. The role of routine patch angioplasty in carotid endarterectomy: a systematic review of the randomised controlled trials. In: Warlow CP, van Gijn J, Sandercock P (eds) Stroke module of the Cochrane Database of Systematic Reviews, 1995 (issue I). London: BMJ Publishing Group.

Cochrane overview showing that routine patching confers significant benefit over routine primary closure of the arteriotomy.

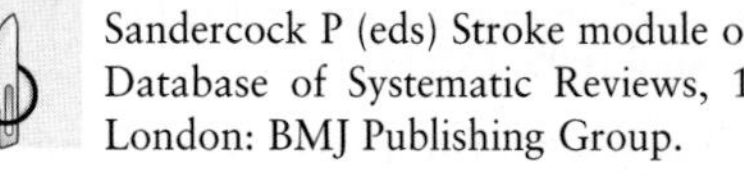

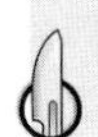

94. Counsell C, Salinas R, Warlow CP, Naylor AR. A comparison of different types of patch in carotid patch angioplasty: a systematic review of the randomized trials. In: Warlow CP, van Gijn J, Sandercock P (eds) Stroke module of the Cochrane Database of Systematic Reviews, 1996 (issue 2). London: BMJ Publishing Group.

Cochrane overview showing that if you choose to patch, it does not matter what patch (vein, prosthetic) you use.

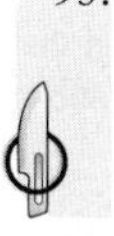

95. Wilkinson JM, Rochestor JR, Sivaguru A et al. Middle cerebral artery velocity, embolisation and neurological outcome during carotid endarterectomy: a prospective study. Eur J Vasc Endovasc Surg 1997; 14:399–402.

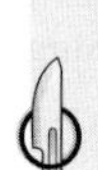

96. Counsell C, Salinas R, Warlow CP, Naylor AR. The role of carotid artery shunting during carotid endarterectomy: a systematic review of the randomised trials of routine and selective shunting and the different methods of intra-operative monitoring. In: Warlow CP, van Gijn J, Sandercock P (eds) Stroke module of the Cochrane Database of Systematic Reviews, 1996 (issue 2). London: BMJ Publishing Group.

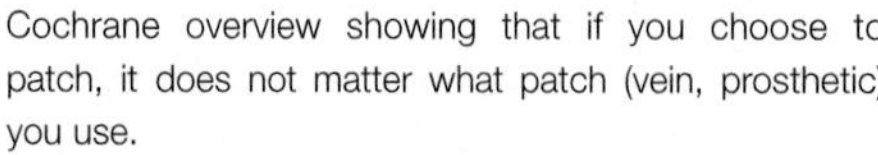

Cochrane overview showing that if you choose to patch, it does not matter what patch (vein, prosthetic) you use.

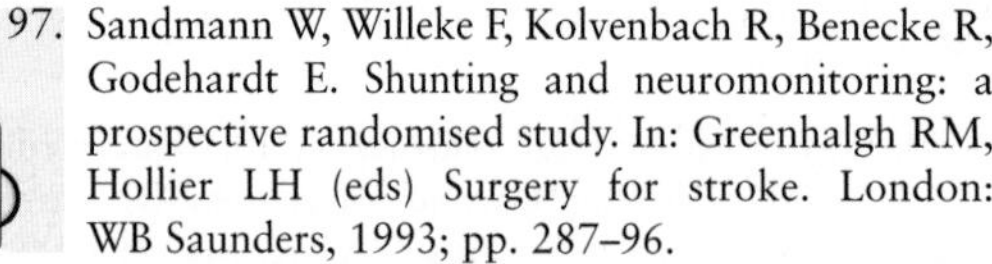

97. Sandmann W, Willeke F, Kolvenbach R, Benecke R, Godehardt E. Shunting and neuromonitoring: a prospective randomised study. In: Greenhalgh RM, Hollier LH (eds) Surgery for stroke. London: WB Saunders, 1993; pp. 287–96.

This trial was flawed because patients randomised to no shunt were then shunted if EEG changes developed during carotid clamping, i.e. it could never be expected to answer the question posed.

98. Mason PF, Dyson EH, Sellars V, Beard JD. The assessment of cerebral oxygenation during carotid endarterectomy utilizing near infrared spectroscopy. Eur J Vasc Surg 1994; 8:590–4.

99. Astrup J, Siesjo BK, Symon L. Thresholds in cerebral ischaemia: the ischaemic penumbra. Stroke 1981; 12:723–5.

100. Naylor AR, Bell PRF, Ruckley CV. Monitoring and cerebral protection during carotid endarterectomy. Br J Surg 1992; 79:735–41.

101. Naylor AR, Hayes PD, Allroggen H et al. Reducing the risk of carotid surgery: a seven year audit of the role of monitoring and quality control assessment. J Vasc Surg 2000; 32:750–9.

102. Blaisdell FW, Lim R, Hall AD. Technical result of carotid endarterectomy: arteriographic assessment. Am J Surg 1967; 114:239–45.

103. Spencer MP, Reid JM. Quantitation of carotid stenosis with continuous wave Doppler ultrasound. Stroke 1979; 10:326–30.

104. Paciaroni M, Eliasziw M, Kappelle J et al. Medical complications associated with carotid endarterectomy. Stroke 1999; 30:1759–63.

105. Forsell C, Bergqvist D, Bergentz SE. Peripheral nerve injuries in carotid artery surgery. In: Greenhalgh RM, Hollier LH (eds) Surgery for stroke. London: WB Saunders, 1993; pp. 217–34.

106. Ferguson GG, Eliasziw M, Barr HWK et al. The North American Symptomatic Carotid Endarterectomy Trial: surgical results in 1415 patients. Stroke 1999; 30:1751–8.

Subgroup analysis of NASCET surgery database documenting the surgical risk. Although quite high risk, the incidence of major complications was extremely low.

107. Naylor AR, Payne D, Thompson MM et al. Prosthetic patch infection after carotid endarterectomy. Eur J Vasc Endovasc Surg 2002; 23:11–16.

108. Krul JMJ, van Gijn J, Ackerstaff RGA et al. Site and pathogenesis of infarcts associated with carotid endarterectomy. Stroke 1989; 20:324–8.

109. Naylor AR, Merrick MV, Ruckley CV. Risk factors for intra-operative neurological deficit during carotid endarterectomy. Eur J Vasc Surg 1991; 5:33–9.

110. Naylor AR, Ruckley CV. The post-carotid endarterectomy hyperperfusion syndrome. Eur J Vasc Endovasc Surg 1995; 9:365–7.

111. Naylor AR, Evans J, Thompson MM et al. Seizures after carotid endarterectomy: hyperperfusion, dysautoregulation or hypertensive encephalopathy? Eur J Vasc Endovasc Surg 2003; 26:39–44.

112. Gaunt ME, London NJM, Smith J et al. Early diagnosis of post-operative carotid occlusion using transcranial Doppler ultrasound. J Vasc Surg 1994; 20:1004–5.

113. Levi CR, O'Malley HM, Fell G et al. Transcranial Doppler detected cerebral embolism following carotid endarterectomy: high microembolic signal loads predict post-operative cerebral ischaemia. Brain 1997; 120:621–9.

114. Spencer MP. Transcranial Doppler monitoring and causes of stroke from carotid endarterectomy. Stroke 1997; 28:685–91.

115. Cantelmo NL, Babikian VL, Samaraweera RN et al. Cerebral microembolism and ischaemia changes associated with carotid endarterectomy. J Vasc Surg 1998; 27:1024–30.

116. Gaunt ME, Smith J, Martin PJ et al. On-table diagnosis of incipient carotid artery thrombosis during carotid endarterectomy using transcranial Doppler sonography. J Vasc Surg 1994; 20:104–7.

117. Laman DM, Wieneke GH, van Duijn H, van Huffelen AC. High embolic rate after carotid endarterectomy is associated with early cerebrovascular complications. J Vasc Surg 2002; 36:278–84.

118. Gaunt ME, Smith JL, Martin PJ et al. A comparison of quality control methods applied to carotid endarterectomy. Eur J Vasc Endovasc Surg 1996; 11:4–11.

119. Naylor AR, John T, Howlett J et al. Fate of the non-operated carotid artery after contralateral endarterectomy. Br J Surg 1995; 82:44–8.

120. Latimer CR, Burnand KG. Recurrent carotid stenosis after carotid endarterectomy. Br J Surg 1997; 84:1206–19.

Systematic review showing that while the prevalence of restenosis was quite high after CEA, it did not seem to matter clinically.

121. Frericks H, Kievit J, van Baalen JM, van Bockel JH. Carotid recurrent stenosis and risk of ipsilateral stroke. A systematic review of the literature. Stroke 1998; 29:244–50.

Further systematic review showing that while the prevalence of restenosis was quite high after CEA, it did not seem to matter clinically.

122. Horrocks M. When should I re-operate for recurrent carotid stenosis. In: Naylor AR, Mackey W (eds) Carotid artery surgery: a problem based approach. London: Harcourt, 2000; pp. 371–4.

123. Moore WS, Kempczinski RF, Nelson JJ, Toole JF. Recurrent carotid stenosis: results of the Asymptomatic Carotid Atherosclerosis Study. Stroke 1998; 29:2018–25.

124. Lauder C, Kelly A, Thompson MM et al. Early and late outcomes following carotid artery bypass using saphenous vein. J Vasc Surg 2003; 38:1025–30.

125. Wholey MW, Mathias K, Roubin GS et al. Global experience in cervical carotid artery stent placement. Cathet Cardiovasc Intervent 2000; 50:160–7.

126. Wholey MH, Al-Mubarak N. Update review of the global carotid stent registry. Cathet Cardiovasc Intervent 2003; 60:259–66.

127. Kastrup A, Groschel K, Krapf H et al. Early outcome of carotid angioplasty and stenting with and without cerebral protection devices. A systematic review of the literature. Stroke 2003; 34:813–19.

128. Castriota F, Cremonesi A, Manetti R et al. Impact of cerebral protection devices on early outcome of carotid stenting. J Endovasc Ther 2002; 9:786–92.

129. McKevitt FM, Macdonald S, Venables GS, Cleveland TJ, Gaines PA. Complications following carotid angioplasty and carotid stenting in patients with symptomatic carotid artery disease. Cerebrovasc Dis 2004; 17:28–34.

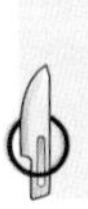

130. Naylor AR, Bolia A, Abbott RJ et al. Randomized study of carotid angioplasty and stenting versus carotid endarterectomy: a stopped trial. J Vasc Surg 1998; 28:326–34.

A small randomised trial of 17 patients stopped because of very poor results in the stent arm.

131. CAVATAS Investigators. Endovascular versus surgical treatment in patients with carotid stenosis in the Carotid and Vertebral Artery Transluminal Angioplasty Study (CAVITAS): a randomised trial. Lancet 2001; 357:1729–37.

The largest randomised study to date showing equivalence between the two treatments but considered by many to have unnacceptable results in the surgical arm.

132. Alberts MJ. Results of a multicenter prospective randomized trial of carotid artery stenting versus carotid endarterectomy (abstract). Stroke 2001; 32:325.

Only available in abstract. Reasons for the trial being stopped unclear. Poor results in the stented patients.

133. Brooks WH, McClure RR, Jones MR, Coleman TC. Carotid angioplasty and stenting versus carotid endarterectomy: randomized trial in a community hospital. J Am Coll Cardiol 2001; 38:1589–95.

Small numbers from one centre showing equivalence.

134. Yadav JS, Wholey MH, Kuntz RE et al. Protected carotid artery stenting versus endarterectomy in high risk patients. N Engl J Med 2004; 351:1493–501.

Much criticised randomised trial essentially showing that if you operate on patients at high risk for surgery, the results are poor and stenting may have a role.

135. Coward LJ, Featherstone RL, Brown MM. Percutaneous transluminal angioplasty and stenting for carotid artery stenosis (Cochrane review). The Cochrane Library. Chichester: John Wiley & Sons, 2003.

Shows equivalent procedural outcomes between the two treatments but wide confidence intervals support further trials.

136. AbuRahma AF, Bates MC, Wulu JT, Stone PA. Early postsurgical carotid restenosis: redo surgery versus angioplasty/stenting. J Endovasc Ther 2002; 9:566–72.

137. Al-Mubarak NR, Gomez CR, Liui MW, Vitek JJ. Carotid stenting for severe radiation-induced extracranial carotid artery occlusive disease. J Endovasc Ther 2000; 7:36–40.

138. Alric P, Branchereau P, Berthet J-P, Mary H, Marty-Ane C. Carotid artery stenting for stenosis following revascularization or cervical irradiation. J Endovasc Ther 2002; 9:14–19.

139. Bowser AN, Bandyk DF, Evans A et al. Outcome of carotid stent-assisted angioplasty versus open surgical repair of recurrent carotid stenosis. J Vasc Surg 2003; 38:432–8.

140. Hobson RW, Goldstein JE, Jamil Z et al. Carotid restenosis: operative and endovascular management. J Vasc Surg 1999; 29:228–38.

141. New G, Roubin GI, Vitek JJ et al. Safety, efficacy and durability of carotid artery stenting for restenosis following carotid endarterectomy: a multicenter study. J Endovasc Ther 2000; 7:345–52.

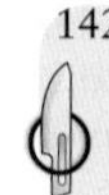

142. Intercollegiate Working Party for Stroke. Secondary Prevention Update, Section 11.3. National Clinical Guidelines for Stroke. London: Royal College of Physicians, 2002.

143 McKevitt FM, Randall MS, Cleveland TJ et al. The benefits of combined antiplatelet treatment in carotid artery stenting. Eur J Vasc Endovasc Surg 2005; 29:522–7.

CHAPTER

Seventeen

Diagnosis and management of complex venous thromboembolic disease of the lower limb

Andrew Platts, Eric Preston and Anthony Watkinson

INTRODUCTION

Venous thromboembolic disease is a common medical problem. The first-episode incidence ranges between 60 and 180 per 100 000 persons per year in the USA. Estimates are that more than 250 000 patients per year in the USA suffer from symptomatic lower limb deep vein thrombosis (DVT). There is considerable associated morbidity and mortality, especially when the proximal leg veins are involved. Pulmonary embolism (PE), the major early complication, is estimated to affect 500 000–600 000 people per year in the USA, with fatal consequences in up to 200 000. PE is estimated to be either the primary or secondary cause in 30 000–40 000 deaths per year in the UK. In a UK study of all admissions to a single district general hospital, 10% of all deaths (i.e. 0.9% of all admissions) were due to PE.[1] DVT is very common in hospitalised patients: up to 30% have asymptomatic non-obstructive calf vein thrombosis as shown by radioactive fibrinogen leg scanning.[2] The clinical significance of these isolated distal thromboses remains debatable. Patients with proximal thrombus propagation have a much higher risk of developing PE. In their original report of 1969, Kakkar et al.[3] found a 10% incidence of PE in patients where there was proximal propagation to the popliteal vein and more proximally. Asymptomatic PE accompanying clinically diagnosed DVT is also common – incidence is roughly 50% in proximal DVT and 30–50% in isolated calf vein thromboses.[4,5]

PATHOPHYSIOLOGY OF THROMBOSIS

The mechanisms that cause thrombosis were first elucidated by Virchow approximately 150 years ago.[6] He postulated that the major pathogenetic factors for the development of thrombosis are abnormalities of the vessel wall, of the constituents of the blood and of the dynamics of blood flow. This prophetic insight has been adequately confirmed and it is now clear that both arterial and venous thrombosis occur predominantly as a result of interplay between these three variables.

Blood coagulation is essentially a series of stepwise reactions in which inactive zymogens are converted into active serine proteases. The final enzyme to be formed in this system is thrombin, which converts soluble fibrinogen into insoluble fibrin that forms the basis of the thrombus, or clot. Clotting factors V and VIII act as cofactors in this process. The word 'clot' is usually used to describe in vitro thrombosis (i.e. in a test tube), while 'thrombus' is used for an in vivo event.

Fibrinolysis is the mechanism whereby insoluble fibrin is digested by plasmin, an enzyme derived from plasminogen and formed by the conversion of inactive zymogens to active serine proteases, i.e. proteolytic enzymes, in a manner analogous to the formation of thrombin. Apart from thrombin formation at sites of vascular injury, in vivo coagulation does not normally occur. This is on account of the antithrombotic properties of the endothelium, the presence of inactive serine protease precursors (zymogens) and coagulation inhibitors.

Activation of coagulation is initiated by vascular injury and/or biochemical events such as the release of cytokines. There are several mechanisms whereby blood coagulation is regulated. These involve not only inhibitors such as tissue factor pathway inhibitor, antithrombin, protein C and protein S but also dilution factors and the rate of blood flow. Clinical support for the vital role of coagulation inhibitors antithrombin, protein C and protein S is evidenced by the increased venous thrombotic risk associated with deficiencies of these proteins.

Risk factors for venous thrombosis

Many factors are associated with an increased risk of venous thrombosis. Some of these are inherited abnormalities of the coagulation cascade and for these the term 'familial thrombophilia' is applied. There are, in addition, numerous acquired risk factors for venous thrombosis. These include not only environmental or lifestyle factors, such as prolonged periods of immobilisation or use of oral contraception, but also other clinical disorders, such as malignancy or the myeloproliferative disorders or the possession of lupus anticoagulant or other antiphospholipid antibody. These non-familial risk factors for venous thrombosis can be grouped together under the term 'acquired thrombophilia'.

Since Egeberg[7] first reported a genetic predisposition to venous thrombosis in 1965, other prothrombotic genetic mutations have been described, and throughout western Europe and the USA a prothrombotic genetic mutation can now be identified in approximately 50% of subjects presenting with venous thrombosis.

FAMILIAL THROMBOPHILIA

The familial thrombophilias comprise a group of inherited disorders in which a predisposition to venous thrombosis is linked to quantitative or qualitative abnormalities of proteins participating in the coagulation cascade (**Box 17.1**). The first to be described were gene mutations affecting the coagulation inhibitors antithrombin, protein C and protein S. These mutations result in loss of function of the affected allele and a corresponding reduction in the plasma concentration of the inhibitor. These abnormalities are rare in the general population (<0.2%) but are strong risk factors for venous thrombosis (relative risk approximately 10).[8]

More recently, so-called 'gain-of-function' abnormalities have been described that are associated with an increased risk of venous thrombosis through alterations in the balance between procoagulants and coagulation inhibitor activity. Gain-of-function abnormalities such as factor V Leiden and prothrombin G20210A mutations are associated with mechanisms for increased procoagulant activity and also elevated plasma concentrations of the clotting factors VIII, IX and XI, for which mechanisms remain to be elucidated.[8] In the general population, gain-of-function disorders are not uncommon but they are relatively weak risk factors for venous thrombosis (relative risk 2–5).[8] Some genetically determined abnormalities of fibrinogen (dysfibrinogenaemia) may also be associated with an increased venous thrombotic tendency. Although there are reports of a possible association between a venous thrombotic tendency and inherited abnormalities of other coagulation proteins, it remains doubtful that such an association exists. This applies to familial abnormalities of plasminogen, heparin cofactor II and tissue plasminogen activator (tPA).

Box 17.1 • Risk factors for venous thromboembolism

Genetic mutations resulting in loss of function of coagulation inhibitors
Antithrombin
Protein C
Protein S
Genetic mutations resulting in gain of function of coagulation inhibitors (increased procoagulant activity)
Factor V Leiden
Prothrombin 20210A
Physiological changes resulting in gain-of-function disorders (mechanism unknown)
Increased concentrations of factor VIII:C, factor IX:C, factor XI:C
Genetic mutations resulting in other disorders (mechanism unknown)
Dysfibrinogenaemia

Antithrombin deficiency

Antithrombin (previously known as antithrombin III) is a single-chain glycoprotein that is synthesised in the liver. It is the major serine protease inhibitor within the coagulation cascade and inactivates not only thrombin but also other serine proteases, including clotting factors XIIa, XIa, IXa and Xa. The association between inherited antithrombin deficiency and venous thrombosis was first reported in 1965 by Egeberg.[7] The estimated prevalence of the disorder is within the range 1 in 2000 to 1 in

40 000 and antithrombin deficiency is observed in approximately 2–5% of individuals under the age of 45 years who present with a first venous thromboembolic event.[9]

Homozygous antithrombin deficiency is extremely rare and is associated with an aggressive clinical course including both venous and arterial thrombotic events.[10] Affected individuals do not usually survive beyond the neonatal period.[11]

Heterozygous antithrombin deficiency is the commonest manifestation of this inherited disorder. By using both activity and antigen assays, familial antithrombin deficiency can be classified into type I and type II defects. Type I defects are characterised by a reduced concentration of a structurally normal protein, whereas type II defects are characterised by a structurally abnormal protein. Type II antithrombin defects can be further subclassified according to whether the structural abnormality is confined to the heparin-binding site or the thrombin (reactive)-binding site of the molecule. The subclassification of type II defects is of more than academic interest because the venous thrombotic risk associated with reactive site defects is marked and approximates to that associated with type I defects. In contrast, the venous thrombotic risk associated with heparin-binding site defects is considerably less.

Protein C deficiency

Protein C is a vitamin K-dependent protein that is synthesised in the liver and plays a vital role in the anticoagulant properties of vascular endothelial cells. Under physiological circumstances protein C is converted to its activated form, activated protein C (APC), on the endothelial cell surface by a thrombin–thrombomodulin complex. Following its activation, APC, a serine protease, inhibits the coagulation activation pathway by inhibiting factors Va and VIIIa, the activated forms of clotting factors V and VIII respectively. The inactivation of factors Va and VIIIa by APC is facilitated by another vitamin K-dependent protein, protein S, which functions as a cofactor in this process. Protein C deficiency from whatever cause will effectively reduce the coagulation inhibitory potential and this will result in increased thrombin formation.

The clinical importance of protein C deficiency was first recognised in 1981 when Griffin et al.[12] reported familial protein C deficiency as a cause of familial thrombophilia. The clinical features of familial protein C deficiency are similar to those described for antithrombin deficiency. Although DVT is the commonest manifestation of familial protein C deficiency, thrombosis in unusual sites may also occur.[13,14] These include involvement of cerebral, renal, mesenteric, portal and hepatic veins. [15,16] Haemorrhagic infarction of the skin is a rare manifestation of familial protein C deficiency. This usually occurs shortly after the commencement of oral anticoagulant therapy with coumarin and is therefore termed 'warfarin-induced skin necrosis'. The lesions, which are microthrombotic in nature, invariably develop over areas of adiposity and are probably caused by a transient period of hypercoagulability consequent upon further reduction of protein C that occurs in advance of the anticoagulant effects of coumarin on the vitamin K-dependent clotting factors II, IX and X.

Homozygous protein C deficiency is rare. Purpura fulminans neonatalis, characterised by extensive purpuric and necrotic skin lesions, disseminated intravascular coagulation and organ infarction, has been reported in neonates with homozygous protein C deficiency, often within 12 hours of birth. The prevalence of heterozygous protein C deficiency in the general population is approximately 0.2%.[17,18] In consecutive patients presenting with venous thrombosis the prevalence is approximately 3% and this figure rises to approximately 6% in selected patients with a family history of venous thrombosis.[19]

As with the general population, the risk of venous thrombosis in those with heterozygous protein C deficiency increases with age. It has been reported that approximately 50% of affected subjects will have had a venous thrombotic event by the age of 40 years.[13,20] This probably overestimates the overall venous thrombotic risk associated with protein C deficiency. Whereas this figure is appropriate when applied to affected subjects presenting with venous thrombosis, the venous thrombotic risk of affected family members is less than that of the index family member.[21] In the same study, the incidence of a venous thrombotic event per 1000 person-years in an affected relative of an index patient was 3.3 compared with 0.3 for the controls.[21] The risk of venous thrombosis is further increased in protein C-deficient individuals with additional inherited risk factors for this disorder.[21,22]

Protein S deficiency

Protein S is a vitamin K-dependent protein that is synthesised in the liver, vascular endothelial cells and megakaryocytes. It binds to protein C on phospholipid surfaces and functions as a cofactor to protein C in the inactivation of the activated clotting factors V and VIII. In plasma, approximately 60% of total protein S is bound to C4b-binding protein. This component has no haemostatic function. The remaining 40% is the physiologically important moiety and circulates as free protein S.

Protein S deficiency was first recognised as an inherited risk factor for venous thrombosis in 1984.[23] It is now recognised that there are three different types of protein S deficiency defined on the basis of results obtained with three different assay systems: (i) total protein S antigen, (ii) free protein S antigen and (iii) functional protein S assay. The different types of protein S deficiency reflect either different genetic mutations of the protein S gene or abnormal concentrations or binding characteristics of C4b-binding protein. Although of academic interest, the different types of protein S deficiency do not appear to influence the phenotypic expression of protein S deficiency and their discussion is outside the scope of this chapter. Difficulties with protein S assays, resulting in large interlaboratory variability, together with the influence of sex, age and hormonal status, have resulted in wide variability in estimates of the prevalence of inherited protein S deficiency in the general population.[24] The prevalence of inherited protein S deficiency in the general population would appear to be approximately 1.3%. This figure rises to approximately 6% in selected thrombophilic families.[19,25]

The clinical manifestations of inherited protein S deficiency are very similar to those associated with protein C deficiency, including warfarin-induced skin necrosis. In addition to DVT and PE, affected individuals may experience thrombosis affecting the cerebral, mesenteric and portal venous systems.[26–28] It has been estimated that by 45 years of age, 50% of individuals with familial protein S deficiency will have experienced a venous thrombotic event.[29] Overall, and as discussed for protein C deficiency, this may be an overestimate. A report of the European Prospective Cohort on Thrombophilia (EPCOT) study showed that the incidence per 1000 years of a venous thrombotic event in affected first-degree relatives of index patients with protein S deficiency is 7.1 compared with the incidence in unaffected controls.[21] As with protein C-deficient subjects, the risk of venous thrombosis is further increased in those with familial protein S deficiency and another independent inherited risk factor for venous thrombosis.[30]

Protein S levels are affected by a variety of physiological and pathophysiological conditions and acquired protein S deficiency is therefore not uncommon. Protein S levels are lower in women than in men and protein S falls progressively during pregnancy.[31,32] It is also reduced in women receiving oestrogen-containing oral contraceptives. Clinical conditions associated with acquired protein S deficiency include coumarin use, liver disease, bacterial and viral infections and disseminated intravascular coagulation.[33] In the context of thrombophilia screening, reports of an association between antiphospholipid antibodies, including lupus anticoagulants, and acquired protein S deficiency are of particular interest,[34] since both abnormalities are associated with thrombosis.

From the above discussion it is clear that great care should be taken when interpreting protein S results and a diagnosis of familial protein S deficiency should not be confirmed until a possible acquired deficiency state has been confidently excluded. The exclusion of antiphospholipid antibodies, including the lupus anticoagulant, in an individual with thrombosis and identified as having protein S deficiency is clearly of paramount importance.

Activated protein resistance/factor V Leiden

In 1993, Dahlbäck et al.[35] reported their findings in a family with dominant thrombophilia but with no evidence of deficiency of antithrombin, protein C or protein S. A consistent abnormality was resistance of the patients' plasma to prolongation of the activated partial thromboplastin time (APTT) following the addition of APC. In the same year the same abnormality was demonstrated in 20% of patients presenting with venous thromboembolism.[36] In 1994, Bertina et al.[37] in Leiden demonstrated that the basis for the phenomenon of familial APC resistance was the presence of an abnormal factor V molecule that was resistant to proteolytic degradation by APC. The abnormality was shown to be a single point mutation at nucleotide 1691 in the factor V gene resulting in the replacement of arginine by glutamine in the factor V protein. This effectively removed one of the three cleavage sites for APC. The genetic abnormality is frequently referred to as factor V Leiden (FVL).

FVL is commonly found in Europe, with a median prevalence of 4.4%.[38] The prevalence of FVL is higher in northern Europe (3.4–7.9%) than in southern Europe (0.6–2.9%). In the USA, there is a higher prevalence in Caucasians (3–7.6%) than in African Americans (0.6%).[33] The mutation is rare in Asia (1.0%) and absent in Africa.[33] Worldwide, FVL is the commonest cause of familial thrombophilia. Published prevalence data are markedly influenced by the method of patient selection. For example, in the UK the prevalence of FVL in the general population is approximately 4%. This figure rises to 20% in consecutive patients with venous thrombosis and to 45% in selected patients with family histories of thrombophilia.[19]

The risk of a venous thrombotic event in an individual heterozygous for FVL is substantially increased in those with an additional genetic risk factor such as protein C or protein S deficiency.[22] In addition, the risk of venous thrombosis recurrence is also greater in those with combined genetic defects[39,40] compared with that in individuals with single defects. Homozygotes for FVL are also at higher risk of venous thrombosis compared with heterozygotes.

DVT and PE are the predominant features of FVL. However, and as with the other types of familial thrombophilia, thrombosis can also occur in more unusual sites, for example within the cerebral venous system.[41]

Prothrombin 20210A mutation

In 1996, Poort et al.[42] reported a new type of familial thrombophilia characterised by a G→A mutation in the 3′ untranslated portion of the prothrombin gene at position 20210 and associated with an increased plasma concentration of prothrombin. The prevalence of the mutation is low in African populations and approximately 1% in Caucasians. In contrast to FVL, the prevalence of prothrombin 20210A is higher in southern Europe than in northern Europe.[43] The reported prevalence of the mutation in a Spanish population was approximately 6%, which represents the commonest form of familial thrombophilia in that country.[44]

The relative risk of venous thrombosis is approximately fourfold compared with that of non-carriers[45] and this becomes higher in individuals with combined FVL and prothrombin 20210A.

Who should be tested for familial thrombophilia?

More and more individuals are being tested for possible familial thrombophilia but unselected patient testing introduces important clinical and cost-effectiveness issues that need to be addressed.[46] Surprisingly, there is no evidence to support the view that the identification of familial thrombophilia is of value in decisions relating to the choice of anticoagulant or to the intensity and duration of treatment. In most instances of venous thrombosis the identification of familial thrombophilia is unlikely to have any impact on the clinical management of that patient.

For these reasons the Haemostasis and Thrombosis Task Force, a subcommittee of the British Society for Haematology, has published the following recommendations in respect of the selection of patients for testing for familial thrombophilia.

- Testing of unselected patients is inappropriate and should be avoided.
- Haematologists must give guidance to clinical colleagues on the selection of patients for testing.
- In respect of familial thrombophilia, in most instances any value of laboratory testing will relate to the possibility of preventing a first venous thromboembolic event in affected relatives.
- Testing for possible familial thrombophilia, and particularly genetic testing, should be avoided in children unless there is a very strong clinical indication for it.

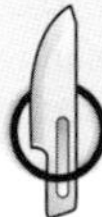

ACQUIRED RISK FACTORS

It is now accepted that venous thrombosis is multifactorial in origin. Causal factors may be genetic, environmental or a combination of the two.[47] Environmental risk factors for venous thrombosis can be demonstrated in approximately 50% of patients presenting with venous thrombosis. These include recent surgery, immobilisation, hospitalisation, application of a plaster cast, pregnancy (including the puerperium) and long-distance travel. Malignancy is a potent risk factor for venous thrombosis and consideration should be given to this possibility when unexpected venous thrombosis occurs in middle-aged or elderly individuals (**Box 17.2**).

The influence of extraneous factors on venous thrombosis is well illustrated by the impact of oral contraceptive use on venous thrombotic risk. Results obtained by the Leiden Thrombophilia Study indicate that the relative risk of venous thrombosis is approximately fourfold for women who do not have FVL but who take oral contraceptives. The relative risk for venous thrombosis is slightly higher (approximately fivefold) for a woman with FVL but who is not taking oral contraceptives. However, if a woman with FVL takes oral contraceptives, then the risk of venous thrombosis increases to approximately 35-fold,[48] which far exceeds the sum of the separate risks and strongly suggests an interaction between FVL and the use of oral contraceptives. A similar interaction is observed with regard to

Box 17.2 • Acquired risk factors for venous thromboembolism

- Immobility
- Trauma
- Surgery
- Oestrogens
- Obesity
- Previous deep vein thrombosis
- Congestive cardiac failure
- Malignancy
- Nephrotic syndrome
- Advancing age
- Hyperviscosity syndrome
- Primary antiphospholipid syndrome
- Behçet's syndrome
- Paroxysmal nocturnal haemoglobinuria
- Heparin-induced thrombocytopenia

cerebral thrombosis in oral contraceptive users with FVL or prothrombin 20210A. Thus, both are known risk factors for cerebral vein thrombosis[49,50] but the risk of cerebral thrombosis in women using oral contraceptives and possessing either prothrombin 20210A or FVL is much greater than the sum of the separate risks associated with these two factors.

Primary antiphospholipid syndrome

In this syndrome, both arterial and venous thrombosis are associated with the persistent presence in the plasma of antiphospholipid antibodies (APAs). Most commonly these antibodies are directed against cardiolipin (i.e. anticardiolipin antibodies) or are manifest as lupus anticoagulant. The latter is a misnomer in that paradoxically it suggests a relationship with a bleeding disorder, whereas in fact it is a risk factor for thrombosis. Initially, the lupus anticoagulant was considered to relate specifically to systemic lupus erythematosus but it is now known that it can be a feature of other autoimmune disorders and can also occur as an isolated abnormality.

Poor pregnancy outcome is also a feature of the primary antiphospholipid syndrome. Recurrent miscarriage characteristically occurs during early pregnancy or in the mid-trimester period.

Since APAs are heterogeneous, a comprehensive laboratory approach is necessary for their diagnosis. Some patients with arterial and/or venous thrombosis have lupus anticoagulant only, others lupus anticoagulant and anticardiolipin antibodies, and others anticardiolipin antibodies only. It is therefore recommended that laboratory screening should include at least two sensitive coagulation assays, usually the kaolin–cephalin clotting time and the dilute Russell's viper venom time for the detection of lupus anticoagulant, as well as solid-phase assays for anticardiolipin antibodies. APAs, including lupus anticoagulant, may interfere with protein S assays, producing apparent acquired protein S deficiency.[51,52] Great care should therefore be taken to exclude the presence of APAs before accepting as confirmed a diagnosis of familial protein S deficiency. An important clinical feature of the primary antiphospholipid syndrome is the high recurrence rate of venous thrombotic events.

DIAGNOSIS OF DVT

The clinical diagnosis of DVT is generally thought to be unreliable but Wells et al.[53] have shown that the use of a clinical model can stratify patients with suspected DVT into high, moderate or low probability groups (**Box 17.3**). The use of such a model can simplify the diagnostic process by excluding low-probability patients with a normal duplex scan or venogram from further testing.

Box 17.3 • Clinical diagnosis of deep vein thrombosis (DVT)

Major criteria
Active cancer
Paralysis or recent plaster immobilisation of leg
Recently bedridden (>3 days) or major surgery (<4 weeks)
Past history of DVT or strong family history
Thigh and calf swelling
Calf swelling 3 cm greater than asymptomatic side
Minor criteria
History of recent leg trauma (<60 days)
Hospitalisation within the last 6 months
Unilateral pitting oedema
Unilateral erythema or dilated superficial veins
CLINICAL PROBABILITY
High
More than three major points and no alternative diagnosis
More than two major points and more than two minor points and no alternative diagnosis
Low
One major point plus more than two minor points and alternative diagnosis
One major point plus more than one minor point and no alternative diagnosis
No major points plus more than three minor points and alternative diagnosis
No major points plus more than two minor points and no alternative diagnosis
Moderate
All other combinations

After Wells PS, Hirsch J, Anderson DR et al. Accuracy of clinical assessment of deep vein thrombosis. Elsevier (The Lancet 1995; 345:1326–30) with permission.

D-dimer assays

In the clotting process, cleavage of a small peptide, fibrinopeptide A, from adjacent fibrinogen molecules results in fibrin monomer formation. This is followed by polymerisation and the production of insoluble fibrin. The fibrin polymers are stabilised through cross-linking, which is catalysed by activated factor XIII. Cross-linked fibrin is the basis of the stable thrombus. Thrombus formation is accompanied by an immediate fibrinolytic response and digestion of the cross-linked fibrin occurs through plasmin cleavage. This results in the formation and release into the plasma of a variety of cleavage fragments. These include D-dimers that retain the γ–γ links derived from the original fibrinogen γ-chains.

Active thrombus formation with accompanying fibrinolysis is therefore characterised by increased plasma D-dimer concentrations. The corollary of this is that normal D-dimer levels argue against ongoing thrombosis. This is the underlying principle for employing sensitive assays for D-dimer determination that have a high negative predictive value for the diagnosis of venous thrombosis. High plasma D-dimer levels should be interpreted with much more caution since levels are frequently increased in hospitalised patients, particularly in those with malignancy and infection and during the immediate postoperative period.

Currently, a variety of quantitative and qualitative methods are available for D-dimer determination. Techniques include turbidimetry, latex particle agglutination, fluorescence immunoassay, immunofiltration and enzyme-linked immunosorbent assay. There is considerable variability in their sensitivity and performance and it is essential that laboratories confine themselves to those assays and test systems that have demonstrated adequate sensitivity and specificity in properly conducted clinical studies. Assays employing latex bead agglutination for the diagnosis of disseminated intravascular coagulation are not suitable for the exclusion of DVT.[54] An assessment of the utility of different D-dimer assays for exclusion of DVT was performed by van der Graaf et al.,[55] who compared the results of 13 different assays in the same group of patients with suspected DVT.

Ultrasonography

B-mode ultrasound is widely available and relatively inexpensive. The lumen of a patent vein is usually anechoic, whereas thrombus within a vein, depending on the age, usually demonstrates internal echoes (**Fig. 17.1**). Static or slow-flowing venous blood may contain echoes and thereby mimic thrombus. However, thrombus is only slightly compressible unlike the lumen of a patent vein, the walls of which are easily opposed by external compression. By using this simple technique, thrombus within the large veins of the thigh and popliteal region can be diagnosed with a sensitivity and specificity of 90% and 99% respectively.[56]

Duplex ultrasound scanning refers to a combination of real-time B-mode grey-scale ultrasound

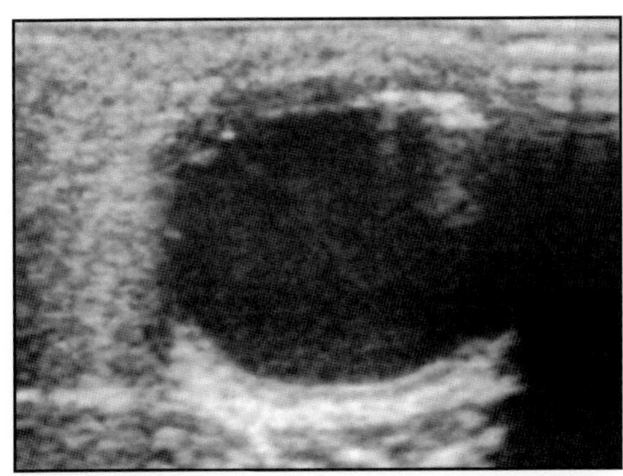

(a)

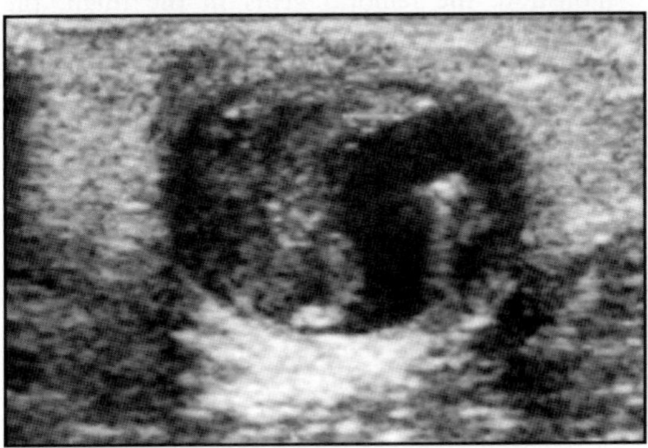

(b)

Figure 17.1 • Grey-scale ultrasound. **(a)** Normal common femoral vein with echo-free lumen. This was freely compressible. **(b)** Common femoral vein with mixed echogenic material consistent with fresh thrombus. This was only partly compressible.

imaging with pulsed Doppler, which provides information on blood velocity. It is most useful for encoding the average frequency shift by superimposing a colour scale onto the image in order to demonstrate the average flow within patent areas of vessels (colour flow Doppler). Areas of no flow due to thrombus show up black against the colour flow.

There are two main strategies employed in ultrasound scanning. The first is simply to identify patients at risk from PE, i.e. those with thrombus in large veins, including popliteal, superficial femoral, and iliac veins. It is common practice in those patients with normal veins above the tibial veins, and who may not receive anticoagulant therapy, to re-scan at 2 weeks to exclude proximal propagation of thrombus. The second strategy involves the extension of these techniques into the calf region in an attempt to demonstrate more localised thrombosis. However, it is often time-consuming to demonstrate all groups of the deep calf vein plexus. Using a combination of colour flow Doppler, real-time scanning and external compression of the veins, or augmentation of flow by other means, a high degree of confidence in the demonstration of calf vein thrombosis can be achieved.

The demonstration of pelvic veins, including the iliac veins, is particularly challenging when bowel gas obscures the retroperitoneum. Isolated common iliac vein thrombosis is likely to be missed by inexperienced operators, particularly if this possibility is not raised on the request form.

Venography

Venography is performed by injection of contrast into a superficial vein on the foot. A single injection of 30–40 mL of contrast may be used to completely demonstrate the femoral veins in the thigh, the external and common iliac veins and the lower inferior vena cava (IVC).[57] If the iliac vessels are not well shown, direct injection into the common femoral vein in the groin will produce a full anatomical demonstration. If direct venography demonstrates occlusion of the iliac system, then contralateral common femoral puncture can be performed to demonstrate the extent, if any, of propagation of thrombus into the IVC (**Fig. 17.2**). Imaging of the iliac veins is a major advantage of venography over duplex scanning. However, venography damages the endothelium of the veins and can itself cause venous thrombosis.

Other diagnostic techniques

COMPUTED TOMOGRAPHY

Although not widely used in the imaging of peripheral venous occlusion, computed tomography (CT), particularly with intravenous contrast enhancement, can be very useful in the diagnosis of central venous occlusion and is being used increasingly in peripheral venous thrombosis. The specific advantages of CT include the ability to demonstrate thrombus within all veins including internal iliac veins, the generation of axial images to demonstrate any extrinsic compressive lesion and the ability to show abdominal tumours associated with venous thrombosis, such as pancreatic cancer. CT may play a role in selection of patients for thrombolysis, those with hyperdense and therefore recent thrombus being more likely to respond rapidly to lytic therapy.[58]

MAGNETIC RESONANCE STUDIES

Magnetic resonance imaging (MRI) and magnetic resonance angiography can be applied to both peripheral and central venous systems. MRI is used to demonstrate the presence of patent veins or the presence of thrombus within vessels. Magnetic resonance venography is solely used to demonstrate the presence of patent vessels. By using a combination of time-of-flight, phase contrast and contrast-enhanced protocols, peripheral and central veins can be shown (**Fig. 17.3**). Multiplanar imaging studies allow diagnosis of extrinsic vascular compression and may show intrinsic venous disease such as damaged valves or venous webs. Magnetic resonance angiography has established a central role in the imaging of veno-occlusive disease, its utility only inhibited by expense and relative scarcity of machines.

PLETHYSMOGRAPHY

Mercury strain gauge and impedance plethysmography demonstrate changes in the volume of the limb

(a)

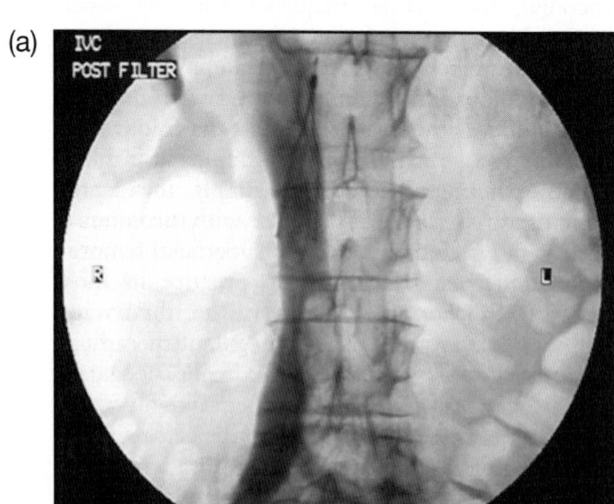

(b)

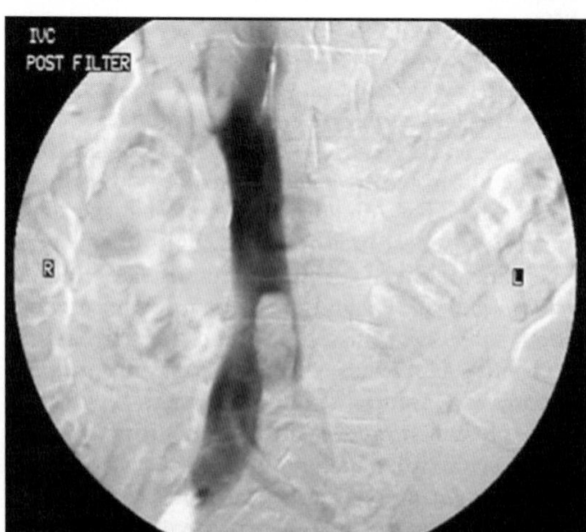

Figure 17.2 • Ascending venogram **(a)** without and **(b)** with digital subtraction. Right common femoral vein injection after a Günther Tulip inferior vena cava (IVC) filter has been deployed. A tongue of non-adherent thrombus is shown propagating into the IVC from the thrombosed left common iliac vein.

(a)

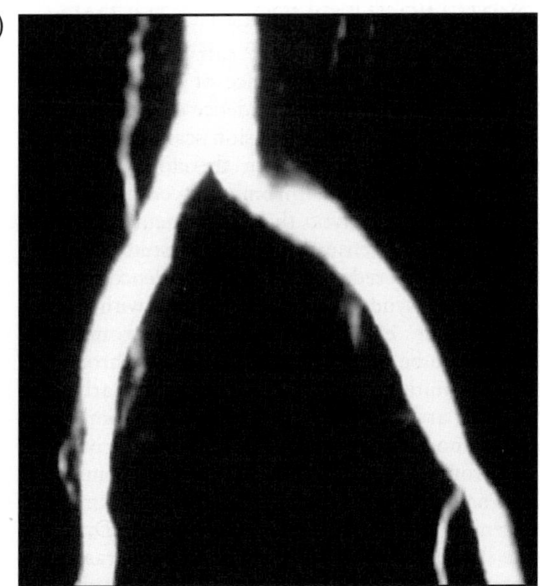

(b)

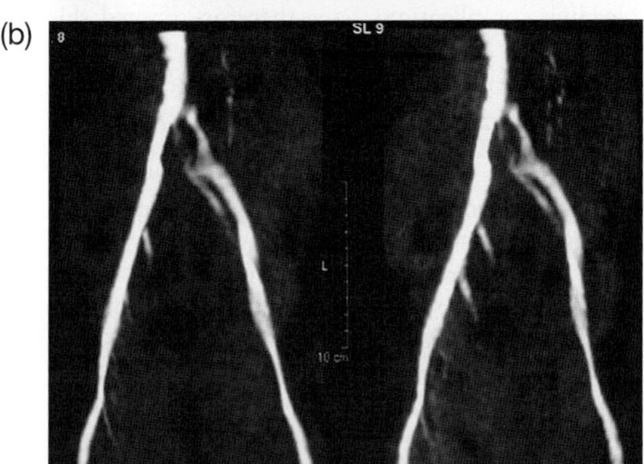

Figure 17.3 • **(a)** Time-of-flight magnetic resonance venogram. A normal study with cranial presaturation to null signal in arteries. A normal minor impression is seen on the left iliac vein and a small right ascending lumbar vein is shown. **(b)** Time-of-flight magnetic resonance venogram with cranial presaturation to null signal in arteries. There is a severe left common iliac stenosis with bridging collateral vein.

during occlusion of venous outflow by a pneumatic tourniquet and after release of the occlusion. They demonstrate the effect of venous obstruction proximal to the detector and thus these methods cannot reliably demonstrate DVT that develops, and remains, below the knee. These techniques are usually employed in studies of populations at increased risk of DVT and are not universally available.[59]

RADIOISOTOPE IMAGING

The demonstration of leg and central venous occlusion has been pursued using isotope labelling of various agents. Isotope-labelled fibrinogen can demonstrate calf thrombus but has been shown to be unreliable in demonstrating more proximal thrombus, particularly when causing complete occlusion. If thrombus is not being actively formed, fibrinogen will not be bound and the study will be falsely negative. Pulmonary emboli are not demonstrated by labelled fibrinogen scans. Labelled platelets suffer from poor specificity but there are great hopes for new agents, which include those that bind to fibrinogen receptors on activated platelets and labelled antibodies that bind to fibrin. It is likely that these agents will have a major role in the investigation of venous thrombosis within the next decade.

NON-LIMB-THREATENING DVT

Calf DVT

Thromboses can form in any part of the venous system but the vast majority arise in the vein valve pockets in the soleal veins of the calf .[60] Proximal extension of isolated calf vein thrombosis occurs in 10–29% of cases. DVT has a clinical spectrum of severity ranging from asymptomatic isolated thrombosis of the tibial veins detectable only with radiolabelled fibrinogen studies to the life- and limb-threatening phlegmasia caerulea dolens (PCD) and venous gangrene. The severity of the clinical syndrome depends on the extent of thrombosis present and the speed of progression. Anticoagulation with heparin and warfarin remains the mainstay of modern treatment. These work by halting clot propagation, reducing the risk of PE and optimising clot resolution by fibrinolysis. The natural history of DVT treated with anticoagulant is of collateral vessel formation with endogenous clot fibrinolysis leading to vessel recanalisation over weeks or months. There is usually damage to the venous valves, with resulting chronic venous incompetence and the post-thrombotic syndrome. There appears to be a relationship between early recanalisation and preservation of venous valvular competence but this is by no means straightforward. Eklov and co-workers have shown by meticulous duplex ultrasound studies that valvular incompetence is common in venous segments adjacent to thrombosed calf veins but not in thrombosed recanalised venous segments.[61] The basic paradox is that early recanalisation and preservation of vein wall and valve function must be accomplished before inflammatory change occurs in the vessel wall. However, before phlebitis and periphlebitis become established, the limb is usually completely asymptomatic and by the time the patient develops symptoms it is already too late.

Iliofemoral DVT

Much confusion surrounds the reporting and outcome of treatment of iliofemoral DVT. There are two forms of iliofemoral DVT. The first occurs when calf vein thrombus propagates centrally to involve the popliteal, femoral and iliac segments and which may then propagate to the IVC. The thrombus is frequently poorly adherent to the vein wall and will often have a free-floating proximal segment. The potential for massive PE is very high.

The second form of iliofemoral DVT occurs when the thrombus originates in the iliac vein with distal propagation into the femoral vein with or without caval extension. This disease is normally the result of extrinsic vein compression, typically by a gravid uterus, nodes or crossing vessel or by intrinsic vein wall disease when there is a venous web or spur (itself usually associated with chronic compression by a crossing vessel).[62] When this latter disease is restricted to the iliac veins, with or without femoral involvement, the potential for PE is small. When there is caval propagation, and particularly when the thrombus is not adherent, the potential for embolisation is high.

Both forms of the disease contain a large volume of thrombus, and recanalisation with restoration of normal vein function is unlikely. However, the iliac venous segment is functionally a simple conduit and restoration of a patent channel without obstruction to flow may be sufficient to re-establish normal venous return from the limb.

Principles of management of DVT

Historically, unfractionated heparin and warfarin form the mainstay of treatment of DVT and prevention of PE. The more recent low-molecular-weight heparins have provided more convenient, reliable and safer alternatives.[63] A course of adequate anticoagulation therapy can reduce the risk of recurrent venous thrombosis from 29–47% to 5–7%. The incidence of fatal PE following DVT on adequate anticoagulation is very low (0.4–1.5%). Conventional anticoagulation is largely ineffective in preventing post-thrombotic syndrome, with valvular insufficiency occurring in 28% at 5 years. Systemic thrombolysis leads to more rapid, more effective venous recanalisation of thrombosed veins than anticoagulants alone. An association has been demonstrated between early recanalisation and preservation of venous valvular competence, with reduction in the severity of post-thrombotic syndrome.

SYSTEMIC THROMBOLYTIC THERAPY

Thrombolytic treatment of calf vein thrombosis does not reduce the incidence of symptomatic PE and in fact increases the incidence of asymptomatic emboli on ventilation–perfusion scanning. The role of thrombolytic therapy is therefore limited to reducing local post-thrombotic complications. Systemic thrombolytic therapy in acute DVT has been studied extensively, with most studies demonstrating some reduction in the incidence of post-thrombotic syndrome when compared with heparin alone. The efficacy of systemic thrombolysis appears to be related to the duration of thrombosis and the initial thrombus burden. Particularly poor results are seen when systemic thrombolysis starts more than 2 weeks after the first onset of symptoms. Despite potential benefits, thrombolysis has had disappointing results in the treatment of extensive iliofemoral thrombosis and PCD, where the large volumes of thrombus can rarely be completely lysed.[64] The associated high risks of bleeding complications have therefore limited this technique.

LOCAL–REGIONAL THROMBOLYTIC THERAPY

This refers to the delivery of pharmacological thrombolytic agents directly into the thrombus. This technique maximises local doses while minimising the systemic thrombolytic effect and therefore haemorrhagic complications. Two approaches have been adopted. The first technique is catheter-directed regional therapy, in which the thrombolytic drug is infused directly into the clot via percutaneous catheters and specialised infusion wires. The delivery catheter is usually placed from the contralateral femoral vein (if patent) or from the internal jugular vein, or frequently both. Because of the high risk of PE during the treatment, it is advisable to place a temporary filter in the infrarenal IVC via one of these approaches, although the internal jugular or brachial vein approach is the most convenient. The infusion catheter can be safely passed through the filter and embedded in the thrombus. One advantage of this method is that the entire venous system may be evaluated prior to starting therapy. The second technique is flow-directed regional therapy, in which high doses of thrombolytic agents are infused into an ipsilateral dorsal foot vein. Most of the flow is directed into the deep venous system via tourniquets. This method is more time-consuming, requires higher doses of thrombolytics but allows more effective treatment of the smaller crural veins.

Historically the most widely used thrombolytic agent has been urokinase, but a number of protocols involving other agents have been evaluated with similar outcome and side-effect profiles. Currently, the most widely used agent is tPA. Thrombolytic therapy seems most effective in the acute thrombus (<3 days) and becomes increasingly less effective in thrombus older than 4 weeks. Early series of catheter-directed thrombolysis reported complete or substantial recanalisation rates of 60–83%. The National Venous Thrombolysis Registry provides the largest published series to date; 287 patients (303 limbs) from multiple centres were followed up at 1 year following catheter-directed thrombolysis.[65] Complete thrombolysis was achieved in 31% and partial (>50%) thrombolysis in 52% of patients. The procedure was more successful in acute DVT and in those with no previous history of DVT. There was an 11% incidence of major bleeding (requiring transfusion) and a 16% incidence of minor bleeding, with a procedure-related mortality of 0.4%. The overall 12-month primary patency rate was 80%, with better results in the iliofemoral than femoro-popliteal segments. The overall rate of valvular reflux was 58%, but was only 28% in those who underwent complete thrombolysis. Other complications include sepsis and traumatic valvular incompetence.

PERCUTANEOUS MECHANICAL THROMBECTOMY

Percutaneous mechanical thrombectomy (PMT) refers to the use of mechanical energy to disperse thrombus using a percutaneous device and includes any combination of mechanical dissolution, fragmentation and aspiration. The combination of catheter-directed pharmacological thrombolytic therapy and PMT has become an effective means of rapid ablation of venous thrombus, particularly in situations where there are contraindications to aggressive or prolonged thrombolytic therapy. In extensive DVT, where rapid venous decompression and restoration of flow is crucial, PMT can restore a venous channel, debulk thrombus and increase the surface area of thrombus exposed to the pharmacological agent.

PMT carries a risk of fragment embolisation, but meticulous aspiration and recirculation techniques, pharmacological thrombolytics and protective IVC filters can reduce the size of particles reaching the lungs. However, PMT devices can themselves cause damage to venous valves, resulting in chronic venous insufficiency and post-thrombotic syndrome. There is evidence that proper technique, such as introducing the device via large conduits and with the direction of flow, can reduce such damage.

Techniques and devices

There are a number of commercially available devices that have been used extensively in both the arterial and venous systems. These can be classified into the following categories.

Percutaneous aspiration thrombectomy In this technique, thrombus is sucked out through a large-lumen aspiration catheter. A vascular sheath is inserted and the thrombus crossed with an appropriate catheter/guidewire combination. The aspiration catheter, which has a large lumen and a non-tapered tip, is then advanced over the wire until it abuts the leading edge of the clot. The wire is then withdrawn and steady suction applied with a large syringe. Soft thrombus will remodel and pass through the catheter, while firmer clot will lodge in the end of the catheter and can be removed by withdrawing the catheter through the sheath while maintaining back-pressure on the syringe. The most extensively researched devices have comparable efficacy to surgical thrombectomy, with lower associated mortality and morbidity.

Pull-back thrombectomy and trapping This technique uses a balloon catheter or basket to pull thrombus back into a trapping device, enabling it to be removed. These devices include the Greenfield transvenous pulmonary embolectomy, which consists of a steerable balloon-tipped catheter with a vacuum cup to hold the thrombus, and the self-expanding tulip sheath, a modified self-expanding wallstent that forms a cone to catch thrombus pulled back by a 4-Fr coaxial Fogarty balloon catheter.

Recirculation mechanical thrombectomy These devices generate a hydrodynamic vortex. An example is the Amplatz rotational thrombectomy device (**Fig. 17.4a**), which comprises a catheter with a rotating coaxial metal impeller housed within a protective cage at its distal end. The impeller rotates at 150 000 rpm, creating a vortex that traps and pulverises thrombus. An example of an alternative approach is the Angiojet device, which employs multiple high-speed retrograde fluid jets to create an area of low pressure that pulls fragments of thrombus into the catheter tip (Venturi effect). In both devices, the pulverised fragments are returned to the circulation via side holes.

Non-recirculation mechanical thrombectomy This technique is similar to recirculation mechanical thrombectomy but there is no recirculation and larger fragments are released into the circulation. This includes the Treratola (Arrow, USA) device (**Fig. 17.4b**, see also Plate 14, facing p. 116).

Other devices These devices use ultrasonic, radiofrequency or laser energy, either directly or indirectly, to fragment clot. There are currently no

(a)

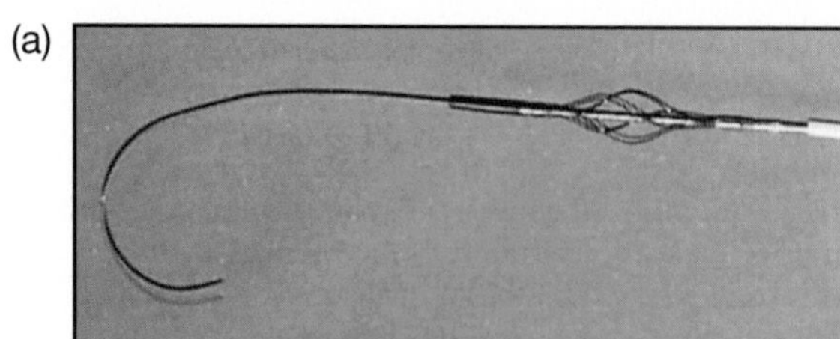

(b)

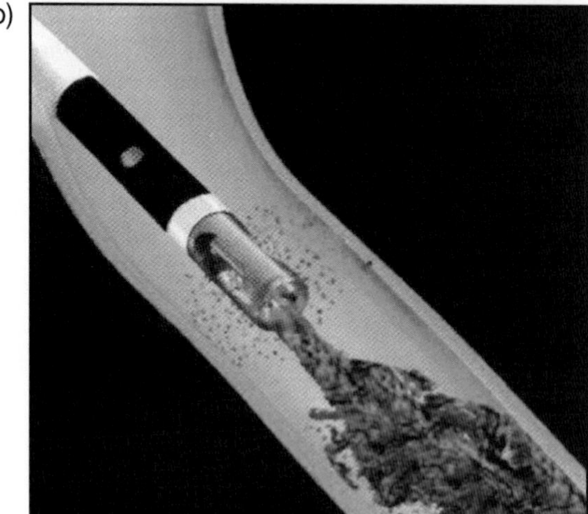

Figure 17.4 • (a) Amplatz rotational thrombectomy device. **(b)** Arrow Treratola mechanical thrombectomy device.

prospective trials comparing the efficacy or complication rates of any of these devices in the venous system.

SURGICAL VENOUS THROMBECTOMY

Venous thrombectomy will successfully clear thrombus from the major veins, relieving the major site of venous occlusion, but will not clear any thromboses involving the venular or capillary circulation. The results of this operation in severe PCD with venous gangrene are therefore poor.[66] Initial enthusiasm for this procedure in the 1960s focused on the benefits of reduction of not only the risks of PE but also acute venous wall damage, with the goal of reducing the incidence of post-thrombotic syndrome. Indeed, impressive early results of venous thrombectomy performed within 10 days of onset of iliofemoral thrombosis (without PCD or venous gangrene) reported 85% patency rates and minimal symptoms of post-thrombotic syndrome.[67] However, later studies found high rethrombosis rates and significant morbidity from late post-thrombotic syndrome on long-term follow-up.[68,69] These poor long-term results and high operative morbidity and mortality has led to reduced enthusiasm in surgical venous thrombectomy. The main indications now are failure of anticoagulant therapy or impending venous gangrene.[70] More recently, improved outcomes of venous thrombectomy have been reported (80% patency of iliac vein), particularly from Europe, with use of adjunctive arteriovenous fistulas and attention to relieving proximal venous obstruction in the common iliac veins.[71]

If the venous occlusion cannot be treated, a cross-over bypass (Palma procedure) can be performed in the presence of a patent contralateral iliac vein and IVC. The tributaries of the contralateral long saphenous vein are ligated and the vein transected just above the knee. The vein is then tunnelled subcutaneously and anastomosed to the ipsilateral common femoral vein. Early patency rates can be improved by performing a side-to-side vein-to-vein anastomosis and temporary end-to-side arterio-venous fistula.[72] Similarly, with long-term anti-coagulation and the use of an arteriovenous fistula, the patency of ring-supported PTFE grafts from the ipsilateral common femoral vein to the contra-lateral iliac vein has been improved.[73,74]

LIMB-THREATENING DVT

Severe and extensive iliofemoral DVT causes a swollen, white, painful leg known as phlegmasia alba dolens (PAD). In contrast, PCD is characterised by an acutely swollen cyanotic limb, classically with an extreme constant bursting pain (**Fig. 17.5a**, see also Plate 15a, facing p. 116). PCD arises when there is extension of thrombosis into the venules and capillaries with secondary development of acute arterial ischaemia. Complete occlusion of the major leg veins alone will often result only in a syndrome of PAD and not PCD.[75] PCD is usually associated with extensive thrombosis that involves the distal limb and progresses proximally. In up to half of cases, PCD will progress to venous gangrene and this invariably starts distally in the toes and foot and progresses proximally.[76] PCD occurs when there is almost total microvascular occlusion of venous outflow from the limb, resulting in a massive increase in capillary hydrostatic pressure with outpouring of fluid and massive interstitial oedema.[77] Pressures in the tissues may increase up to fivefold, with major plasma sequestration into an affected limb of up to 6–10 L, accounting for the shock commonly seen in this condition.[78]

Where there is either little or moderate compromise of the arterial circulation, a reversible syndrome of PCD without venous gangrene develops. Typically, after a period of 1–2 days and in up to 50% of patients, venous gangrene will supervene secondary to arterial impairment. The mechanism of this arterial compromise seems to be mainly hydrostatic.

(a)

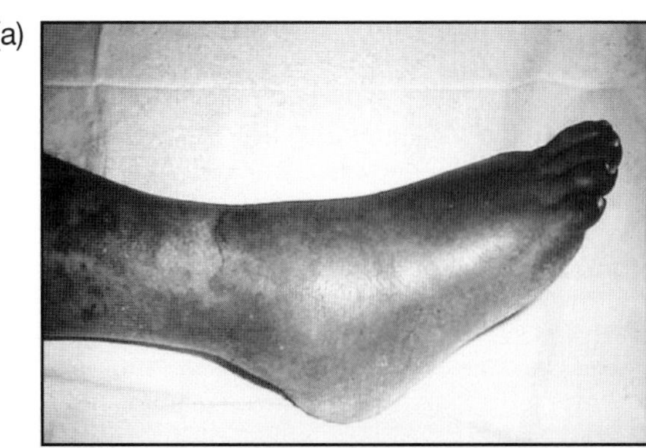

(b)

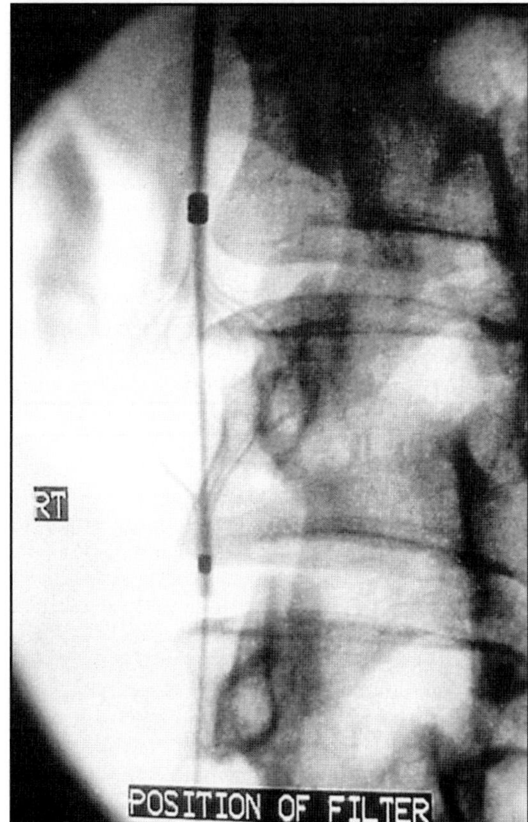

(c)

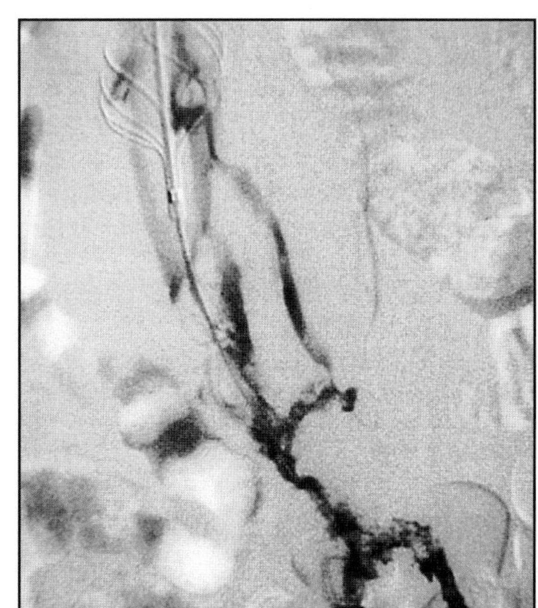

(d)

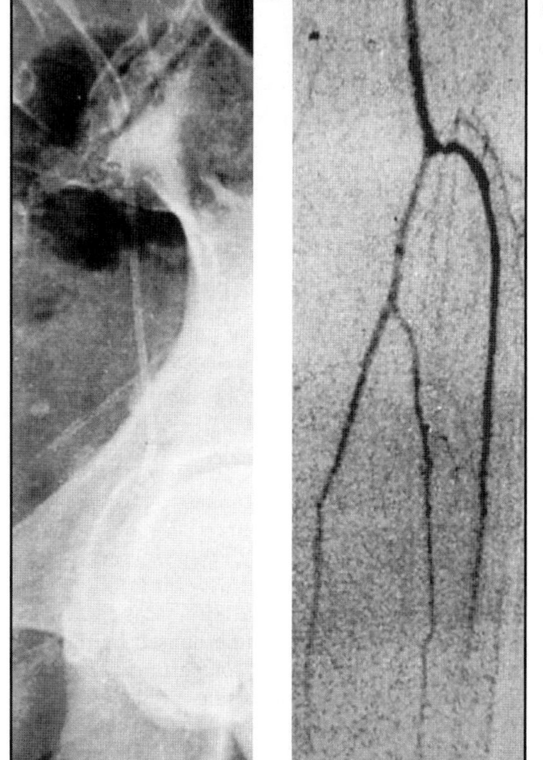

Figure 17.5 • **(a)** Acutely swollen cyanotic limb of phlegmasia caerulea dolens (PCD) before treatment in a patient with carcinoma of the colon. **(b,c)** Venous thrombolysis. A temporary filter has been introduced via a jugular approach and a venogram demonstrates extensive inferior vena caval and left iliac venous thrombus. An infusion of tissue plasminogen activator was commenced at 0.5 mg/hour. **(d)** Concomitant arterial thrombolysis (0.5 mg/hour) via a catheter in the left femoral artery using a contralateral femoral approach has been administered to lyse the capillary bed. Initial flow to the lower limb was very sluggish, taking 35 seconds to reach the calf.

(e)

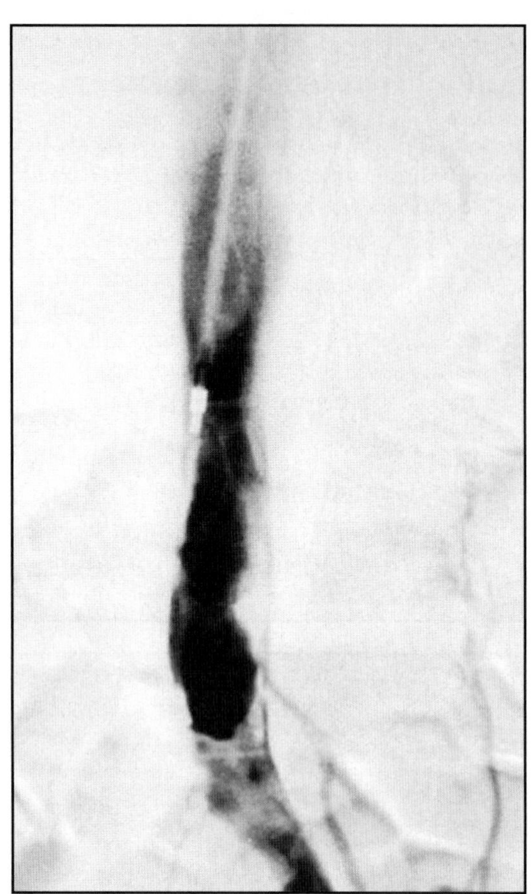

(f)

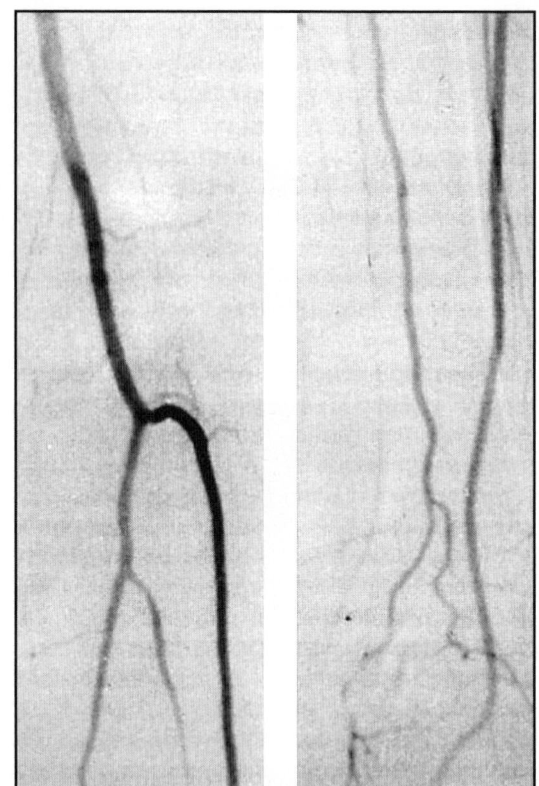

(g)

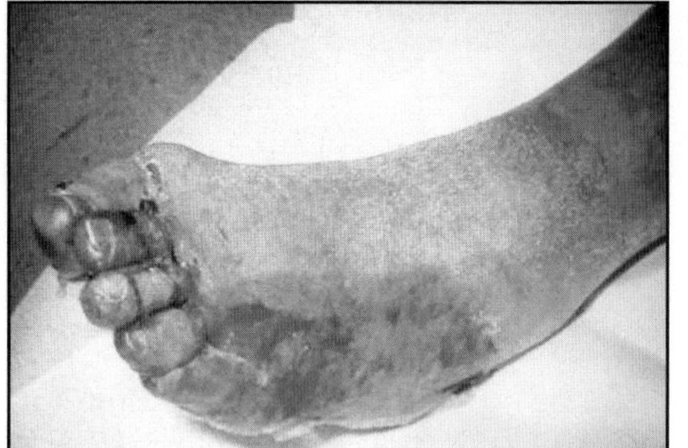

Figure 17.5 • (*cont.*) **(e,f)** After 24 hours of arterial and venous thrombolysis, the inferior vena cava has improved flow and the capillaries have opened up; there is also more rapid flow to the calf, with vessel filling at 7 seconds. **(g)** Limb salvage has been achieved at 3 days.

Capillary flow is further compromised by the high interstitial (intramuscular or compartment) pressures overcoming the critical closing pressures of the arterioles and small peripheral arteries resulting in their collapse.[79] This probably explains the late development of venous gangrene commonly seen in untreated PCD. Arterial spasm has been implicated but there is little evidence to support this as an important pathophysiological mechanism.

PCD develops in hypercoagulable states, with an underlying cause being found in 90% of cases.[80] Underlying malignant disease is the major cause of hypercoagulability, particularly where there is venous gangrene, and this may be the presenting symptom of a previously unsuspected malignancy.[81] In the absence of a malignant cause, an underlying thrombophilia should be suspected, particularly APC resistance and/or antiphospholipid syndrome. PCD can complicate the secondary hypercoagulable states after major surgery or trauma, the puerperal period, radiotherapy, prolonged immobilisation and in chronic inflammatory conditions, particularly relapse of ulcerative colitis.[82,83]

PCD is most common in the fifth and sixth decades of life. There is an equal sex distribution and the left leg is involved almost three times more often than the right, probably as a result of the left iliac vein compression syndrome.[83] There is usually a progression of symptoms in the lower limb from PAD to the cyanosis and extreme pain of PCD over 1–2 days (but this may be more rapid). The affected limb becomes massively swollen and very tense, with distal cyanosis a constant feature. The skin often develops cutaneous bullae and in venous gangrene there is a striking non-blanching purplish/black mottling of the skin. The pain involves the entire limb and is typically intense and bursting in nature. Peripheral pulses are extremely difficult to feel because of the oedema but may be detected with the Doppler probe. Arterial hypotension secondary to hypervolaemia can be severe. The literature overall reports an amputation rate of 50% with a mortality of 20%. PE is common, particularly in venous gangrene, with an incidence of 12–40%.[70]

Diagnosis is largely clinical, although duplex venography is extremely useful in documenting the extent of venous thrombosis and is now the investigation of choice. Venography is technically extremely difficult and meaningful information in the presence of extensive iliofemoral thrombosis can only be obtained by descending venography via a contralateral femoral or brachial approach. Angiography is of little diagnostic value, usually showing only peripheral arterial constriction in severe cases, but is often performed where the diagnosis of PCD and venous gangrene has not been considered or where there is doubt.

Management of PCD

PCD is a medical emergency. Initial management is directed at improving tissue perfusion by resuscitation with intravenous fluids to treat the hypovolaemic shock, and bed rest with aggressive limb elevation to reduce limb oedema and thus the high interstitial pressures. This is best achieved by elevating the leg on a wedge or by some form of gallows traction to optimise venous and lymphatic drainage. The simple use of pillows is not adequate. Immediate anticoagulation with intravenous heparin to achieve and maintain an APTT of 1.5–2.0 will prevent further thrombus propagation. Simple conservative treatment along these lines together with investigation for any underlying cause will suffice in early cases without progression to venous gangrene, and in many of these cases there will be evident clinical improvement within 12–24 hours.

However, conservative treatment alone is not effective in severe PCD, particularly with gangrene, and more definitive treatments must be employed.[84] In addition to anticoagulation, the use, either singly or combined, of thrombolysis and thrombectomy may be necessary. More recently the delivery of thrombolytic agents via intra-arterial catheters to the affected limb has been reported, with excellent results in severe PCD.[82,85] This approach delivers thrombolysis to the capillary and venular thrombus as previously discussed. In the small number of patients so treated, relief from pain, swelling and hypotension was rapid (within 6–12 hours) and dramatic. Thus thrombolytic delivery tailored to both components of PCD, namely the large venous occlusions via intravenous catheters and the microvenous occlusions via intra-arterial catheters, is a logical advance and appears to have promising results (**Fig. 17.5**, see also Plate 15b, facing p. 116). Further experience with this combined approach is required to confirm these initial good results and good clinical outcomes.

Malignant iliocaval obstruction is a common cause of refractory DVT and may benefit from stent placement after thromboablation.[86] Various endovascular stents have been used effectively in the treatment of post-thrombotic iliocaval stenoses.[87] Self-expanding stents seem the best suited to this application (**Figs 17.6** and **17.7**). They can be oversized and left to passively expand and will recoil and re-expand if temporarily deformed or compressed (see Chapter 18).

IVC FILTERS

PE remains a major killer in its own right, ranking with cardiovascular and malignant disease as the most common cause of death.[88] Overall deaths from PE have been estimated at 200 000 per year in the USA and 30 000–40 000 per year in the UK.[89]

Anticoagulation remains the most effective primary treatment for diagnosed venous thromboembolic disease, with good outcomes in 90% of cases. In a minority of patients, however, anticoagulation will be contraindicated, will fail or will result in complications. Before the advent of caval filters, treatment was by open surgical interruption of the IVC below the renal veins by variations of suture plication (sieving) and external clip placement. These procedures to prevent PE in an invariably high-risk patient population carried high morbidity and mortality. Over the last 30 years these surgical approaches have been superseded by the development of endovascularly placed vena caval filters, which are not only convenient but much safer.

History of IVC interruption

The first femoral vein ligation was performed in 1874 by John Hunter, but resulted in frequent recurrent PE.[90] IVC ligation was performed in the 1940s by DeBakey, Ochsner and O'Neal to prevent emboli passing from the lower limbs and pelvis to

(a)

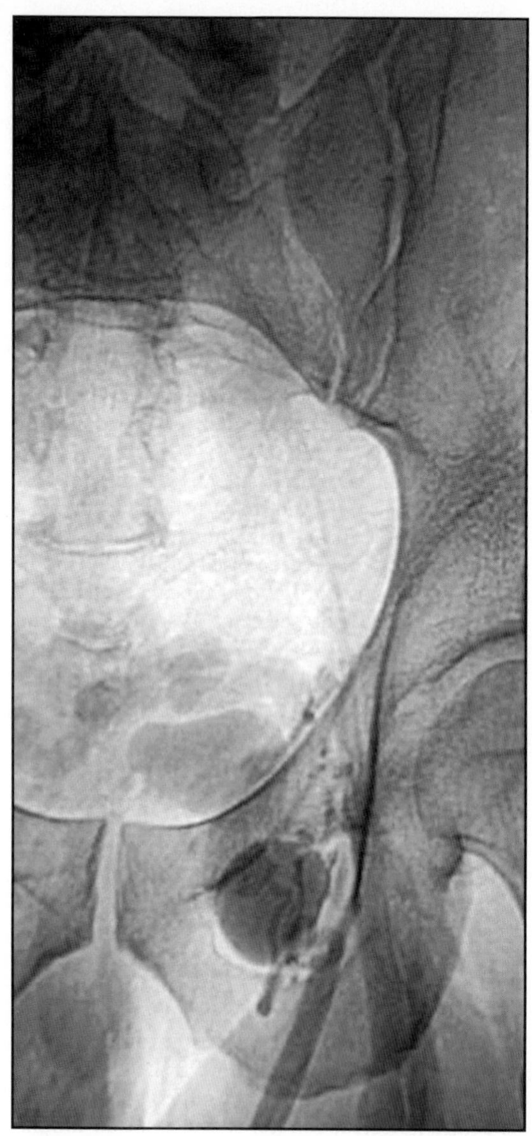

(b)

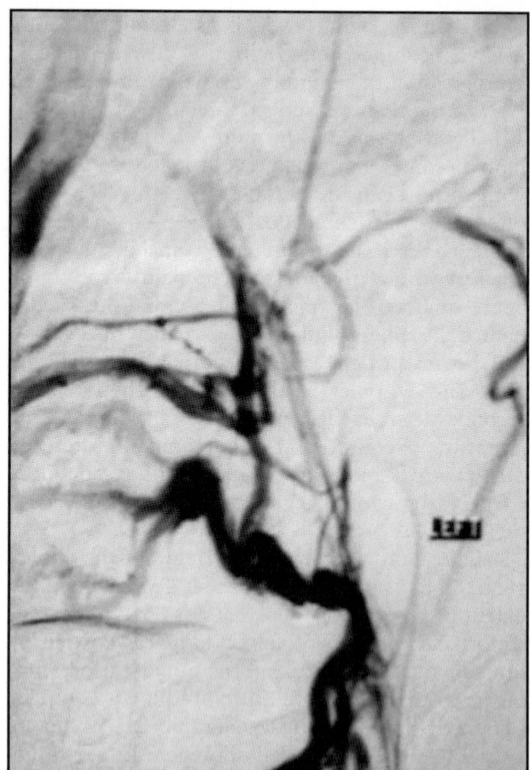

Figure 17.6 • A 37-year-old male with a 13-year history of chronic pain and lower limb swelling following a motorcycle accident. **(a)** A venogram performed via a foot vein demonstrates left common femoral and pelvic vein occlusion with cross-pelvic flow. **(b)** Via a left upper thigh venous puncture a catheter has been advanced into the occluded left common iliac vein.

the lungs.[91] This method had an operative mortality of 14% and a recurrent PE rate of 6% (2% fatal) and chronic venous stasis occurred in 33% of cases.[92,93] The recurrent PE was thought to occur via the large collateral vessels demonstrated post-operatively on venography or from thrombus in the cava above the ligation site. As a further development, sutures, staples and clips were used to compartmentalise the IVC but rates of operative mortality, recurrent PE and IVC thrombosis remained high (12%, 4% and 33%, respectively).[94–97] The first endoluminal filter was devised in 1967: the Mobin-Uddin umbrella filter.[98] A structure composed of six stainless steel struts coated with a heparin-impregnated fenestrated Silastic membrane, the filter was inserted via venotomy with its apex pointing inferiorly. The major problems with this device were IVC thrombosis (60%) and migration (0.4%). The Greenfield filter, first described in 1974, was a conical filter introduced via venotomy through a 29.5 Fr sheath.[99] It had superior flow characteristics and hence lower rates of associated IVC thrombosis. The first percutaneous insertion of a Greenfield filter was performed in 1984.[100] The initial percutaneous transvenous filters were delivered by large (24 Fr) delivery systems that resulted in insertion-site haemorrhage or thrombosis. These complications resulted in the development of the modern generation of low-profile filters delivered by 9–10 Fr introducers, dramatically reducing the incidence of insertion-site complications. Because of concerns about movement of these

(c)

(d)

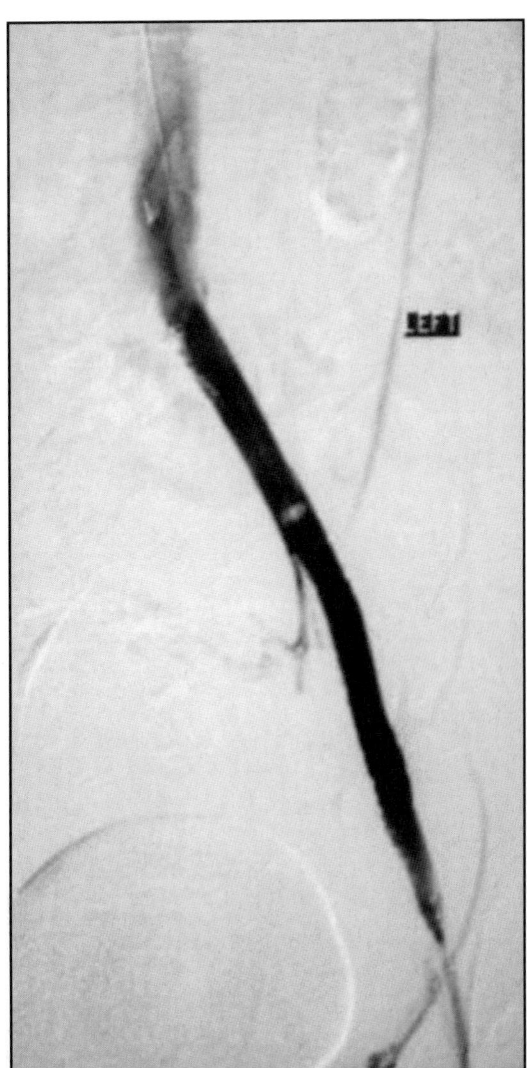

Figure 17.6 • (*cont.*) A 37-year-old male with a 13-year history of chronic pain and lower limb swelling following a motorcycle accident. **(c)** The occluded vein has been traversed and after access to the inferior vena cava, two overlapping 12-mm mesh nitinol stents (Memotherm, Bard UK) have been placed with post-placement balloon expansion. **(d)** Post-placement venogram demonstrating good flow. The patient has been warfarinised and at 1-year follow-up is asymptomatic, with resumption of normal activities and stents remaining patent.

devices when subjected to strong magnetic fields during magnetic resonance scanning, most of the newer models are made of titanium or nitinol (nickel–titanium alloy), which are non-ferromagnetic.

IVC filter design

The main desirable attributes of an IVC filter are ease of insertion, efficacy of capturing emboli, maintenance of IVC patency and secure fixation. Currently, there is a range of commercially available IVC filters. Most modern filter devices can be inserted through small delivery systems via a jugular or femoral vein approach and a few can also be inserted via brachial vein approaches (e.g. ALN filter).

The Titanium Greenfield filter (Boston Scientific/Meditech, Natick, MA), introduced in 1988, consists of six titanium MRI-compatible struts compressed into a 12 Fr carrier (outside diameter of sheath, 14.3 Fr). Its conical design means that it will only begin to obstruct flow after 70% of the cone is filled with thrombus and it will effectively trap emboli 3 mm or more in diameter. Its stainless steel predecessor had been troubled by tilting or migration, which led to modified hooks on the legs of the

(a)

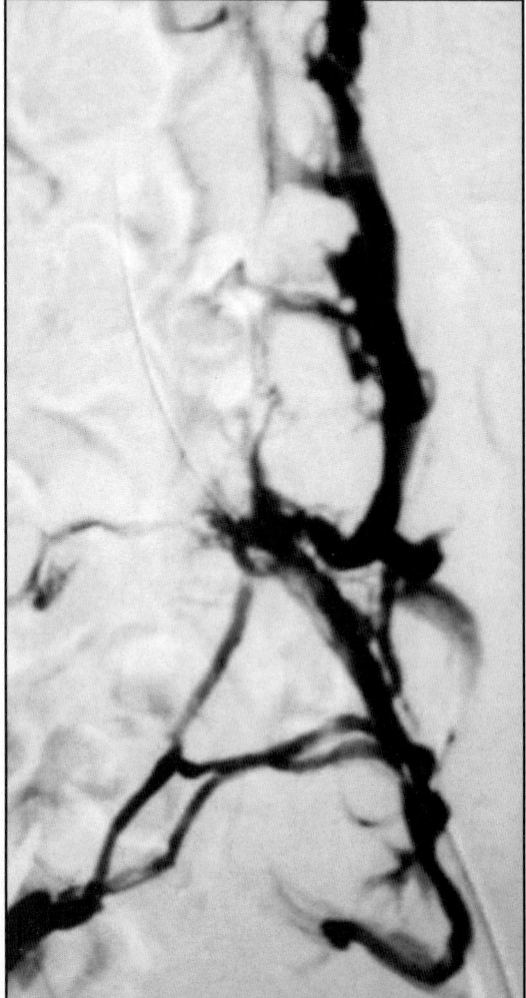

(b)

Figure 17.7 • A 45-year-old female with a history of left-sided deep vein thrombosis partially resolved with heparin complaining of left leg swelling and unsightly vulval and upper thigh varices. **(a)** A venogram performed via a left foot vein demonstrates a small-calibre left external iliac vein with preferential flow via the azygous system. **(b)** A digital subtraction venogram via a sheath in the left common femoral vein demonstrates a tight stenosis at the origin of the left common iliac vein consistent with a May–Thurner lesion.

titanium device. The filter is designed for IVC diameters smaller than 28 mm and comes in femoral and jugular versions.[101]

The Gianturco-Roehm Bird's Nest filter (Cook, Bloomington, IN), introduced in 1982, consists of four stainless steel wires attached to two V-shaped struts, which have small barbs to fix to the IVC wall.[102] It compresses into an 11 Fr carrier (outside diameter 14 Fr) and comes in femoral and jugular versions. It deploys a tangled mesh of wires that act as an effective filter. Its advantages are that it is suitable for IVC diameters up to 40 mm and that its delivery system is flexible enough to allow deployment from left-sided approaches. It creates a large

(c)

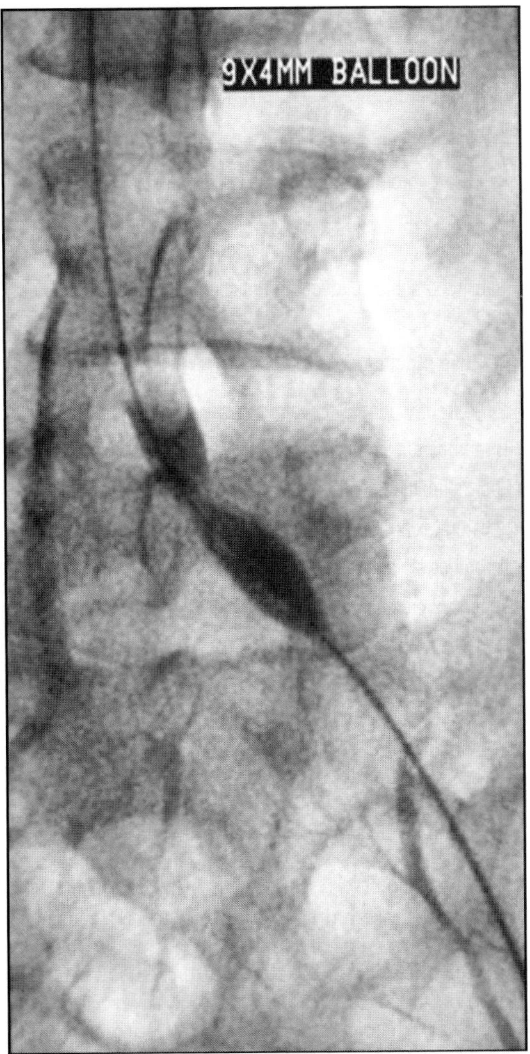

(d)

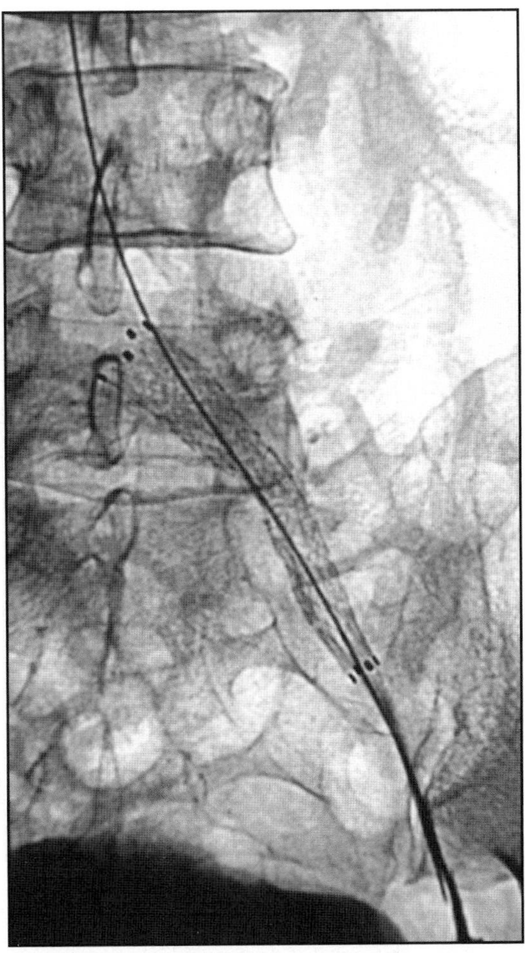

Figure 17.7 • (*cont.*) A 45-year-old female with a history of left-sided deep vein thrombosis partially resolved with heparin complaining of left leg swelling and unsightly vulval and upper thigh varices. **(c)** The left common iliac venous stenosis has been traversed with a guidewire and balloon dilated to 12 mm. A tight waist is visible in the balloon at the site of the stenosis. **(d)** A 12-mm self-expanding nitinol stent (Memotherm, Bard UK) has been positioned across the stenosis.

artefact on MRI but is thought to be safe from displacement in a 1.5-T magnet.[103]

The Günther Tulip filter (Cook), introduced in Europe in 1993, is made from the MRI-compatible compound Elgiloy arranged as four struts in a conical fashion with a small retrieval hook on its cephalad portion and small anchoring hooks at the ends of the struts. It can be deployed by a jugular or femoral approach via a much smaller 8.5 Fr introducer sheath. It has the further advantage of being retrievable.[104]

Other devices include the LGM or VenaTech filter (B. Braun/VenaTech, Evanston, IL), the Simon Nitinol filter (Bard, Covington, GA) and the TrapEase filter (Cordis, Europa N.V., L.J. Roden, The Netherlands).

There are currently no prospective data that compare the efficacy and complications of these various devices. There are many retrospective case series for each device but meaningful comparison is difficult due to wide variations in study methods and quality of follow-up.[88] The Society of Interventional Radiology has recently published reporting guidelines for these devices in an attempt to standardise future studies and allow valid meta-analysis.[105]

(e)

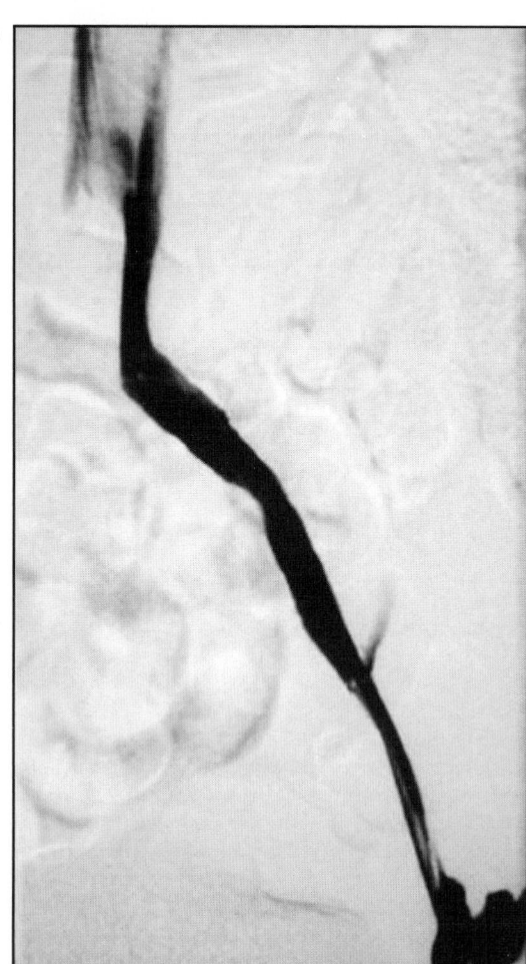

Figure 17.7 • (*cont.*) A 45-year-old female with a history of left-sided deep vein thrombosis partially resolved with heparin complaining of left leg swelling and unsightly vulval and upper thigh varices. **(e)** A completion venogram demonstrates rapid flow into the inferior vena cava through a patent stent. At 9-month follow-up the patient had marked improvement in her symptoms and the stent remains patent.

Indications and contraindications

Strict criteria should be applied when assessing patients for caval filter insertion, as there are significant associated risks. These can be divided into absolute and relative indications (**Box 17.4**). Patients with a contraindication to anticoagulation should be managed with a caval filter alone. In certain cases, a combination of a filter and anticoagulation may be desirable, such as in patients with severe cardiopulmonary compromise. Each case should be considered on an individual basis. There is evidence to suggest that the presence of large free-floating iliocaval thrombus is associated with a much higher risk of PE (50%) compared with occlusive thrombus (15%), despite anticoagulation.[106]

The use of IVC filter protection during DVT thrombolysis remains contentious, but is routinely practised in our institution. The only absolute contraindications to IVC filter insertion are complete IVC thrombosis and lack of access to the IVC. The absence of long-term performance data should make clinicians reluctant to place permanent devices in young patients.

Box 17.4 • Indications and contraindications for IVC filter insertion

Absolute indications
Contraindication to anticoagulation
Recurrent thromboembolic disease despite anticoagulant therapy
Significant complication of anticoagulant therapy
Inability to achieve adequate anticoagulation (despite patient compliance)
Relative indications
Large free-floating iliocaval thrombus
Thromboembolic disease with poor cardiopulmonary reserve
Poor compliance with medications
Severe ataxia; at risk of falls on anticoagulant therapy
Thrombolysis for deep vein thrombosis
Renal cell cancer with renal vein or IVC involvement

RECENT IVC FILTER TRIALS

In 1998, Decousus et al.[107] performed the first prospective, randomised, controlled trial using IVC filters; 400 patients with venography-proven DVT were randomised to receive anticoagulants alone (unfractionated or low-molecular-weight heparin followed by oral anticoagulants for at least 3 months) or anticoagulants with placement of one of four types of IVC filter. The rates of recurrent venous thromboembolism (DVT or PE), death and major bleeding were analysed at 12 days and 2 years. The results are summarised in **Table 17.1**. The results demonstrate that IVC filters are effective in preventing PE but there is no improvement in the overall mortality rate, possibly because fatal PE is quite rare. There was a significant twofold increase in risk of recurrent DVT with IVC filter at 2 years. No comparison was made

Table 17.1 • Results of PREPIC (Prevention du Risque d'Embolic Pulmonaire par Interruption Cave) Study

	Anticoagulation alone (*N* = 200)	Anticoagulation and IVC filter (*N* = 200)	Odds ratio (95% CI)	*P* value
At 12 days				
Recurrent PE	9 (4.8%)	2 (1.1%)	0.22 (0.05–0.90)	0.03*
Recurrent fatal PE	4 (2.1%)	0 (0.0%)	–	0.12
Mortality	5 (2.5%)	5 (2.5%)	0.99 (0.29–3.42)	0.99
Cumulative at 2 years				
Recurrent PE	12 (6.3%)	6 (3.4%)	0.5 (0.19–1.33)	0.16
Recurrent fatal PE	5 (2.6%)	1 (0.6%)	0.22	0.22
Recurrent DVT	21 (11.6%)	37 (20.8%)	1.87 (1.10–3.20)	0.02*
IVC filter thrombosis	–	16 (9.0%)	–	–
Mortality	40 (20.1%)	43 (21.6%)	1.10 (0.72–1.70)	0.65

*Significant.
DVT, deep vein thrombosis; IVC, inferior vena cava; PE, pulmonary embolism.

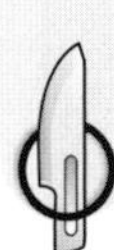

between the four different types of IVC filter used. However, the data may not apply to the use of IVC filters without anticoagulation in the large group of patients in whom anticoagulant therapy cannot be effectively used.

A number of large, population-based, multicentre studies in the USA have retrospectively examined the outcomes of IVC filter placement. The Veterans Affairs Medical Centres study in 1999 examined 157 filter placements in a group of 4882 patients admitted with PE between 1990 and 1995, finding a non-significant reduction in unadjusted in-hospital mortality from 16.0% to 13.4%.[108]

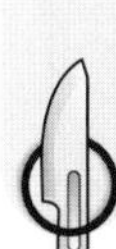

In 2000, a study of Californian hospitals discharge data of 3622 patients treated with filters and 64 333 control patients admitted with venous thromboembolism found no significant difference in readmission rates for PE between filter and non-filter groups.[109]

Like the study by Decousus et al., filter insertion was associated with a significantly higher relative risk of readmission with venous thrombosis in patients initially admitted with PE. Also in 2000, a Massachusetts General Hospital study reviewed their 26-year experience of 1765 filter insertions, finding a prevalence of 5.6% post-filter PE and 3.7% fatal post-filter PE.[110] IVC thrombosis occurred in 2.7% and major complications in 0.3% of patients after filter insertion. The conclusion was that IVC filters provided protection from life-threatening PE with minimal morbidity and few complications. In 2001, Greenfield used the Michigan filter registry to examine the incidence of recurrent DVT in 465 patients with IVC filters.[111] The overall incidence of DVT was 13.3%, with no significant difference between the 241 given anticoagulants (12%) and the 224 who were not (15%). However, leg swelling was twice as common in the patients who received no anticoagulation ($P = 0.006$).

SUPRARENAL FILTERS

There are a number of situations in which placement of the filter in the normal infrarenal position is impossible or potentially hazardous (**Box 17.5**). These include thrombosis in the infrarenal IVC or renal veins and pregnancy (or female of childbearing age). Small series of superior vena cava (SVC) filter placements have been reported with varying success. SVC thrombosis has complicated some of these and large studies are necessary to further evaluate this application.

Box 17.5 • Indications for suprarenal placement of IVC filters

- Infrarenal vena cava thrombosis
- Thrombus propagating proximal to infrarenal IVC filter
- Renal vein thrombosis
- Large patent ovarian vein (pregnancy or childbearing age)

TEMPORARY AND RETRIEVABLE FILTERS

Some patients require only temporary protection against thromboembolic events and the indications for this are listed in **Box 17.6**. The long-term effects of permanent IVC filters are untested. This has led to the development of filters that can be safely removed once the risk of emboli has passed. Certain temporary filters, such as the Tempofilter (B. Braun), remain attached to an accessible transcutaneous catheter or wire. They have a similar design to the permanent filters but have modified caval attachment sites. The disadvantages are that these require a second procedure to remove them and that the transcutaneous catheter or wire is a potential pathway for infection. Alternatively, attempts have been made to remove permanent filters before there is endothelialisation of the filter struts to the IVC wall. The Günther Tulip filter (Cook) is widely used in Europe and can be successfully retrieved from the right internal jugular vein using a retrieval snare through an 11 Fr sheath (**Fig. 17.8**). The manufacturers recommend removal within 14 days of insertion of the device. In a 2002 study from the multicentre Canadian registry, 52 of 53 Günther Tulip filters were successfully retrieved between 2 and 25 days from their insertion.[112] In 2002,

Box 17.6 • Indications for temporary or retrievable IVC filter

- Treatment of iliofemoral deep vein thrombosis (DVT) with catheter thrombolysis
- Known DVT with a short period of contraindication to anticoagulant therapy
- Prophylaxis after major trauma
- High-risk free-floating DVT

(a)
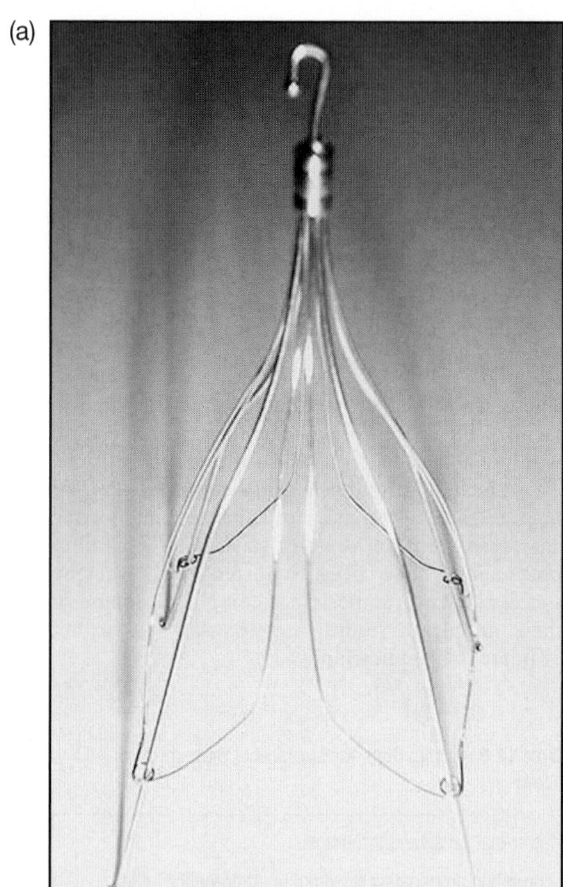

(b)
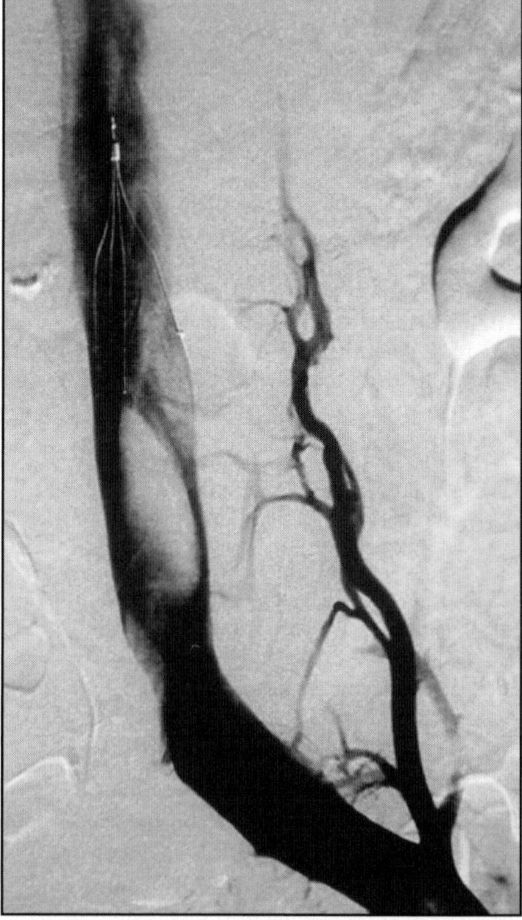

Figure 17.8 • **(a)** Günther Tulip Retrievable Filter (Cook UK Ltd); **(b)** free-floating thrombus in the inferior vena cava with a filter above.

(c)

(d)

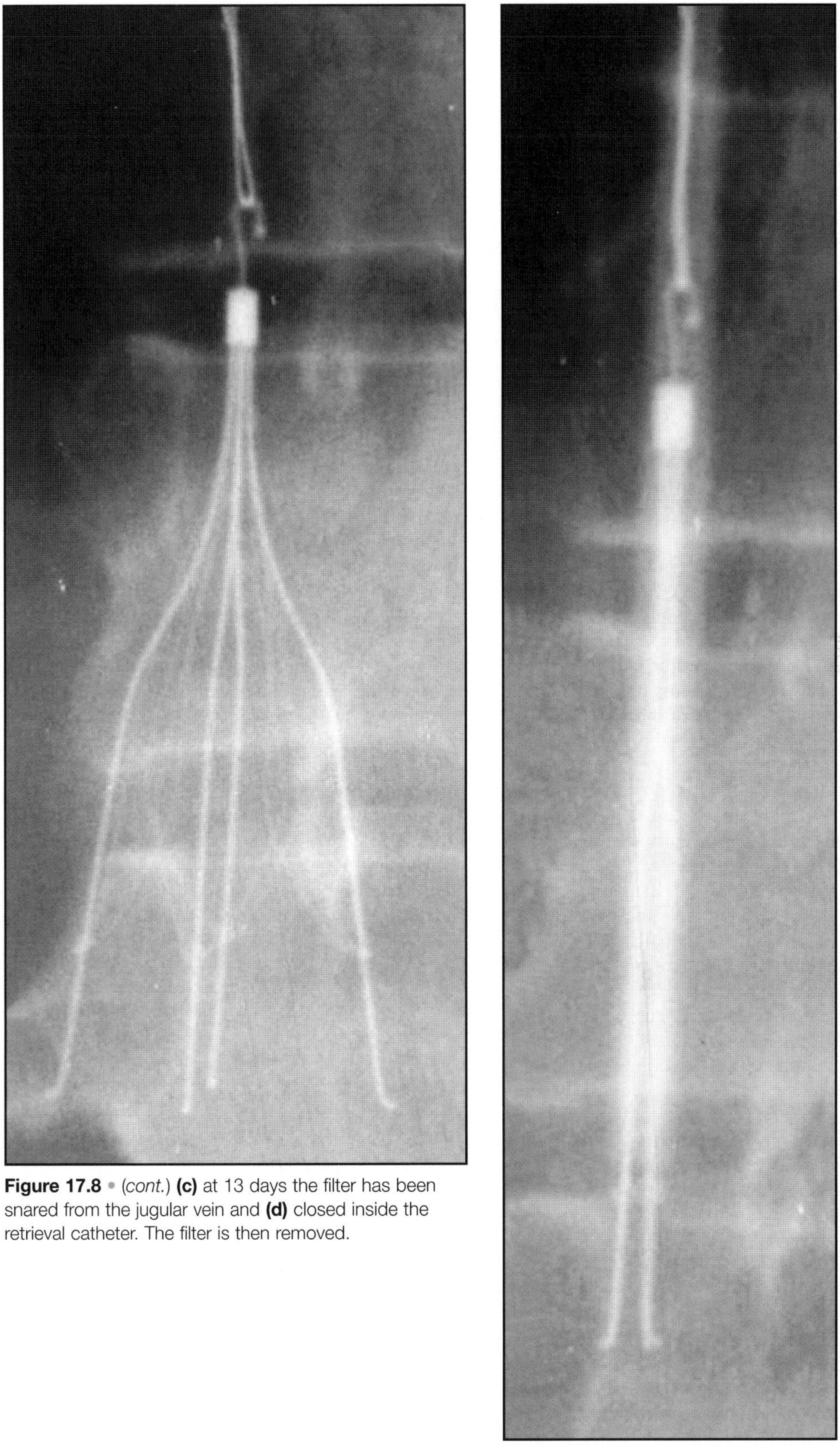

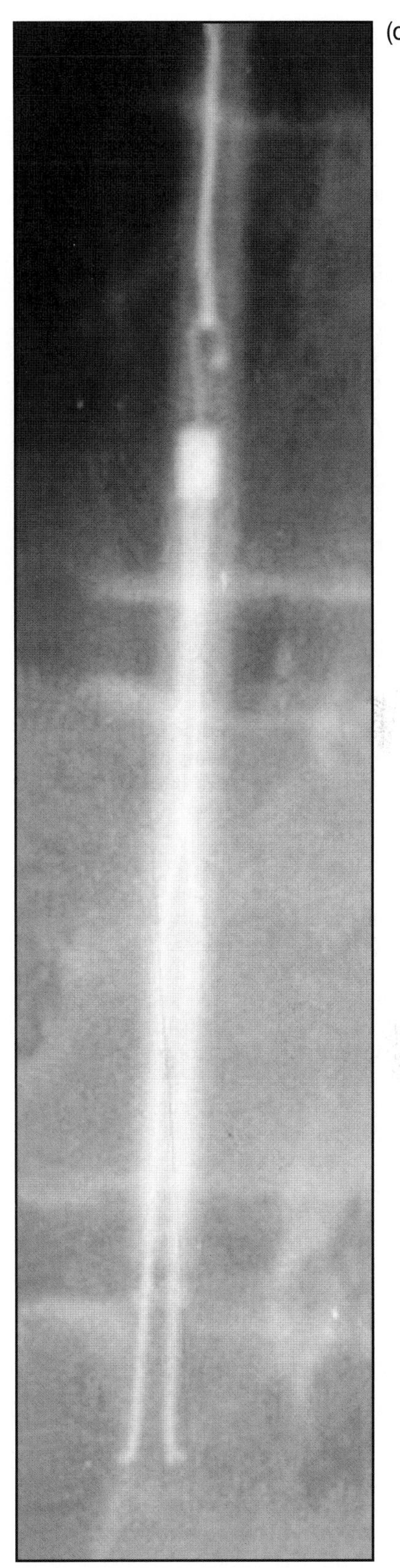

Figure 17.8 • (*cont.*) **(c)** at 13 days the filter has been snared from the jugular vein and **(d)** closed inside the retrieval catheter. The filter is then removed.

Asch[113] reported successful retrieval of all 24 nitinol Recovery filters (Bard UK) via the right internal jugular vein using a novel retrieval device composed of a cone with nine metal claws. Problems encountered with filter retrieval are deciding when the filter can be safely removed and what should be done if a large clot is found on the filter at the time of planned removal. The options for the latter include thrombolysis prior to filter removal or leaving the filter in place.

Other more recently introduced retrievable IVC devices include the ALN filter (Pyramed UK) and the Recovery Filter (Bard UK), both of which can be left in situ for up to 60–90 days prior to removal.

PROPHYLACTIC IVC FILTERS

Definitions of prophylactic IVC filters have evolved.[114] Previously, situations considered to be prophylactic would include patients with large 'high-risk' proximal or free-floating DVT where anticoagulation alone was considered inadequate, particularly if there was poor cardiorespiratory reserve. Currently there is a trend, particularly in the USA, to place prophylactic IVC filters in patients who do not yet have thromboembolism but who are at very high risk by virtue of associated medical conditions, such as traumatic injury or malignancy. Most malignancies render patients hypercoagulable and thromboembolic events are more common.[115] These patients also suffer higher rates of complications from anticoagulation, due to comorbidity and cancer therapy. There is an argument for prophylactic IVC filter placement but results are conflicting and inconclusive, with some reduction in PE but higher mortality rates.[116,117] Similarly, multiply injured patients have increased risk of thromboembolic events due to a combination of venous stasis, venous damage and a hypercoagulable state. Anticoagulants are often contraindicated and in addition the usual conservative measures such as venous compression devices and surveillance ultrasound are often impossible. Studies have identified a subgroup of trauma patients who may be at a 50-fold increased risk of thromboembolic events compared with other trauma patients. These include brain- or spinal cord-injured patients and those with pelvic or lower limb long-bone fractures.[118] There have been some favourable results but again they remain inconclusive.[119–121]

Complications of IVC filter insertion

Recurrent PE is effectively failure of the primary function of the IVC filter and occurs relatively infrequently, approximately 2–5% in reported series.[122,123] However, many recurrent PEs will be subclinical and the true incidence is likely to be higher. There are a variety of potential mechanisms for recurrent PE, which should be considered in the work-up for filter placement. Unusual sites of the embolic source include the upper limb veins (often associated with central venous catheters) and the right atrium. Most IVC filters will trap large life-threatening clots, but smaller clots may pass through unhindered. Clot within the filter itself may also become the source of emboli and this should be considered when imaging recurrent PE. This thrombus may result from de novo thrombus, trapped emboli from the lower limb veins or thrombus propagating up the IVC. Technical failures, such as incomplete expansion, filter tilting or migration, or failure to appreciate clot above the position of the filter at time of deployment, may also account for recurrent PE.

The incidence of filter-related IVC thromboses varies from 0 to 28% in reported series.[117] The range is likely to reflect a number of methodological variations. Some researchers have examined thromboses in all patients while others only looked at symptomatic patients. IVC thrombosis can be asymptomatic in a minority of patients. Some groups considered non-occlusive clot within the filter as IVC thrombosis while others did not. Timing may also be important since IVCs occluded at one point may later recanalize. Insertion-site thrombosis has been reported at 2–28%. The incidence may be lower in lower-profile systems.

Procedural complications are reported at 4–11% and include bleeding, infection, pneumothorax, air embolism, delivery system complications (such as guidewire entrapment) and suboptimal filter deployment. Reported delayed complications include filter migration into the heart, IVC penetration and filter fracture. The reported incidences of these are listed in **Box 17.7**.

Box 17.7 • Complications reported with use of IVC filters

- Pulmonary embolism (2–5%)
- Fatal pulmonary embolism (0.7%)
- Death linked to insertion of IVC filter (0.12%)
- Procedural complications (4–11%)
- Venous access site thrombosis (2–28%)
- Migration of filter (3–69%)
- Penetration of IVC (9–24%)
- Obstruction of IVC (6–30%)
- Venous insufficiency (5–59%)
- Filter fracture (1%)
- Guidewire entrapment (<1%)

Key points

- The familial thrombophilias comprise a group of inherited disorders in which a predisposition to venous thrombosis is linked to quantitative or qualitative abnormalities of proteins participating in the coagulation cascade.
- The familial thrombophilias comprise factor V Leiden (FVL), prothrombin 20210A and abnormalities of the coagulation inhibitors antithrombin, protein C and protein S.
- Worldwide, FVL is the commonest cause of familial thrombophilia. It is rare in Asia and absent in Africa.
- Testing of unselected patients is inappropriate and should be avoided.
- Great care should be taken when interpreting protein S results since acquired protein S deficiency is not uncommon.
- DVT and PE are the commonest clinical manifestations of familial thrombophilia. Venous thrombosis in unusual sites may also occur, including thrombosis of cerebral, renal, mesenteric, portal and hepatic veins.
- The risk of thrombosis is greater in those with combined genetic defects (e.g. FVL and protein C deficiency) compared with those with single defects.
- Venous thrombosis is a multifactorial disorder. Environmental risk factors can be found in approximately 50% of patients presenting with venous thrombosis.
- In the primary antiphospholipid syndrome, both arterial and venous thrombosis are associated with the persistent presence of APAs, e.g. lupus anticoagulant, anticardiolipin antibodies.
- There is a high rate of recurrent venous thrombosis in patients with primary antiphospholipid syndrome.
- Iliofemoral DVT, particularly with PCD or venous gangrene, is a limb- and life-threatening condition.
- Early and aggressive treatment will achieve the goals of restored venous patency, limb viability and reduce mortality in comparison with standard conservative treatment alone.
- Surgical venous thrombectomy is highly effective but has higher associated morbidity and mortality.
- Catheter-directed thrombolysis and PMT yield similar results but with fewer associated complications.
- Results are particularly good when treatment begins close to the onset of thrombosis and before phlebitis and periphlebitis remove any possibility of restoring normal venous function.
- Endovascular stents appear to have an emerging role in treating underlying May–Thurmer lesions in acute thrombosis post pharmacological lysis and/or mechanical thrombectomy and in the management of longstanding chronic venous occlusions.
- The current generation of IVC filters are relatively safe and easy to insert. Although they do not confer total protection, they seem to be effective in reducing the risk of PE in both the short and longer term.
- There appears to be a higher incidence of both IVC thrombosis and recurrent lower limb DVT with IVC filters.
- There have been no studies directly comparing the different available filters, and at present there is no evidence to choose one filter over another.
- The long-term performance of filters is unknown and therefore strict adherence to the indications for insertion is recommended, particularly in the younger age group. Potential for filter retrieval should be considered in each case.

REFERENCES

1. Sandler DA, Martin JF. Autopsy proven pulmonary embolism in hospital patients: are we detecting enough deep thrombosis? Br Med J 1989; 82: 203–5.
2. Flanc C, Kakkar VV, Clarke MD. Detection of venous thrombosis of the legs using ^{125}I-labelled fibrinogen. Br J Surg 1968; 55:742–7.
3. Kakkar VV, Howe CT, Flanc C, Clarke MD. Natural history of post-operative deep vein thrombosis. Lancet 1969; ii:230–2.

4. Huisman MV, Buller HR, ten Cate JW et al. Unexpected high prevalence of silent pulmonary embolism in patients with deep venous thrombosis. Chest 1989; 95:498–502.
5. Doyle DJ, Turpie AGG, Hirsh J et al. Adjusted subcutaneous heparin or continuous intravenous heparin in patients with acute deep vein thrombosis: a randomised trial. Ann Intern Med 1987; 107: 441–5.
6. Virchow R. Phlogose und Thrombose im Gefässystem. Gesammelte Abhandlungen zur Wissenschaftlichen Medizin. Frankfurt: Staatsdruckerei, 1856.
7. Egeberg O. Inherited antithrombin deficiency causing thrombophilia. Thromb Diath Haemorrh 1965; 13:516–30.
8. Rosendaal FR, Bovill EG. Heritability of clotting factors and the revival of the prothrombotic state. Lancet 2002; 359:638–9.
9. Greaves M, Preston FE. Pathogenesis of thrombosis: antithrombotic therapy. In: Hoffbrand AV, Lewis SM, Tuddenham EG (eds) Postgraduate haematology, 4th edn. Oxford: Butterworth Heinemann, 1999; pp. 653–74.
10. Aiach M, Gandrille S, Emmerich J. A review of mutations causing deficiencies of antithrombin, protein C and protein S. Thromb Haemost 1995; 74:81–9.
11. Murin S, Marelich GP, Arroliga AC et al. Hereditary thrombophilia and venous thromboembolism. Am J Respir Crit Care Med 1998; 158:1369–73.
12. Griffin JH, Evatt B, Zimmerman TS et al. Deficiency of protein C in congenital thrombotic disease. J Clin Invest 1981; 68:1370–3.
13. Bovill EG, Bauer KA, Dickerman JD et al. The clinical spectrum of heterozygous protein C deficiency in a large New England kindred. Blood 1989; 73:712–17.
14. Tollefson DF, Friedman KD, Marlar RA. Protein C deficiency. A cause of unusual or unexplained thrombosis. Arch Surg 1988; 123:881–4.
15. Vieregge P, Schwieder G, Kompf D. Cerebral venous thrombosis in hereditary protein C deficiency. J Neurol Neurosurg Psychiatry 1989; 52:135–7.
16. Prat F, Ouzan D, Trecziak N et al. Portal and mesenteric thrombosis revealing constitutional protein C deficiency. Gut 1989; 30:416.
17. Miletich J, Sherman L, Broze G Jr. Absence of thrombosis in subjects with heterozygous protein C deficiency. N Engl J Med 1987; 317:991–6.
18. Tait RC, Walker ID, Reitsma PH et al. Prevalence of protein C deficiency in the healthy population. Thromb Haemost 1995; 73:87–93.
19. Bertina RM. Genetic approach to thrombophilia. Thromb Haemost 2001; 86:92–103.
20. Allaart CF, Poort SR, Rosendaal FR et al. Increased risk of venous thrombosis in carriers of hereditary protein C deficiency defect. Lancet 1993; 341: 134–8.
21. Vossen CY, Conard J, Fontcuberta J. Familial thrombophilia and lifetime risk of venous thrombosis. J Thromb Haemost 2004; 2:1526–32..
22. Koeleman BP, Reitsma PH, Allaart CF et al. Activated protein C resistance as an additional risk factor for thrombosis in protein C-deficient families. Blood 1994; 84:1031–5.
23. Comp PC, Nixon RR, Cooper MR et al. Familial protein S deficiency is associated with recurrent thrombosis. J Clin Invest 1984; 74:2082–8.
24. Liberti G, Bertina RM, Rosendaal FR. Hormonal state rather than age influences cut-off values of protein S: reevaluation of the thrombotic risk associated with protein S deficiency. Thromb Haemost 1999; 82:1093–6.
25. Mateo J, Oliver A, Borrell M et al. Laboratory evaluation and clinical characteristics of 2,132 consecutive unselected patients with venous thromboembolism: results of the Spanish Multicentric Study on Thrombophilia (EMET-Study). Thromb Haemost 1997; 77:444–51.
26. Koeleman JH, Bakker CM, Plandsoen WC et al. Hereditary protein S deficiency presenting with cerebral sinus thrombosis in an adolescent girl. J Neurol 1992; 239:105–6.
27. Broekmans AW, van Rooyen W, Westerveld BD et al. Mesenteric vein thrombosis as presenting manifestation of hereditary protein S deficiency. Gastroenterology 1987; 92:240–2.
28. Sas G, Blasko G, Petro I et al. A protein S deficiency family with portal vein thrombosis. Thromb Haemost 1985; 54:724.
29. Aiach M, Borgel D, Gaussem P et al. Protein C and protein S deficiencies. Semin Hematol 1997; 34:205–16.
30. Bertina RM. Hereditary protein S deficiency. Haemostasis 1985; 15:241–6.
31. Edson JR, Vogt JN, Huesman DA. Laboratory diagnosis of inherited protein S deficiency. Am J Clin Pathol 1990; 94:176–86.
32. Faught W, Garner P, Jones G et al. Changes in protein C and protein S levels in normal pregnancy. Am J Obstet Gynecol 1995; 172:147–50.
33. Marder VJ, Matei DE. Hereditary and acquired thrombophilic syndromes. In: Colman RW, Hirsh J, Marder VJ, Clowes AW, George JN (eds) Hemostasis and thrombosis: basic principles and clinical practice, 4th edn. Philadelphia: Lippincott Williams & Wilkins, 2001; pp. 1243–75.
34. Ginsberg JS, Demers C, Brill-Edwards P et al. Acquired protein S deficiency is associated with antiphospholipid antibodies and increased thrombin generation in patients with systemic lupus erythematosus. Am J Med 1995; 98:379–83.

35. Dahlbäck B, Carlsson M, Svensson PJ. Familial thrombophilia due to a previously unrecognized mechanism characterized by poor anticoagulant response to activated protein C: prediction of a cofactor to activated protein C. Proc Natl Acad Sci USA 1993; 90:1004–8.

36. Koster T, Rosendaal FR, de Ronde H et al. Venous thrombosis due to poor anticoagulant response to activated protein C: Leiden Thrombophilia Study. Lancet 1993; 342:1503–6.

37. Bertina RM, Koeleman BP, Koster T et al. Mutation in blood coagulation factor V associated with resistance to activated protein C. Nature 1994; 369:64–7.

38. Rees DC, Cox M, Clegg JB. World distribution of factor V Leiden. Lancet 1995; 346:1133–4.

39. De Stefano V, Martinelli I, Mannucci PM et al. The risk of recurrent deep venous thrombosis among heterozygous carriers of both factor V Leiden and the G20210A prothrombin mutation. N Engl J Med 1999; 341:801–6.

40. Margaglione M, D'Andrea G, Colaizzo D et al. Coexistence of factor V Leiden and factor II A20210 mutation and recurrent venous thromboembolism. Thromb Haemost 1999; 82:1564–6.

41. Martinelli I, Landi G, Merati G et al. Factor V gene mutation is a risk factor for cerebral venous thrombosis. Thromb Haemost 1996; 75:393–4.

42. Poort SR, Rosendaal FR, Reitsma PH et al. A common genetic variation in the 3′-untranslated region of the prothrombin gene is associated with elevated plasma prothrombin levels and an increase in venous thrombosis. Blood 1996; 88:3698–703.

43. Rosendaal FR, Doggen CJ, Zivelin A et al. Geographic distribution of the 20210 G to A prothrombin variant. Thromb Haemost 1998; 79:706–8.

44. Souto JC, Coll I, Llobet D et al. The prothrombin 20210A allele is the most prevalent genetic factor for venous thromboembolism in the Spanish population. Thromb Haemost 1998; 80:366–9.

45. Rosendaal FR. Risk factors for venous thrombotic disease. Thromb Haemost 1999; 82:610–19.

46. Greaves M, Baglin T. Laboratory testing for heritable thrombophilia: impact on clinical management of thrombotic disease. Br J Haematol 2000; 109:699–703.

47. Bertina RM, Rosendaal FR. Venous thrombosis: the interaction of genes and environment. N Engl J Med 1998; 338:1840–1.

48. Vandenbrouke JP, Kaster T, Briet E et al. Increased risk of venous thrombosis in oral-contraceptive users who are carriers of factor V Leiden mutation. Lancet 1994; 344:1453–7.

49. de Bruijn SF, Stam J, Vandenbrouke JP. Increased risk of cerebral venous thrombosis with third-generation oral contraceptives. Cerebral Venous Sinus Thrombosis Study Group. Lancet 1998; 351:1404.

50. Martinelli I, Sacchi E, Landi G et al. High risk of cerebral vein thrombosis in carriers of a prothrombin gene mutation and in users of oral contraceptives. N Engl J Med 1998; 338:1793–7.

51. Ginsberg JS, Demers C, Brill-Edwards P et al. Acquired free protein S deficiency is associated with antiphospholipid antibodies and increased thrombin generation in patients with systemic lupus erythematosus. Am J Med 1995; 98:379–83.

52. Tomas JF, Alberca I, Tabernero MD et al. Natural anticoagulant proteins and antiphospholipid antibodies in systemic lupus erythematosus. J Rheumatol 1998; 25:57–62.

53. Wells PS, Hirsch J, Anderson DR et al. Accuracy of clinical assessment of deep vein thrombosis. Lancet 1995; 345:1326–30.

54. Bounameaux H, de Moerloose P, Perrier A et al. D-dimer testing in suspected venous thromboembolism: an update. Q J Med 1997; 90:437–42.

55. van der Graaf F, van den Borne H, van der Kolk M et al. Exclusion of deep vein thrombosis with D-dimer testing: comparison of 13 D-dimer methods in 99 outpatients suspected of deep vein thrombosis using venography as reference standard. Thromb Haemost 2000; 83:191–8.

56. Rajhavendra BN, Hori SC, Hilton S et al. Deep venous thrombosis: detection by probe compression of veins. J Ultrasound Med 1986; 5:89–95.

57. Lea-Thomas M, MacDonald L. The accuracy of bolus ascending phlebography in demonstrating the ilio-femoral segment. Clin Radiol 1997; 28:165.

58. Roh BS, Park KH, Kim EA et al. Prognostic value of CT before thrombolytic therapy in iliofemoral deep venous thrombosis. J Vasc Intervent Radiol 2002; 13:71–6.

59. Criado E , Farber M, Marston W et al. The role of air plethysmography in the diagnosis of chronic venous insufficiency. J Vasc Surg 1998; 27:660–70.

60. Nicolaides AM, Kakkar VV, Remmey JTG. The soleal sinuses: origin of deep vein thrombosis. Br J Surg 1971; 58:307.

61. Masuda EM, Kessler DM, Kistner RL et al. The natural history of calf vein thrombosis: lysis of thrombi and development of reflux. J Vasc Surg 1998; 28:67–73.

62. Hurst DR, Forauer AR, Bloom JR et al. Diagnosis and endovacular treatment of iliocaval compression syndrome. J Vasc Surg 2001; 34:106–13.

63. Breddin HK, Hach-Wunderle V, Nakov R et al. Effects of low-molecular-weight heparin on thrombus regression and thromboembolism in patients with deep venous thrombosis. N Engl J Med 2001; 344:626–31.

64. Hill SL, Martin D, Evans P. Massive vein thrombosis of the extremities. Am J Surg 1989; 158:131–6.

65. Mewissen MW, Seabrook GR, Meissner MH. Catheter-directed thrombolysis for lower extremity deep venous thrombosis: report of a national multicenter registry. Radiology 1999; 211:39–49.

66. Haimovici H. The ischaemic forms of venous thrombosis. J Cardiovasc Surg (Torino) 1986; 1(suppl.):164–73.

67. Haller JA Jr, Abrams BL. Use of thrombectomy in the treatment of acute iliofemoral venous thrombosis in 45 patients. Ann Surg 1963; 158:561–9.

68. Karp RB, Wykie EJ. Recurrent thrombosis after iliofemoral venous thrombectomy. Surg Forum 1966; 17:147.

69. Lansing AM, Davis WM. Five year follow up study of iliofemoral venous thrombectomy. Ann Surg 1968; 168:620–8.

70. Weaver FA, Meacham PW, Adkins RB, Dean RH. Phlegmasia caerulea dolens: therapeutic considerations. South Med J 1988; 81:306–12.

71. Eklof B, Kistner RL. Is there a role for thrombectomy in iliofemoral venous thrombosis? Semin Vasc Surg 1996; 9:34–45.

72. Halliday P, Harris J, May J. Femoro-femoral crossover grafts (Palma opertion), a long term follow up study. In: Bergan JF, Yao JST (eds) Surgery of the veins. New York: Grune & Stratton, 1985; p. 241.

73. Husni EA. Venous reconstruction in post-phlebitic disease. Circulation 1971; 43(suppl. 1):147–50.

74. Leizorovic A. Long-term consequences of deep venous thrombosis. Haemostasis 1998; 28(suppl. 3): 1–7.

75. Haller JA Jr, May ST. Experimental studies on iliofemoral venous thrombosis. Am Surg 1963; 29:567–71.

76. Haimovici H. Gangrene of the extremities of venous origin. Review of the literature with case reports. Circulation 1950; 1:225–40.

77. Qvarfordt P, Eklof B, Ohlin P. Intramuscular pressure in the lower leg in deep vein thrombosis and phlegmasia caerulea dolens. Ann Surg 1983; 197:450–3.

78. Haller JS Jr. Effects of deep femoral thrombophlebitis on the circulation of the lower extremities. Circulation 1963; 27:693–8.

79. Perkins JMT, Magee TR, Galland RB. Phlegmasia caerulea dolens and venous gangrene. Br J Surg 1996; 83:19–23.

80. Adamson AS, Littlewood TJ, Poston GJ et al. Malignancy presenting as peripheral venous gangrene. J R Soc Med 1988; 81:609–10.

81. Woolling KR, Lawrence K, Rosenak BD. Phlegmasia caerulea dolens and ulcerative colitis. Report of a case. Angiology 1967; 18:556–64.

82. Wlodarczyk ZK, Gibson M, Dick R, Hamilton G. Low-dose intra-arterial thrombolysis in the treatment of phlegmasia caerulea dolens. Br J Surg 1994; 81:370–2.

83. Elliot MS, Immelman EJ, Jeffry P et al. The role of thrombolytic therapy in the treatment of phlegmasia caerulea dolens. Br J Surg 1979; 66: 422–4.

84. Comerota AJ, Aldridge SC, Cohen G et al. A strategy of aggressive regional therapy for acute iliofemoral venous thrombosis with contemporary venous thrombectomy or catheter directed thrombolysis. J Vasc Surg 1994; 20:244–54.

85. Bjarnason H, Kruse JR, Asinger DA et al. Iliofemoral deep venous thrombosis: safety and efficacy outcome during 5 years of catheter-directed thrombolytic therapy. J Vasc Intervent Radiol 1997; 8:405–18.

86. Razavi MK, Hansch EC, Kee ST et al. Chronically occluded inferior venae cavae: endovascular treatment. Radiology 2000; 214:133–8.

87. AbuRahma AF, Perkins SE, Wulu JT et al. Iliofemoral deep venous thrombosis: conventional therapy versus lysis and percutaneous transluminal angioplasty and stenting. Ann Surg 2001; 233:752–60.

88. Kinney TB. Update on inferior vena cava filters. J Vasc Intervent Radiol 2003; 14:425–40.

89. Ansari A. Acute and chronic pulmonary thromboembolism: current perspectives. Part I: glossary of terms, historic evolution and prevalence. Clin Cardiol 1986; 9:398–402.

90. Greenfield LJ. Evolution of venous interruption for pulmonary thromboembolism. Arch Surg 1992; 127:622–6.

91. Ochsner A, Ochsner JL, Saunders HS. Prevention of pulmonary embolism by caval ligation. Ann Surg 1970; 171:923–38.

92. Amador E, Ting KL, Crane C. Ligation of the inferior vena cava for thromboembolism. JAMA 1968; 206:1758–60.

93. Garner AMN. Inferior vena cava interruption in prevention of fatal thromboembolism. Am J Surg 1972; 84:537.

94. Nasbeth DC, Moran JM. Reassessment of the role of inferior vena cava ligation in thromboembolism. N Engl J Med 1965; 273:1250–3.

95. Miles RM. Prevention of pulmonary embolism by the use of a plastic vena caval clip. Ann Surg 1966; 163:192–8.

96. Moretz W, Rhode C, Shepard M. Prevention of pulmonary emboli by partial occlusion of the inferior vena cava. Ann Surg 1959; 25:617.

97. Adams JT, DeWeese JA. Experimental and clinical evaluation of partial vein interruption in the prevention of pulmonary embolism. Surgery 1965; 57:82–102.

98. Mobin-Uddin K, Smith PE, Martines LO, Lombardo CR, Jude JR. A vena caval filter for the prevention of pulmonary embolus. Surg Forum 1967; 18:209–11.

99. Greenfield LJ, McCrudy JR, Brown PP, Elkins RC. A new intracaval filter permitting continued flow and resolution of emboli. Surgery 1973; 73: 599–606.

100. Tadarthy SM, Castaneda-Zuniga W, Salomonowitz E et al. Kimray–Greenfield vena cava filter: percutaneous introduction. Radiology 1984; 151: 525–6.

101. Greenfield LJ, Cho KJ, Pais SO, Van Aman M. Preliminary clinical experience with the titanium Greenfield vena cava filter. Arch Surg 1989; 124: 657–9.

102. Roehm JOF, Gianturco C, Barth MH, Wright KC. Percutaneous transcatheter filter for the inferior vena cava: a new device for treatment of patients with pulmonary embolism. Radiology 1984; 150:255–7.

103. Watanabe AT, Teitelbaum GP, Gomes AS, Roehm JOF. MR imaging of the bird's nest filter. Radiology 1990; 177:578–9.

104. Millward SF, Bhargava A, Aquino J et al. Gunther tulip filter: preliminary experience with retrieval. J Vasc Intervent Radiol 2000; 11:75–82.

105. Grassi CJ, Swan TL, Cardella JF. Quality improvement guidelines for percutaneous permanent inferior vena cava filter placement for the prevention of pulmonary embolism. J Vasc Intervent Radiol 2003; 14:S271–S275.

Suggested guidelines for standardised reporting for IVC filter studies that should allow comparisons between independent series.

106. Ranomski JS, Jarrel BE, Carabasi TA, Yang SL, Koolpe H. Risk of pulmonary embolus with inferior vena caval thrombosis. Am J Surg 1987; 53:97–101.

107. Decousus H, Leizorovicz A, Parent F et al. A clinical trial of vena caval filters in the prevention of pulmonary embolism in patients with proximal deep-vein thrombosis. N Engl J Med 1998; 338:409–15.

A randomised trial of anticoagulants alone or with IVC filter in 400 patients. This shows a reduction in non-lethal PE with filter use and an increase in recurrent leg vein thrombosis.

108. Kazmers A, Jacobs LA, Perkins AJ. Pulmonary embolism in veterans affairs medical centers: is vena cava interruption underutilized? Am Surg 1999; 65:1171–5.

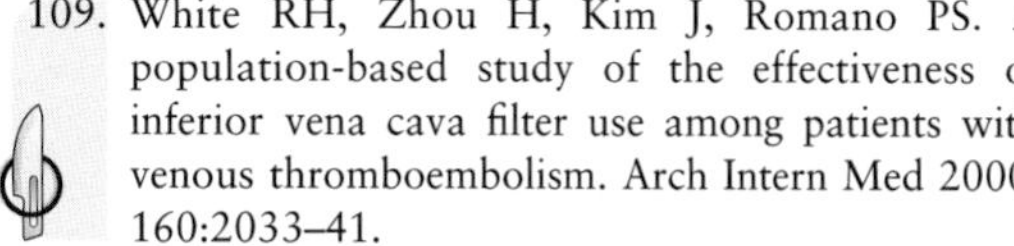

109. White RH, Zhou H, Kim J, Romano PS. A population-based study of the effectiveness of inferior vena cava filter use among patients with venous thromboembolism. Arch Intern Med 2000; 160:2033–41.

110. Athanasoulis CA, Kaufman JA, Halpern EF et al. Inferior vena caval filters: review of a 26-year single-center clinical experience. Radiology 2000; 216:54–66.

111. Greenfield LJ, Proctor MC. Recurrent thromboembolism in patients with vena cava filters. J Vasc Surg 2001; 33:510–14.

112. Millward SF, Oliva VL, Bell SD et al. Gunther tulip retrievable vena cava filter: results from the registry of the Canadian interventional radiology association. J Vasc Intervent Radiol 2001; 12:1053–8.

113. Asch MR. Initial experience in humans with a new retrievable inferior vena cava filter. Radiology 2002; 225:835–44.

114. Proctor MC. Indications for filter placement. Semin Vasc Surg 2000; 13:194–8.

115. Falanga A, Donati MB. Pathogenesis of thrombosis in patients with malignancy. Int J Haematol 2001; 73:137–44.

116. Rosen P, Porter DH, Kim D. Reassessment of vena caval filter use in patients with cancer. J Vasc Intervent Radiol 1994; 5:501–6.

117. Streiff MB. Vena caval filters: a comprehensive review. Blood 2000; 95:3669–77.

118. Shackford SR, Davis JW, Hollingsworth-Fridlung P et al. Venous thromboembolism in patients with major trauma. Am J Surg 1990; 159:365–9.

119. Khansarinia S, Dennis JW, Veldenz HC, Butcher JL, Hartland L. Prophylactic Greenfield filter placement in selected high-risk trauma patients. J Vasc Surg 1995; 22:231–6.

120. Rogers FB, Strindberg G, Shackford SR et al. Five-year follow-up of prophylactic vena cava filters in high risk trauma patients. Arch Surg 1998; 133:406–12.

121. McMurty AL, Owings JT, Anderson JT et al. Increased use of prophylactic caval filters in trauma patients failed to decrease overall incidence of pulmonary embolism. J Am Coll Surg 1999; 189:314–20.

122. Rousseau H, Perreault P, Otal P et al. The 6-F Nitinol TrapEase inferior vena cava filter: results of a prospective multicentre trial. J Vasc Intervent Radiol 2001; 12:299–304.

123. Greenfield LJ, Proctor MC. The percutaneous Greenfield filter: outcomes and practice patterns. J Vasc Surg 2000; 32:888–93.

CHAPTER

Eighteen

Chronic venous insufficiency and lymphoedema

Timothy A. Lees and
Nicholas F.W. Redwood

CHRONIC VENOUS INSUFFICIENCY

Chronic venous insufficiency encompasses disease of the lower limb veins in which venous return is impaired, usually over a number of years, by reflux, obstruction or calf muscle pump failure. This leads to sustained venous hypertension and ultimately clinical complications including oedema, eczema, lipodermatosclerosis and ulceration.

Clinical features

The clinical features of chronic venous insufficiency include swelling, skin changes, ulceration, varicose veins and pain.

SWELLING

Severe swelling is uncommon in chronic venous insufficiency compared with lymphoedema. Most of the swelling is due to oedema fluid, which is initially pitting, but as the disease progresses subcutaneous fibrosis and induration occur. If there is any skin defect, this leads to copious exudation of fluid.

SKIN CHANGES

Varicose eczema commences as dry scaly skin leading to pruritus. The skin becomes friable and may become infected following scratching. Pigmentation, due to the deposition of haemosiderin in the tissues, produces a brown discoloration characteristic of chronic venous insufficiency, which together with fibrosis leads to the clinical picture of lipodermatosclerosis around the ankle (**Fig. 18.1**).

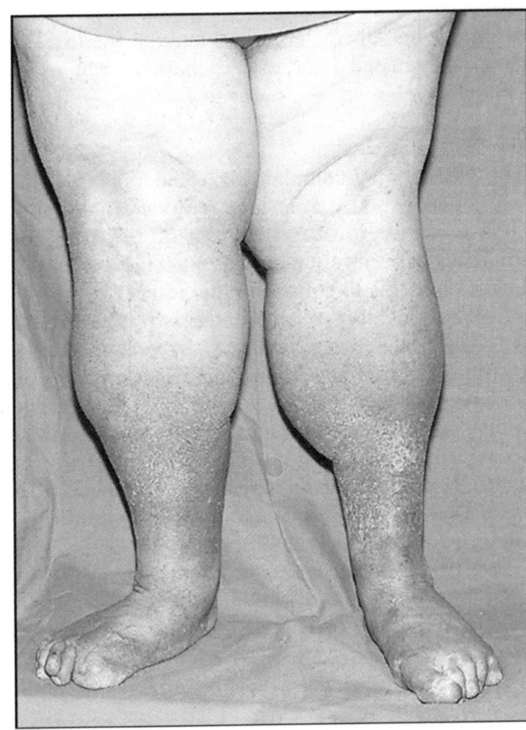

Figure 18.1 • Bilateral chronic venous insufficiency with pigmentation and severe lipodermatosclerosis resulting in the typical 'inverted champagne bottle' shape.

ULCERATION

Ulceration is often precipitated by minor trauma and venous ulcers occur predominantly on the lower leg, more commonly on the medial aspect. These are usually surrounded by eczema or pigmentation and exude fluid that can cause maceration of the surrounding skin. In patients presenting with lower limb ulceration, approximately 80%[1,2] will have evidence of venous disease and 10–25% of limbs will have Doppler-verified arterial disease, with an ankle–brachial pressure index (ABPI) less than 0.9.[2,3]

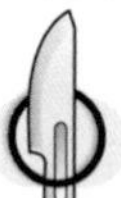

Approximately 12% will have coexisting diabetes or rheumatoid arthritis.[4]

Therefore, assessment of these patients requires a careful history, physical examination and further investigation to elucidate the aetiological factors. Although immobility is often a contributory cause, in isolation it can cause stasis ulceration.

VARICOSE VEINS

It may be obvious that the patient has varicose veins, and a history of previous varicose vein treatment should be sought. However, the absence of visible varicose veins does not exclude the presence of significant superficial reflux, making the investigations discussed later in the chapter even more important.

PAIN

The patient may complain of a general ache and heaviness in the leg after long periods of standing. This is worse towards the end of the day but improves with elevation or bed rest. The occupation of the patient is important in this respect.

A history of deep vein thrombosis (DVT) should be sought, along with a history of venous claudication. The latter is not common and is usually due to extensive iliofemoral vein occlusion in more active individuals. The symptoms may be distinguished from arterial claudication because the increase in arterial inflow during exercise combined with decreased outflow results in acute distension of the limb, giving rise to generalised pain in the leg and a severe bursting sensation. The pain does not stop immediately on cessation of exercise and often requires elevation for 10–20 minutes for relief.

Differential diagnosis

Any diseases or disorders causing lower limb swelling, ulceration or skin changes of lipodermatosclerosis must be considered in the differential diagnosis of chronic venous insufficiency. The more common of these are listed in **Box 18.1**.

Epidemiology

The prevalence of chronic venous insufficiency in the adult population lies between 2 and 9%.[5,6] A

Box 18.1 • Differential diagnosis of chronic venous insufficiency

Venous disease
Primary varicose veins
Primary deep venous incompetence
Post-thrombotic syndrome
Arterial disease
Atheroma
Arteritis
Arteriovenous fistulas
Connective tissue disorders
Rheumatoid arthritis
Systemic lupus erythematosus
Scleroderma
Sarcoid
Behçet's disease
Lymphoedema
Primary
Secondary
Metabolic
Diabetes
Pretibial myxoedema
Inflammatory bowel disease
Nephrotic syndrome
Hepatic failure
Haematological
Sickle cell disease
Thalassaemia
Leukaemia
Polycythaemia rubra vera
Infective
Bacterial
Fungal
Tumours
Basal cell carcinoma
Squamous cell carcinoma
Drugs
Burns
Cardiac failure
Frostbite
Factitious
Dependency

recent study has indicated that it may be higher in males than females (9% vs. 7%).[5] The most serious feature of chronic venous insufficiency is ulceration, which is a distressing and debilitating condition. It has been demonstrated that approximately 50% of ulcers have been present for more than 12 months and 72% are recurrent.[7] Determination of the point prevalence helps health-care planning but accurate assessment of the prevalence of venous ulcers is difficult. Despite this, published reports show similar results. Bobek et al.[8] in Czechoslovakia and Widmer[9] in Switzerland found 1% of subjects had evidence of active ulceration or a history of previous ulceration. Within the UK, Australia, Sweden and Italy, overall rates for active ulceration range from 0.15 to 0.5%, and increase with age.[10–14] More importantly, approximately half the men and one-quarter of the women with ulceration are below retirement age. It has been estimated that in Belgium in 1995, 2–2.5% of the total healthcare budget was spent on the treatment of chronic venous insufficiency.[6] In the UK, the total cost to the National Health Service has been estimated to be £230–600 million a year.[15,16] Combined with the cost of working days lost, this represents a significant burden to the taxpayer.

Aetiology

To understand chronic venous insufficiency, one must consider the changes that occur in both the larger veins (macrocirculation) and the capillary bed (microcirculation).

MACROCIRCULATION

During exercise in the normal individual, effective contraction of the calf muscles combined with vein patency and valvular competence aids venous return and reduces venous pressure in the lower leg from about 90 mmHg to 30 mmHg. Failure of any of these mechanisms may result in postambulatory venous hypertension, which is accepted as the underlying haemodynamic abnormality in chronic venous insufficiency. The recognised causes are outlined in **Box 18.2**.

Box 18.2 • Causes of venous hypertension

Superficial venous reflux
Long saphenous vein reflux
Short saphenous vein reflux
Deep venous reflux and occlusion
Primary (idiopathic)
Secondary to deep venous thrombosis or injury
Perforating vein reflux
Abnormal calf pump
Neurological
Musculoskeletal
Combination of the above

Deep and superficial reflux

Historically, most venous ulcers have been considered secondary to previous DVT. However, with the advent of duplex scanning it has become apparent that there is also a group with primary deep venous reflux and that the superficial systems are more important than previously thought. Isolated superficial venous incompetence without deep venous incompetence has been shown to occur in between 31%[17] and 57%[18] of patients with venous ulceration. In the latter study, in patients with more than one site of reflux, 77% had involvement of the superficial venous system and deep venous reflux was present in 39%. Using ascending and descending venography, superficial reflux has been found in 39% and deep reflux in 57%.[19] It has also been suggested that reflux accounts for up to 95% of the deep venous abnormalities.[20] Of the possible sites of reflux, the iliofemoral, long saphenous and popliteal veins have the greatest effect on haemodynamics and skin changes as opposed to the superficial femoral, profunda femoris and short saphenous veins.[21]

Perforating vein reflux

The contribution of incompetent perforating veins to the development of chronic venous insufficiency remains an area of controversy. Much of the evidence for this is based on healing rates after treatment. However, in most studies of perforator surgery this is combined with other venous surgery and therefore its benefit is difficult to evaluate.[22] The studies which have looked at the patterns of reflux (discussed above) show that isolated perforator incompetence occurs in only 2–4% of limbs with skin changes, and perforator incompetence is usually associated with reflux in the superficial or deep systems. However, the prevalence of incompetent calf-perforating veins and their calf to thigh ratio increase linearly with the clinical severity of chronic venous insufficiency.[23] Whereas ambulatory venous pressures normalise after correction of reflux in the superficial venous systems, no change is seen after perforator surgery and the pressures are very similar to those seen in deep venous reflux.[24] In those cases where superficial and perforator reflux coincide, treating only the former results in healing rates of 95%.[19]

MICROCIRCULATION

The pathophysiological pathway from venous hypertension through lipodermatosclerosis to ulceration is still not fully understood and debate continues on the possible mechanisms.[25] The two most popular current explanations for this process are the white cell trapping hypothesis and the fibrin cuff hypothesis.

1. *White cell trapping hypothesis.* White blood cells are larger and less deformable than red blood cells. The haemodynamic effect of this is that the white cell has a greater effect on blood flow through a narrow channel such as a capillary.[26] If the perfusion pressure across the capillary bed is reduced because of an increase in venous pressure, white cells plug the capillaries and red cells build up behind. On reaching the postcapillary venule, the white cells are forced to marginate by the red cells.[27] Adherence of white cells to the endothelium is then stimulated by (i) decreased shear force[28] and (ii) up-regulation of adhesion molecules by the endothelium as a response to venous hypertension.[29] The trapped white cells release proteolytic enzymes and oxygen free radicals, causing endothelial and tissue damage. As a consequence there is a release of vascular endothelial growth factor. This increases microvascular permeability, which may explain the presence of a fibrin cuff, and also produces excessive amounts of nitric oxide. This in turn damages tissues.[30] Trapping, by reducing perfusion, also has the effect of generating local ischaemia,[31] which may be a trigger to white cell activation.
2. *Fibrin cuff hypothesis.* A rise in venous pressure is directly transmitted to the capillary bed.[32] Associated with this is capillary elongation[33] and widening of the pores between endothelial cells.[34] This results in an increase in the endothelial surface area available for exchange and allows the passage of larger molecules out of the intravascular compartment into the tissues. Fibrinogen is one such molecule that is deposited in the presence of capillary hypertension[35] and polymerises to form fibrin. Patients with chronic venous insufficiency also appear to have a defective interstitial fibrinolytic system within the lower limb,[36] and therefore fibrin accumulates. This may act as a barrier to oxygen, resulting in local tissue ischaemia and cell death, producing ulceration.[37]

There is good evidence to support white cell-mediated damage, with the initiating event being endothelial derangement secondary to venous hypertension. However, neither hypothesis accounts for how lipodermatosclerosis becomes frank ulceration. A possible explanation lies with matrix metalloproteinases. These enzymes help remodel the extracellular matrix by protein degradation, and enhanced matrix metalloproteinase activity has been demonstrated in lipodermatosclerosis. An imbalance in matrix turnover then exists, leading to unrestrained degradation and ulceration.[38] Therefore it is not unreasonable to propose that matrix metalloproteinases finish what the white cells have started.

Other possible mechanisms for the development of ulceration include:

- arteriovenous communications;[39]
- the trap hypothesis[40] (trapping of growth factors and other stimulatory substances by macromolecules leaking from the circulation);
- increased tissue pressure;[41]
- cutaneous iron overload.[42]

Classification

Chronic venous insufficiency involves a variety of anatomical and physiological abnormalities and so a standardised system is required to allow uniformity of reporting.

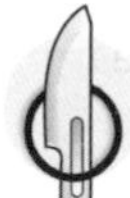

A classification was developed in 1994 by an international consensus conference under the auspices of the American Venous Forum.[43]

This includes clinical signs (C), aetiology (E), anatomical distribution (A) and pathophysiological condition (P), and is therefore known by the acronym CEAP. The CEAP system is helpful in comparing limbs for the purposes of research, although it is rather unwieldy for everyday use (**Box 18.3**).

Investigation

Patients with isolated arterial disease or mixed arterial and venous disease may require arterial intervention. Duplex scanning and arteriography should be considered in these patients. Investigation of venous disease is discussed below.

HAND-HELD DOPPLER

Continuous-wave hand-held Doppler using an 8-MHz probe is a useful tool in screening for arterial and venous disease. Its limitations are that the exact vein being insonated is unknown, it is operator dependent and the significance of reflux of short duration may be uncertain.

Box 18.3 • CEAP classification

Clinical signs (C_{0-6})
Limbs are placed into one of seven clinical classes according to objective signs as follows:
Class 0, no visible or palpable signs of venous disease
Class 1, telangiectases, reticular veins, malleolar flare
Class 2, varicose veins
Class 3, oedema without skin changes
Class 4, skin changes ascribed to venous disease, e.g. lipodermatosclerosis
Class 5, skin changes as above with healed ulceration
Class 6, skin changes as above with active ulceration
Each limb is further classified as asymptomatic (A) or symptomatic (S)
Aetiology (E_C, E_P, E_S)
This classification refers to congenital (C), primary (P) (unknown cause but not congenital) and secondary (S) (acquired) aetiologies. These groups are mutually exclusive
Anatomical distribution ($A_{S,D,P}$)
This refers to superficial (S), deep (D) and perforating (P) veins. More than one system may be involved
Pathophysiological condition ($P_{R,O}$)
This refers to reflux (R) or obstruction (O), or both may be present

DUPLEX SCANNING

This combines a B-mode grey-scale ultrasound image with Doppler ultrasound, which allows the user to accurately select vessels for insonation and to determine the direction of flow. The Doppler flow information can also be incorporated onto the B-mode image as a colour, providing real-time images of blood flow within a vessel. This allows assessment of flow direction and is called colour flow imaging. Very low flow rates can also be detected with power Doppler.

Duplex is an important investigation of lower limb venous disease and is rapidly becoming the gold standard. Modern equipment allows easy identification of normal and abnormal venous anatomy,[44] along with the presence of venous reflux[45] (**Fig. 18.2**). It is also extensively used for the diagnosis of DVT.[46]

VENOGRAPHY

Venography is invasive and to a large extent has been superseded by duplex scanning for the investigation of venous disease. Nevertheless, it can provide useful anatomical and functional information, particularly when the duplex findings are equivocal or duplex is limited, for example in the obese leg.

Varicography

Injection of contrast directly into a varicose vein gives anatomical information and may be of benefit in locating sites of deep to superficial venous connections in recurrent varicose veins and in peri-operative localisation of the sapheno-popliteal junction.[47]

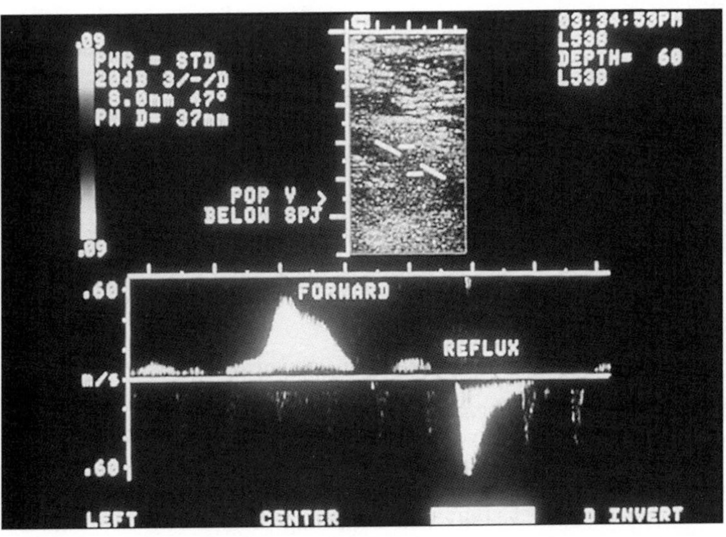

Figure 18.2 • Duplex scan of an incompetent popliteal vein with normal forward flow on squeezing the calf but abnormal reflux on calf release.

Ascending venography

Injection of contrast into a superficial foot vein with a tourniquet occluding the superficial veins at the ankle fills the deep veins. This provides anatomical information regarding occlusion, and can identify perforating vein incompetence.[48] The presence of reflux in deep veins cannot be directly diagnosed by this investigation (**Fig. 18.3**).

Descending venography

Valvular incompetence can be diagnosed by descending venography performed via a cannula inserted into the common femoral vein in the groin.

FUNCTIONAL CALF VOLUME MEASUREMENTS

The investigations described above provide anatomical and functional information on individual veins but do not examine the overall function of the venous system in the lower limb, which is also influenced by the calf muscle pump.[49] The ultimate factor leading to skin changes and ulceration is venous hypertension or, more accurately, lack of venous hypotension on exercise.[50] The venous pressure at the ankle can be measured directly and this remains the gold standard, although it is invasive. Plethysmographic methods indirectly measure venous filling and emptying. These provide an overall measurement of venous function and can help to predict the development of skin changes but are by no means precise for this purpose. Foot volumetry[46] may be used in a similar manner to measure venous filling and emptying.

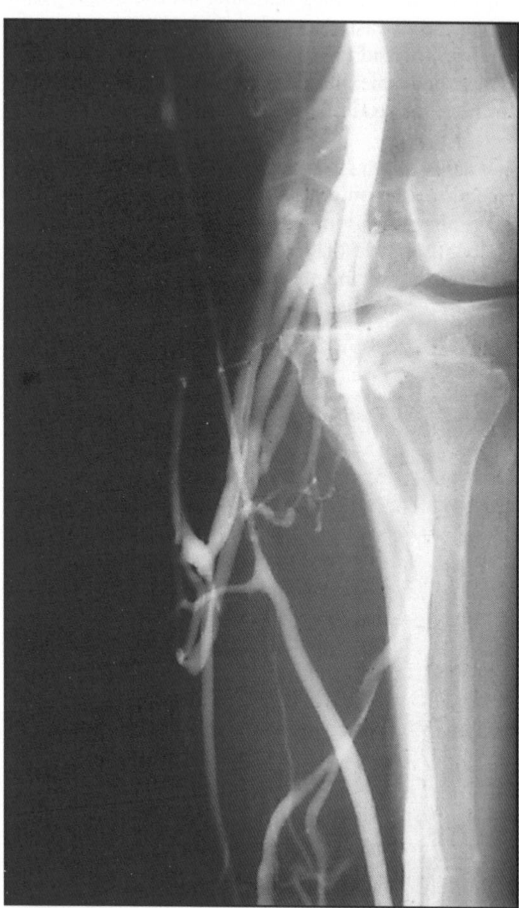

Figure 18.3 • Ascending venogram demonstrating reflux of the sapheno-popliteal junction at the level of the knee. However, reflux in the deep veins cannot be assessed by this technique.

Ambulatory venous pressure measurement

This provides direct measurement of the superficial venous pressure at the ankle.[51] This is achieved by cannulation of a vein on the dorsum of the foot connected to a pressure transducer, amplifier and recorder. The pressure changes recorded in the long saphenous vein in the foot during and after ten tiptoe exercises are shown in **Fig. 18.4**. This investigation is an indicator of overall lower limb venous function including calf muscle pump function.

Plethysmography

There are many different types of plethysmography and these measure either alterations in calf volume directly or other parameters that indirectly reflect volume change. These include photoplethysmography,[52] strain gauge plethysmography[53] and air plethysmography.[54]

Treatment

Management of patients with chronic venous insufficiency may be divided into the prevention or treatment of clinical complications such as lipodermatosclerosis and ulceration. Correcting the underlying cause will help to stop or reverse these complications. In addition, vigorous treatment of conditions known to lead to chronic venous insufficiency, particularly acute DVT, may reduce the incidence of this problem in the long term (see Chapter 17). Management of patients with ulcers of mixed aetiology will require treatment aimed at each specific cause but this section deals predominantly with the treatment of isolated venous disease.

GENERAL MEASURES

These should include elevation of the legs at rest above the level of the heart. This helps to reduce oedema, decrease exudate from ulcers and accelerate regression of skin changes.[4] Immobility, occupation, obesity and coexisting disease may also influence

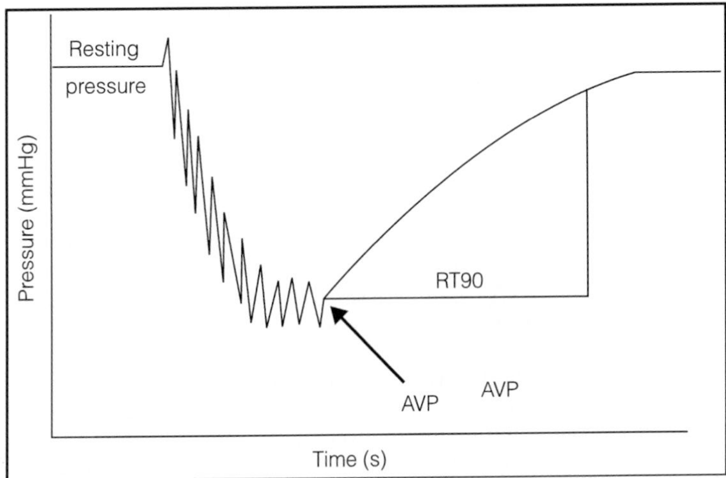

Figure 18.4 • Venous pressure trace recorded from a superficial vein on the dorsum of the foot during ten tiptoe exercises and return to the resting value after exercise. AVP, ambulatory venous pressure; RT90, time for 90% refilling.

the development of skin complications and should be addressed. Placing the patient in bed reduces the venous pressure at the ankle to about 12–15 mmHg and will therefore usually lead to ulcer healing. However, this is not a treatment enjoyed by most patients and may increase the risk of DVT. It is therefore generally reserved for ulcers that have failed to heal by all other methods.

GRADUATED ELASTIC COMPRESSION

Applying a sustained graduated compressive force that is highest at the ankle and decreases proximally has been shown to reduce venous pressure at the ankle,[55] increase femoral vein blood flow[56] and increase venous refilling time.[57] This improves venous function and can heal up to 93% of venous ulcers.[58] Graduated elastic compression may be applied using either bandages or stockings. It is important that these are applied by experienced staff as inexpertly applied compression can do more harm than good.[59]

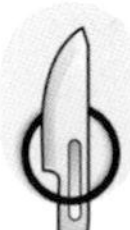

A Cochrane systematic review of compression in the treatment of venous leg ulcers provides a useful summary of the benefits of elastic stockings and bandaging systems.[60]

This demonstrates that in the healing of leg ulcers: (i) compression is more effective than no compression; (ii) elastic compression is more effective than non-elastic compression; (iii) multilayered high compression is more effective than single-layer compression; and (iv) there is no significant difference between four-layer bandaging and other high-compression multilayered systems.

In the prevention of ulcer recurrence, there are no randomised trials comparing compression with no compression.

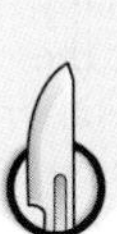

However, a review of trials comparing different grades of compression stocking concludes that higher grades of compression are associated with lower recurrence rates, but at a cost of lower patient compliance[61] (approximately one-third of patients do not comply with the long-term use of compression hosiery).[62]

Stockings are classed according to the pressure they exert at the ankle and are designed to provide a linear graduated decrease in pressure above this, although in practice this may not always be the case.[57] Pressures of up to 60 mmHg may be produced by elastic stockings and conventional pressure classes and indications are given in **Table 18.1**.[62,63]

For the majority of patients with chronic venous insufficiency or mild lymphoedema, a knee-length class 2 compression stocking is ideal, but this will be influenced by how well they tolerate the stocking and their ability to apply them. Thigh-length stockings seem to confer little benefit over knee-length ones and as shorter stockings are easier to put on, compliance with these tends to be better. Stocking applicators may also aid patient compliance.

INTERMITTENT PNEUMATIC COMPRESSION

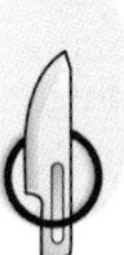

There is some evidence that intermittent pneumatic compression may provide accelerated ulcer healing when used either alone or in combination with elastic compression, although there is a need for further trials in this area.[64,65]

PHARMACOTHERAPY

Dressings

For those patients with venous ulceration, there is a wide variety of topical dressings available. Trials to identify which of these produce the best healing rates

Table 18.1 • Conventional pressure classes of compression stockings

Class	Pressure at ankle (mmHg)	Indications
I	<25	Mild varicosis, venous thrombosis prophylaxis
II	25–35	Marked varicose veins, oedema, chronic venous insufficiency
III	35–45	Chronic venous insufficiency, lymphoedema, following venous ulceration to prevent recurrence
IV	45–60	Severe lymphoedema and chronic venous insufficiency

have been difficult to construct because of many other treatment variables and therefore most of the dressings in everyday use have not been directly compared in the treatment of venous ulceration. Whatever dressing is chosen should be used in conjunction with treatment of the underlying venous insufficiency, usually by adequate graduated elastic compression. Simple non-adherent dressings are all that is required for many ulcers.

Emollients

These soothe, smooth and hydrate the skin and are indicated for all dry or scaling disorders. Therefore they may be of benefit in treating the skin changes associated with chronic venous insufficiency, such as varicose eczema. Their effects are short-lived and frequent application is necessary. Preparations containing an antibacterial should be avoided unless infection is present.

Oxpentifylline (pentoxifylline)

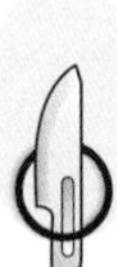

There have been several randomised controlled trials of oxpentifylline compared with placebo, with or without compression, in the healing of venous leg ulcers.[66] These have demonstrated that this drug is more effective than placebo in ulcer healing.

Nutrition

Adequate nutrition is important for ulcer healing, and protein, vitamins A and C, zinc and other trace elements are all important. It may be appropriate to consider dietary supplements if these are deficient.

SURGICAL INTERVENTION

Superficial venous surgery

Superficial surgery may be of benefit in healing ulcers in situations of isolated superficial venous incompetence[67] or combined superficial and deep venous incompetence.[68] Surgery for isolated superficial venous incompetence may also reduce long-term recurrence rates.[69]

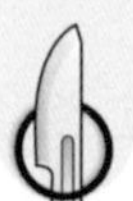

A recent randomised controlled trial comparing superficial venous surgery plus elastic compression with compression alone for venous ulceration has demonstrated no difference in initial healing rates but a reduction in recurrence rates at 12 months in the surgical group, apart from ulcers due to combined superficial and total deep reflux.[70]

Perforating vein surgery

Recently, there has been renewed interest in medial calf-perforating vein incompetence with the advent of subfascial endoscopic perforating vein surgery.[71] This new type of surgery is associated with less morbidity than open perforator surgery[72] and ulcer healing rates in the region of 90% at 1 year have been reported.[73] However, although there have been many studies on this new technique, it is usually carried out in combination with other reflux corrective surgery and the precise indications and benefit of perforator surgery remain unclear.

Deep venous reconstruction

Worldwide experience of deep venous valvular reconstruction is limited as most patients with chronic venous insufficiency can be managed very adequately with superficial venous surgery and the conservative measures described above. Therefore, in most published series it is reserved for those patients with severe symptoms that prove resistant to conservative treatment.[74]

The benefit of deep venous reconstructive surgery is unclear as many of the published series have included ancillary procedures such as high saphenous ligation and stripping, and in the few series where the influence of these procedures has been excluded the numbers involved tend to be small or the follow-up short. A number of different procedures have been described and these are shown in **Box 18.4**.

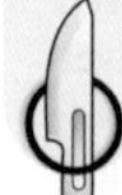

A recent Cochrane review has found only one randomised trial of deep venous reconstructive surgery.[75] This trial compared external valvuloplasty plus superficial venous ligation with superficial venous ligation only. There was a moderate improvement in clinical outcome in the valvuloplasty plus ligation group compared with mild clinical improvement in the ligation-only group. A useful review of non-randomised results of surgery for deep venous incompetence is available.[74]

Venous bypass

Following DVT, recanalisation will occur in all affected venous segments in over 50% of limbs by

Box 18.4 • Procedures for correction of deep venous valvular incompetence

Valvular repair
Valvuloplasty
Valve transposition
Valve transplantation
External support of vein wall
Dacron cuff
Vein wall plication

90 days.[76] However, occasionally there is a failure in recanalisation that leaves a functional venous outflow obstruction (**Fig. 18.5**). If severe, this gives rise to a swollen leg and ultimately skin changes associated with chronic venous insufficiency, and may also cause venous claudication. Surgical bypass of an obstructed vein may be possible, but this should be reserved for those patients in whom there is measured evidence of outflow obstruction and in whom there are severe symptoms. As spontaneous improvement may occur due to the development of collaterals up to 4 years after DVT,[77] surgery should not usually be considered before this time. Two principal surgical procedures have been described.

1. The femoro-femoral crossover graft for iliac obstruction (Palma operation; **Fig. 18.6**).[78] Only a small number of patients are suitable for this procedure, but in these patients long-term patency and relief of symptoms may be achieved in up to 70% of cases.[79] The long saphenous vein on the unaffected side is used as a crossover graft.
2. Limbs with functional outflow obstruction due to stenosed or occluded deep thigh veins may be suitable for sapheno-popliteal bypass, which uses the long saphenous vein as a bypass channel. The theoretical difficulty with this procedure is that the long saphenous vein may already be acting as a collateral channel and to interfere with this may make matters worse should thrombosis occur. However, good long-term patency rates have been reported.[80]

Skin grafting

Large ulcers may be usefully treated with a split-skin graft or pinch grafts, which, if successful, will reduce the healing time. Before this is undertaken, it is important that the ulcer bed is clear from slough and not infected (particularly β-haemolytic

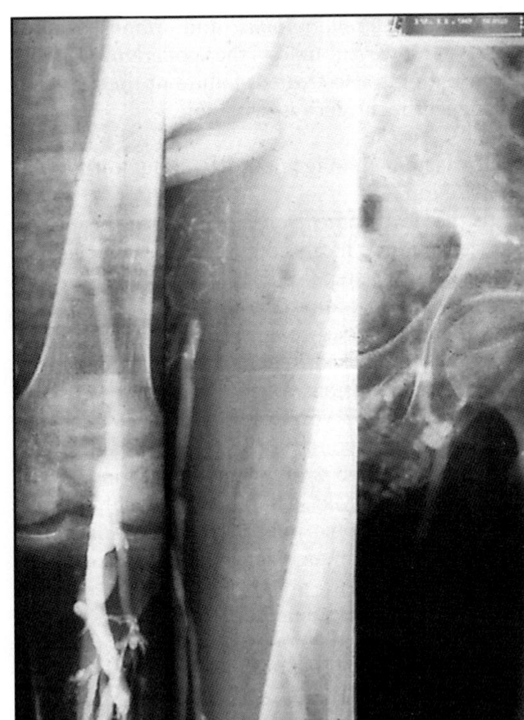

Figure 18.5 • Ascending venogram demonstrating severe disease/occlusion of the superficial femoral vein above the knee. The long saphenous vein is acting as a collateral and refilling the iliac vein at the groin.

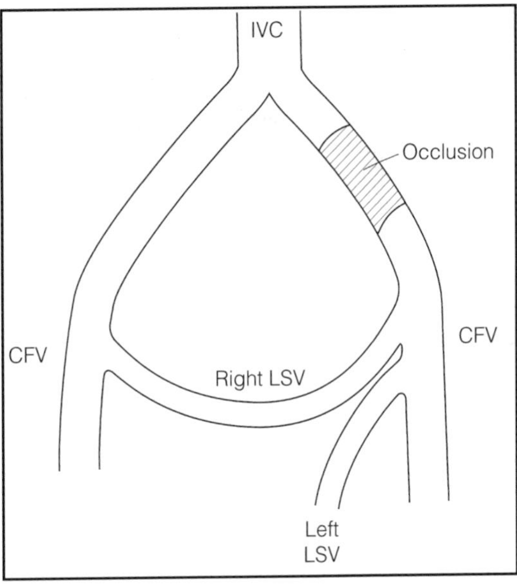

Figure 18.6 • Femoro-femoral crossover graft using long saphenous vein (LSV) to bypass unilateral iliac obstruction. IVC, inferior vena cava; CFV, common femoral vein.

streptococci, *Pseudomonas* and *Staphylococcus aureus*). However, unless the underlying venous abnormality is also treated, failure of the graft and subsequent recurrence is inevitable.

Endovascular management of venous outflow obstruction

With the development of endovascular treatments in recent years it has become clear that iliac venous occlusions and stenoses may be treated by endoluminal stenting, although the long-term results have not been directly compared with surgery. Raju et al.[81] have reported treating a small series of long iliac venous occlusions, with primary and secondary patency rates at 2 years of 49% and 76% respectively. Further studies have reported patency rates in the region of 90% at 1 year for stenting of iliac venous stenoses (May–Thurner syndrome).[82,83] This refers to the chronic pulsatile compression of the proximal left common iliac vein by the overlying right common iliac artery or aortic bifurcation, resulting in an intraluminal venous spur web or membrane. This common lesion (20% of the adult population) is an increasingly well-recognised cause of left iliac vein thrombo-occlusive disease, particularly in young patients. The clinical picture is of left leg venous hypertension or DVT and is likely to explain the preponderance for left-sided DVT in general.

Preventing the post-thrombotic limb

Chronic venous insufficiency developing secondary to previous DVT is commonly referred to as post-thrombotic syndrome (PTS) or post-phlebitic syndrome. The management of DVT has historically been directed at preventing thrombus extension and pulmonary embolus in the acute phase. There has been little focus on long-term treatment in order to prevent the development of PTS.

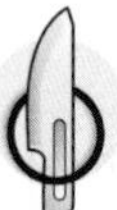

The risk of developing severe chronic venous insufficiency with ulceration following DVT is in the order of 2–10% at 10 years.[84–86]

However, 30% or more will develop features of mild or moderate PTS.[86–88] This risk increases with more proximal DVT and recurrent thrombosis, the latter occurring in approximately 30% of patients at 8 years.[89] Even with isolated calf vein thrombosis there is a risk of development of PTS, although this risk is lower than with popliteal or more proximal thromboses.

The causes of PTS related to previous DVT are either valvular incompetence or residual outflow obstruction with eventual calf muscle pump failure. Therefore treatment of the primary DVT should be aimed not only at preventing thrombus propagation and pulmonary embolism but also at preventing venous damage and preserving or restoring venous function. This may include anticoagulation, limb elevation, elastic compression therapy and, in some cases, thrombolysis. Patients who have had DVT should be considered for long-term elastic compression hosiery, in particular those patients with residual reflux and who are on their feet all day or travel long journeys.[85] They should be encouraged to take regular exercise to stimulate the calf muscle pump. These simple measures may be required for life but are often all that is needed to prevent a lifetime of debility due to PTS.

Mixed arterial and venous disease

Ulcers with a mixed arterial and venous aetiology are becoming increasingly recognised, possibly because of improved diagnostic techniques but also because of the ageing of the population. It has been demonstrated that venous disease only is present in approximately 60% of lower limb ulcers,[90,91] pure arterial disease in approximately 15%, and combined arterial and venous disease in approximately 13%.[91,92]

In patients with severe arterial disease (ABPI <0.5), there is little doubt that this should be treated first. Successful revascularisation may then be followed by elastic compression therapy. Patients with an ABPI greater than 0.85 can usually be treated with compression therapy without arterial intervention,[93] although it should be remembered that some patients with calcified vessels may have falsely elevated ankle pressures. In patients with an ABPI between 0.5 and 0.85, traditional teaching is that these patients should undergo arterial revascularisation before compression therapy. However, there is some evidence that many of these patients may achieve ulcer healing with compression therapy alone.[58,93,94] The degree of compression may need to be reduced, for example a three-layer bandage utilising only one elastic layer instead of two in the conventional four-layer bandage. Patients treated in this manner should be carefully monitored for signs of deterioration in the ulcer, as in this circumstance arterial intervention may be necessary.

Summary

Investigation and treatment must be tailored to the individual patient but a simplified everyday management plan is shown in **Fig. 18.7**.

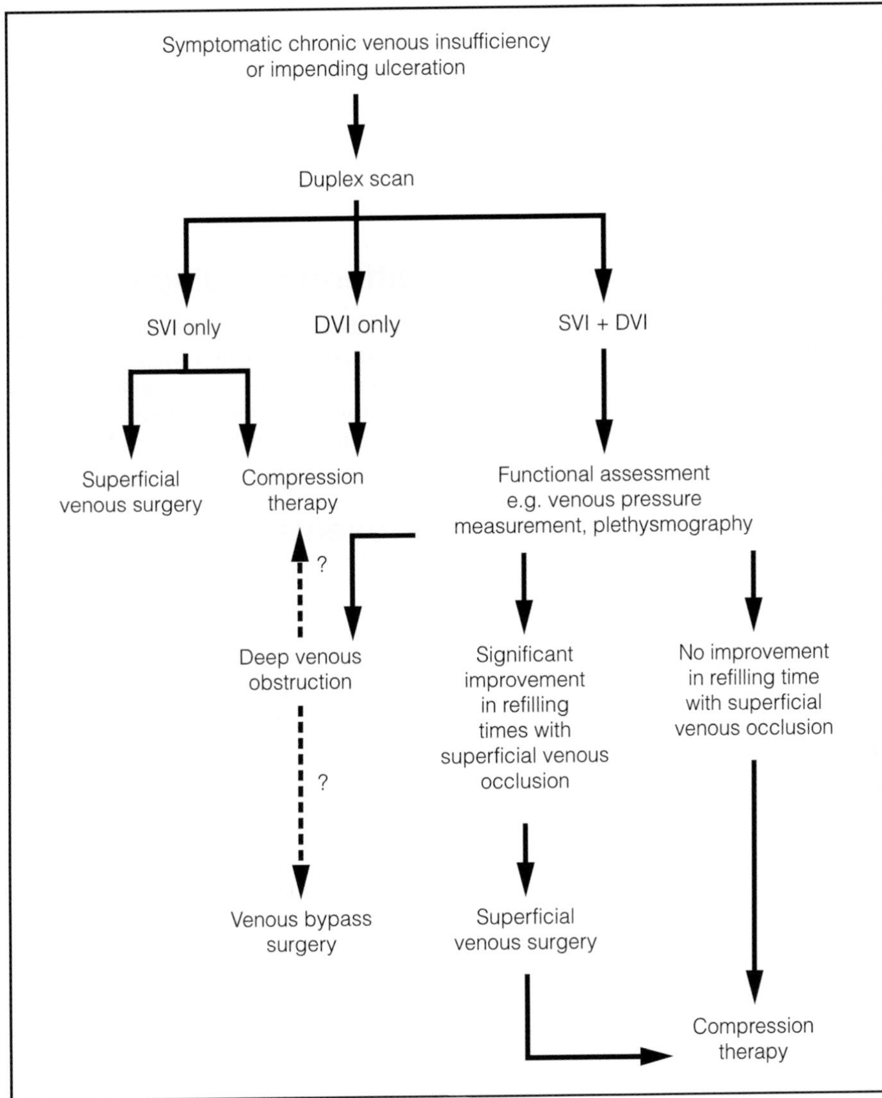

Figure 18.7 • Flow diagram for the management of chronic venous insufficiency. DVI, deep venous incompetence; SVI, superficial venous incompetence.

LYMPHOEDEMA

Lymphoedema is the progressive swelling of a limb that occurs when the lymphatic system fails to transport fluid via the lymphatic vessels and lymph nodes.

Aetiology

Lymphoedema can be primary or secondary.

PRIMARY

The traditional classification of primary lymphoedema is shown in **Box 18.5**. Congenital lymphoedema occurs at or soon after birth and in some rare cases is autosomally inherited (Milroy's disease[95,96]). Lymphoedema praecox[97] presents up to the age of 35 years and is more common in women than men. Lymphoedema tarda[98] presents over the age of 35 years. It is likely that these three groups represent different parts of the same spectrum of disease, which has been attributed to aplasia, hypoplasia or hyperplasia of the lymph vessels during development. However, a fibrotic obstruction in the lymph nodes has also been described.[99,100]

In addition to this, a functional classification more oriented to the treatment of these conditions

Box 18.5 • Causes of lymphoedema

Primary
Congenital (age <1 year)
Familial (Milroy's disease)
Non-familial
Praecox (age <35 years)
Familial
Non-familial
Tarda (age >35 years)
Secondary
Malignant disease
Surgery
Radical mastectomy
Radical groin dissection
Radiotherapy
Infection
Parasitic (filariasis)
Pyogenic (β-haemolytic streptococci, *Staphylococcus aureus*)
Tuberculosis
Impairment
Arterial surgery
Venous disease and venous surgery

may be used. This type of classification was first described by Browse.[101]

- Obliterative (80%): the distal lymphatics undergo progressive obliteration. This occurs predominantly in females and is often bilateral.
- Proximal obstruction (10%): proximal occlusion occurs in the abdominal, pelvic or inguinal lymph nodes. This is predominantly unilateral.
- Lymphatic valvular incompetence and hyperplasia (10%): development of the valve system is incomplete and lymphatic dilatation and hyperplasia occur. This is usually bilateral.

SECONDARY

Secondary lymphoedema occurs when the lymphatic channels become occluded due to an acquired cause. The lymphatic channels distal to the obstruction become dilated and the valves secondarily incompetent. The commonest cause worldwide is filarial infestation but in the UK the commonest cause is neoplasia and its treatment, for example post-mastectomy lymphoedema. Impairment of lymphatic drainage can also be demonstrated after arterial[102] and venous[103] surgery. The causes of secondary lymphoedema are also listed in **Box 18.5**.

Differential diagnosis

Any cause of chronic swelling of the leg must be considered in the differential diagnosis of lymphoedema. This is very similar to the differential diagnosis of chronic venous insufficiency and the commoner causes are listed in **Box 18.1**.

Presentation

Initial presentation is with peripheral oedema. History and examination will usually be able to differentiate lymphoedema from other causes of limb swelling and may distinguish between primary and secondary causes.

HISTORY

The patient complains of a slowly progressive swelling of the limb, and as the oedema progresses skin complications develop. Limb swelling usually commences distally and may progress during the day, particularly on standing. Although rarely painful, the leg may feel heavy and uncomfortable and there may be a history of recurrent lymphangitis. Primary lymphoedema occurs predominantly in females in their early teens, especially around puberty,[104] whereas patients with secondary lymphoedema will commonly have a history of previous surgery, neoplastic disease or radiotherapy.

EXAMINATION

Examination reveals swelling of the limb, which may be unilateral or bilateral. Initially it will pit like other types of oedema but with time the swelling becomes non-pitting due to fat and increasing subcutaneous fibrosis, although pitting can usually be demonstrated with prolonged pressure. The swelling is uniform and as it progresses the leg becomes like a tree-trunk (**Fig. 18.8**). The skin, which is initially pinkish-red, develops a 'peau d'orange' appearance with hyperkeratosis of the toes and skin fissuring with secondary fungal infection. The skin gradually thickens, becoming less elastic until it is not possible to pick up a fold in the lower leg. The dorsum of the foot is usually involved, producing the characteristic 'buffalo hump' appearance, and chylous vesicles may occur on the pretibial area.

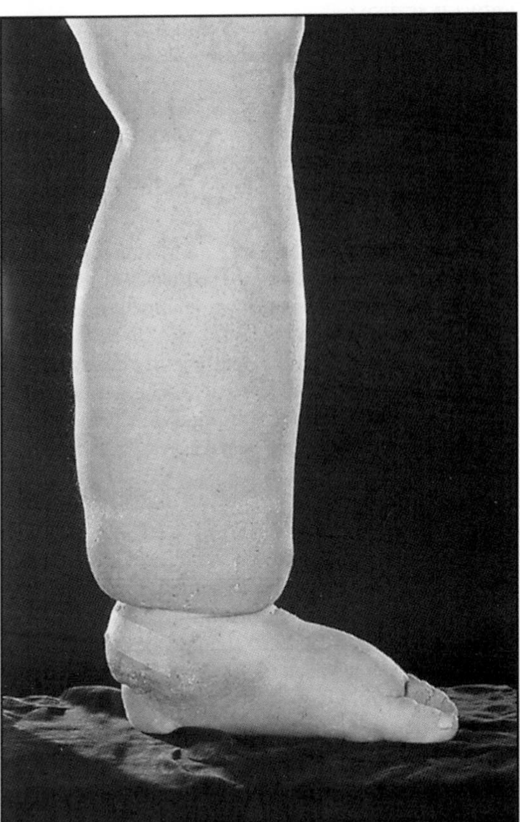

Figure 18.8 • Chronic lymphoedema of the leg with tree-trunk appearance and 'buffalo-hump' of the foot.

Ankle ulceration is not usually found with lymphoedema. It has been suggested that the reason for this is that the skin remains more elastic than in venous disease, allowing expansion to occur without increased tension.[105] The presence of surgical scars or skin telangiectasia following radiotherapy should be noted and may indicate a cause of secondary lymphoedema.

Investigation

The diagnosis of lymphoedema can usually be made clinically. Investigation is needed to exclude sinister underlying causes such as a mass in the pelvis or if surgery is being considered in order to confirm the diagnosis and plan treatment. The investigations are listed in **Box 18.6**.

DUPLEX ULTRASONOGRAPHY

This is useful to exclude chronic venous insufficiency. The B-mode image will also detect the changes in the dermis and subcutaneous layers and can therefore be used as a means of monitoring the disease.

Box 18.6 • Investigations that aid the diagnosis of lymphoedema

- Duplex ultrasonography
- Lymphangioscintigraphy
- Computed tomography
- Magnetic resonance imaging
- Contrast lymphangiography
- Volumetry

LYMPHANGIOSCINTIGRAPHY (ISOTOPE LYMPHOGRAPHY)

This is now one of the most frequently performed investigations as it provides an overall assessment of lymphatic drainage and in the majority of cases avoids the need for conventional lymphangiography (**Fig. 18.9**). Radiolabelled (usually technetium) colloid is injected into the interdigital space between the second and third toes on both sides and gamma-camera pictures are taken at 5-minute intervals to assess transit through the lymph channels. Scintigraphy has been demonstrated to have a sensitivity of 92% and a specificity of 100% for the diagnosis of lymphoedema,[106] such that a negative investigation effectively excludes the

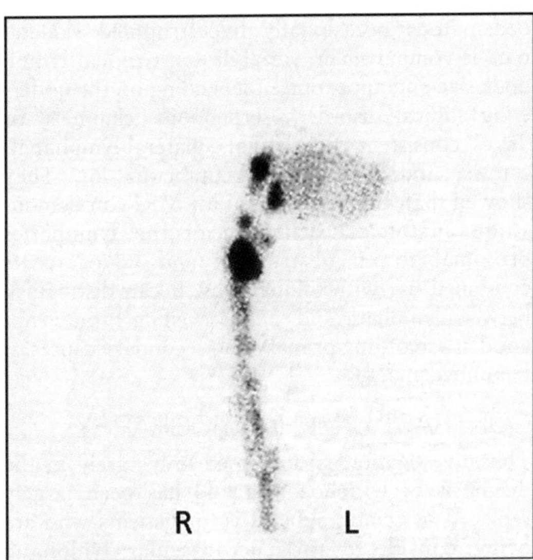

Figure 18.9 • Lymphangioscintigram confirming left-sided lymphoedema. On the right, the isotope is travelling up the lymphatics of the leg with concentration in the ilioinguinal nodes (normal). On the left, the isotope has remained in the foot (not seen).

diagnosis. Primary and secondary lymphoedema are frequently associated with similar scintigraphic appearances, including delayed transit, the presence of collaterals, a cutaneous pattern in the distal limb (dermal backflow), and reduced uptake in one or more groups of lymph nodes. However, it can be used to distinguish between a venous and lymphatic cause of limb swelling[107] and is a good method to assess treatment responses.

COMPUTED TOMOGRAPHY

Computed tomography will show the presence of dilated lymphatic channels, thereby aiding the diagnosis of obstructive lymphoedema and lymphatic valvular incompetence. It will also provide evidence of lymphoedema by the presence of a honeycomb appearance of fluid in the subcutaneous tissues, and has been used to monitor the response to compression therapy by measuring the cross-sectional area of limb compartments.[108] Patients with a previous history of pelvic or abdominal malignancy should be scanned for recurrent disease in order to diagnose enlarged lymph nodes or pelvic masses that may be compressing the lymphatic channels.

MAGNETIC RESONANCE IMAGING

In patients with chronic lymphoedema, magnetic resonance imaging (MRI) has been shown to demonstrate circumferential subcutaneous oedema with a fibrotic honeycomb pattern.[109,110] Case et al.[111] examined 32 patients with peripheral lymphoedema using both scintigraphy and MRI. They found that MRI characteristically showed diffuse dermal and subcutaneous oedema, a non-oedematous occasionally hypertrophied skeletal muscle compartment, variability in regional lymph node size and appearance (depending on the underlying clinical disorder), serpiginous 'channels' or 'lakes' consistent with dermal collateral lymphangiectasis, and increased subcutaneous fat. They showed that, unlike scintigraphy, MRI can demonstrate anatomical definition of the lymphatics proximal to an obstruction and advocate its combined use with scintigraphy. It can distinguish between lymphatic and venous swelling[112] but is not good at separating primary and secondary causes of lymphoedema.[113]

CONTRAST LYMPHANGIOGRAPHY

This investigation is now used only rarely in the diagnosis of lymphoedema and has been largely replaced by scintigraphy. It is for patients who are being considered for microvascular lymphatic reconstruction and remains the best investigation for imaging the thoracic duct and for identifying lymphatic fistulas in the chest, abdomen and pelvis. In addition, it can distinguish reactive lymph glands from tumour-containing glands.[114]

VOLUMETRY

This is not a diagnostic test but is used as a reliable method of measuring upper or lower limb volume by water displacement, allowing an objective assessment of treatment [115,116]

Treatment

The aim of treatment is to reduce limb swelling, reduce the risk of infection and improve function. If management begins early in the disease process when pitting oedema is present, conservative measures should be successful. Once achieved the improvement must be maintained. Surgical options are available in a few centres for resistant and severely symptomatic cases.

GENERAL MEASURES

Once the diagnosis is made, a clear explanation of the condition and its non-life-threatening nature is given to the patient. Information leaflets help to reassure the patient and encourage good compliance, which is needed for a lifetime of careful attention. Simple elevation of a lymphoedematous limb while resting during the day and sleeping at night reduces oedema by increasing venous return and reducing the production of interstitial fluid, thus allowing the lymphatics to catch up. The muscle contraction of exercise, such as on an exercise bicycle, encourages movement of lymph along non-contractile vessels and increased contractility of collecting lymph vessels.[117]

MANUAL LYMPHATIC DRAINAGE

This can be initiated by the physiotherapist. It involves manipulating the leg by squeezing just above the most proximal area of oedema and then working from proximal to distal. This enhances lymphatic flow.

GRADUATED ELASTIC COMPRESSION

Compression stockings are worn to cover the extent of the lymphoedema and have been shown to be effective.[118] A pressure of approximately 50 mmHg is recommended or a pressure as high as can be tolerated. The advantage of the stocking is that it can be used for maintenance of the limb after oedema reduction but compliance is low in the summer months, and the elderly and frail find them difficult to apply. Compression can also be achieved by multilayer bandaging with wool and short stretch bandages.

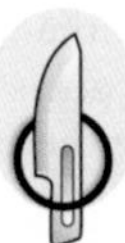

If graduated elastic compression is used initially followed by a stocking for maintenance, a greater and more sustained limb volume reduction is achieved than if stockings alone are used throughout.[119]

INTERMITTENT PNEUMATIC COMPRESSION

More sophisticated methods include sequential external pneumatic compression. The limb is placed in a multicompartmental sleeve. Each compartment consists of an air cell connected separately to a compressor. The cells are sequentially inflated to a pressure of about 80 mmHg and deflated from distal to proximal, thus massaging the lymph centrally. Patients use this for 4 hours a day and it can be done at home. It is necessary to wear a long sock to collect the moisture that develops and prevent skin maceration. If the lymphatic system is obliterated or obstructed more proximally, massaging the lymph centrally can precipitate collections elsewhere, such as the genitals, and high pressures may injure peripheral lymphatics. Reports combining pneumatic compression with stockings have given figures of 90% for immediate benefit and long-term maintenance.[120] The poor responders have usually had oedema for more than 10 years. In these chronic patients, compression using the hydrostatic pressure of mercury has had some effect.[121] The leg is placed in a cylinder and is covered by two membranes, which are filled and emptied with mercury in cycles. Pressures of up to 800 mmHg are generated at the foot and this linearly decreases towards normal atmospheric pressure at the surface. This is well tolerated and improvement is even seen in those with brawny (fibrosclerotic) oedema. Despite its theoretical simplicity, the application and safety precautions are complex.

THERMAL TREATMENT[122]

Hyperthermia of the leg is produced by microwave heating or immersion in hot water. There is no change to the flow of lymph but it does reduce the local inflammatory infiltrate and extracellular protein matrix. A reduction in limb volume follows, along with a decrease in the rate of recurrent infections.

COMPLEX DECONGESTIVE PHYSIOTHERAPY (COMPLEX PHYSICAL THERAPY)

Complex decongestive physiotherapy initially combines compression bandaging, manual lymphatic drainage, exercise and skin care for about 2 weeks. This is followed by wearing a stocking, wrapping at night and continued exercise. With good compliance a 65–67% reduction in limb volume can be achieved, with 90% of the reduction being maintained at 9 months.[123,124] As an added benefit the incidence of infection almost halves.

PREVENTION OF INFECTION

The lymphatic system transports lymphocytes, enabling rapid response to foreign antigens. Stagnation of lymph prevents this and so increases the risk and severity of infection. The common pathogens are β-haemolytic streptococci and *Staph. aureus*. With each attack of cellulitis or erysipelas the organisms further obliterate the lymph channels, making the oedema worse. Well-fitting comfortable shoes prevent small cracks in the skin that may act as a portal of entry. The affected limb should be washed daily with a mild soap and the feet must be dry before putting on shoes. If the skin is moist and macerated, fungal infection occurs and allows secondary infection. The patient must keep a very careful eye on the foot and any early signs of infection must be treated aggressively with antibiotics. Failure to control recurrent infection can be managed by long-term, prophylactic, low-dose antibiotics such as amoxicillin, flucloxacillin or a cephalosporin.

DRUGS

Benzopyrones are thought to reduce oedema by activating extralymphatic absorption of tissue proteins by increasing the number of macrophages. The onset of action is slow but in a meta-analysis of 20 trials in early lymphoedema, mean volume reductions of 55% were seen.[125] In four trials, reduction was even seen in elephantitic legs. When used in conjunction with complex decongestive physiotherapy in a multicentre trial, an increased volume reduction of between 150 and 300% at 1 year was reported.[126]

Diuretics may help for a short time in early oedema in combination with other modalities, but long-term therapy is of no value. Underlying filarial infection should be treated with diethylcarbamazine.

Lymphangiogenesis is mediated through the vascular endothelial growth factor (VEGF)-3 receptor on lymphatic endothelia.[127] Some early work on animal models has shown that stimulation of this receptor by VEGF-C will improve lymphatic function.[128]

SURGICAL TREATMENTS

These can be divided into debulking operations and bypass procedures. Surgery is only indicated if conservative measures have failed and there is monstrous lymphoedema, inability to work or walk, lymphorrhagia or recurrent lymphangitis. The surgical approach depends on the underlying lymphatic abnormality. Obliterative causes, which form the majority of cases, are best treated by debulking procedures, whereas in lymphatic obstruction physiological bypass is recommended.

Debulking operations

The principle in these procedures is to excise variable amounts of the excess skin and subcutaneous tissue from the affected limb. The techniques range from removal of ellipses of tissue and primary closure (Homan's operation) (**Fig. 18.10**) to the radical Charles' operation, which excises all the skin and subcutaneous tissues of the calf down to and sometimes including the deep fascia. Primary skin grafting is then required. Good functional results have been obtained with this method[129] but cosmesis is poor and it may be complicated by warts, resistant ulceration, lymph weeping and pantalooning of the thigh. Suction lipectomy, which has good results in the postmastectomy arm,[130] has been advocated in order to overcome these problems but only in the less severe situation[131] because there is a tendency for greater fibrosis in the lower limb.

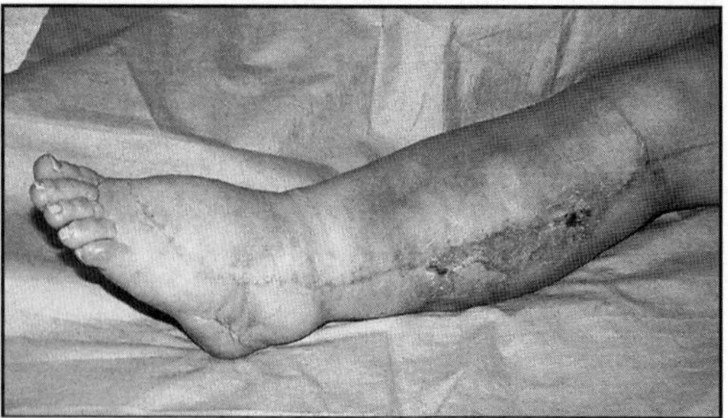

Figure 18.10 • Homan's operation. A long ellipse of skin and subcutaneous tissue has been excised from the lateral side of the leg after a previous procedure on the medial side. Poor wound healing is common.

Bypass procedures

These are reserved for regional blockage of the lymphatics, which could be due to either primary obstructive or secondary causes. If an iatrogenic secondary cause is suspected, a period of 6 months should elapse to allow any procedural swelling to subside before embarking on a lymphatic bypass. The bypass procedures are listed in **Box 18.7**.

Box 18.7 • Bypass procedures for lymphoedema

- Skin and muscle flaps
- Omental bridges
- Enteromesenteric bridges
- Lymphatico-lymphatic anastomosis
- Lymphatico-venous anastomosis

Skin, muscle and omentum have been used to bypass regional obstructions but these tissues tend to have a paucity of lymphatics and as the technique relies on the development of new channels, high levels of success have not been reported. The more sophisticated technique of enteromesenteric bridging was designed to overcome this problem.[132] A 10-cm segment of ileum is resected on its mesentery and opened along its antimesenteric border. The mucosa is dissected off, leaving a submucosal area rich in lymphatics and blood vessels. The uppermost normal nodes are identified and bisected. The submucosal patch is then stitched in place over the top. Investigation has shown the early development of a lymphatic bridge and follow-up for 6 years has demonstrated a maintained improvement in 75% of legs, but the numbers are very small.[133]

Autologous lymphatic vessels harvested from the contralateral normal limb are used to perform lymphatico-lymphatic anastomoses[134] and bypass obstruction. A lymphatic vessel suitable as a conduit is identified in the thigh after the injection of patent blue dye into the interdigital spaces. The recipient vessels are found by searching with the operating microscope. In the presence of an iliac block, the graft is crossed over to the contralateral groin. The anastomosis requires 40× magnification and 11-0 interrupted sutures, making the operation technically demanding. Despite this, animal models have shown 100% patency rates. Assessment by measuring limb volumes reveals initial improvements in 66% of cases but this falls to about 50% at 1 year. Data are now available showing that lower limb bypasses maintain improvement to 8 years and those in the upper limb for 10 years.[135,136]

Lymphatico-venous anastomosis is physiological if one considers the termination of the thoracic duct at the subclavian vein. Where possible, the lymphatics are identified as above and anastomosed end to side to an adjacent vein allowing lymph to return centrally. The best results are obtained if the lymphoedema is not chronic and multiple anastomoses are performed with a leash of lymphatic vessels. Excellent long-term results have been published, with volume reductions on average of 67% lasting more than 7 years in the 85% of patients followed up.[137] After the microsurgery, an 87% reduction in the incidence of cellulitis was seen.

Key points

- Chronic venous insufficiency affects 2–9% of the adult population.
- The risk of mild to moderate chronic venous insufficiency after DVT is 30% at 10 years.
- The risk of severe chronic venous insufficiency after DVT is 2–10% at 10 years.
- Superficial venous reflux alone may cause chronic venous insufficiency.
- Graduated elastic compression is effective in healing ulcers and preventing recurrence.
- Superficial venous surgery may be of benefit in isolated superficial venous incompetence and combined superficial and deep venous incompetence.
- There is only limited evidence for the benefit of deep venous reconstructive surgery and endovascular therapy.
- Lymphoedema may be classified as primary or secondary.
- A further functional classification of obliterative, proximal obstruction, and valvular incompetence and hyperplasia may be used.
- The commonest cause of lymphoedema worldwide is filariasis.
- In the UK the commonest cause is malignancy and its treatment.
- Oedema is initially pitting, but becomes non-pitting due to subcutaneous fat deposition and fibrosis.
- Ulceration is rare.
- Diagnosis is usually confirmed by isotope lymphangioscintigraphy.
- Satisfactory treatment can usually be achieved by conservative measures, including manual drainage, elastic compression, complex decongestive therapy and prevention of infection.

REFERENCES

1. Ruckley CV, Callam MJ, Dale JJ. Causes of chronic leg ulceration. Lancet 1982; ii:615–16.
2. Cornwall JV, Lewis JD. Leg ulcers: epidemiology and aetiology. Br J Surg 1986; 73:693–6.
3. Callam MJ, Harper DR, Dale JJ et al. Arterial disease in chronic leg ulceration: an underestimated hazard? Lothian and Forth Valley leg ulcer study. Br Med J 1987; 294:1389–91.

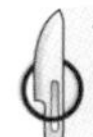

4. The Alexander House Group. Consensus paper venous leg ulcers. J Dermatol Surg Oncol 1992; 18:592–602.

   A condensed consensus report summarising the status of various aspects of epidemiology, diagnosis and treatment of venous ulcers. Various investigational and treatment approaches are summarised and recommendations given. Level 2 evidence.

5. Evans CJ, Fowkes FG, Ruckley CV, Lee AJ. Prevalence of varicose veins and chronic venous insufficiency in men and women in the general population: Edinburgh Vein Study. J Epidemiol Community Health 1999; 53:149–53.
6. Van den Oever R, Hepp B, Bebbaut B, Simon I. Socio-economic impact of chronic venous insufficiency. An underestimated public health problem. Int Angiol 1998; 17:161–7.
7. Nelzen O, Bergqvist D, Lindhagen A. Venous and non-venous leg ulcers: clinical history and appearance in a population study. Br J Surg 1994; 81:182–7.
8. Bobek K, Cajzl L, Cepalek V et al. Etude de la frequence des maladies phlebologiques et de quelques facteurs etiologiques. Phlebologie 1966; 19:217–30.
9. Widmer LK. Peripheral venous disorders: prevalence and sociomedical importance. Bern: Hans Huber, 1978.
10. Callam MJ, Ruckley CV, Harper DR et al. Chronic ulceration of the leg: extent of the problem and provision of care. Br Med J 1985; 290:1855–6.
11. Cornwall JV, Dore CJ, Lewis JD. Leg ulcers: epidemiology and aetiology. Br J Surg 1986; 73:693–9.
12. Baker SR, Stacey MC, Jopp-McKay AG et al. Epidemiology of chronic venous ulcers. Br J Surg 1991; 78:864–7.
13. Lees TA, Lambert D. Prevalence of lower limb ulceration in an urban health district. Br J Surg 1992; 79:1032–4.
14. Cesarone MR, Belcaro G, Nicolaides AN et al. 'Real' epidemiology of varicose veins and chronic venous disease: the San Valentino Vascular Screening Project. Angiology 2002; 53:119–30.
15. Harding K. Wound management in general practice. In: Royal College of General Practice Members' Reference Book. London: Sabre-crown, 1991; pp. 313–16.

16. Bosanquet N. Costs of venous ulcers: from maintenance therapy to investment programmes. Phlebology 1992; 7:44–6.
17. Ruckley CV, Evans CJ, Allan PL et al. Chronic venous insufficiency: clinical and duplex correlations. The Edinburgh Vein Study of venous disorders in the general population. J Vasc Surg 2002; 36:520–5.
18. Lees TA, Lambert D. Patterns of venous reflux in limbs with skin changes associated with chronic venous insufficiency. Br J Surg 1993; 80:725–8.
19. Darke SG, Penfold C. Venous ulceration and saphenous ligation. Eur J Vasc Surg 1992; 6:4–9.
20. McEnroe CS, O'Donnell TF, Mackay WC. Correlation of clinical findings with venous hemodynamics in 386 patients with chronic venous insufficiency. Am J Surg 1988; 156:148–52.
21. Payne SPK, London NJM, Jagger C et al. Clinical significance of venous reflux detected by duplex scanning. Br J Surg 1994; 81:39–41.
22. Negus D, Friedgood A. The effective management of venous ulceration. Br J Surg 1983; 70:623–7.
23. Delis KT, Ibegbuna V, Nicolaides AN et al. Prevalence and distribution of incompetent perforating veins in chronic venous insufficiency. J Vasc Surg 1998; 28:815–25.
24. Burnand KG, O'Donnell TF, Lea Thomas M et al. The relative importance of incompetent communicating veins in the production of varicose veins and venous ulcers. Surgery 1977; 82:9–14.
25. Coleridge Smith PD. The microcirculation in venous hypertension. Vasc Med 1997; 2:203–13.
26. Chien S, Schmalzer EA, Lee MML et al. Role of white blood cells in filtration of blood cell suspension. Biorheology 1983; 20:11–27.
27. Schmid-Schonbein GW, Usami S, Skalak R et al. The interaction of leukocytes and erythrocytes in capillary and postcapillary vessels. Microvasc Res 1980; 19:45–70.
28. Lawrence MB, McIntire LV, Eskin SG. Effect of flow on polymorphonuclear leukocyte/endothelial cell adhesion. Blood 1987; 70:1284–90.
29. Sahary M, Shields DA, Georgiannos SN et al. Endothelial activation in patients with chronic venous disease. Eur J Vasc Endovasc Surg 1998; 15:342–9.
30. Shoab SS, Scurr JH, Coleridge Smith PD. Increased plasma vascular endothelial growth factor among patients with chronic venous disease. J Vasc Surg 1998; 28:535–40.
31. Coleridge Smith PD, Thomas P, Scurr JH et al. Causes of venous ulceration: a new hypothesis. Br Med J 1988; 296:1726–7.
32. Landis EM. Micro-injection studies of capillary blood pressure in human skin. Heart 1930; 15:404–53.
33. Vanscheidt W, Laaf H, Weiss JM et al. Immunohistochemical investigation of dermal capillaries in chronic venous insufficiency. Acta Derm Venereol (Stockh) 1991; 71:17–19.
34. Wenner A, Leu HJ, Spycher M et al. Ultrastructural changes of capillaries in chronic venous insufficiency. Exp Cell Biol 1980; 48:1–14.
35. Leach RD, Browse NL. Effect of venous hypertension on canine hind limb lymph. Br J Surg 1985; 72:275–8.
36. Gajraj H, Browse NL. Fibrinolytic activity of the arms and legs of patients with lower limb venous disease. Br J Surg 1991; 78:853–6.
37. Browse NL, Burnand KG. The cause of venous ulceration. Lancet 1982; ii:243–5.
38. Herouy Y, Nockowski P, Schopf E, Norgauer J. Lipodermatosclerosis and the significance of proteolytic remodeling in the pathogenesis of venous ulceration. Int J Mol Med 1999; 3:511–15.
39. Gius JA. Arteriovenous anastomoses and varicose veins. Arch Surg 1960; 81:299–309.
40. Falanga V, Eaglstein WH. The 'trap' hypothesis of venous ulceration. Lancet 1993; 341:1006–8.
41. Chant A. Tissue pressure, posture, and venous ulceration. Lancet 1990; 336:1050–1.
42. Ackerman Z, Seidenbaum M, Loewenthal E et al. Overload of iron in the skin of patients with varicose ulcers. Arch Dermatol 1988; 124:1376–8.
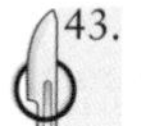
43. Porter JM, Moneta GL. Reporting standards in venous disease: an update. J Vasc Surg 1995; 21:635–45.

This is an international consensus document produced under the auspice of the American Venous Forum that provides a classification for chronic venous insufficiency.

44. Vasdekis SN, Clarke GH, Hobbs JT et al. Evaluation of non-invasive and invasive methods in the assessment of short saphenous vein termination. Br J Surg 1989; 76:929–32.
45. Szendro G, Nicolaides AN, Zukowski AJ et al. Duplex scanning in the assessment of deep venous incompetence. J Vasc Surg 1986; 4:237–42.
46. Hobbs JT. Peroperative venography to ensure accurate saphenopopliteal vein ligation. Br Med J 1980; 280:1578–9.
47. Lea Thomas M, McAllister V, Rose DH et al. A simplified technique for phlebography for the localisation of incompetent perforating veins of the legs. Clin Radiol 1972; 23:486–91.
48. Stegall HF. Muscle pumping in the dependent leg. Circ Res 1966; 19:180–90.
49. Michell CC. Microcirculation in the limbs in venous hypertension. Medicographia 1989; 11:40–2.
50. Norgren L. Non-invasive investigation of chronic venous insufficiency with special reference to foot volumetry. Acta Chir Scand Suppl 1988; 544:39–43.

51. Nicolaides AN, Zukowski AJ. The value of dynamic venous pressure measurements. World J Surg 1986; 10:919–24.

52. Abramowitz HB, Queral LA, Flinn WT et al. The use of photoplethysmography in the assessment of venous insufficiency. A comparison to venous pressure measurements. Surgery 1979; 86:434–41.

53. Barnes RW, Collicott PE, Mozersky D et al. Non-invasive quantitation of venous reflux in the postphlebitic syndrome. Surg Gynecol Obstet 1973; 136:769–74.

54. Christopoulos D, Nicolaides AN. Non-invasive diagnosis and quantitation of popliteal reflux in the swollen and ulcerated leg. J Cardiovasc Surg (Torino) 1988; 29:535–9.

55. Somerville JJF, Brow GO, Byrne PJ et al. The effects of elastic stockings on superficial venous pressures in patients with venous insufficiency. Br J Surg 1974; 61:979–81.

56. Sigel B, Edelstein AL, Felix WR et al. Compression of the deep venous system of the lower leg during inactive recumbency. Arch Surg 1973; 106:38–43.

57. Cornwall JV, Dore CJ, Lewis JD. Graduated compression and its relation to venous refilling time. Br Med J 1987; 295:1087–90.

58. Mayberry JC, Moneta GL, Taylor LM Jr et al. Fifteen year results of ambulatory compression therapy for chronic venous ulcers. Surgery 1991; 109:575–81.

59. Cornwall J. Compression therapy for venous leg ulcers. Wound Manage 1991; 1:10–13.

60. Cullum N, Nelson EA, Fletcher AW, Sheldon TA. Compression for venous leg ulcers (Cochrane review). In: The Cochrane Library, issue 4. Chicester: John Wiley & Sons, 2003.

This is a meta-analysis of 22 trials comparing compression with no compression and various types of compression in the healing of venous leg ulcers. Six trials compared compression with no compression, five trials compared elastic with non-elastic compression, three trials compared four-layer bandaging with other multilayered systems, four trials compared healing rates between elastomeric multilayered systems, and four trials compared multilayered high compression with single-layer compression. Results are given in the text.

61. Nelson EA, Bell-Syer SEM, Cullum NA. Compression for preventing recurrence of venous ulcers (Cochrane review). In: The Cochrane Library, issue 4. Chicester: John Wiley & Sons, 2003.

This is a review of two randomised controlled trials, one of which compared class 3 stockings with class 2 stockings and the other compared two different makes of class 2 stocking in the prevention of ulcer recurrence. Higher grades of compression are associated with lower recurrence rates. Also, not wearing stockings is strongly associated with ulcer recurrence.

62. Ruckley CV. Treatment of venous ulceration: compression therapy. Phlebology Suppl 1992; 1:22–6.

63. Partsch H. Do we need firm compression stockings exerting high pressure? Vasa 1984; 13:52–7.

64. Coleridge Smith P, Sarin S, Hasty J et al. Sequential gradient pneumatic compression enhances venous ulcer healing: a randomized trial. Surgery 1990; 108:871–5.

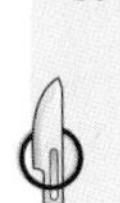

65. Mani R, Vowden K, Nelson EA. Intermittent pneumatic compression for treating venous leg ulcers (Cochrane review). In: The Cochrane Library, issue 4. Chicester: John Wiley & Sons, 2003.

This is a review of four randomised controlled trials; three compared intermittent pneumatic compression (IPC) plus compression with compression alone. One of these found increased ulcer healing with IPC, while two found no evidence of benefit. One trial compared IPC without additional compression with compression alone and found no difference.

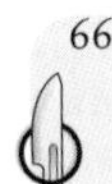

66. Jull AB, Waters J, Arroo B. Pentoxifylline for treating venous leg ulcers (Cochrane review). In: The Cochrane Library, issue 4. Chicester: John Wiley & Sons, 2003.

This is a meta-analysis of nine trials, eight of which compared pentoxifylline (oxpentifylline) with placebo. Oxpentifylline is more effective than placebo in terms of complete ulcer healing or significant improvement. The relative risk of ulcer healing with oxpentifylline compared with placebo is 1.41.

67. Bello M, Scriven M, Hartshorne T et al. Role of superficial venous surgery in the treatment of venous ulceration. Br J Surg 1999; 86:755–9.

68. Adam DJ, Bello M, Hartshorne T, London NJ. Role of superficial venous surgery in patients with combined superficial and segmental deep venous reflux. Eur J Vasc Endovasc Surg 2003; 25:469–72.

69. Barwell JR, Taylor M, Deacon J et al. Surgical correction of isolated superficial venous reflux reduces long-term recurrence rates in chronic venous leg ulcers. Eur J Vasc Endovasc Surg 2000; 20:363–8.

70. Barwell J, Davies C, Taylor M et al. The ESCHAR venous ulcer study: a randomized controlled trial assessing venous surgery in 500 leg ulcers. Br J Surg 2003; 90:497.

Although only published in abstract form at present, this is a well-conducted study in a large number of patients that assesses the role of superficial venous surgery in the healing and prevention of recurrence of leg ulcers. There was no difference in initial healing rates but a reduction in recurrence at 12 months in the surgical group, apart from those ulcers due to superficial and total deep reflux.

71. Pierik EGJM, Wittens CHA, van Urk H. Sub-fascial endoscopic ligation in the treatment of incompetent perforating veins. Eur J Vasc Endovasc Surg 1995; 9:38–41.

72. Stuart WP, Adam DJ, Bradbury AW et al. Subfascial endoscopic perforator surgery is associated with significantly less morbidity and shorter hospital stay than open operation. Br J Surg 1997; 84:1364–5.

73. Gloviczki P, Bergan JJ, Rhodes JM et al. Mid-term results of endoscopic perforator vein interruption for chronic venous insufficiency: lessons learned from the North American subfascial endoscopic perforator surgery registry. The North American Study Group. J Vasc Surg 1999; 29:489–502.

74. Eriksson I. Reconstructive surgery for deep vein valve incompetence in the lower limb. Eur J Vasc Surg 1990; 4:211–18.

This is a useful review of non-randomised results of surgical procedures for deep venous incompetence. Level 3 evidence.

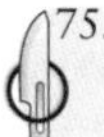

75. Abidia A, Hardy SC. Surgery for deep venous incompetence. In: The Cochrane Library, issue 4. Chicester: John Wiley & Sons, 2003.

This is a review of randomised trials of surgical treatment of patients with deep venous incompetence. Only one trial was found comparing superficial venous ligation and limited deep anterior valve plication with superficial ligation alone, with moderate improvement in clinical outcome in the former group compared with mild improvement in the latter group.

76. Killewich LA, Bedford GR, Beach KW et al. Spontaneous lysis of deep venous thrombi: rate and outcome. J Vasc Surg 1989; 9:89–97.

77. Darke SG. Venous reconstruction. In: Bell PRF, Jamieson CW, Ruckley CV (eds) Surgical management of vascular disease. London: WB Saunders, 1992; pp. 1221–38.

78. Palma EC, Esperon R. Vein transplants and grafts in the surgical treatment of the post-phlebitic syndrome. J Cardiovasc Surg (Torino) 1960; 1:94–107.

79. Halliday P, Harris J, May J. Femoro-femoral cross-over grafts (Palma operation), a long term follow up study. In: Bergan JF, Yao JST (eds) Surgery of the veins. New York: Grune & Stratton, 1985; p. 241.

80. Husni EA. Venous reconstruction in postphlebitic disease. Circulation 1971; 43(suppl. 1):147–50.

81. Raju S, McAllister S, Neglen P. Recanalisation of totally occluded iliac and adjacent venous segments. J Vasc Surg 2002; 36:903–11.

82. O'Sullivan GJ, Semba CP, Bittner CA et al. Endovascular management of iliac vein compression (May–Thurner syndrome). J Vasc Intervent Radiol 2000;11:823–36.

83. Raju S, Owen S Jr, Neglen P. The clinical impact of iliac venous stents in the management of chronic venous insufficiency. J Vasc Surg 2002; 35:8–15.

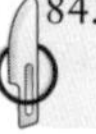

84. Leizorovicz A. Long-term consequences of deep venous thrombosis. Haemostasis 1998; 28(suppl. 3): 1–7.

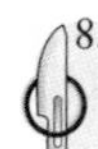

85. McCollum C. Avoiding the consequences of deep venous thrombosis. Br Med J 1998; 517:696.

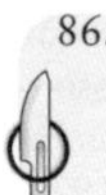

86. Janssen MC, Haenen JH, van Asten WN et al. Clinical and haemodynamic sequelae of deep venous thrombosis: retrospective evaluation after 7–13 years. Clin Sci 1997; 93:7–12.

In this study, 81 patients with venographically confirmed lower-extremity DVT were clinically and haemodynamically re-examined 7–13 years after DVT (mean 10 years) to assess PTS; 7–13 years after DVT 31% of the patients had moderate and 2% had severe clinical PTS, while 57% of the patients had abnormal haemodynamic findings. Level 2 evidence.

87. Franzeck UK, Schalch I, Bollinger A. On the relationship between changes in the deep veins evaluated by duplex sonography and the post-thrombotic syndrome 12 years after deep venous thrombosis. Thromb Haemost 1997; 77:1109–12.

88. Johnson BF, Manzo RA, Bergelin RO et al. Relationship between changes in the deep venous system and the development of the postthrombotic syndrome after an acute episode of lower limb deep vein thrombosis: a one- to six-year follow up. J Vasc Surg 1995; 21:307–12.

89. Piovella F, Barone M. Long-term management of deep vein thrombosis. Blood Coagul Fibrinolysis 1999; 10(suppl. 2):S117–S122.

90. Bello YM, Phillips TJ. Management of venous ulcers. J Cutan Med Surg 1998; 3(suppl. 1):S1–S12.

91. Nelzen O, Bergqvist D, Lindhagen A. Leg ulcer aetiology: a cross sectional population study. J Vasc Surg 1991; 14:557–64.

92. Liew I, Sinha S. A leg ulcer clinic. J Wound Care 1998; 7:405–7.

93. Ghauri AS, Nyamekye I, Grabs AJ et al. The diagnosis and management of mixed arterial/venous leg ulcers in community based clinics. Eur J Vasc Endovasc Surg 1998; 16:350–5.

94. Bowering CK. Use of layered compression bandages in diabetic patients. Experience in patients with lower leg ulceration, peripheral oedema, and features of venous and arterial disease. Adv Wound Care 1998; 11:129–35.

95. Milroy WF. Chronic hereditary oedema: Milroy's disease. JAMA 1928; 91:1172–5.

96. Salem AH, Mulhim AM, Grant C, Khaja MS. Milroy's disease in a Saudi family. J R Coll Surg Edinb 1986; 31:143–6.

97. Allen EV. Lymphoedema of the extremities: classification, aetiology and differential diagnosis: study of 300 cases. Arch Intern Med 1934; 54:606–24.

98. Kinmonth JB. The lymphoedemas. General considerations. In: Kinmonth JB (ed.) The lymphatics. Surgery, lymphography and diseases of the chyle and lymph systems. London: Edward Arnold, 1982; pp. 83–104.

99. Kinmonth JB, Wolfe JH. Fibrosis in the lymph nodes in primary lymphoedema. Histological and clinical studies in 74 patients with lower limb oedema. Ann R Coll Surg Engl 1980; 62:344–54.

100. Browse NL, Stewart G. Lymphoedema: pathophysiology and classification. J Cardiovasc Surg (Torino) 1985; 26:91–106.

101. Browse NL. The diagnosis and management of primary lymphoedema. J Vasc Surg 1986; 3:181–4.

102. Suga K, Uchisako H, Nakanishi T et al. Lymphoscintigraphic assessment of leg oedema following arterial reconstruction using a load produced by standing. Nucl Med Commun 1991; 12:907–17.

103. Foldi M, Idiazabal G. The role of operative management of varicose veins in patients with lymphoedema and/or lipedema of the legs. Lymphology 2000; 33:167–71.

104. Wright NB, Carty HM. The swollen leg and primary lymphoedema. Arch Dis Child 1994; 71:44–9.

105. Chant ADB. Hypothesis: why venous oedema causes ulcers and lymphoedema does not. Eur J Vasc Surg 1992; 6:427–9.

106. Gloviczki P, Calcagno D, Schirger A et al. Noninvasive evaluation of the swollen extremity: experiences with 190 lymphoscintigraphic examinations. J Vasc Surg 1989; 9:683–98.

107. Brautigam P, Vanscheidt W, Foldi E, Krause T, Moser E. The importance of the subfascial lymphatics in the diagnosis of lower limb edema: investigations with semiquantitative lymphoscintigraphy. Angiology 1993; 44:464–70.

108. Collins CD, Mortimer PS, D'Ettorre H et al. Computed tomography in the assessment of response to limb compression in unilateral lymphoedema. Clin Radiol 1995; 50:541–4.

109. Haaverstad R, Nilsen G, Myhre HO et al. The use of MRI in the investigation of leg oedema. Eur J Vasc Surg 1992; 6:124–9.

110. Duewell S, Hagspiel KD, Zuber J et al. Swollen lower extremity: role of MR imaging. Radiology 1992; 184:227–31.

111. Case TC, Witte MH, Unger EC et al. Magnetic resonance imaging in human lymphoedema: comparison with lymphangioscintigraphy. Magn Reson Imaging 1992; 10:549–58.

112. Werner GT, Scheck R, Kaiserling E. Magnetic resonance imaging of peripheral lymph oedema. Lymphology 1998; 31:34–6.

113. Idy-Peretti I, Bittoun J, Alliot FA et al. Lymphedematous skin and sub cutis: in vivo high resolution magnetic resonance imaging evaluation. J Invest Dermatol 1998; 110:782–7.

114. Kinmonth JB. Lymphography in man: a method of outlining lymphatic trunks at operation. Clin Sci 1952; 11:13–20.

115. Megans AM, Harris SR, Kim-Sing C, McKenzie DC. Measurement of upper extremity volume in women after axillary dissection for breast cancer. Arch Phys Med Rehabil 2001; 82:1639–44.

116. Vignes S, Boursier V, Priollet P et al. Quantitative evaluation and qualitative results of surgical lymphovenous anastomosis in lower limb lymphedema. J Mal Vasc 2003; 28:30–5.

117. Mortimer PS. Swollen lower limb. 2. Lymph oedema. Br Med J 2000; 320:1527–9.

118. Yasuhara H, Shigematsu H, Muto T. A study of the advantages of elastic stockings for leg lymphoedema. Int Angiol 1996; 15:272–7.

119. Badger CM, Peacock JL, Mortimer PS. A randomised, controlled, parallel-group trial comparing multilayer bandaging followed by hosiery versus hosiery alone in the treatment of patients with lymphedema of the limb. Cancer 2000; 88:2832–7.

This is a randomized, controlled, parallel-group trial in which 90 women with unilateral lymphoedema (of the upper or lower limbs) underwent 18 days of multilayer bandaging followed by elastic hosiery or hosiery alone, each for a total period of 24 weeks. The reduction in limb volume due to multilayer bandaging followed by hosiery was approximately double that from hosiery alone and was sustained over the 24-week period. The mean overall percentage reduction at 24 weeks was 31% (N = 32) for multilayer bandaging versus 15.8% (N = 46) for hosiery alone, for a mean difference of 15.2% (95% CI 6.2–24.2) (P = 0.001). Level 1 evidence.

120. Pappas CJ, O'Donnell TF. Long-term results of compression treatment for lymphedema. J Vasc Surg 1992; 16:555–64.

121. Palmer A, Macchiaverna J, Braun A et al. Compression therapy of limb oedema using hydrostatic pressure of mercury. Angiology 1991; 42:533–42.

122. Liu NF, Olszewski W. The influence of local hyperthermia on lymphedematous skin of the human leg. Lymphology 1993; 26:28–37.

123. Cheville AL, McGarvey CL, Petrek JA et al. Lymphedema management. Semin Radiat Oncol 2003; 13:290–301.

124. Ko DS, Lerner R, Klose G, Cosimi AB. Effective treatment of lymphedema of the extremities. Arch Surg 1998; 133:452–8.

125. Casley-Smith JR. Benzo-pyrones in the treatment of lymph oedema. Int Angiol 1999; 18:31–41.

126. Casley-Smith JR, Casley-Smith JR. Treatment of lymphedema by complex physical therapy, with and without oral and topical benzopyrones: what should therapists and patients expect? Lymphology 1996; 29:76–82.

127. Saaristo A, Karkkainen MJ, Alitalo K. Insights into the molecular pathogenesis and targeted treatment of lymphedema. Ann NY Acad Sci 2002; 979:94–110.

128. Szuba A, Skobe M, Karkkainen MJ et al. Therapeutic lymphangiogenesis with human recombinant VEGF-C. FASEB J 2002; 16:1985–7.

129. Dellon AL, Hoopes JE. The Charles procedure for primary lymphedema. Long term clinical results. Plast Reconstr Surg 1977; 60:589–95.

130. Brorson H, Svenson H. Liposuction combined with controlled compression therapy reduces arm lymphedema more effectively than controlled compression therapy alone. Plast Reconstr Surg 1998; 102:1058–67.

131. Sando WC, Nah F. Suction lipectomy in the management of limb lymphedema. Clin Plast Surg 1989; 16:369–73.

132. Kinmonth JB, Hurst PA, Edwards JM et al. Relief of lymph obstruction by use of a bridge of mesentery and ileum. Br J Surg 1978; 65:829–33.

133. Hurst PAE, Stewart G, Kinmonth JB et al. Long-term results of the enteromesenteric bridge operation in the treatment of primary lymphoedema. Br J Surg 1985; 72:272–4.

134. Baumeister RG, Siuda S. Treatment of lymphedemas by microsurgical lymphatic grafting: what is proved? Plast Reconstr Surg 1990; 85:65–74.

135. Weiss M, Baumeister RG, Hahn K. Post-therapeutic lymphedema: scintigraphy before and after autologous vessel transplantation: 8 years of long-term follow up. Clin Nucl Med 2002; 27:788–92.

136. Baumeister RG, Frick A. The microsurgical lymph vessel transplantation. Handchir Mikrochir Plast Chir 2003; 35:202–9.

137. Campisi C, Boccardo F, Zilli A, Napoli F. Long-term results after lymphatic–venous anastomoses for the treatment of obstructive lymphedema. Microsurgery 2001; 21:135–9.

CHAPTER

Nineteen

Varicose veins

Rachel C. Sam and
Andrew W. Bradbury

INTRODUCTION

Lower limb venous disease causes major socioeconomic and health problems. Most of the adult population in developed countries is affected by 'varicose veins' (VV); in the UK, for example, the treatment and complications of VV consume about 2% of total NHS spending.[1] Because VV rarely presents as an acute life-threatening condition, it is generally given a low priority both clinically and in terms of research funding. However, it does have a significant impact upon quality of life, which can be improved by surgery. VV remains the single largest cause of medicolegal claims against surgeons,[2] and up to 20% of all operations for VV are performed for recurrent disease.[3] Patient satisfaction is paramount and depends on a thorough understanding of anatomy and pathophysiology, awareness of the patient's expectations and a knowledge of the techniques applicable in each case.[4]

VENOUS RECIRCULATION

In patients with VV there is often recirculation of venous blood within the leg.[5] During calf relaxation, large volumes of blood enter the muscle pump from the superficial varices. The muscle pump expels blood from the leg only for it to re-enter the leg via superficial varices. This blood re-enters the muscle pump through perforating veins, and so on. Patients with mild superficial reflux and/or an efficient calf pump are able to compensate by increasing their calf muscle pump 'stroke volume' and output, allowing them still to reduce ambulatory venous pressure (AVP) to (near) normal levels on walking. However, severe reflux and/or a weak muscle pump may overwhelm the deep system and lead to the development of sustained venous hypertension and the skin changes of chronic venous insufficiency (CVI). This accounts for two important clinical observations:

- CVI and ulceration can develop without primary deep venous pathology;
- in some patients with both VV and deep venous reflux on duplex, the latter disappears following superficial surgery.

EPIDEMIOLOGY

Classification

The lack of a universally accepted and validated classification of VV or CVI has hampered attempts to describe the natural history.

Prevalence

The Edinburgh Vein Study, a cross-sectional survey of a random sample of the Edinburgh population, showed that 40% of men and 30% of women aged 18–64 years had 'trunk' varices and approximately 80% (both sexes) had 'reticular' or 'hyphenweb' varices.[6]

Gender

Most clinical series comprise an excess of women (male to female ratio 1.5–3.5:1), possibly because their veins are more symptomatic. Female patients often relate their VV to pregnancy and childbirth. The rapidly increasing levels of female sex hormones together with the increased blood volume observed during the first trimester of pregnancy almost certainly affect venous tone and function. However, there is little epidemiological evidence of an association between (multi)parity and venous disease. It seems more likely that pregnancy aggravates an underlying predisposition to VV.

Age

The prevalence of VV increases with age in both sexes. However, on objective testing, 12% of schoolchildren can be shown to have saphenous incompetence.

Hereditary factors

A genetic element to the condition seems likely but is difficult to define. VV is more commonly found in developed than in developing countries but it is difficult to know whether this is 'nature' or 'nurture'. Thus, white and black Americans appear equally affected.

Lifestyle

Obesity and occupation may aggravate the condition as well as making presentation to medical services more likely. Numerous other lifestyle and social factors have been mooted as predisposing factors for the development of VV but none, except possibly the consumption of a low-fibre diet, are supported by robust epidemiological data.

TYPES OF VARICOSE VEIN

Primary trunk varicose veins

These are derived from the long saphenous vein (LSV) and/or short saphenous vein (SSV) and/or their major tributaries. In young patients, the superficial veins may be prominent but these 'athletic' veins are physiological and, unlike trunk varicose veins, are usually uniformly dilated and exhibit no tortuosity or elongation.

Secondary trunk varicose veins

Dilated superficial trunk veins may be acting as collateral venous return in the presence of deep venous disease. The presence of the skin changes of CVI should alert the clinician to this possibility. Although such veins are dilated, they may show little in the way of varicosity. They should not be removed unless testing confirms that they are hindering the venous haemodynamics of the leg.[7]

Reticular varices

These veins lie just beneath the skin and, even when normal, may form a highly visible 'reticular' pattern of dark blue veins, especially in those with thin pale skin. The owners of such veins may find them unsightly and seek their ablation, even though they are physiological and cause no symptoms. Reticular veins may become dilated, often in association with back-pressure from mainstem or tributary reflux, although this may not be visible.

Hyphenweb veins

These dilated intradermal venules (also called thread veins, spider veins, telangiectasia, venectasia, phlebectasia, and venous 'flares') can be associated with trunk or reticular varices. They often appear on the legs of women after pregnancy and in those approaching menarche, and may be related to hormonal changes.

Venous malformations

These may be purely venous or associated with an arterial component, often with a pulsation or thrill on palpation, while a stethoscope may detect a continuous 'hum'. The commonest venous malformation of the leg is Klippel–Trenaunay syndrome, where the deep venous system of the leg is often hypoplastic or absent such that the malformation acts as the primary venous outflow from the leg.

PATHOGENESIS

Primary VV is due to valvular failure, the cause of which remains unclear in most cases. There are two main hypotheses.

1. Primary valve failure: primary degenerative changes in the valve annulus and leaflets.
2. Secondary valve failure: developmental weakness in the vein wall leads to secondary widening of the valve commissures and incompetence.

It is likely that both mechanisms are involved, but to a variable extent in different patients.

CLINICAL PRESENTATION

Patients with VV fall into two groups.

1. Uncomplicated group: patients in whom venous disease is confined to the superficial system and/or who have compensated mixed deep and superficial disease such that AVP is near normal.
2. Complicated group: patients who have combined superficial and deep venous disease and/or isolated superficial disease that has decompensated leading to high AVP and the risk of skin changes.

Uncomplicated VV

COSMESIS

Many patients express dissatisfaction with the cosmetic appearance of their legs and different factors determine whether this leads an individual to seek medical treatment. There is a general consensus that 'cosmetic' surgery should not normally be funded from the public purse. However, it is suspected that some will attribute symptoms to their cosmetic varices, fearing that they will not otherwise receive treatment.

SYMPTOMS

Many symptoms have been attributed to uncomplicated VV. The Edinburgh Vein Study showed an inconsistent and gender-dependent relationship between a range of lower limb 'venous' symptoms (heaviness/tension, feeling of swelling, aching, restless leg, cramps, itching, tingling) and the presence and severity of trunk, reticular and hyphenweb varices.[8] Clinical experience also suggests little concordance between symptoms and signs because some small varices are painful while many large varices are asymptomatic. Some interpret these discrepancies as implying that uncomplicated VV almost never causes lower limb symptoms and, as such, surgery is always 'cosmetic' and should not be provided by the NHS. However, several studies have shown that surgery is associated with significant improvements in quality of life.[9] This suggests that assessment and investigation does allow the genuinely symptomatic patients to be distinguished. In these, discomfort in the leg is often worse at the end of the day or after prolonged standing or, in women, around menstruation. Swelling can be associated with VV but is also caused by other conditions, particularly in older patients.

REASSURANCE

Many patients attending clinic have concerns about the subsequent risk of venous ulceration and deep vein thrombosis (DVT). Despite considerable literature on the subject, the relationship between simple VV and chronic venous ulceration remains controversial. The majority of patients with uncomplicated VV never develop skin changes and, in the absence of other venous pathology, can be confidently reassured. Other patients, particularly young women on the oral contraceptive pill, attend because of concerns that VV will put them at risk of DVT. Although VV is frequently cited as a risk factor for thromboembolic disease, there is little evidence and the vast majority of young patients with VV will not develop DVT. However, in older patients undergoing surgery or prolonged immobilisation, the presence of VV (which in this age group may indicate previous DVT), together with other risk factors, must be taken into account when deciding upon thromboembolic prophylaxis.

SUPERFICIAL THROMBOPHLEBITIS

This is a sterile inflammation of the vein wall and surrounding tissues secondary to thrombosis and is a painful and (rarely) life-threatening complication of VV. Treatment includes analgesia and anti-inflammatory agents. Compression may prevent propagation but the leg is often too tender for this. Early local evacuation/aspiration of semiliquid haematoma may help. Where phlebitis involves the main saphenous trunks, duplex should be performed to ensure that thrombus is not propagating into the deep system. If such thrombus is found, patients should be anticoagulated as for DVT and some surgeons recommend surgical removal of the thrombus. Recurrence is common and the affected segments of vein should be removed once the inflammation has settled. If thrombophlebitis is migratory or occurs in the absence of VV, then there is likely to be an underlying condition (e.g. malignancy, thrombophilia).[10]

Complicated VV

The complications of VV include the following.

- *Corona phlebectatica*. This is also called malleolar flare and is one of the earliest skin manifestations of CVI. It comprises a leash of prominent, dilated, intradermal or subdermal veins at the medial malleolus. The overlying skin is thin and fragile leading to a 'blue bleb' appearance. Trauma can lead to haemorrhage, and sometimes ulceration.
- *Lipodermatosclerosis*. Increased venous pressure can lead to extravasation of blood, with resulting inflammation and skin staining due to haemosiderin deposition. This may develop insidiously or can present acutely with severe pain and discoloration that mimics cellulitis.
- *Atrophie blanche*. Scar-like tissue that is thin and pale as a result of the reduction in papillary capillaries and collagen; occurs at the site of previous ulceration.

- *Varicose eczema.* Itchy, scaly, dry skin over a varicose vein.
- *Oedema.* Other non-venous causes of oedema should be considered. A degree of lymphoedema may coexist with CVI.
- *Pain.*
- *Haemorrhage.* This is often alarming, even life-threatening, and frequently occurs following trauma. Direct pressure and elevation of the limb will always arrest venous haemorrhage.

CLINICAL ASSESSMENT

When assessing the patient with VV, three important questions need to be answered.

- Are the symptoms due to venous disease?
- Is the presentation complicated or uncomplicated?
- Is there any other significant pathology, such as arterial disease?

History

Orthopaedic, neurological and arterial causes of leg symptoms must be excluded. Particular attention must be paid to a history of previous DVT and any previous venous surgery. A family history of venous disease, particularly early-onset, recurrent or unusual thrombotic events, should be sought.

General examination

The patient should be examined in a warm room, standing with the hip and knee flexed to allow venous filling. The examiner must see the whole leg and lower abdominal wall to define the presence of scars and the pattern of varices. In addition, the following should be recorded:

- oedema;
- skin changes of CVI;
- arterial pulses with or without ankle–brachial pressure index (ABPI).

Virtually all varicose veins are dilated. Athletic veins and secondary varicose veins carry increased amounts of venous blood, *but in the correct physiological direction and without reflux*, and do not show varicosity. Reflux, leading to subvalvular turbulence, is necessary to produce varicosity, i.e. elongation, tortuosity and sacculation.[4] A cough impulse and thrill are often palpable.

In those with the advanced skin changes of CVI there may be few visible varicose veins, despite the presence of marked superficial reflux, because of fibrosis of the vein wall and surrounding tissues. In such patients it is easy to underestimate the severity of venous disease on inspection alone. The presence of varicose veins can sometimes be inferred by the development of grooves on elevating the leg.

Hand-held Doppler examination

Common sites of deep to superficial reflux give rise to typical distributions of varices. Tourniquet tests may help to define the source of incompetence but these and other clinical tests have largely been supplanted by hand-held Doppler (HHD) (continuous-wave Doppler).[11]

With the patient standing, the probe is placed over the sapheno-femoral junction (SFJ), which is found by insonating the femoral artery and moving medially. Squeezing the calf results in a prograde signal. In the presence of SFJ incompetence, release of calf compression results in a retrograde signal (>0.5 seconds) that is abolished by LSV compression. Reflux down the LSV should also be assessed at the medial side of the knee. Continuous prograde flow should raise the possibility of deep venous occlusion.

Reflux in the popliteal fossa may be detected by finding the arterial signal, moving laterally, and using the calf-squeeze manoeuvre. Although reflux at the sapheno-popliteal junction (SPJ) cannot be distinguished from popliteal and/or gastrocnemius vein incompetence, HHD provides a useful screening test. The absence of reflux in the popliteal fossa provides good evidence that the SSV system is competent.[12] The technique of HHD venous assessment can be learnt reliably for primary uncomplicated long saphenous varicose veins,[13] with an accuracy of greater than 95% in this situation.[14]

INVESTIGATIONS

Duplex ultrasonography

Ideally, all patients being considered for surgery should undergo preoperative duplex examination as a proportion of patients (even those with primary VV) will have an inappropriate and/or incomplete operation if it is based purely on clinical assessment.[15,16] In addition to mapping out reflux within the saphenous systems, duplex will detect SSV disease, locate the SPJ and incompetent non-junctional perforators, and diagnose deep venous disease (**Fig. 19.1**).

There is debate as to what should be considered pathological reflux, with duration of reflux of 0.5 or 1 second as a cut-off. However, the dimension of the vein affects the amount of reflux, with a grossly

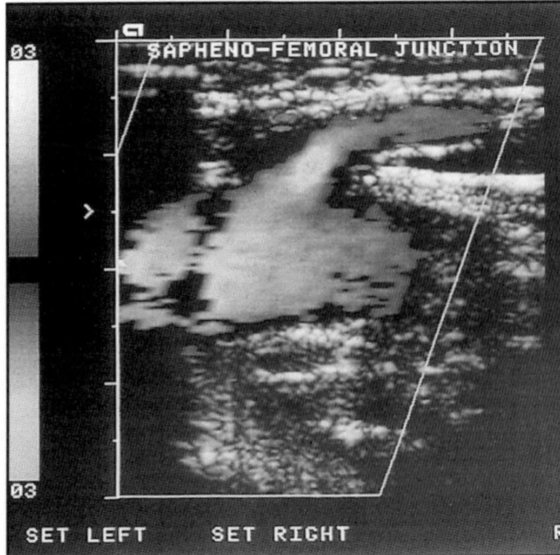

Figure 19.1 • Duplex scan clearly defining the sapheno-femoral junction (SFJ) in a patient with 'recurrent' varicose veins. In this case the SFJ was intact.

enlarged vein permitting a large volume of blood to pass over a short duration. More heed should perhaps be paid to volume of reflux. The lack of association between patterns and duration of reflux on duplex and symptoms in the Edinburgh Vein Study serve to illustrate this point.

Duplex scanning has also identified a group of patients in whom there is LSV mainstem and/or tributary reflux without SFJ incompetence,[17] challenging the view that reflux progresses from the SFJ downwards; this probably represents VV 'in evolution'. The finding of limited segmental incompetence has led to the concept of selective surgery for VV, where the surgeon deals with only those refluxing segments seen on duplex. This is said to reduce morbidity and preserve healthy vein for possible arterial bypass later in life and is popular in North America. The drawback with limited duplex-directed surgery is that, on one hand, the reflux may not be clinically significant whereas, on the other, one might perform an inadequate operation causing the patient to return with reflux a few years later.

Pragmatically, at least in terms of most UK surgical practice, economics and availability limit the role of duplex to the assessment of VV where clinical examination is equivocal:

- recurrence of varicose veins following previous surgery;
- where HHD has detected reflux in the popliteal fossa;
- suspected deep venous disease in patients with VV and skin changes suggesting CVI.

Other investigations

Plethysmography and varicography have been replaced mainly by duplex scanning. Plethysmography provides functional information and may be useful for patients with complicated VV where deep venous disease often coexists. Varicography can be performed on-table and is particularly useful for determining the anatomy of recurrent varicose veins and the location of the SPJ (**Fig. 19.2**). Ovarian vein reflux and pelvic varices can be visualised by placing a catheter into the ovarian and/or internal iliac veins via a common femoral vein (CFV) approach. As well as being diagnostic, the ovarian vein can be embolised.

TREATMENT

Reassurance

In order to provide a clinically effective and cost-efficient service, the surgeon must identify those patients whose varicose veins seem likely to be the cause of the symptoms. During pregnancy, treatment is normally conservative using compression hosiery, although for severe or recurrent thrombophlebitis SFJ ligation under local anaesthesia may be considered. Patients with uncomplicated VV with concerns about future thrombosis, bleeding and/or ulceration can usually be reassured and discharged. Patients who request treatment purely for cosmetic reasons pose a potentially difficult problem in the present healthcare environment. In the absence of guidelines from the employing authority, surgeons have to make up their own minds on the merit of intervention in these cases.

Compression hosiery

Compression hosiery may relieve symptoms, conceal veins and prevent deterioration of the skin changes associated with venous hypertension. However, stockings may be uncomfortable and their beneficial effect lasts only as long as they are worn. Compression must be strong (20–30 mmHg at the ankle), graduated (maximal at the ankle reducing to 75% at the calf and 50% at the thigh) and replaced regularly (every 6 months). Although most patients require only a below-knee stocking, compliance remains a major problem.

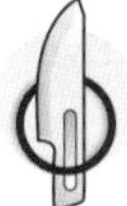

Some authorities believe that stockings reduce the recurrence of varicose veins after surgery for uncomplicated VV.[18]

It remains unclear how stockings might achieve these effects and further studies seem necessary.

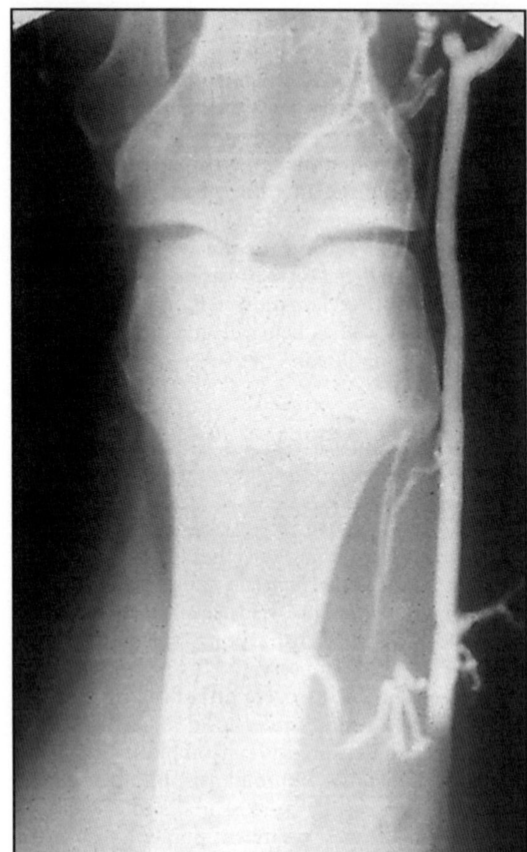

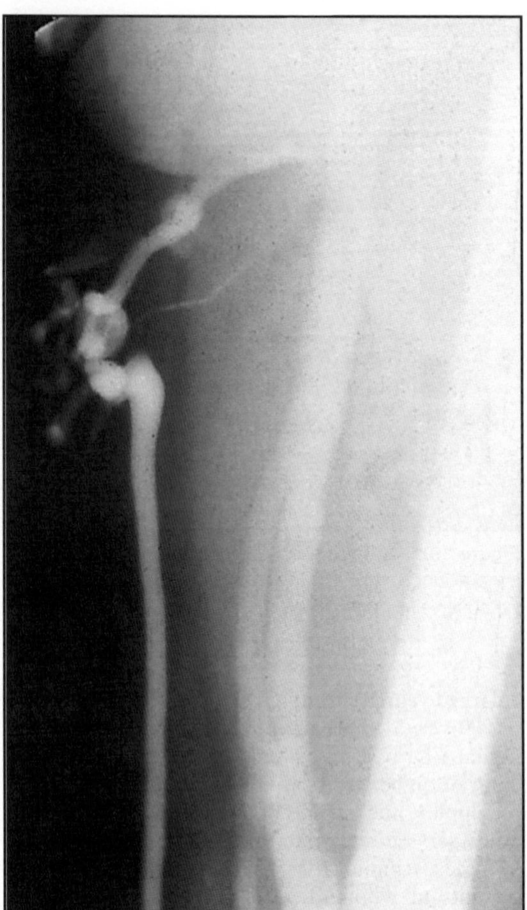

Figure 19.2 • Varicogram of two patients with recurrent varicose veins demonstrating an intact long saphenous vein with an incompetent lower thigh perforating vein **(a)** and a residual connection with the common femoral vein in the groin **(b)**.

There seems little doubt that class II, or preferably class III, stockings retard the progression of skin changes and prevent recurrent ulceration in patients with complicated VV. Such patients should be encouraged to wear their stockings for life. Stockings are a useful diagnostic test when there is uncertainty about the extent to which leg symptoms are attributable to varices.

Sclerotherapy

Opinions vary greatly as to whether injection sclerotherapy or surgery is the most appropriate first-line therapy for VV. These views are usually based on a practitioner's professional background and country of origin rather than comparative studies.

THE SCLEROTHERAPISTS' VIEW

All varicose veins can be treated successfully with repeated courses of injection sclerotherapy. Although the long-term results of sclerotherapy are not as good as surgery in the presence of SFJ or SPJ incompetence, for many patients repeated injections seems preferable to an operation, with its risks and inevitable scarring. It is also worth noting that to follow surgery with injection sclerotherapy subjects the patient to the worst of both worlds.

THE SURGEONS' VIEW

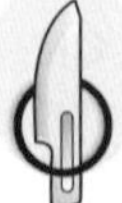

Only two randomised studies have compared surgery with sclerotherapy and both indicated the long-term superiority of the former in the presence of mainstem disease.[19,20]

Sclerotherapy can also be associated with significant morbidity.

THE BALANCED VIEW

Both modalities appear appropriate in different circumstances depending on the nature of the condition and the patient's preference. In the UK, trunk varicose veins are usually treated surgically, whereas non-mainstem varicose veins and isolated thread veins are usually treated with sclerotherapy.[21]

TECHNIQUE

The aim of sclerotherapy is to place a small volume of sclerosant in the lumen of a vein empty of blood, and then appose the walls of that vein with appropriate compression. The vein then undergoes fibrosis in a closed position without the formation of clot. The major salient aspects are as follows.

- The sclerosant must remain localised within the treated segment of vein.
- The vein must be kept empty of blood both during and after the injection. One method is to insert the needles into the veins with the legs dependent, tape the syringes to the patient's leg, elevate the leg to empty the vein, isolate the segment of vein to be treated with the fingers, inject, and then apply local compression with pads and bandages or stockings.
- Patients should mobilise immediately afterwards and walk on a daily basis until review in clinic.

SCLEROSANTS

Sclerosants fall into three categories:

1. detergent solutions, e.g. sodium tetradecyl sulphate (STD) and polidocanol (popular in the UK);
2. osmotic solutions, e.g. hypertonic saline (used in Europe and the USA);
3. chemical irritants, e.g. chromated glycerine.

The strength of sclerosant depends on the clinical circumstance, and the following is a rough guide for STD:

- trunk, 1–3%;
- tributaries, 0.5–1%;
- reticular veins <3 mm, 0.2–0.5%;
- hyphenwebs <1 mm, 0.1–0.3%.

The maximum recommended dose during any one treatment session is 3 mL of 3% STD. Polidocanol is roughly half as strong. In general it is better to err on the side of caution, using small volumes with low concentrations until the patient's response to the sclerosant, which varies greatly between individuals, can be assessed.

COMPLICATIONS

Patients should be specifically warned about the complications of sclerotherapy and this fact should be recorded in the case records. Information leaflets are helpful.

Anaphylaxis

A rare event (<0.3%) but has been responsible for the handful of deaths associated with sclerotherapy. Use of a small test dose is recommended and resuscitation facilities must be available, with hydrocortisone, adrenaline (epinephrine) and oxygen.

Allergic reactions

Lesser reactions are also rare but may occur from 2 minutes to 48 hours after injection. Symptoms include urticaria, periorbital and oral swelling, bronchospasm and migraine. Antihistamines are used for treatment as well as future prophylaxis.

Ulceration

This usually, but not always, occurs following extravascular injection. In other cases, sclerosant may enter an arteriole. Immediately after injecting, the skin blanches due to intense vasoconstriction. Infiltrating the area with normal saline or dilute local anaesthetic, or rubbing the skin surface with nitrate, have all been recommended. However, in some cases an ulcer appears over the next 7–14 days. It is usually painful and has a necrotic core surrounded by inflamed skin. A scab gradually forms over the eschar and healing is usually complete, with or without scarring, at 6–8 weeks. Treatment is symptomatic.

Arterial injection

A serious complication, accompanied by severe pain distal to the injection site. The most vulnerable artery appears to be the posterior tibial at the ankle. Treatment includes analgesia, cooling of the foot, and infusion of heparin and dextran in a hospital setting with monitoring by a vascular surgeon.

Pigmentation

This occurs in 1–30% of injections and is due to the deposition of haemosiderin, often following superficial thrombophlebitis. It is probably unavoidable in some cases but every effort should be made to minimise bleeding, and ensure adequate compression. Fortunately, most staining fades with time, although it may never disappear completely.

Superficial thrombophlebitis

This occurs when clot remains in the lumen of the sclerosed vein and is due to inadequate compression (**Fig. 19.3**). Localised haematoma is particularly painful and may be eased by aspiration with a needle or scalpel under local anaesthesia.

Deep venous thrombosis

The risk is reduced by careful patient selection and by advice with regard to immediate and regular mobilisation.

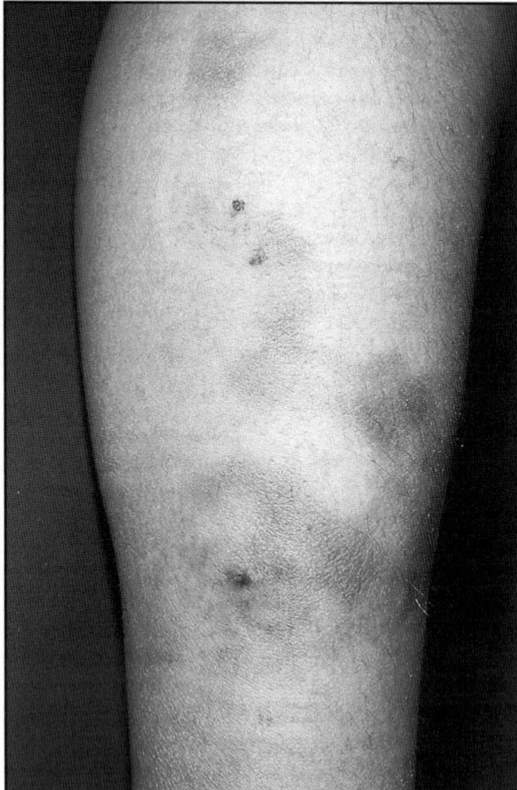

Figure 19.3 • Superficial thrombophlebitis following injection sclerotherapy. Inadequate compression may cause this problem.

Nerve damage

This can occur as a result of approximate injection and/or pressure from bandaging.

Operative treatment

GENERAL POINTS

Surgery for VV is one of the commonest sources of litigation in the UK. Much can be done during preoperative assessment to minimise this risk, particularly with informed consent.

The patient should be warned about the common, almost inevitable, consequences of surgery as failure to do so may lead the patient to conclude that an unsatisfactory operation has been performed. These include bruising, small areas of paraesthesia, and the fact that it is sometimes impossible to remove all prominent veins with a stab avulsion technique. Any small residual veins can be dealt with by means of injection sclerotherapy, which should be viewed as an integral part of the overall treatment. The risk of recurrence, inevitable in a proportion of patients, should be discussed openly with the patient and documented in the case records. Information leaflets and specific consent forms may be useful but do not guarantee legal protection.

The operating surgeon must take personal responsibility for preoperative marking. Whether single lines or tramlines are used, incisions should not cut through markings to avoid tattooing. After marking, the patient should be asked if any varices have been missed. Some patients will point out prominent veins on the dorsum of the foot. Although these are usually physiological, many patients will express disappointment if these are still present when they return to the clinic. It is therefore worth discussing with the patient what should be done with these veins preoperatively, as their removal appears to carry no detriment to the patient (but beware tendons and nerves).

WHAT CONSTITUTES AN ADEQUATE PREOPERATIVE ASSESSMENT?

In the UK it is clear from a recent survey[22] that, compared with literature ideals, the preoperative assessment of patients with VV falls short of suggested guidelines. In this study, 62% of vascular surgeons supplemented clinical examination with HHD and only 17 of 71 performed preoperative localisation of the SPJ. However, it has never been proved that a more thorough investigation actually improves outcome. Furthermore, with respect to LSV varices, if the 'typical' surgeon performs the same operation for every case treated, i.e. 'high tie', thigh strip and avulsions, then it could be argued that all the experienced surgeon has to do prior to surgery is make the diagnosis by examining the leg, any further assessment being viewed as unnecessary. Similarly, if the surgeon's approach to recurrent VV is always to re-explore the SFJ, then further assessment of this area may also be unnecessary.

The same arguments cannot be applied so easily to those patients with SSV varices as it seems inevitable that, because the SPJ is highly variable, 'blind' exploration of the popliteal fossa will lead to suboptimal results in many patients. The SPJ is most commonly situated about 2 cm above the knee crease, but this actually applies to less than half of all patients. In up to 25% of patients, the SSV does not enter the popliteal vein but continues uninterrupted up the thigh to connect with either (i) the deep system via a high posterior thigh perforator or (ii) the posteromedial branch of the LSV (Giacomini vein). For these reasons, accurate preoperative marking of the course and termination of the SSV is essential if SPJ ligation is to be carried out satisfactorily.

DAY-CASE SURGERY

Patient fitness and suitability is assessed in the clinic and confirmed by means of a questionnaire, usually completed by an experienced day-care nurse.[23]

Some surgeons would consider bilateral varicose vein surgery or recurrent groin/popliteal fossa surgery a contraindication to day-case surgery. Obviously, practice depends on many factors, such as the experience of the surgeon and anaesthetist, patient age and fitness and the availability of inpatient facilities, but it is essential to take account of the patient's wishes.[24] In a prospective study, 84% were suitable for day-case surgery.[25] Of 00 patients who underwent day surgery, 90 were willing to have the same procedure again. Only 12 patients contacted their GP and three their district nurse; 28 took no analgesia following hospital discharge and 81 felt their pain was less than, or as, they had expected. Factors germane to these excellent results included operation by experienced surgeons, avoidance of opiates, infiltration of the wound with local anaesthetic, and insertion of a non-steroidal anti-inflammatory suppository. Patients were also given careful verbal post-operative advice supplemented by a written advice sheet and contact telephone number.

ANAESTHESIA

Surgery for VV can be performed under general, regional or local anaesthesia. The LSV can be stripped using a femoral nerve block but this inevitably leads to motor loss that prevents walking for several hours. Others inject along the course of the vein with a large volume of dilute local anaesthetic ('tumescent' anaesthesia) and stress the value of using adrenaline to reduce blood loss and bruising. When using local anaesthetic it is important not to exceed the toxic dose.

POSITIONING

- Supine for LSV surgery, usually prone for SSV surgery. Some experienced surgeons perform SSV surgery with the patient on one side but it is not recommended as the important anatomical relationships can be obscured.
- A head-down position reduces venous bleeding and the risk of air embolism but can lead to facial and laryngeal oedema and ventilatory problems.

SAPHENO-FEMORAL LIGATION

- In a patient of normal build the SFJ lies directly beneath the groin crease; in the obese it lies above.
- Do not divide any vein until the SFJ has been unequivocally identified.
- The superficial external pudendal artery usually passes between the LSV and CFV but passes superficial to the LSV in 5–10% of cases.
- Follow and divide all tributaries beyond secondary branch points (**Fig. 19.4**).
- Ligate the LSV flush with the CFV using either a transfixion suture or double tie. Some authorities recommend a non-absorbable suture with a view to reducing neovascularisation.
- Divide the deep external pudendal vein as it comes off the CFV (optional if small).
- Directly ligate the posteromedial and anterolateral thigh branch of the LSV, reducing the risk of haematoma and thigh recurrence.
- If the LSV is not stripped, then as much as possible should be removed to minimise recurrence.

STRIPPING

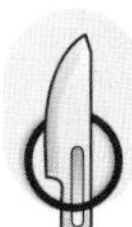

Studies including randomised trials have clearly shown that routinely stripping the LSV reduces the risk of recurrence and has a positive impact on quality of life.[26–30]

Stripping markedly reduces the risk of recurrence by (i) disconnecting the thigh perforators and saphenous tributaries and (ii) preventing any neovascularisation arising from the saphenous stump reconnecting with the LSV. Some argue that the LSV should be preserved for subsequent bypass surgery. However, long-term studies have shown that this is rarely required.[31]

Stripping from above downwards has been shown to cause less nerve damage. However, as in this study stripping was to ankle level, the situation with regard to above-knee stripping remains unclear.[32]

Full-length stripping is associated with a significant incidence of saphenous nerve injury (4–23%).[32–34] In about 1% of patients this can cause saphenous neuralgia, leading to a chronic pain syndrome and dysaesthesia that is difficult to treat. For this reason, many now recommend stripping to approximately one hand's breadth below the knee. At this level the below-knee perforator (Boyd) will have been crossed but the saphenous nerve will not yet have joined the vein.

Many still use a commercial stripping device with an 'acorn' head (e.g. Babcock). This tends to cut a tunnel around the LSV, causing unnecessary tissue trauma and bleeding and requiring a large incision for its removal. The PIN (perforation-invagination) stripper is a steerable rod with an offset head. This is used to perforate the vein at the lower extent of the segment to be stripped and is then retrieved through the skin via a small 2–3 mm cut-down. The proximal end of the vein is tied to the stripper, leaving a long 'tail' in case the vein breaks. Traction on the lower end of the stripper invaginates the vein during stripping.

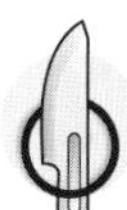

The suggested advantages of less nerve injury and bleeding and a smaller exit wound have not been demonstrated in two randomised controlled trials.[35,36]

Sequential avulsion of the LSV is believed by some to be more complete and less likely to damage the

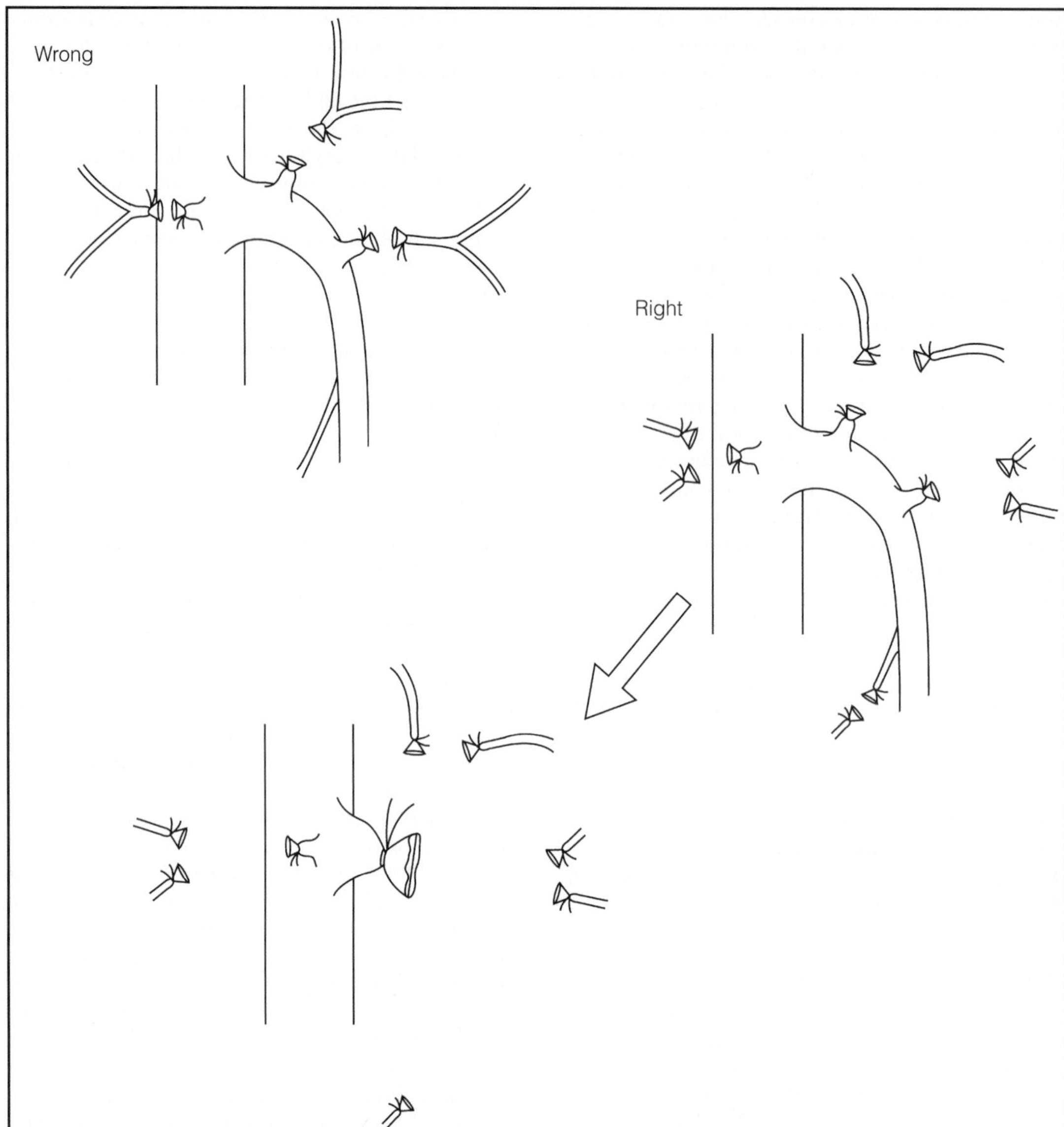

Figure 19.4 • At the sapheno-femoral junction, small feeding tributaries should be divided beyond secondary branch points in order to minimise the chances of reconnection and subsequent recurrence.

saphenous nerve.[37] However, it is less cosmetically acceptable and takes longer.

Whatever method is used, safe stripping requires that the groin anatomy is clearly displayed and that the stripper is passed from above downwards (minimising the danger of passage through a perforator into the deep system) and is palpated subcutaneously throughout its course.

SAPHENO-POPLITEAL LIGATION

SPJ ligation can prove to be a challenging procedure, especially when performed for recurrent disease. Beware the following pitfalls.

- Failure preoperatively to mark the SPJ (see above) will lead to a misplaced incision in a significant number of cases, necessitating blind incisions or abandonment of the procedure. Insist on a duplex or varicogram.
- If there is difficulty in recognising the SPJ, look for the upward continuation of the SSV (Giacomini vein), which usually joins the LSV or the profunda system.
- Traction on the SSV can tent up and damage the mobile and thin-walled popliteal vein. Palpation of the artery gives an indication of the depth of dissection.

- The common peroneal nerve runs adjacent to and then around the medial edge of biceps femoris and is at risk from lateral retraction or a careless stitch when closing the popliteal fascia.
- Flush ligation of the SPJ, generally thought to reduce recurrence, can be difficult to achieve, especially in the obese. The anatomy may also be obscured by large gastrocnemius veins joining the SSV just before the junction. There is no consensus about whether to ligate these (we do not). Therefore, in some patients, the possible benefits of a flush SPJ ligation (as opposed to one 1–2 cm distal to the junction) are outweighed by the risks of nerve and vascular injury.
- Stripping the SSV is said to run a significant risk of damage to the sural nerve and is therefore generally not performed. However, the evidence for this is poor and must be balanced against the risks of recurrent disease and surgery. The results of ongoing trials are awaited.
- Failure to close the popliteal fascia as a definite layer will result in a rather unattractive 'bulge' at the back of the knee that is difficult to treat.

TOURNIQUETS

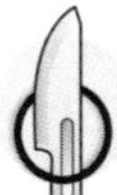

The main advantage of a tourniquet is reduction of blood loss, confirmed by a recent randomised trial.[38]

For large varicose veins of the LSV, the Lofqvist or Boazul pneumatic tourniquet is inflated to 40 mmHg above systemic systolic blood pressure and then rolled on to the leg over the prepared foot. The device acts both as an exsanguinator and a tourniquet and is held in the high thigh position with a small rubber wedge (**Fig. 19.5**). A stripper can be passed beneath the tourniquet if required. Postoperatively, the bandage must not be applied too tightly as the leg will swell significantly once the tourniquet is removed.

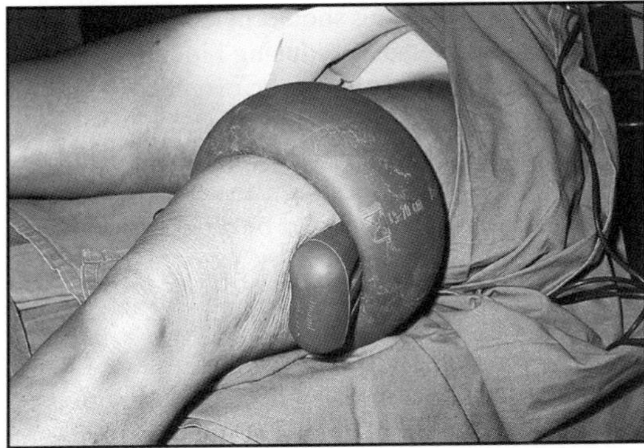

Figure 19.5 • Exsanguination tourniquet for bloodless varicose vein surgery. The sterile inflatable tourniquet is rolled up the leg and held in place with a rubber wedge.

AVULSIONS

Some non-venous structures are at risk during avulsions: the lateral popliteal (common peroneal) nerve at the neck of fibula, the tibial nerves and vessels behind the medial malleolus, the sural nerve in the median line of the posterior calf or behind the lateral malleolus, and the saphenous nerve on the medial calf. Using a variety of hooks, veins can be removed through tiny stab incisions, requiring no suture. Stab incisions should normally be made vertically as these are closed naturally by the compression bandage.

PERFORATOR LIGATION

There is no evidence that interrupting calf perforating veins by either open surgery or subfascial endoscopic perforator surgery alters the natural history of primary or recurrent VV.

BANDAGING

When bandaging the leg, the surgeon should be aware of any arterial impairment and ensure the presence of good capillary return to the toes. Traditional crepe bandages quickly lose any compression and become soaked with blood, whereas cohesive acrylic bandages maintain compression and are non-absorbent. However, there is no good evidence that any one bandaging system is superior.[39]

REPEAT GROIN DISSECTION

The CFV and SFJ are approached through non-operated tissues, usually laterally. The CFV can then be skeletonised for 1–2 cm above and below the junction, which is then divided flush and repaired with non-absorbable suture. The LSV is often still present and its upper end can be difficult to locate, in which case it can be located at the knee, aided by preoperative duplex marking. The stripper is passed up to the groin and then stripped in the normal way. If the duplex scan shows large connections in the groin, then a formal groin redissection is performed. However, if the scan shows only neovascularisation with tiny channels, then groin dissection and its associated morbidity can be avoided; simply passing a stripper upwards from below removes the remaining LSV.

PERIOPERATIVE CARE

Although surgery for VV is 'clean' surgery, a single dose of prophylactic antibiotic may be used in repeat surgery and other 'high-risk' groins. The use of thromboembolism prophylaxis is variable.[40]

In the absence of other thrombotic risk factors, hormonal therapy can be continued.[41]

Precise postoperative instructions and adequate analgesia should be given and the patient warned to return to hospital immediately if the operated leg becomes excessively painful. The bandage can be removed after 24–48 hours and replaced with a full-length stocking worn continuously for 1 week. It is often said that the stockings should be worn during the daytime for 6 weeks, although there is no evidence that this is necessary.[39]

ALTERNATIVE TECHNIQUES

In an attempt to reduce the morbidity of surgery and improve results, a number of new techniques have been devised to treat VV.

Endovenous techniques

A percutaneously placed catheter is used to thermally ablate the LSV using radiofrequency energy or, less commonly, laser energy. In isolation this can be done under local anaesthesia or, if combined with sapheno-femoral ligation,[42] under regional or general anaesthesia. Additional avulsions are also required. The stated benefits are reduced haematoma and improved postoperative recovery. A number of case series and registries have reported excellent results, with complete ablation of the LSV in up to 85% at 2 years.[43] However, complications include skin burns and paraesthesiae. In addition, it is recommended that the LSV must not be 'too tortuous' and must be less than 12 mm in the supine position.[44] The cost of implementing these techniques is considerable and further assessment with randomised controlled trials is necessary to compare performance against current surgical techniques.

Duplex-guided foam sclerotherapy

A controlled mixture of gas and sclerosant is used to produce relatively stable foam, which can then be injected under ultrasound guidance into the superficial veins of the lower limb. The advantage of this technique over traditional sclerotherapy is that the foam displaces any blood from the vein, increasing the surface area of sclerosant in contact with the endothelium. Ultrasound guidance allows the cannulation of the LSV, usually at the knee, to be confirmed, thus reducing the chance of extravasation. The foam bubbles are visible and progress can be followed and directed to treat tributaries of the LSV. This treatment is given in an outpatient setting, with no need for any anaesthesia. Recent studies have shown promise, with one series of 500 legs achieving obliteration of the LSV in 81% and of the superficial tributaries in about 97% at 3 years and no major complications.[45] However, comparison with surgery in a randomised controlled trial is awaited.

Venocuff

This is a reinforced band that is applied around a dilated valve annulus to control the maximal diameter of the ring.[46] At present there is little clinical experience or long-term follow-up with this device.

OUTCOME

Surgery for VV is carried out to improve quality of life rather than to save life or limb. However, until recently, little work has examined the success or otherwise in achieving this aim. Use of quality of life as an outcome measure has become standard practice in many diseases.[47] Typically, a generic measure is used that enables comparisons with the healthy population, and a disease-specific measure allows details of the condition to be assessed. A number of validated and reliable disease-specific measures have been devised for the assessment of patients with VV and CVI.[48–51] Several studies have shown that patients with VV score worse than a healthy population on generic measures of quality of life,[47,52] particularly in those domains relating to physical problems.[53] In addition, surgery for both uncomplicated and complicated VV is associated with significant improvements in both disease-specific and the physical domains of generic quality of life.[9,51] Ongoing studies will attempt to determine the relationship between this improvement in quality of life and objective measures of venous disease.

COMPLICATIONS

Major complications following surgery for VV seem relatively rare. However, up to 20% of patients suffer some form of minor morbidity.

1. Major venous damage: complete division of the CFV occurs in about 1 in 10 000 operations. Bleeding should be controlled with direct local pressure, reducing blood loss and allowing the dissection to be extended as required; the bleeding point should be repaired accurately with fine monofilament suture. Any suspicion that the deep system has been compromised should be quickly investigated and repaired by a vascular surgeon, as delay reduces the likelihood of a successful outcome.
2. Arterial damage: division and stripping of the superficial femoral artery have been reported and are made more likely by attempts to perform the operation through inappropriately small incisions.
3. Nerve damage (see above).

4. Haematoma: this is the commonest cause of discomfort after surgery and can be minimised as described above.
5 Venous thromboembolism.

RECURRENT VARICOSE VEINS

Approximately 20% of patients attending vascular clinics have 'recurrent' VV. For the purposes of understanding how recurrence can occur and how it can be prevented, the problem can be categorised into one or more of three subgroups.

New varicose veins The patient has developed 'new' VV, often in a second system, since the time of the original operation, for example in the popliteal fossa.[54] In this case, the so-called recurrent SSV varices were due to one of the following causes: (i) failure to recognize their presence initially due to inadequate examination or (ii) development of reflux in the SSV subsequently.

Persistent varicose veins The varices for which the patient was originally treated were never adequately removed at the time of operation. These can be tested by subsequent sclerotherapy or avulsions under local anaesthesia.

True recurrent varicose veins This is the development of further varicose veins in the same system originally operated upon and is the largest group of patients with recurrent VV. Objective assessment of such a group of patients resulted in the following subdivision.[55]

- Type 1: 31% recurrence through thigh perforators.
- Type 2: 11% incompetence through a second saphenous system.
- Type 3: 48% recurrent SFJ (11% SPJ) incompetence, with more than 50% due to neovascularisation.

A persistent thigh LSV was present in approximately two-thirds of types 1 and 3. In a series of patients undergoing repeat groin dissection, only 28% had a ligated SFJ, 44% had intact major tributaries and 73% had an intact LSV in the thigh. There was a strong association between the presence of a mid-thigh perforator leading to recurrent VV and failure to strip the LSV at the first operation [56]

Assessment

In patients with recurrent VV emanating from a previously operated groin, the fundamental question to be answered is whether the SFJ is still patent and therefore requires redissection and flush ligation on the CFV. Redissection can be difficult and is associated with morbidity in terms of wound healing, infection, nerve damage (paraesthesia), lymph leak and possibly lymphoedema. The pattern of recurrence should therefore be defined preoperatively with a duplex scan. Clinical and HHD examination alone have been shown to be inadequate and in some cases where scarring is significant, varicography may be the preferred method of assessment.[56]

Following a study reviewing the varicograms of 128 legs in order to define the pattern of recurrent VV,[57] a new classification of recurrent groin VV was presented (**Fig. 19.6**). This illustrated that the majority of recurrent VV are due to failure to carry out a flush SFJ ligation and/or remove the LSV as a source of perforator incompetence at the first operation.

Neovascularisation

A number of experts believe that most groin recurrence is due to so-called neovascularisation, pointing to the appearance of numerous venous channels on duplex, varicography and histological sections that join the LSV stump in the groin with recurrent varices in the thigh. Several different manoeuvres, such as mersiline mesh, PTFE patch and pectineus flap, have been employed in an attempt to prevent the SFJ 'sprouting' these new vessels, with variable success.[58–60]

Non-absorbable suture for SFJ ligation has been recommended by some in the belief that this will prevent vascular smooth muscle and endothelial cells entering the scar tissue and acting as a source of new vessels. Neovascularisation certainly occurs in a proportion of patients but its relative importance in producing significant recurrent VV remains disputed. In particular, it is pointed out that if the SFJ tributaries are taken back beyond their secondary branch points, and the LSV is stripped, even if new vessels do form in the vicinity of the scar they are unlikely to be able to connect up with vessels down the leg. It is also debatable whether significant volumes of blood could reflux through these numerous tiny channels because of their considerable resistance to flow.

VULVAL VARICES

Vulval varices may arise in women as a complication of pregnancy or following pelvic vein thrombosis (surgery, trauma or pelvic inflammatory disease) and are a consequence of ovarian and internal iliac venous valve incompetence. They typically extend down the medial aspect of the

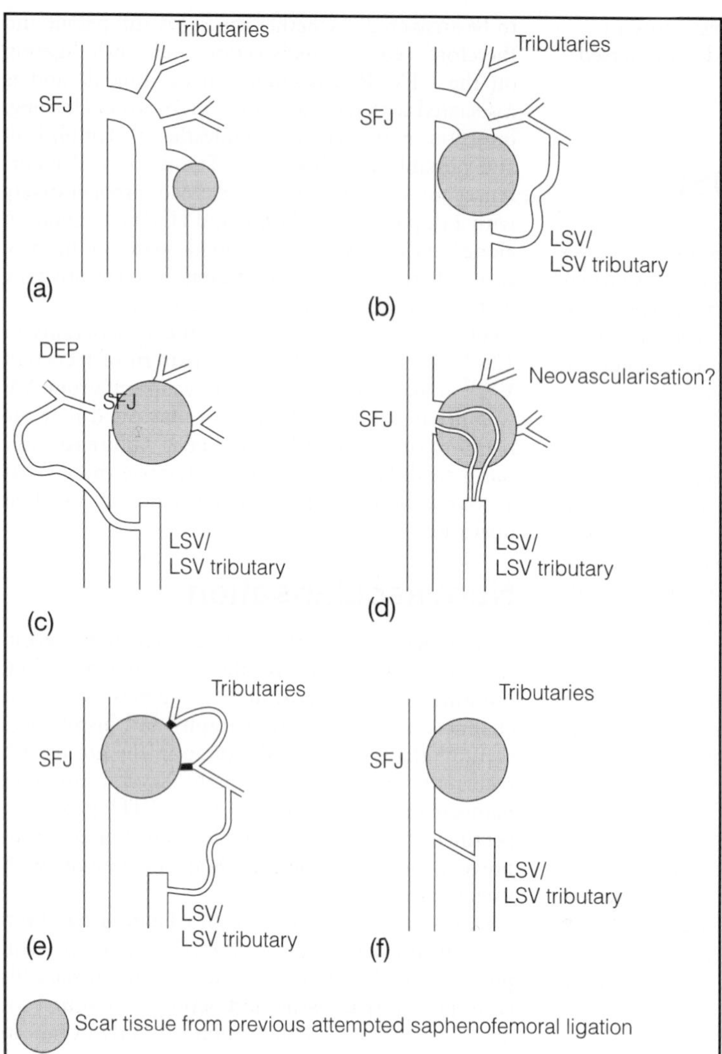

Figure 19.6 • Anatomical patterns of recurrent varicose veins in the groin. **(a–d)** Type I, sapheno-femoral venous complex intact. **(e, f)** Type II, sapheno-femoral venous complex obliterated. SFJ, sapheno-femoral junction; LSV, long saphenous vein; DEP, deep external pudendal.

thigh, and may join the saphenous system, which may also be incompetent. Treatment is carried out in two phases:

1. reflux in the ovarian vein is abolished;
2. the varicose veins themselves are dealt with locally by means of stab avulsions, sclerotherapy, with or without standard saphenous surgery.

Ovarian vein interruption was originally accomplished surgically through a loin incision and retroperitoneal approach. More recently, radiological ovarian vein embolisation has been successfully practised.[61] Ovarian vein reflux may be associated with the 'pelvic congestion syndrome', characterised by pelvic pain, backache, dysmenorrhoea, menorrhagia, dyspareunia and urological symptoms including dysuria.

Key points

- Patients with asymptomatic uncomplicated VV can generally be reassured as they are at low risk of developing complications.
- Surgery for symptomatic uncomplicated VV clearly improves quality of life and should be publicly funded.
- Adequate training and supervision should be provided to junior surgeons to prevent complications and high recurrence rates.[62]
- Thorough preoperative counselling is essential to provide informed consent.
- Duplex scanning is recommended for all patients. If this is not possible, duplex should certainly be used when there has been previous surgery, where there is suspicion of deep venous disease, and preoperatively in SSV surgery to mark the SPJ.
- Injection sclerotherapy should be reserved for small varices or reticular and hyphenweb veins in the absence of truncal or major junction reflux.
- Primary VV of the LSV is generally treated with sapheno-femoral ligation, stripping of the LSV to below the knee, and avulsions.
- Inversion stripping is popular, makes sense but is not based on evidence.
- Surgery in the popliteal fossa is potentially very difficult and adequate preoperative assessment is paramount. The place of SSV stripping has yet to be fully evaluated.
- Tourniquets have been shown to reduce blood loss significantly.
- Novel techniques require assessment in randomised controlled trials with long-term outcome assessment to determine their place in the treatment repertoire.

REFERENCES

1. Laing W. Chronic venous diseases of the leg. London: Office of Health Economics, 1992.
2. Tennant WG, Ruckley CV. Medicolegal action following treatment for varicose veins. Br J Surg 1996; 8:291–2.
3. Ruckley CV, Bradbury AW. How do we prevent recurrence of varicose veins? In: Ruckley CV, Fowkes FGR, Bradbury AW (eds) Venous disease. London: Springer-Verlag, 1999; pp. 239–45.
4. Tibbs DJ. Disordered venous function. In: Tibbs DJ, Sabiston DC, Davies MG, Mortimer PS, Scurr JH (eds) Varicose vein, venous disorders, and lymphatic problems in the lower limbs. Oxford: Oxford University Press, 1997; pp. 13–19.
5. Tretbar LL. Venous disorders of the leg. London: Springer-Verlag, 1999; p. 29.
6. Evans CJ, Fowkes FGR, Ruckley CV, Lee AJ. Prevalence of varicose veins and chronic venous insufficiency in men and women in the general population: Edinburgh Vein Study. J Epidemiol Community Health 1999; 53:149–53.
7. Raju S, Easterwood L, Fountain T et al. Saphenectomy in the presence of chronic venous obstruction. Surgery 1998; 126:637–44.
8. Bradbury AW, Evans CJ, Allan PL et al. What are the symptoms of varicose veins? Edinburgh vein study cross sectional population survey. Br Med J 1999; 318:353–6.
9. MacKenzie RK, Lee AJ, Paisley A et al. Patient, operative and surgeon factors influencing the effect of superficial venous surgery on disease-specific quality of life. J Vasc Surg 2002; 36:896–902.
10. Hanson JN, Ascher E, DePippo P et al. Saphenous vein thrombophlebitis (SVT): a deceptively benign disease. J Vasc Surg 1998; 27:677–80.
11. Campbell WB, Niblett PG, Ridlow BMF, Peters AS, Thompson JF. Hand-held Doppler as a screening test in primary varicose veins. Br J Surg 1997; 84:1541–3.
12. Kent PJ, Weston MJ. Duplex scanning may be used selectively in patients with primary varicose veins. Ann R Coll Surg Engl 1993; 80:388–9.
13. Bladin C, Royle JP. Acquisition of skills for use of Doppler ultrasound and the assessment of varicose vein. Aust NZ J Surg 1987; 57:225–6.
14. Dawke SG, Vetrivel S, Foy DMA, Smith S, Baker S. A comparison of duplex scanning and continuous wave Doppler in the assessment of primary and uncomplicated varicose veins. Eur J Vasc Endovasc Surg 1997; 14:457–61.
15. Mercer KG, Scott DJA, Berridge DC. Preoperative duplex imaging is required before all operations for primary varicose veins. Br J Surg 1998; 85:1495–7.

16. Wills V, Moylan D, Chambers J. The use of routine scanning in the assessment of varicose veins. Aust NZ J Surg 1998; 68:41–4.

17. Labropoulos N, Kang SS, Mansour MA et al. Primary superficial vein reflux with competent superficial trunk. Eur J Vasc Endovasc Surg 1999; 18:201–6.

18. Travers JP, Makin GS. Reduction of varicose vein recurrence by use of post-operative compression stockings. Phlebology 1994; 9:104–7.

Patients undergoing surgery for VV were randomised preoperatively to either postoperative full-length class II stockings or no stockings. Of those patients allocated stockings, 50% declined to wear them, abandoned them after 3 months or were lost to follow-up. However, at 12 months only 6% of the stocking group had recurrent VV compared with 71% in those without.

19. Hobbs JT. Surgery and sclerotherapy in the treatment of varicose veins. A random trial. Arch Surg 1974; 109:793–6.

Patients with VV were randomized to either surgery or sclerotherapy. Incompetent lower leg perforators and dilated venous tributaries were found to be better treated by sclerotherapy. For mainstem and junctional disease, sclerotherapy was better than surgery for 2–3 years, after which operated patients did better.

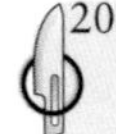

20. Hamilton Jacobsen B. The value of different forms of treatment for varicose veins. Br J Surg 1979; 66:182–4.

This study comparing surgery with sclerotherapy for the treatment of saphenous varicosities found surgery to be more successful (97%) than sclerotherapy (37%) at 3-year follow-up.

21. Galland RB, Magee TR, Lewis MH. A survey of current attitudes of British and Irish vascular surgeons to venous sclerotherapy. Eur J Vasc Endovasc Surg 1998; 16:43–6.

22. Lees TA, Holdsworth ID. Assessment and treatment of varicose veins in the Northern Region. Phlebology 1995; 10:56–61.

23. Lane IF, Bourantas NE. What is the scope of day care for venous surgery? In: Ruckley CV, Fowkes FGR, Bradbury AW (eds) Venous disease. London: Springer-Verlag, 1999; pp. 216–21.

24. Ramesh S, Umeh HN, Galland RB. Day case varicose vein operations: patient suitability and satisfaction. Phlebology 1995; 10:103–5.

25. Onuma OC, Beam PE, Khan U, Malluci P, Adiseshiah M. The influence of effective analgesia and general anaesthesia on patients' acceptance of day case varicose vein surgery. Phlebology 1993; 8:29–31.

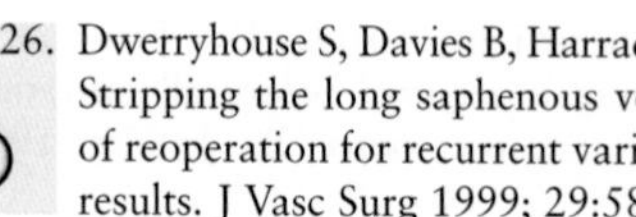

26. Dwerryhouse S, Davies B, Harradine K, Earnshaw JJ. Stripping the long saphenous vein reduces the rate of reoperation for recurrent varicose veins: five-year results. J Vasc Surg 1999; 29:589–92.

In this randomised trial comparing sapheno-femoral ligation and LSV stripping (to knee level) with sapheno-femoral ligation alone, stripping of the LSV reduced the reoperation rate from 20% to 6% after 6 years.

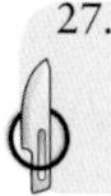

27. Munn SR, Morton JB, Macbeth WAAG, McLeish AR. To strip or not to strip the long saphenous vein. A varicose vein trial. Br J Surg 1981; 68:426–8.

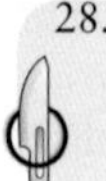

28. Rutgers PH, Kitslar PJEHM. Randomised trial of stripping versus high ligation combined with sclerotherapy in the treatment of the incompetent greater saphenous vein. Am J Surg 1994; 168:311–15.

29. Sarin S, Scurr JH, Coleridge-Smith PR. Stripping of the long saphenous vein in the treatment of primary varicose veins. Br J Surg 1994; 81:1455–8.

30. MacKenzie RK, Paisley A, Allan PL et al. The effect of long saphenous vein stripping on quality of life. J Vasc Surg 2002; 35:1197–203.

31. Hammarsten J, Pedersen P, Cederlund CC, Campanello M. Long saphenous vein-saving surgery for varicose veins. A long-term follow-up. Eur J Vasc Surg 1990; 4:361–4.

32. Docherty JG, Morrice JJ, Ben G. Saphenous neuritis following varicose vein surgery. Br J Surg 1994; 81:695–8.

33. Cox S J, Wellwood JM, Martin A. Saphenous nerve injury caused by stripping of the long saphenous vein. Br Med J 1974; 1:415–17.

34. Negus, D. Should the incompetent saphenous vein be stripped to the ankle? Phlebology 1986; 1:33–6.

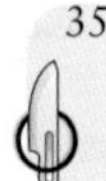

35. Durkin MT, Turton EP, Scott DJ, Berridge DC. A prospective randomised controlled trial of PIN versus conventional stripping in varicose vein surgery. Ann R Coll Surg Engl 1999; 81:171–4.

Patients were randomised to either conventional or PIN stripping and assessed 1 week postoperatively. There was no difference in area of bruising or presence of paraesthesia and the only advantage to PIN stripping was a smaller exit wound.

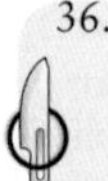

36. Lacroix H, Nevelstein A, Suy R. Invagination versus classic stripping of the long saphenous vein. A randomised prospective study. Acta Chir Belg 1999; 99:22–5.

In this comparison, again no difference was found between PIN and conventional stripping in terms of pain score, haematoma size and nerve injuries.

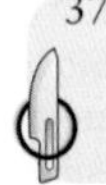

37. Khan RBN, Khan SN, Greavey MG, Blair SD. Prospective randomized trial comparing sequential avulsions with stripping of the long saphenous vein. Br J Surg 1996; 83:1559–62.

38. Sykes TCF, Brookes P, Hickey NC. A prospective randomised trial of tourniqet in varicose vein surgery. Br J Surg 1999; 86:A44.

This randomised trial assessing the additional benefit of tourniquet use in patients undergoing primary sapheno-femoral ligation and LSV stripping found a significant reduction in preoperative blood loss, bruising and operative time in the tourniquet group.

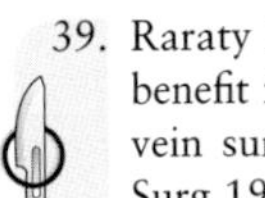

39. Raraty MGT, Greavey MG, Blair SD. There is no benefit from 6 weeks of compression after varicose vein surgery: a prospective randomised trial. Br J Surg 1997; 84:A574.
40. Campbell WB, Ridler BM. Varicose vein surgery and deep vein thrombosis. Br J Surg 1995; 82:1484–97.
41. Drugs in the peri-operative period. Part 3. Hormonal contraceptives and hormone replacement therapy. Drug Ther Bull 1999; 37:78–80.
42. Chandler JG, Pichot GO, Sessa C et al. Defining the role of extended saphenofemoral junction ligation: a prospective comparative study. J Vasc Surg 2000; 32:941–53.
43. Merchant RF, dePalma RG, Kabnick LS. Endovascular obliteration of saphenous reflux: a multicentre study. J Vasc Surg 2002; 35:1190–6.
44. Rautio T, Ohinmaa A, Perala J et al. Endovenous obliteration versus conventional stripping operation in the treatment of primary varicose veins: a randomised controlled trial with comparison of costs. J Vasc Surg 2002; 35:958–65.

    In this comparison of endovenous ablation with conventional LSV stripping, 85 of 121 patients were excluded, the majority due to bilateral disease or large-calibre LSV. Postoperatively, those who underwent conventional surgery scored higher on pain scores and had significantly more sick leave than the endovenous group.

45. Cabrera J, Cabrera J Jr, Garcia-Olmedo MA. Treatment of varicose long saphenous veins with sclerosant in microfoam form: long-term outcomes. Phlebology 2000; 15:19–23.
46. Lane RJ, McMahon C, Cuzzina M. The treatment of varicose veins using the venous valve cuff. Phlebology 1994; 9:136–45.
47. McDaniel MD, Nehler MR, Santilli SM et al. Extended outcome assessment in the care of vascular diseases: revising the paradigm for the 21st century. J Vasc Surg 2000; 32:1239–50.
48. Garratt AM, Ruta DA, Abdalla MI, Russell IT. Responsiveness of the SF-36 and a condition-specific measure of health for patients with varicose veins. Quality of Life Res 1996; 5:223–34.
49. Smith JJ, Guest, GA, Greenhalgh MA, Davies AH. Measuring quality of life in patients with venous ulcers. J Vasc Surg 2000; 31:642–9.
50. Kurz X, Lamping DL, Khan SR et al. Do varicose veins affect quality of life? Results of an international population-based study. J Vasc Surg 2001; 34:641–8.
51. Lamping DL, Schroter S, Kurz X, Kahn SR, Abenheim L. Evaluation of outcomes in chronic venous disorders of the leg: development of a scientifically rigorous, patient-reported measure of symptoms and quality of life. J Vasc Surg 2003; 37:410–19.
52. Smith JJ, Garratt GA, Guest M, Greenhalgh MA, Davies AH. Evaluating and improving health-related quality of life in patients with varicose veins. J Vasc Surg 1999; 30:710–19.
53. Kaplan H, Criqui MH, Denenberg J, Bergan JJ, Fronek A. Quality of life in patients with chronic venous disease: San Diego population study. J Vasc Surg 2003; 37:1047–53.
54. Bradbury AW, Stonebridge PA, Ruckley CV, Beggs I. Recurrent varicose veins: correlation between preoperative clinical and hand-held Doppler ultrasonographic examination, and anatomical findings at surgery. Br J Surg 1993; 80:849–51.
55. Darke SG. The morphology of recurrent varicose veins. Eur J Vasc Surg 1992; 6:512–17.
56. Bradbury AW, Stonebridge IPA, Callam MJ et al. Recurrent varicose veins: assessment of the saphenofemoral junction. Br J Surg 1994; 81:373–5.
57. Stonebridge PA, Chalmers N, Beggs I, Bradbury AW, Ruckley CV. Recurrent varicose veins: a varicographic analysis leading to a new practical classification. Br J Surg 1995; 82:60–2.
58. Glass GM. Prevention of recurrent saphenofemoral incompetence after surgery for varicose veins. Br J Surg 1989; 76:1210.
59. Earnshaw JJ, Davies B, Harradine K, Heather BP. Preliminary results of PTFE patch. Saphenoplasty to prevent neovascularization leading to recurrent varicose veins. Phlebology 1998; 13:10–13.
60. Gibbs P, Foy DMA, Darke SG. Recurrent varicose veins: to patch or not to patch. Br J Surg 1999; 86:A112–A113.
61. Cordts PR, Eclavea A, Buckley PJ et al. Pelvic congestion syndrome: early clinical results after transcatheter ovarian embolisation. J Vasc Surg 1998; 28:862–8.
62. Turton EP, Whitely MS, Berridge DC, Scott DJ. Calman, venous surgery and the vascular trainee. J R Coll Surg Edinb 1999; 44:172–6.

Index

Notes

Page numbers followed by 'f' indicate figures, those followed by 't' indicate tables or boxes.
vs. indicates a comparison or differential diagnosis.